aim
FOR WELLBEING!

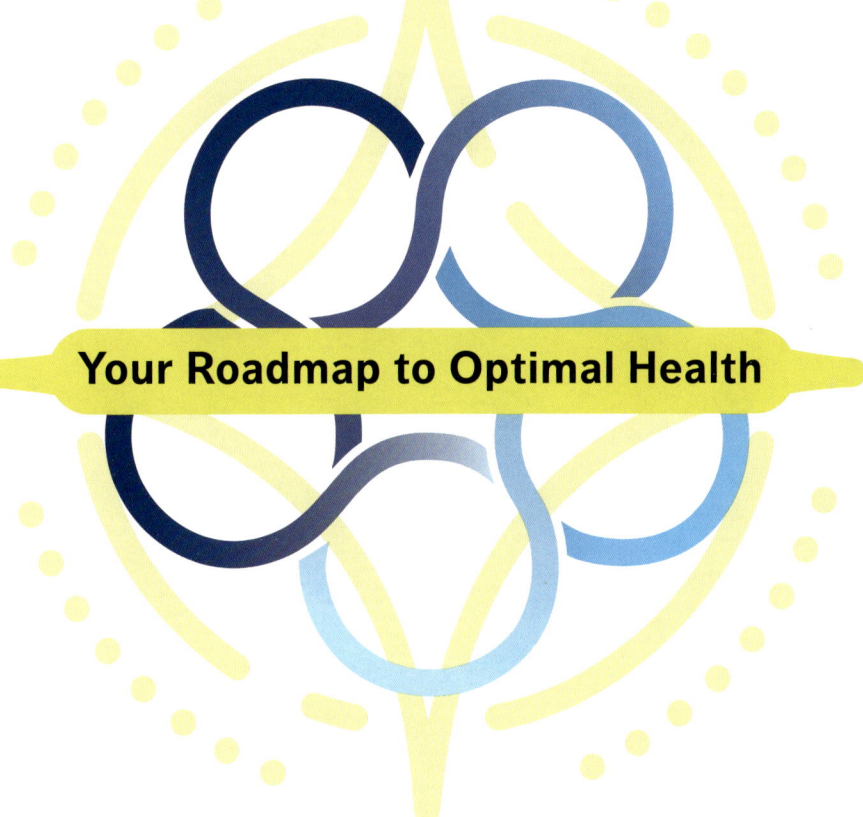

Your Roadmap to Optimal Health

Steve Amoils, M.D. & Sandi Amoils, M.D.

The information in this book is designed to help you make informed decisions about your health. It is not intended as a substitute for medical treatment. This information should be used in conjunction with the guidance and care of your physician. If you think you have a medical problem, seek competent professional help.

Transformational Medicine is a registered trademark of Steve and Sandi Amoils, M.D.s.

ACE Healing Treatment is a registered service mark of the Alliance Institute for Integrative Medicine.

Copyright © 2024 by
The Christ Hospital Foundation –
Integrative Medicine Division.
All rights reserved.

Library of Congress Control Number: 2024917711

ISBN: 979-8-218-47445-4

Cover design by Grannan Design Ltd., www.grannandesign.com
Cover painting "Open Sky" by Natasha Barnes, www.natashabarnes.com
Internal design by Grannan Design Ltd.
Artwork by Brenda Grannan, Kristin Luther and Abbey Urbas, www.abbeyurbas.com

Manufactured in the United States of America

Printed by Sheridan, www.sheridan.com

Second edition

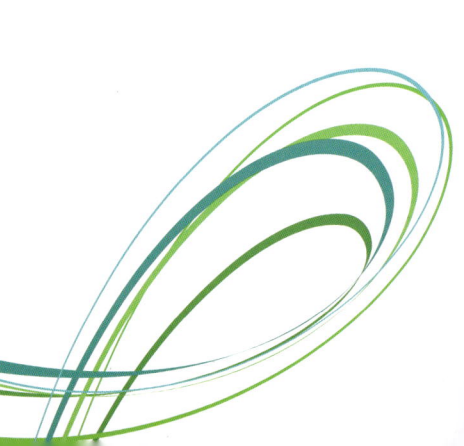

AIM for Wellbeing

Dr. Steve and Dr. Sandi Amoils are long-time pioneers in integrative and functional medicine. In **AIM for Wellbeing** they share their decades of experience helping patients discover the transformational power of this type of medical wisdom in order to personalize their healthcare and achieve lasting improvements. This book offers a fresh perspective on common medical problems, supplying a tailored approach that transports the reader from illness toward wellbeing. Whether you're a healthcare professional or someone on a health journey, this is your blueprint to achieve optimal health.

—**Brian Berman**, MD, President of the Nova Institute for Health, Professor Emeritus at the University of Maryland School of Medicine, where he was Founding Director of the Center for Integrative Medicine, co-founder of the Cochrane Complementary Medicine Field, inaugural Chair of the Academic Consortium for Integrative Medicine and Health

Drs. Steve and Sandi Amoils have been blessed by the ability to explain complex medical theories in simple terms. Yet, as their words penetrate into our consciousness, they guide us strategically toward wellbeing, piercing our misinterpretations about illness. They gently open us up to the possibility of living a life free from trauma on all levels. Steve and Sandi inspire us to live up to our potential, evoking possibilities for us to evolve, to reap the benefits of who and what we are, physically, mentally, and emotionally. This book unlocks all that is available to all of us, offering us treasures of vibrant health and nudging us on a journey that inspires vitality. It is a work that has taken a lifetime of study, working with thousands of patients, and a relentless commitment to heal and improve lives. I highly recommend it!

—**Johnny G**, inventor and founder, Spinning®, Kranking®, and In-Trinity®

The Amoils are holistic and functional medicine pioneers. Their experience and protocols transform lives. We are lucky to have this book as a valuable educational resource.

—**Mimi Guarneri**, MD, integrative cardiologist, President, Academy of Integrative Health and Medicine

Drs. Steve and Sandi Amoils have continued to synthesize the best of conventional medicine, functional medicine, and medical acupuncture into a truly healing approach. The result points to an entirely new way of thinking, where we may in fact begin to reverse aging and eradicate many of the common illnesses we encounter.

—**Joseph M. Helms**, MD, Founding President, American Academy of Medical Acupuncture

AIM for Wellbeing is a complete guidebook to the why, what, and how of healthy living based on the big hearts, keen minds, and life-long experience of physicians, Drs. Steve and Sandi Amoils. It's a compelling read that takes layered, complicated, cutting-edge medical concepts from many disciplines and distills them into memorable explanations, insightful infographics, and action steps so people can get started immediately on their transformational healing journey. Truly, this book provides the best of solid, sound information with the delivery of creative, soulful inspiration – a must-have for every person who is committed to wellness and is seeking answers!

—**Deanna Minich**, PhD, nutrition scientist, author, and educator

In *AIM for Wellbeing*, Drs. Steve and Sandi Amoils, the power couple of integrative health, share their years of experience to masterfully bridge the gap between conventional medicine and the transformative power of integrative and functional approaches. This book is a crucial guide for anyone looking to not just manage illness but to thrive throughout their lives. With its engaging visuals and insightful chapters, it empowers readers to harness their body's innate ability to heal and maintain wellbeing. A must-read for those seeking to age gracefully and transform their approach to health.

—**Melinda Ring**, MD, FACP, ABOIM, Executive Director, Osher Center for Integrative Health at Northwestern University, Drs. Pat and Carl Greer Distinguished Physician in Integrative Medicine, Clinical Associate Professor of Medicine and Medical Social Sciences, Northwestern University Feinberg School of Medicine

At long last, an inspiring book that serves as an invaluable roadmap for both healthcare professionals and patients seeking a comprehensive understanding of integrative and functional medicine approaches to healthcare. The authors are pioneers in the field of integrative medicine who seamlessly blend scientific rigor and therapeutic interventions that go beyond the standard western model with real-world applications, making it an essential resource for anyone interested in optimizing health outcomes through a holistic lens. I am thrilled to recommend this "must-read" to my patients and healthcare colleagues

—**Christopher J. Suhar**, MD, integrative cardiologist, Medical Director, Scripps Center for Integrative Medicine

In the more than 50 years of my career specializing in immunology and autoimmunity, I have become very familiar with how frustrating and mystifying complex diseases can be. This is why this book strikes a chord with me. In their book, **AIM for Wellbeing**, Steve and Sandi Amoils discuss the best features of functional and integrative medicine to demystify complex medical issues for patients and practitioners alike, making them more comprehensible for everyone. They describe how they use a myriad of techniques including functional immunology to diagnose, treat and prevent disease, working toward a future where personalized medicine is better understood and given its proper value. They also offer a fresh perspective on wellness and aging, creating their own blueprint to achieve optimal health and wellness, and even, somehow, offering the tantalizing prospect of the reversal of aging. This book could be a catalyst for change in the world of healthcare, and I give it my recommendation.

—**Aristo Vojdani**, PhD, Clinical Professor, Department of Preventive Medicine, Loma Linda University, Technical Director, Immunosciences Lab, Chief Scientific Advisor, Cyrex Labs

Steve and Sandi's driving force is an insatiable urge to continually learn and synthesize the best of all medical therapies, including medical acupuncture, into a comprehensive program that improves their patients' lives. This book is a comprehensive approach to healing, in all its forms. It has been an honor to witness their dedication to this endeavor.

—**Professor Nadia Volf**, MD, PhD, Founder and Director of the Scientific Acupuncture Postgraduation Program, University of Paris-Saclay, former lecturer, International Structural Acupuncture Course, Harvard Medical School

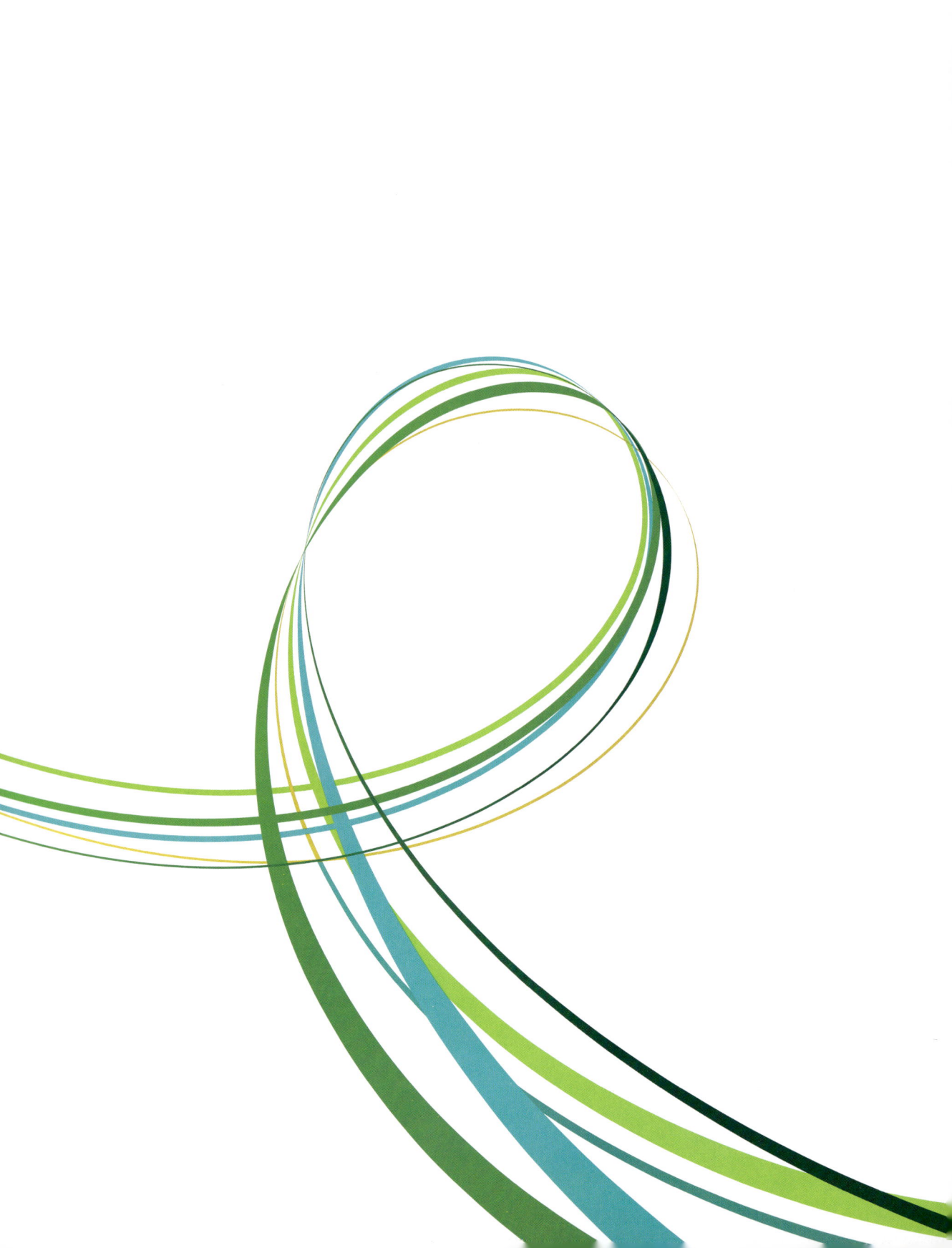

Contributing Authors

Teresa Esterle, MD, PhD
- Director of Education and Fellowship Program, AIM for Wellbeing
- Board-certified in pediatrics, integrative medicine, and acupuncture
- Institute of Functional Medicine certified practitioner
- Graduate, Integrative Medicine Physician of Excellence Program at AIM for Wellbeing
- Treats both adults and children; interests include treatment of complex medical illnesses

Claudia Harsh, MD
- Integrative gynecologist; board-certified in obstetrics and gynecology
- Board-certified in integrative and holistic medicine (ABIHM)
- Graduate, Bravewell Fellow, University of Arizona Integrative Medicine Program
- Long-term practitioner of medical acupuncture, functional medicine, and integrative medicine
- Registered yoga teacher
- Currently in practice in Charlotte, North Carolina
- Interests include women's hormonal health

Caylin Holmes, DC, DACRB
- Chiropractic physician
- Graduate, Integrative Medicine Chiropractor of Excellence Program fellowship at AIM for Wellbeing
- Diplomate, American Chiropractic Rehabilitation Board since 2019
- Interests include rehabilitation and shockwave therapy

Carrie Jones, ND, FABNE, MPH
- Naturopathic physician
- Board-certified in naturopathic endocrinology
- NAMS certified
- Internationally recognized speaker, consultant, and educator
- Expert educator at Rupa Health, DUTCH Test and Lifestyle Matrix Resource Center
- Co-host, *Root Cause Medicine* podcast

Travis McClain, DO, RMSK
- Board-certified physical medicine and rehabilitation physician
- Registered in Musculoskeletal® (RMSK®) sonography certification
- Interests include diagnostic musculoskeletal ultrasound, ultrasound-guided procedures, interventional spine procedures, regenerative medicine/orthobiologics, sports medicine and spine care, non-operative orthopedic care

Katie Peeden, MD
- Board-certified in family medicine, integrative medicine, and acupuncture
- Completed training in functional medicine through the Institute of Functional Medicine
- Graduate, Integrative Medicine Physician of Excellence Program at AIM for Wellbeing
- Interests include metabolic health, stress management, laser therapy, and whole-person care

Colleen Swayze, MD, FACOG
- Board-certified in obstetrics and gynecology and integrative medicine
- Graduate, Integrative Medicine Physician of Excellence Program at AIM for Wellbeing
- Board-eligible in medical acupuncture
- Completed training in functional medicine through the Institute of Functional Medicine
- Specializes in women's health, but treats both men and women

Liz Woolford, MD
- Board-certified family physician
- Founding member of AIM for Wellbeing
- Practicing medical acupuncture and functional medicine since 1999; prolotherapy and perineural injection therapy since 2005
- Interests include pain management, restoring patients back to health, and teaching

---

With special thanks to:

John Bartsch, DC
- Chiropractic physician
- Former Director of Chiropractic, Jewish Hospital, Cincinnati
- Interests include FSM, shockwave therapy and AAT

Steve Bleser, DC (retired)
- Former senior chiropractor at AIM for Wellbeing
- Past president, Ohio State Chiropractic Association; Past President and Board Member Emeritus, Ohio State Board of Chiropractic Examiners; Fellow, International Board of Chiropractic Examiners; Fellow, International College of Chiropractic Examiners, National Board of Chiropractic Examiners

Valerie Bullock, MD
- Board-certified in family medicine and integrative medicine
- Integrative Medicine Physician of Excellence at AIM for Wellbeing
- Trained in medical acupuncture and functional medicine
- Passionate about helping patients explore what it means to live well

Eric Dieffenbaugher, DC
- Chiropractic physician, AAT practitioner
- Head of AAT at AIM for Wellbeing
- Interests include treatment of allergies and sensitivities, pain management, shockwave therapy

Katherine Mattox, RDN
- Functional medicine dietitian
- Interests include weight loss, anti-aging, and metabolic health

Jaime Sanzere, MS, RDN
- Functional medicine dietitian and health coach
- Interests include women's health, PCOS, insulin resistance, and social media

Melissa Van Tassel, MD
- Board-certified in family medicine
- Integrative Medicine Physician of Excellence at AIM for Wellbeing
- Institute of Functional Medicine Certified Practitioner
- Medical acupuncturist
- Interests include preventing and reversing dementia

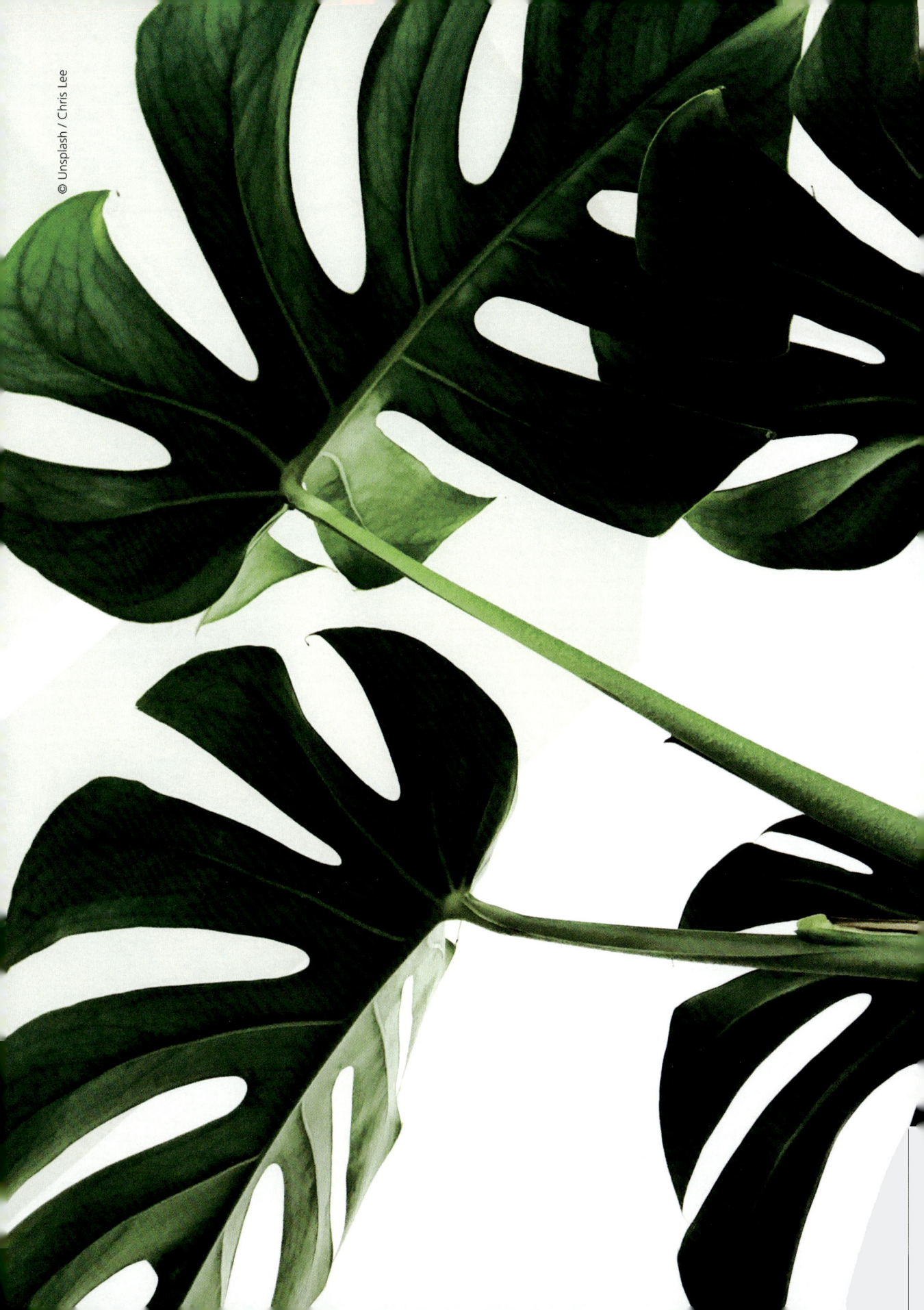

How and why to read this book

This book is not designed to be a compendium of the latest and greatest treatments in medicine. It is based on over forty years of treating thousands of patients from all walks of life. What we aim to provide is an evergreen approach on how to attain wellness. What you will find in this book is a practical distillation of a complex approach. You can read it from front to back, or just cherry-pick the parts you need or want to read.

<mark>Important points are emphasized in YELLOW</mark>

<mark>Medical data is added in ORANGE, for those who are interested</mark>

<mark>There are occasional case reports in BLUE</mark>

We hope you can keep this book on your shelf and access it whenever you need it. There may be times you just want to reference a certain section or idea.

Proceeds from this book will go toward the following nonprofits:
The Integrative Medicine Fund at The Christ Hospital Foundation. This fund:
- Supports the training of fellows in integrative medicine.
- Provides free or low-cost integrative medicine for those who cannot afford it.
- Helps conduct research in integrative medicine.

Maya's Way Fund at The Christ Hospital Foundation. This fund provides free integrative medical care to patients under 40 with cancer.

This book is printed on green paper.

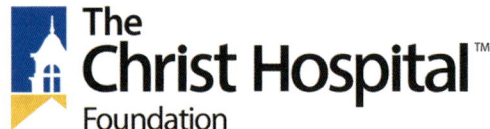

Dedication

To you, the reader:
May this book inspire you to improve your health and wellbeing. May your newfound vitality inspire you to make positive changes in your world.

And to our beloved daughters, who have taught us so much:
- Misha, an ENT surgeon, her husband Dean, and their beautiful children, Rowan and Charlie
- Maya, whose legacy continues to inspire us all

Contents

Foreword

Transformational Medicine: Patient-Focused Care by Dean J. Kereiakes, MD, FACC, MSCAI

Page	Chapter	Title
1	Chapter 1	It's Time to AIM for Wellbeing
11	Chapter 2	Integrating Best Practices – The Development of Transformational Medicine
25	Chapter 3	Using Illness and Dis-ease as a Fulcrum to Transform Your Life
35	Chapter 4	How to Approach an Illness
55	Chapter 5	Stress and the Road to Illness
69	Chapter 6	The Persistent Effects of Trauma – A Sad Situation
79	Chapter 7	How to Transform Stress into Success
95	Chapter 8	Your Body on Fire
111	Chapter 9	The Gut: from Top to Bottom
125	Chapter 10	Food Is Medicine; Food as Medicine
155	Chapter 11	Understanding Immunity and Allergy
171	Chapter 12	Decoding Immunity and Treating Allergies and Sensitivities
183	Chapter 13	Understanding Your Hormones
199	Chapter 14	Optimizing Your Hormone Balance
217	Chapter 15	Understanding Insulin
233	Chapter 16	The Legacy of Our Standard American (SAD) Diet and Lifestyle: The SAD Diseases
239	Chapter 17	Understanding Pain
275	Chapter 18	Treating Pain and Healing the Body Simultaneously
303	Chapter 19	Reversing Cardiovascular Risk
319	Chapter 20	Tackling Cancer: Maya's Way
331	Chapter 21	Is It Possible to Heal a Nation?
339	Chapter 22	Aging As You Know It Is About to Change … the Allure of Modern Wellness
345		**Acknowledgments**
347		**References**
354		**Index**
363		**Appendix**

Transformational Medicine: Patient-Focused Care

> A man need not have grown old in the practice of medicine to bear witness to its having undergone considerable changes.

—Peter Mere Latham (1789–1875), **Remarks on the Practice of Medicine**

These prescient words from the nineteenth century are even more applicable today. The diagnostic and therapeutic aspects of traditional medical practice have reflected both the science (choice of names, causes, or explanations for ailments) and the art (decisions regarding treatment) of medicine. This demarcation of art and science in traditional medicine has several inaccuracies. First, the science component is challenged to go beyond mere explanation to the patient regarding what is wrong. We must also predict what may happen in the future (prognosis) and how that prophecy might be altered. Second, although diagnosis is important, the selection and appraisal of therapy requires more intricate analysis.

Through most of recorded history, medicine was dominated by empiricism and shrouded by dogma with little basis in science. Diagnoses were inexact, the causes of disease were poorly understood, and therapies were, at times, frivolous or haphazard. Interventions such as bleeding, purging, cupping, infusions of plant extracts, or solutions of metals were empirically based on anecdotal experience without scientific foundation. Change emerged in the nineteenth century when pathologists correlated anatomic observations with features of disease and bacteriologists identified specific organisms in the pathogenesis of specific diseases, laying the foundation for future therapies. Still, physicians could do very little for most illnesses beyond providing a diagnosis, prognosis, and common-sense supportive measures. Indeed, most therapeutic interventions of that time were largely useless or even harmful. The dawn of modern medicine arrived starting in the 1920s, with the advent of the antibacterial sulfonamides and gathering speed in the 1940s with the advent of penicillin. Previously fatal diseases were now curable. Biological science and molecular biology became the focus of modern medicine, and major medical advances, based on the scientific understanding of disease mechanisms, revolutionized the care and outlook for many diseases.

The veritable explosion in modern basic science discoveries was, in large part, prompted by a shift in the process of medical education that occurred in the early 1900s. The Flexner Report of 1910 transformed the process of medical education in America from a haphazard collection of often substandard schools to the full-time academic model, where physicians focused primarily on research and teaching and less on patient care. Increased access to philanthropic and, later on, federal funding spurred basic science research, at times without specific clinical objectives in mind. Critics of this shift in focus for medical education rightly voiced concerns that it "overlooked the ethos of medicine in its blind passion for science," and that unintended consequences included both loss of diversity and access to many therapeutic modalities that helped patients. Excellence in science was not balanced by excellence in clinical care or equity.

As modern medicine evolved in the twentieth century, technological advances in both diagnostic and therapeutic measures progressed exponentially. Physicians began to become subspecialists just to keep up with the changes. Medicine became increasingly technical, impersonal, and high volume. The patients' role in their own treatment was increasingly lost to new drugs, new imaging and surgical techniques, and specialist siloing.

In contradistinction, the body-mind-spirit focus of integrative medicine grew out of frustration with the purely physical approach to patients. In integrative medicine, patients are active participants in their healing. Their emotional, intellectual, and spiritual needs and beliefs are considered along with their physical needs. This approach, building on centuries of experience with therapeutic interventions that go beyond the standard western model, provides a deeper understanding of disease processes and effective treatments. Despite the clear value of modalities such as acupuncture, yoga, meditation, mindfulness-based stress reduction, and nutritional/dietary supplements to enhance immune competence and cognitive health or suppress inflammation, they are largely not taught in traditional medical schools.

Many of these well-established integrative measures may provide salutary impact on a patient's perception of and ability to cope with an illness, in addition to more actively engaging the patient's specific interests. The integrative approach more often involves a patient's volitional commitment to therapy, rather than a passive submission to imposed treatment. As a more global, patient-focused approached, integrative medicine may be contrasted with the more limited, disease-focused and targeted approach often taken by traditional medicine. Pain management is an excellent example of how the approaches differ. In traditional medicine, pain management usually means drug treatment, including treatment with narcotics, a strategy that has, in part, led to the current opioid crisis. In integrative medicine, pain management uses conventional treatment approaches along with effective nontraditional treatments such as acupuncture and massage. The outcomes are generally equivalent, but the risks to the patient are far less using the integrative approach—and patient satisfaction is improved as well. The combination of both integrative and traditional or conventional approaches to medical care predictably provides the most comprehensive totality of patient care.

As Dr. Steve and Dr. Sandi Amoils have shown at Alliance Integrative Medicine (AIM), the fusion of integrative and conventional care is the genesis of Transformational Medicine. They combine best practices from both approaches in the best interest of total patient care. Transformational Medicine applies disease-targeted therapies derived from basic science research and proven through randomized controlled clinical trials.

But then Transformational Medicine adds in therapies directed toward the multiple biologic systems that contribute to the disease process and that materially impact the patient's journey through illness. Transformational Medicine represents an "everything it takes" approach to restoring health and well-being.

Doctors Steve and Sandi and their excellent physicians and staff at AIM are now part of The Christ Hospital Health Network, bringing Transformational Medicine to more patients and helping Christ Hospital practitioners incorporate integrative principles into all our practice areas. In time this brand will become AIM for Wellbeing, and we look forward to integrating integrative medicine into what we do at The Christ Hospital Health Network. As the Amoils' say, "There should in time be no more 'integrative medicine!'" Ultimately, we need to incorporate what works into Good Medicine.

In this context, I sincerely hope that you enjoy your journey into their brand of integrative medicine known as Transformational Medicine. I hope this inspiring book both enhances your understanding of wellness and disease and provides a greater awareness of the therapeutic options available to help you heal.

Dean J. Kereiakes, MD, FACC, MSCAI
Chairman, The Christ Hospital Heart and Vascular Institute, Medical Director of the Christ Hospital Research Institute, Professor of Clinical Medicine at Ohio State University, Professor of Medicine at the University of Cincinnati, College of Medicine

CHAPTER 1

It's Time to AIM for Wellbeing

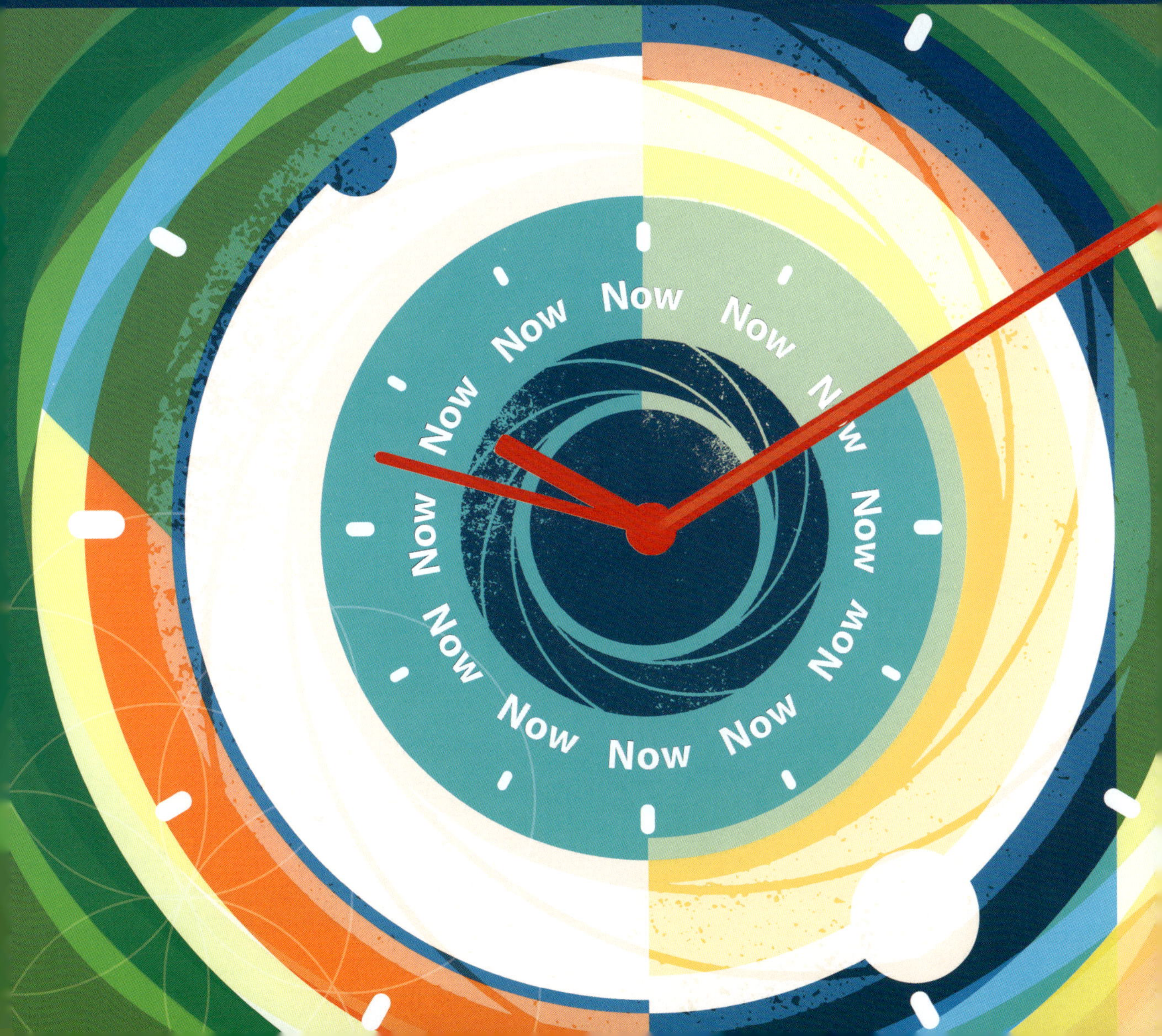

Wishing you the **best of health!**

If you ask someone why they go for a massage or take a nutritional supplement, they'll tell you they're trying to feel better. If you then ask that same person why they see a doctor, they'll reply that they're feeling sick or trying to treat an illness. They've divided two opposing health trajectories: promoting wellbeing or being sick.

They are correct. If we look at our health, there are two opposing forces. One force contains factors that make us sick, such as genetic defects, poor living or working conditions, stress, viruses, bacteria, poor nutrition, smoking, and other aspects of lifestyle. The other force is less understood: it's our body's own ability to heal and to recover. This latter force we take for granted. When we get a cut or scrape, for example, we simply watch and wait as the wound heals and the scar eventually fades or even disappears. When we get seriously ill or injured, the body still wants to heal, even if it needs some help from modern medicine. When we're psychologically bruised or hurt, it is that loving, nurturing force that helps us get rid of the pain and feel "ourselves" again. Our bodies become whole again.

This book is about dealing with these two opposing forces at the same time. We want to mitigate the forces that make us sick, while at the same time promoting the factors that make us heal.

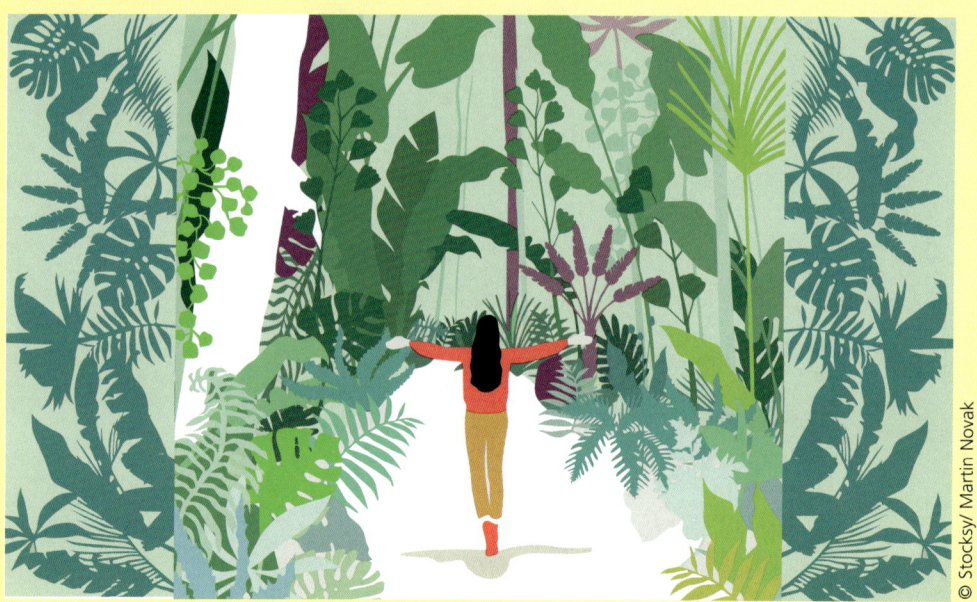

The Future of **Wellbeing**

We have seen the future of medicine, and it's happening now!

While at medical school in South Africa in the late 1970s, we learned much about modern medicine's value but also saw firsthand some of its failures. Although medicine and surgery were preeminent, they clearly didn't help a large proportion of patients. We started to see how profit in medicine could supersede the care of the patient. Today medical care has become so expensive that it has the potential to make medical care inaccessible to many of the very people who need it.

While studying medicine, we came into contact with patients with serious illnesses who had gone outside of the usual medical channels and had received great healing benefits. They had used alternative therapies to the point that their diseases had disappeared. We became fascinated with these patients, who had achieved what we termed "miracle cures." In other words, they had defied conventional medicine's logic by recovering from often incurable diseases like cancer, autoimmune diseases, chronic pain, and more. We realized we had a lot to learn, but there were no textbooks or courses to teach us. All we had were anecdotal stories from inspirational patients who used diverse and non-uniform measures to get better. We wanted to know more!

After graduating from medical school, we set out on a seemingly insurmountable mission: to travel the world and observe and study indigenous healing systems such as traditional African healers, traditional Chinese and Tibetan medicine, Japanese acupuncture, Philippine "psychic surgeons," Hawaiian kahunas, Native American shamans, and others. We met and learned from both medical doctors and healers, herbalists, naturopaths, chiropractors, and osteopaths. Our goal was to seek out more miracle patients, find out what treatments they had used, then synthesize this into something we could all use. We had little money, no insurance, no cell phones, and often no good way of staying in touch with our families. Call us crazy! Many people did.

Fast forward to 1999, when we were medical doctors in America. We were asked by the Health Alliance, a large healthcare system in Cincinnati, to open a large integrative medical clinic, the Alliance Institute for Integrative Medicine. Many naysayers let us know this would never work, especially in Cincinnati. Not our patients, though. They said, "You're way ahead of everyone in understanding that this is what the public wants." In 2004, our clinic was chosen as one of the top six integrative clinical centers in the U.S. by McKinsey & Company, a large consulting firm hired by a group of philanthropists collectively called The Bravewell Collaborative.

This experience allowed us to meet regularly with the top minds in the country as we put in place best practices and continued to refine the techniques we use. The Health Alliance disbanded and we spun off as a private center, Alliance Integrative Medicine (AIM), in 2007. In 2018 we were admitted as one of 14 accredited programs to train physicians as fellows of Integrative Medicine. Today, the number of training sites continues to grow. We were lucky to be surrounded by stellar physicians and adjunct medical staff, all amazing healers in their own right, as we did this. (Many co-authored this book. All are co-authors of this story.) We average about 30,000 patient visits per year and have amassed a large amount of experience. In 2021, our clinic was taken over by a superb hospital system, The Christ Hospital Health Network (interestingly, the founder member of the Health Alliance). Our clinic is now titled the same as this book, AIM for Wellbeing, for reasons you will soon discover.

Today, we once again feel as we did when we opened our clinic in 1999 . . . and what we are about to tell you may once again feel like a stretch. The type of medicine we practice has continued to evolve and grow and is doing so now at what feels like breathtaking speed. We always said that if Integrative Medicine worked, it should and would become part of mainstream medicine. This is happening. We see chiropractors working alongside neurosurgeons, acupuncture and meditation replacing drugs for chronic pain, and doctors more comfortable in using nutritional supplements. Life is changing, fast. We need to move with it. This book is our observation of where medicine has come from, and where it is going. We hope it will be a blueprint for those who wish to follow.

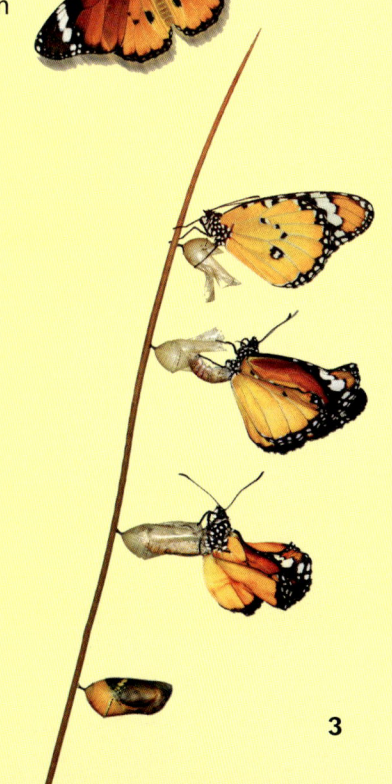

Your Health and Wellbeing
Is Your Highest Good!

Think of the changes that have happened to society since the birth of the iPhone in 2007. We feel the speed of change is now accelerating even faster. Artificial intelligence, nanotechnology, gene editing, systems biology and multi-omics, mass data interpretation, and a host of new technologies are about to radically transform how we see and do almost everything.

These technologies hold great promise, for both good and bad! *It is up to us to use them for good!* How do we do this? *What needs to be the driving principle?* We feel that it is Optimal Health and Wellbeing for ALL! Why? Because if this is the *highest principle*, everything forms underneath it. Our optimal health and wellbeing means we must make continual choices that will help us. To do this, we must by inference also help our families, our societies, our countries, and our planet. In this book we will explain how and why.

We have the good fortune to take care of patients from all walks of life. What do people want when they have everything that money can buy? You got it . . . health and wellbeing! And people struggling to survive financially also know that this survival depends on their health and wellbeing. Although we all seek happiness, health and wellbeing is a higher goal—and true health and wellbeing includes being happy.

Interestingly, health and wellbeing seems to have a fantastic side effect: reversing illness and aging! People around the world are now researching and doing what once seemed impossible: aging themselves backward. When we discuss this with friends, they typically say, "Why would I want to live longer? Being old is just being decrepit." *But what if you could age chronologically but feel and look as you did when you were much younger?* This is a conundrum of Modern Wellness that we will discuss later in the book. It requires us to think differently about how we live in the world, and how we want the world in which we live to be.

Read on as we show you why and how you need to become your best self.

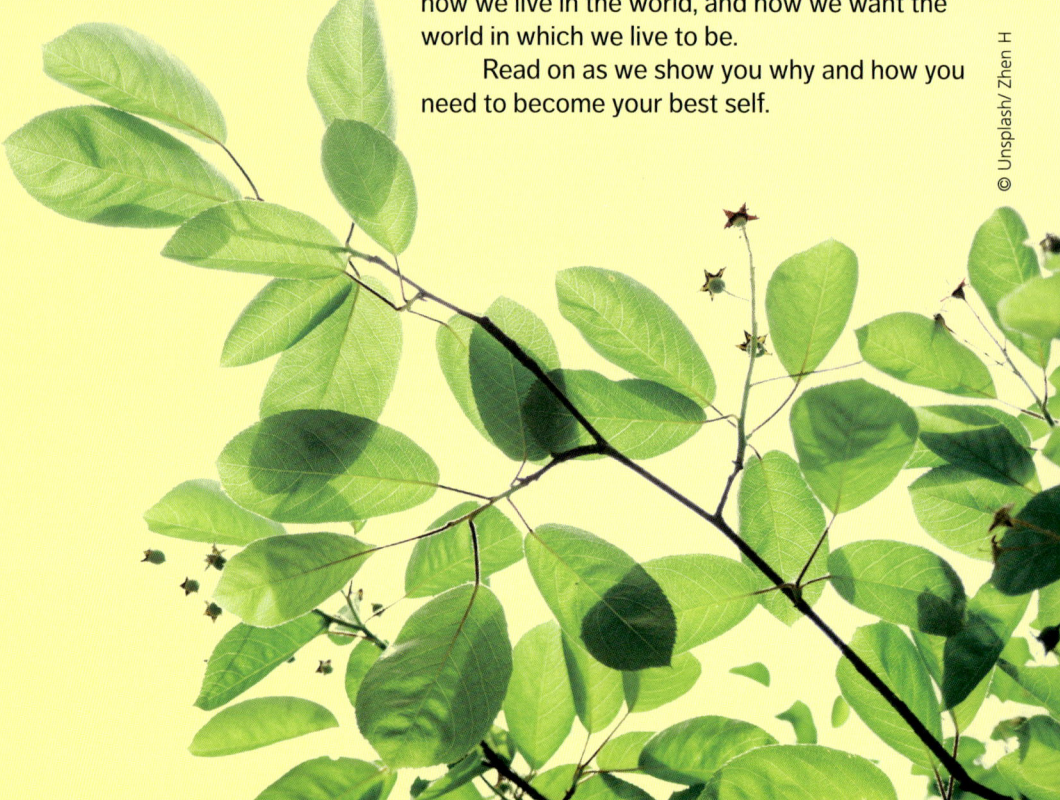

© Unsplash/ Zhen H

CHAPTER 1 | It's Time to AIM for Wellbeing

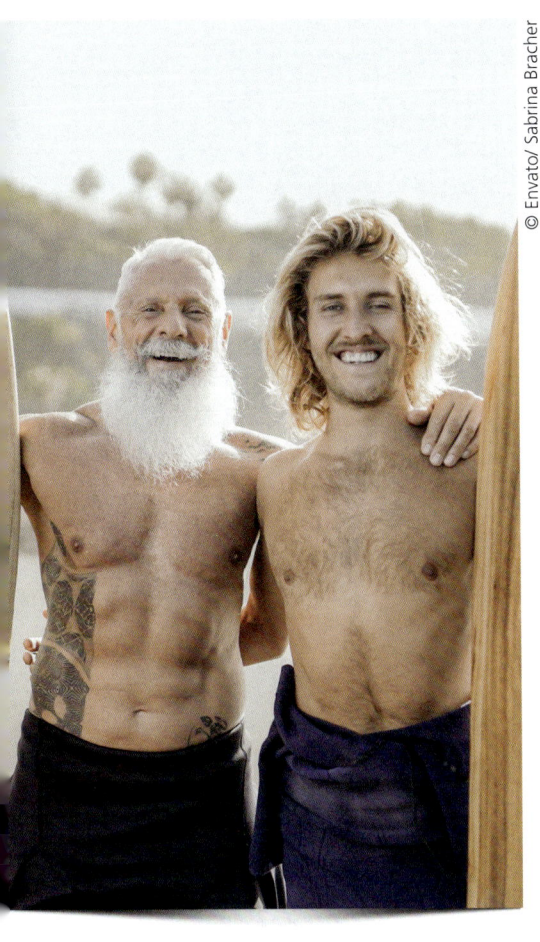

When you consider your long-term health, what are you thinking about? Is it about the number of years you will live, or *lifespan*? Or are you really thinking about your *healthspan*, the number of those years you remain healthy and free of disease? Our goal for you is both: a long lifespan in a state of abundant health and wellbeing.

What Is **Wellbeing?**

To us, wellness means physical, mental, and emotional good health. Wellbeing starts there and goes beyond—it's a subjective state of happiness, positivity, vitality and resilience. We want you to achieve both wellness and wellbeing.

What is **True Wellness?**

True wellness includes:
- Physical health and vitality
- Emotional stability
- A state of wellbeing
- Intellectual acuity
- An ability to express and receive love
- A sense of openness
- The ability to embrace change
- The ability to speak your own truth
- A sense of intuition
- A feeling of spiritual wellbeing, including alignment with your own purpose and meaning in the world
- Creating and building a harmonious community
- A safe and healthy environment

The **Balance** of Health

We tend to think that we navigate through life on a seesaw, where counteracting forces make us sick or well, and balance is only temporary. In the diagram below, we look at this concept.

The seesaw doesn't have to swing up and down all the time—it can stay balanced. To remain healthy and achieve long-term balance, we need to do two things simultaneously:

1. *Reduce the impetus to disease and illness.* Throughout this book, we'll discuss how we do this using the combination of conventional medicine, integrative medicine, and functional medicine.

2. *Promote resilience and vitality* through lifestyle improvements, stress reduction, nutrition, and integrative medicine techniques.

When we do this, we alter our trajectory toward health and wellbeing and away from disease. The changes that lead to an altered trajectory mostly come as small steps—but occasionally as quantum leaps. We call this process Transformational Medicine™.

Our hope is that you too will become optimistic about transforming your health trajectory to one that is positive and reinforces health, vitality, and an improved long-term outlook for your health.

Our aim is to give you options that enable you to change your health for the better by developing your own personalized, proactive Transformational Wellness Plan™.

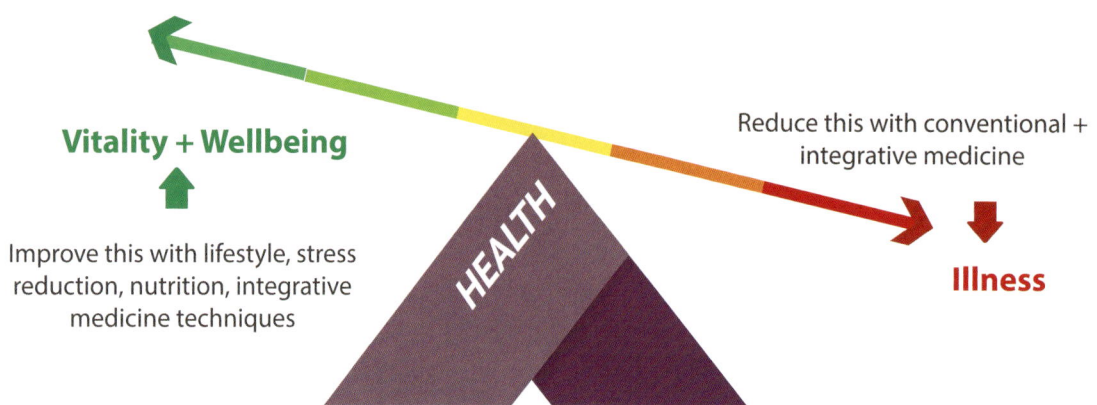

FIGURE 1.1 | Taking Control of Your Health

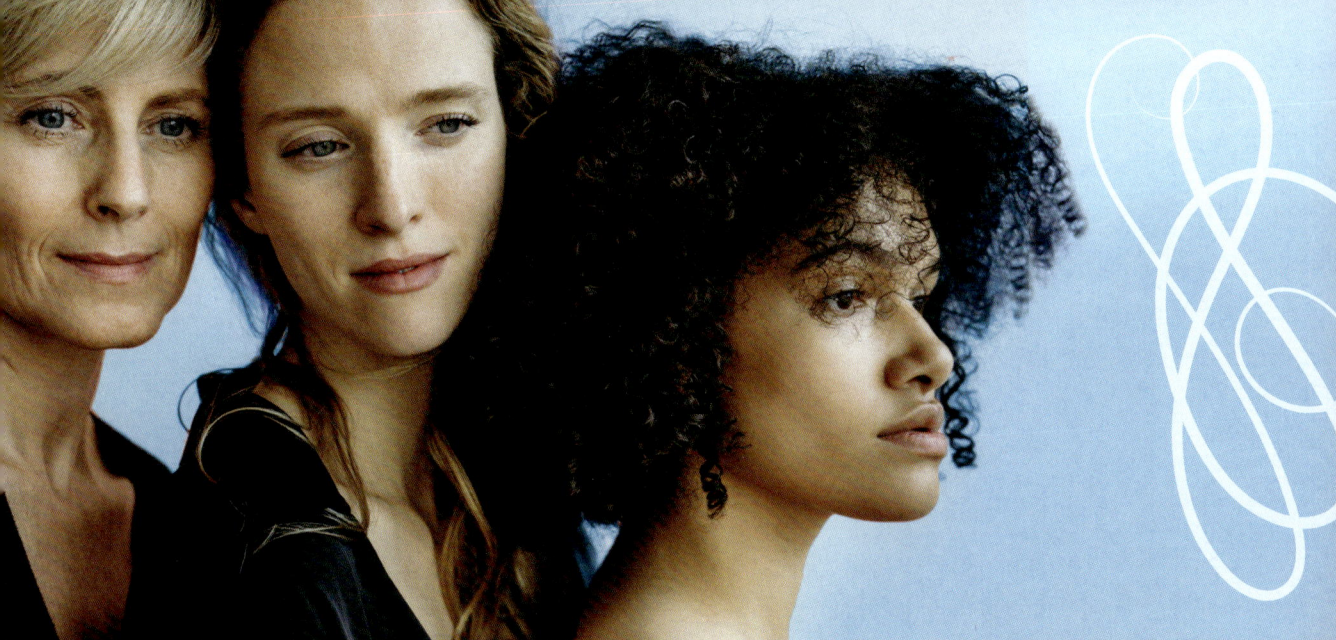

Guiding Principles to Both **Wellness** and **Wellbeing**

❦ Acknowledge the beauty and uniqueness of every person.

While we all share many similarities, we are also all unique. Even identical twins have different fingerprints. Each patient is biochemically unique and will respond differently to medications, nutrients, and stress of all types. To understand what's best for each individual patient, we need to understand what happened to them on their path to illness, and then bring out their strengths as they move toward healing.

❦ Promote mental wellbeing and a sense of empowerment.

Disease can sneak up on us as a silent marauder, often sabotaging our plans and ideas. We like to say that this is often the time when the Disney movie life script changes to that of a slasher film. This is when patients may feel powerless, helpless, and afraid, which often further impacts their illness. At this juncture, we help our patients understand how best to navigate both their illness and its impact on their life and help them regain a sense of control. We give them options—tools for their toolbox—and help them understand that they are a critical part of their own healthcare team. Patients need to understand that while they may have an illness, they are not an illness!

We want you to feel connected to your own sense of life purpose and develop a life of meaning, no matter what age or stage of life you are in.

❦ Boost metabolic resilience and flexiblilty.

As people age, they may feel that their energy has been permanently diminished. Physiologically, they begin to lose resilience. Their capacity to respond to physical and mental stress in a healthy way is diminished. They feel they can't bounce back like they did before.

In our experience, lost resilience can be regained.

As we help patients optimize their nutri-

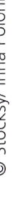
© Stocksy/ Irina Polonina

tion, change their exercise protocols, and look at life differently, their lives begin to change, and they begin to repair themselves. After a while, they notice their health returning. Their bodies are more forgiving. In fact, their entire physiology and outlook are more flexible. Things that were too much for them—like long walks without pain or exhaustion—now are possible again. They've gained insight into what makes them feel well and vibrant.

Metabolically, patients can regain flexibility too. We often see this in our patients with insulin resistance. Once we help them learn how to change their diet, exercise, alter their stress levels, and perhaps take some supplements or medications, they notice that their metabolism begins to function more normally.

We need Real Food!

We cannot overemphasize this. Food is a signal to our cells. Each time we eat, we give our body a message: get healthy, or get sick! Modern food technology means that today more than 60 percent of the Standard American Diet is ultraprocessed foods that have been manufactured in factories. These foods are so refined, modified, and filled with chemicals that they are barely recognizable to our bodies. We need to consume real foods that nature, not food industry factories and fast-food chains, has made. If your great-grandmother wouldn't recognize it, or if it has chemicals that you can't pronounce or don't recognize, it's not *real food*.

Augment nutritional and physiologic reserves.

By reserves, we mean your body's ability to function well even when you're experiencing stresses such as illness, surgery, or a difficult period in your life. The greater your reserves, the better your mind and body can cope and the faster you can bounce back. Although reserves tend to decline with age, we see many younger patients whose reserves are already low. Regardless of the status of your reserves, building them up so you can thrive in trying times is a worthwhile goal.

Have you ever been that person who is so run down that everything seems to go wrong? Do you catch colds more easily, feel angry or tearful at silly things, struggle to get out of bed, or generally feel that life is conspiring against you? This is when your reserves are all used up. Your batteries are low.

A lack of reserves is often difficult to quantify. Patients know they feel bad, yet conventional lab tests say they're normal. (We'll discuss this more in the later chapters of this book.) For now, just know there are ways to build up your nutritional and physiologic reserves.

Encourage physical activity and proprioceptive exercises.

In areas of the world where people live healthy lives into their nineties and beyond, the type of exercise they do doesn't involve a gym. Instead, they incorporate exercise into their daily living. They walk, they do chores, they work in their gardens, they care for animals and children—they move almost as much as they did when they were younger. In most of our suburban and urban lives, we drive or sit much more than we walk, so we have to make a conscious effort to incorporate more activity into our daily living. That may mean using a gym or a remote exercise class a couple of times a week. However, it's also easy to incorporate other forms of activity into our daily lives. Housework, walking with our pets, playing with children and grandchildren, parking further away, taking the stairs instead of the elevator, walking for at least ten minutes after each meal, stretching for a few minutes as we get up or go to sleep—all these activities add up over the course of a day. As we age, we tend to lose our sense of proprioception (knowing where our body is in space). This can lead to poor balance, falls, and even fractures and concussions, which can start a downward spiral of poor health. As we get older, however, we need to fight against sarcopenia (muscle loss) and osteoporosis (thinning bones). That may require adding regular weight-bearing exercise to our daily schedule. To combat this, we need to maintain strong muscles and bones and add daily activity that helps us keep our sense of proprioception intact. Walking, tai chi, dancing, yoga, and balance exercises all help slow or even reverse this loss.

While we promote fitness, being fit doesn't always mean being healthy. We see athletes with many kinds of illnesses. We want to encourage you to be both fit and healthy!

Reduce environmental toxicity.

Every day in modern society, we're exposed to industrial and environmental chemicals in the air we breathe, the water we drink, the foods we eat, and the products we put on our bodies. Vehicle exhaust, air pollution, plastic microparticles, pesticides, agricultural fertilizers, household cleaning products, flame retardants, fabric softeners, personal care products, and thousands of other toxins are almost inescapable. Many of these are "forever chemicals" that don't degrade in our bodies or in the environment. Our bodies are under constant assault—and they can't fight back. These chemicals are new and we haven't evolved the chemical pathways to clear or degrade them. The compounding effect of multiple chemicals in low doses can cause serious health issues that are hard to detect and define, and even harder to treat. While we can't completely eliminate environmental toxins, minimizing our exposures means less stress on our detoxification systems.

It's not just biochemical toxicity that concerns us. Emotional toxicity can have a profound effect on our health too. Physical, verbal, emotional, and sexual abuse permeate up to one in three households and are common in work environments. In recent years, we've gained a lot of clarity on the damaging effects of abuse, sexism, ageism, racial and ethnic intolerance, and hostile work environments. We recognize how these emotionally toxic environments can manifest as physical illness. Seeking help to overcome these situations is vital to creating the love and connection we all need to be our best selves.

We need to change our minds.

In recent years we have seen an unprecedented rise in mental health problems, gun violence, and political discord. These issues are fueling societal stress in a much more interconnected world. Even the U.S. Surgeon General, typically involved in public health matters such as smoking cessation, has now warned about the effect of social media on mental health. Our challenge as a society is to heal the discontent and create harmony and the true sense of belonging that most people desperately crave.

Increase the innate vitality of your body to foster self-healing.

Innate vitality is more than mental wellbeing. It correlates with increased strength, better immunity, higher resilience, and generally improved physiologic function. Have you ever watched your body heal a wound, cut, or scrape? This little miracle happens without our

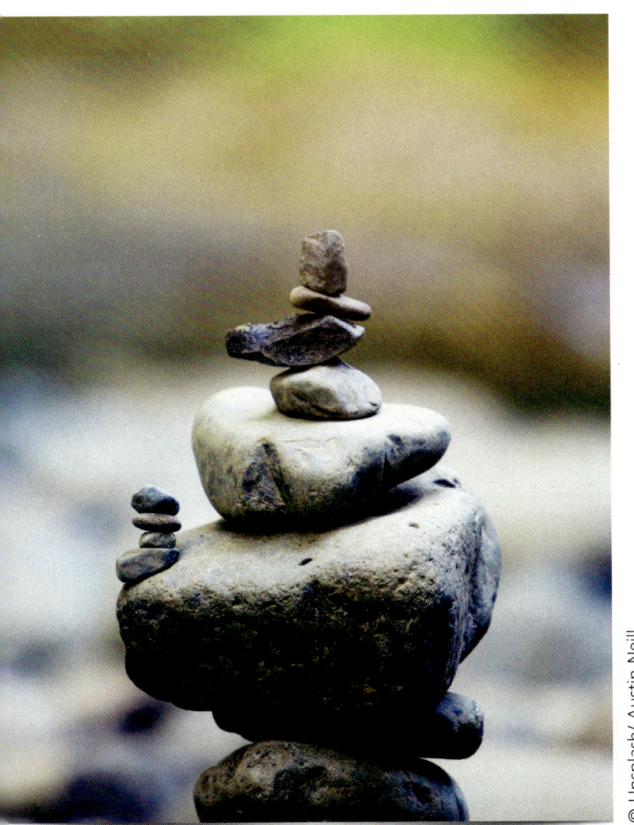

© Unsplash/ Austin Neill

help. The body just knows what to do! This is self-healing in action. Good nutrition, the ability to manage stress, and fitness from regular physical activity all help maintain vitality across a lifetime.

When we lived in China and Japan, we learned how important this innate vitality, called "chi" or "qi" in China and "ki" in Japan—was to good health. In many workplaces, a bell would ring a few times a day and all employees would go outside together for a short period of simple breathing, stretching, and mind-body exercises. Similarly, retired adults would get together in parks and other public places for short exercise periods. The result was an immediate restoration of energy and glow. It's similar to how you would feel after a gym session or exercise class. Throughout this book, we will show you ways to reclaim your sense of vitality.

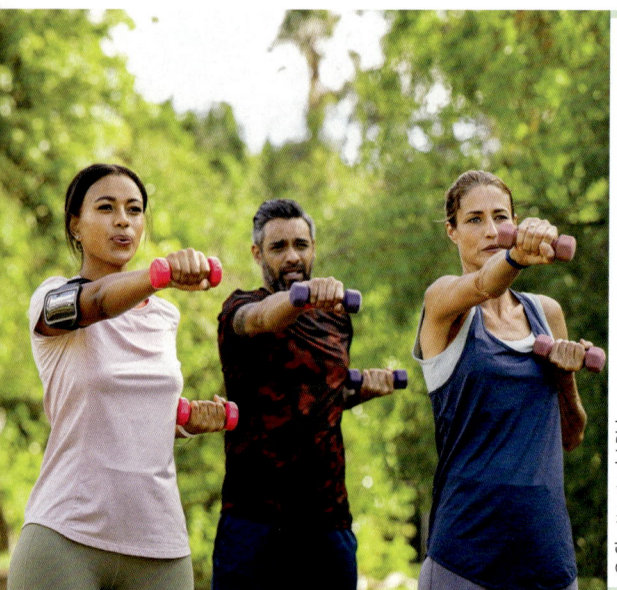

As you read this book, you will learn more about allaying illness, while simultaneously promoting a sense of wellbeing and vitality. In fact, many patients who follow these principles find that while their chronological age (their age in years) is increasing, their biological age (how old their body really is) can decrease.

**You too can
Get Well,
Be Well and Stay Well!**

CHAPTER 2

Integrating Best Practices: The Development of Transformational Medicine®

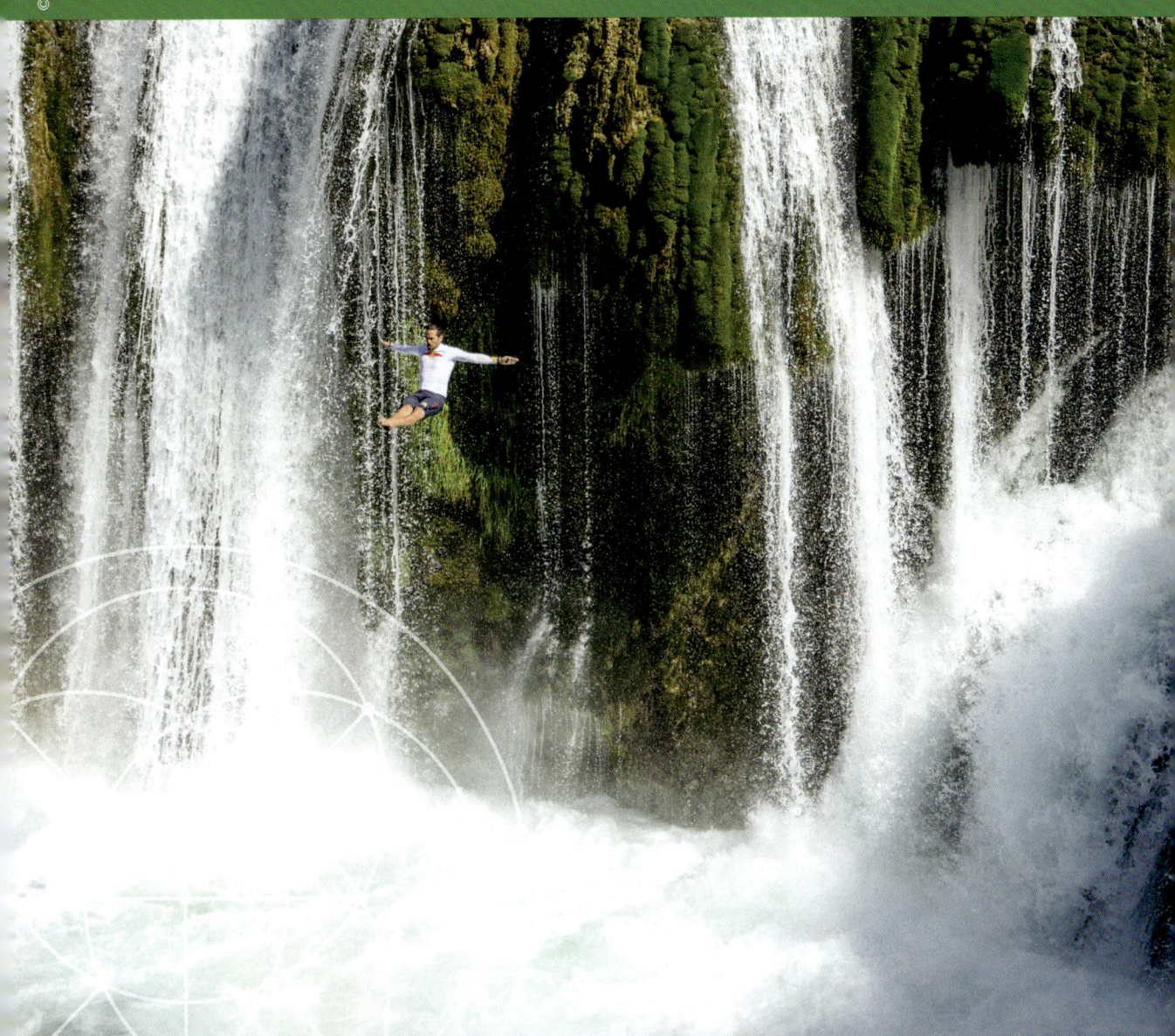

Synergistic Goals and Complementary Talents: **The Evolution of a Philosophy**

We are fortunate to have been influenced and taught by astute philosophers, physicians, and healers who can think outside of the box. Over the past few decades, the ability to produce data is often confused with science. The law of gravity was present long before Newton "discovered" it. Similarly, our bodies behave in ways that have been observed for centuries, even though scientific techniques or theories may not yet have validated them. Diagnostic and therapeutic techniques will continue to evolve, and we will continue to incorporate that progress into our practice. This book is based upon what we have learned from centuries of medical tradition and science but includes evergreen principles distilled from wise teachers, worldwide experience, decades of clinical experience, and the insight gained from treating thousands of patients. These unchanging concepts give you insight into your body's hardware and software—and help you view your health and life in a new way.

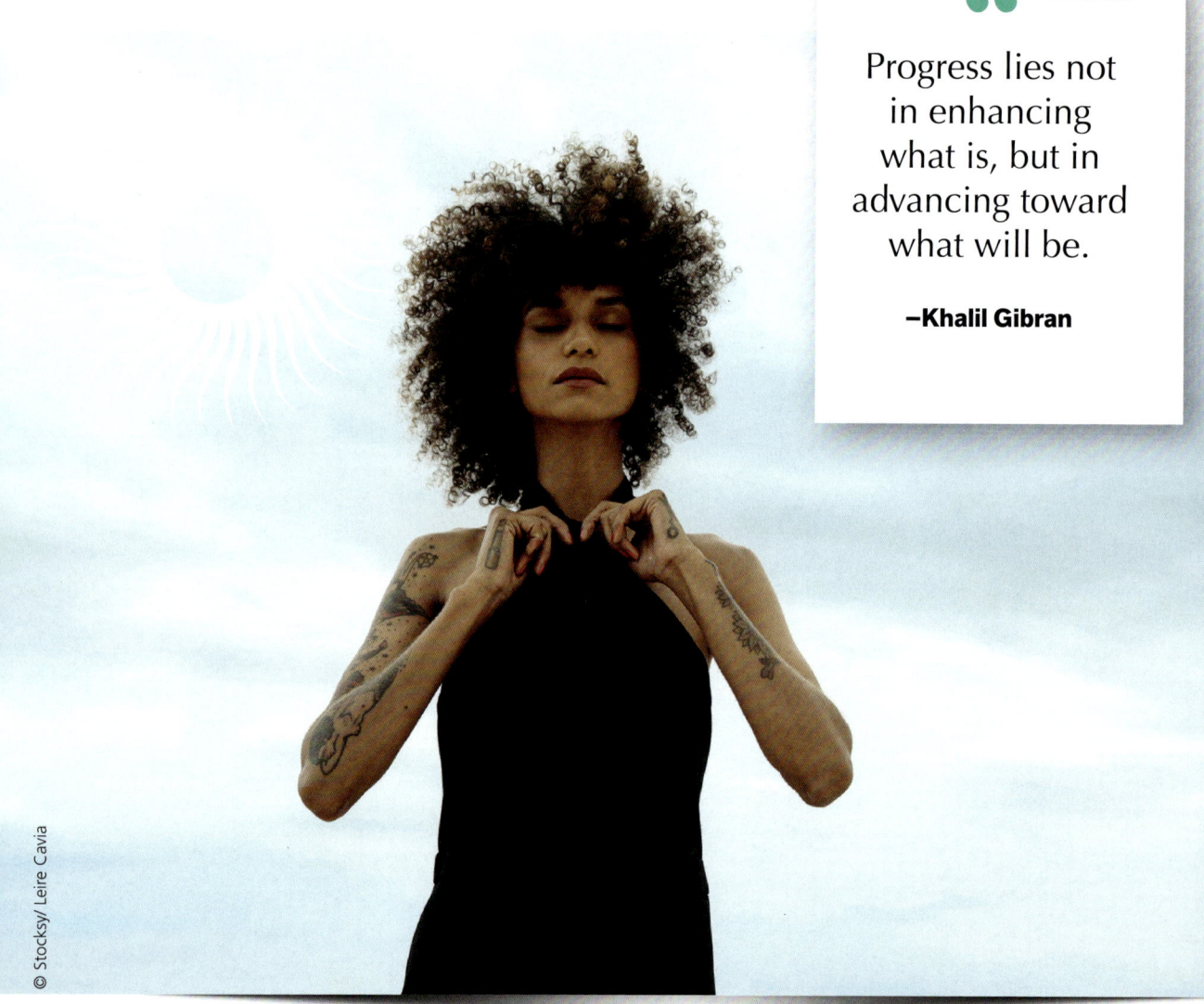

> Progress lies not in enhancing what is, but in advancing toward what will be.
>
> **–Khalil Gibran**

Transforming Your Life

We have seen the ability to bounce back from extreme stress in many of our most successful mentors, friends, and patients. When they do, they come out stronger, wiser, and more successful. They can take a problem that would otherwise devastate most people and use it to make themselves—and the world—a better place. To use a well-known phrase, they turn lemons into lemonade.

Our goal in Transformational Medicine is to optimize physical function, psychological transformation, and spiritual growth to attain true healing. Healing is a dynamic process. Often the starting point is the diagnosis of a disease or the persistence of symptoms even after treatment.

Transformational Medicine usually means working with a health care team. At the center is a physician with whom you can openly discuss both your symptoms and your fears—a doctor you can trust to do an appropriate medical workup and who will refer you to appropriate medical specialists if necessary. However, Transformational Medicine also means looking at other options beyond conventional medicine. Depending on your needs, other health care providers may become part of your team. In our practice, we work with chiropractors, acupuncturists, energy healers, massage therapists, and others who provide healing care.

We have come to realize that we all can move toward wellbeing by transforming our symptoms of dis-ease or dis-comfort into a new state of better health—and this is an approach we can apply to life every day.

In other words, we would like you to reinterpret your illness as a reminder that you may need to change. This approach will enable you to use the challenges in your life as turning points or inflection points to self-correct. We all have the option of changing our trajectory toward either wellbeing or disease. With this book, we would like to give you the tools to expand your options to create healing and achieve positive change in your life.

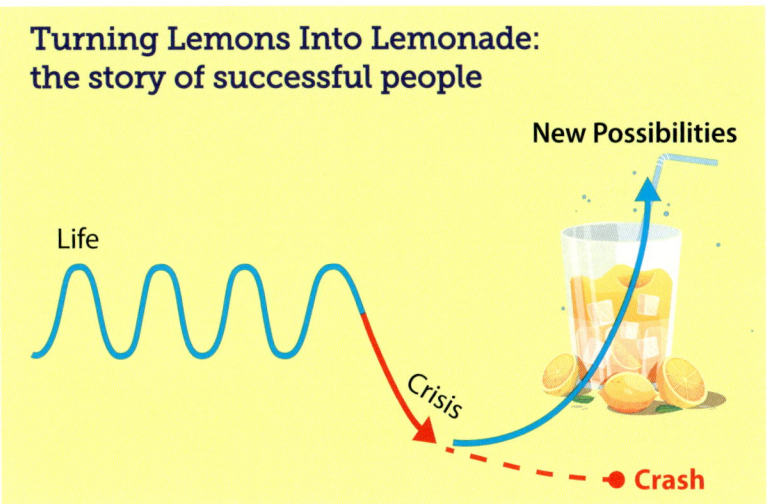

FIGURE 2.1 | Crisis and Transformation

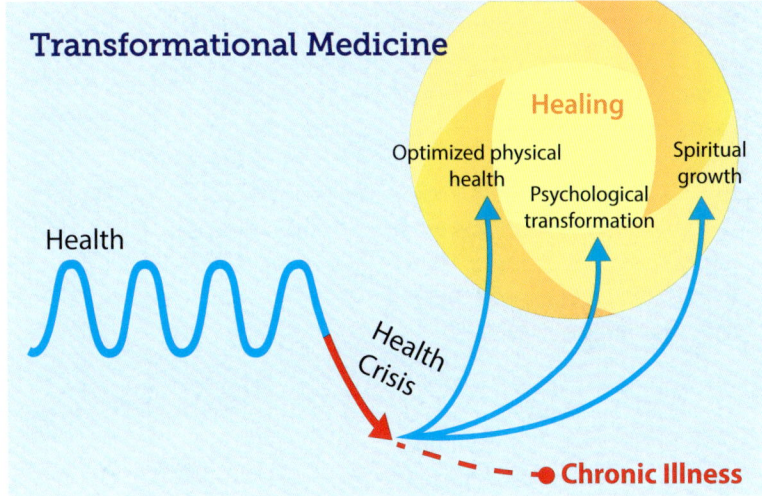

FIGURE 2.2 | The Healing Goals of Transformational Medicine.

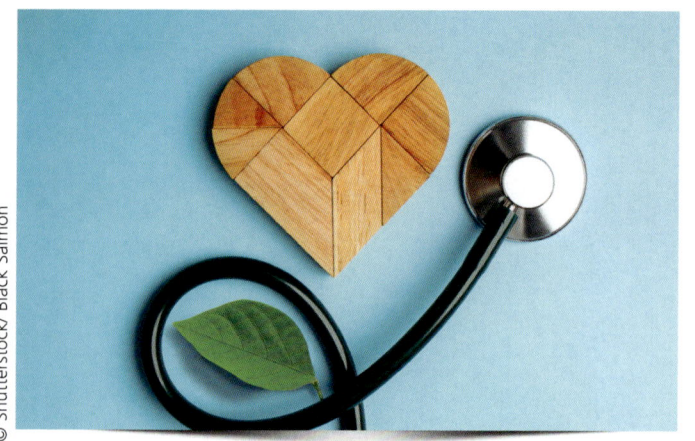

Transformational Medicine: A Solution to the Escalating Burden of Chronic Illness

To explain how and why we want you to change your life, we need you to understand how medicine arrived at its current status. Patients today—especially those with chronic conditions—get a lot of medical treatment: office visits, diagnostic tests of all sorts, many prescriptions for drugs, physical therapy, weight-loss counseling, and more. Yet often their health is no better. How is it possible that we as a society have so much medicine, while at the same time we see more and more people with chronic conditions that only get worse despite aggressive treatment?

The Development of Modern Medicine and the Legacy of Flexner

More than a century ago, there was a need for standardization in medicine. At the time, there were a multitude of approaches to medicine. Many were worthless and others were harmful. It was the time of snake-oil salesmen and charlatans. There was no FDA, there were no national standards, and there were no protections against medicines that were contaminated or ineffective. Medical schools varied widely in how well and how much they taught their students; in some schools, students who didn't even have a high school education could get a diploma after just two years.

To rectify the problem, the Carnegie Foundation commissioned Abraham Flexner, a professional educator, to study medical schools and the drug industry and make recommendations for improvements. The recommendations in the Flexner Report of 1910 set high standards and established a level of consistency within medicine and the emerging pharmaceutical industry. The report set the stage for safer medical protocols and standards of practice as we know them today. It also eliminated proprietary medical schools and established the biomedical model as the gold standard of medical training. Sadly, the report also had sexist and racist elements. It set back the education of women in medicine and led to the closure of five out of seven historically Black medical schools.

This internal housecleaning within American medicine also resulted in over-standardization. Many disciplines focusing on prevention and health promotion were eliminated—they were seen as backward and unscientific. As these other forms of medicine began to fade away, the concept of healing became associated with the top-down biomedical model of drugs and surgery.

The scientific model used as the basis for medical training relied on the Cartesian logic of separation of mind and body, as if there were no link between them. Only in recent decades has science begun to understand the link between these different systems. Hence, we have words like "psychoneuroimmunobiology" or "the gut-brain connection" as we adopt a whole-body systems approach.

The Age of the Silver Bullet

The era of antibiotics began soon after World War II, when penicillin became widely available. The focus of medicine then became finding the correct microbe that was causing the disease and killing it with the correct antibiotic. This quest for a singular cause extended to other areas of medicine as well. Scientists learned to break down a problem into its smallest components and look for a way to remedy these. It became a system of "anti"-dotes—hence our emphasis today on antibiotics, anti-inflammatories, anticancer agents, and other "anti" treatments. As a result, patients nowadays want that silver bullet and expect a quick fix when it comes to their health.

Medical Silos

As medicine became more scientific and our understanding of disease grew, different specialties arose, treating independent parts of the body. The presumption is that with higher specialization comes improved care. This is true if your problem calls for someone who is highly specialized in one area. But what if a specialist acts in a silo, with a narrow vision that can't see the other aspects of your health and excludes your other physicians? That's when problems arise. An orthopedist may prescribe anti-inflammatories without knowing—or even asking—if a patient has kidney problems. The results can be disastrous. In some areas of the United States, the average patient takes six to seven prescription drugs, often prescribed by different doctors who may not know about the other drugs. Adverse drug events from drug interactions to side effects are so common that they cause approximately 1.3 million emergency department visits each year. In addition, patients often use herbal remedies or supplements without telling their doctors, risking potentially dangerous drug interactions. And while there are good studies on the effects of single drugs, there are few good studies on what happens when patients take multiple drugs at the same time.

Where Medicine Succeeds

You don't need to look far to be impressed by the miracles of modern medicine. What is working well is working very well. The benefits of Western medicine range from newer, better medications and less invasive surgeries to high-tech trauma centers and state-of-the-art intensive care units.

If you pause to think about these advances, though, you realize that most of them deal with acute care, highly technical care, less invasive and safer surgery, and the effect of blockbuster drugs on conditions like high cholesterol, heart disease, depression, heartburn, hypertension, inflammation, and psychosis. Western medicine especially excels in acute conditions such as infection, trauma, or heart attacks. The medications and techniques developed to treat these conditions are fast-acting and can be life-saving. Modern trauma care is without parallel in the history of medicine. In acute situations, there is no better place to be than in the hands of a physician who has made a correct diagnosis and is prescribing the correct treatment.

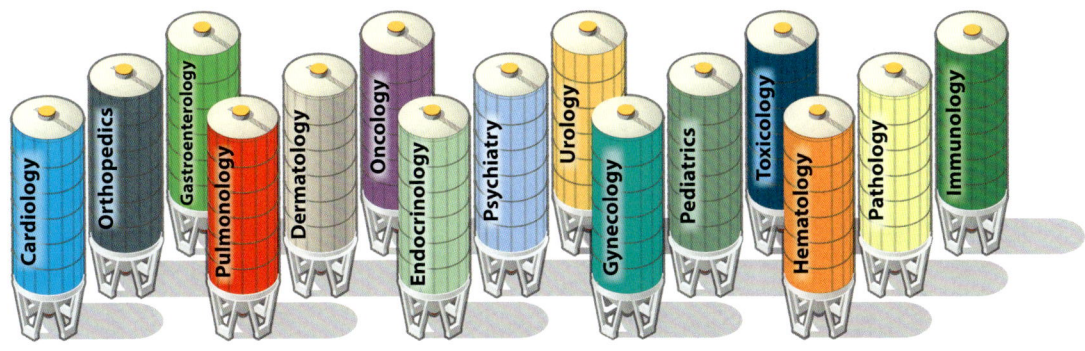

FIGURE 2.3 | Medical Specialization Leads to a Silo Mentality

Chronic Illness and Conventional Medicine

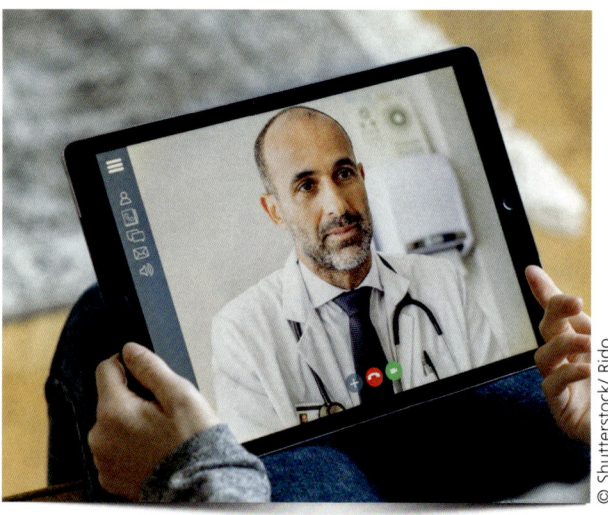

The Western medical approach works well in areas that deal with acute conditions. By accurately defining a problem, medical practitioners can provide the best treatment to save lives.

The problem is that this approach isn't working as well for chronic health issues such as obesity, type 2 diabetes, high blood pressure, chronic pain conditions such as arthritis and back pain, gastrointestinal disorders, and autoimmune diseases, especially if someone has more than one condition.

Chronic health problems are seldom easy to treat. As a result, they are crippling our medical system. More than half of all adults in the United States have some form of chronic illness. In addition, nearly 75 percent of Americans are overweight or obese and at serious risk of type 2 diabetes if they don't have it already. The need for a system of health care that addresses chronic conditions has become more important than ever.

In a medical system built around the use of specific drugs for specific disorders, treating chronic disorders can be extremely frustrating for both physicians and patients. The economic and time constraints placed on primary care physicians in mainstream medicine force them to become technicians, relying on algorithms and guidelines instead of spending time with patients. As a result, patients may feel that they are not being heard, and doctors may inadvertently dismiss important complaints and concerns. Also, treatments tend to focus on symptoms that are the expression of underlying problems, rather than on the problems themselves. For example, high cholesterol is not a disease but an expression of an underlying malfunction that may or may not lead to heart disease. Rather than look upstream for the source of the problem, however, physicians often prescribe a statin drug and give some generic advice about a low-fat diet.

The puzzle of chronic illness has not been easy to decipher. In 1989, Kurt Kroenke, MD, a medical researcher, tracked the progress of one thousand patients in an US Army outpatient medical clinic over a three-year period. He looked at the fourteen most common chronic complaints: chest pain, fatigue, dizziness, headache, edema, back pain, shortness of breath, insomnia, abdominal pain, numbness, impotence, weight loss, cough, and constipation. Kroenke found that patients dealing with three or more concurrent health conditions for at least three months had only one chance in six of getting well. The likelihood that conventional medical treatment would resolve the problem was less than 16 percent.

Unresolved Health Issues

In Kroenke's study of common chronic problems, 55 percent of the patients received symptomatic treatment, and this treatment was often ineffective. The conditions most likely to improve were those that had lasted less than four months in patients with a history of two or fewer symptoms, or whose symptoms turned out to have a specific cause. Among patients with vague, nonspecific, or difficult-to-treat complaints, such as chronic fatigue, frequent insomnia, or dizziness, only 39 percent reported relief from conventional therapies.

Although the study was performed in 1989, the findings are still valid. In fact, in our experience, the problems seem to have magnified. The care provided for these types of chronic conditions is often both expensive and ineffective. It simply treats symptoms rather than getting at the underlying cause. According to Ralph Snyderman, MD, chancellor emeritus of the Duke University School of Medicine, "What we have now is a 'sick-care' system that is reactive to problems. The integrative approach flips the system on its head and puts the patient at the center, addressing not just symptoms, but the real causes of illness. It is care that is preventive, predictive, and personalized." We need to change the system and adopt this integrative approach.

The Best of Medicine

Integrative medicine offers a solution. Simply defined, integrative medicine provides the best of conventional medicine in tandem with the best of complementary therapies. It is a synergistic, real-world, evidence-based approach to treatment.

We fully support the ethic described by Marcia Angell, MD, former editor of the prestigious *New England Journal of Medicine,* who said, "There cannot be two kinds of medicine—conventional and alternative. There is only medicine that has been adequately tested and medicine that has not, medicine that works and medicine that may or may not work." However, complementary therapies are often not easy to study in a controlled trial. It is difficult to perform sham acupuncture, for example, so that the results can be compared to similar patients who get real acupuncture. Furthermore, an integrative approach often uses several less invasive treatments simultaneously, making a study on this type of approach even more complicated. In addition, there is limited research data on herbal, nutritional, and supplement-based therapies because there is no financial support for such studies, as the pharmaceutical industry cannot make money on these therapies.

The Goals of Integrative Medicine

As practitioners of Integrative Medicine, we aim for a new approach that emphasizes health and wellbeing. In Integrative Medicine, care is:

- **Personalized.** Health care customized to your genetics, body chemistry, stress level, and lifestyle.
- **Proactive.** An approach that involves you in your own care, focusing on practical action steps.
- **Preventive.** Treatment that not only resolves current problems, but also reduces the risks of future health problems before they develop.
- **Patient-centered.** Treatment that includes you as the primary member of your health care team, acknowledging that you know your symptoms better than anyone does.
- **Empowering.** Care that provides you with an expanded range of tools that support your health and wellbeing, helping you to become more responsible for your health outcome.

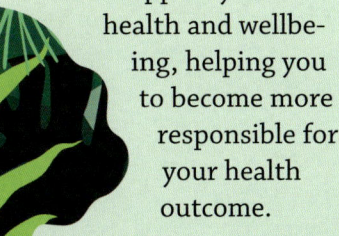

A Systems Biology Approach to Understanding Health and Disease

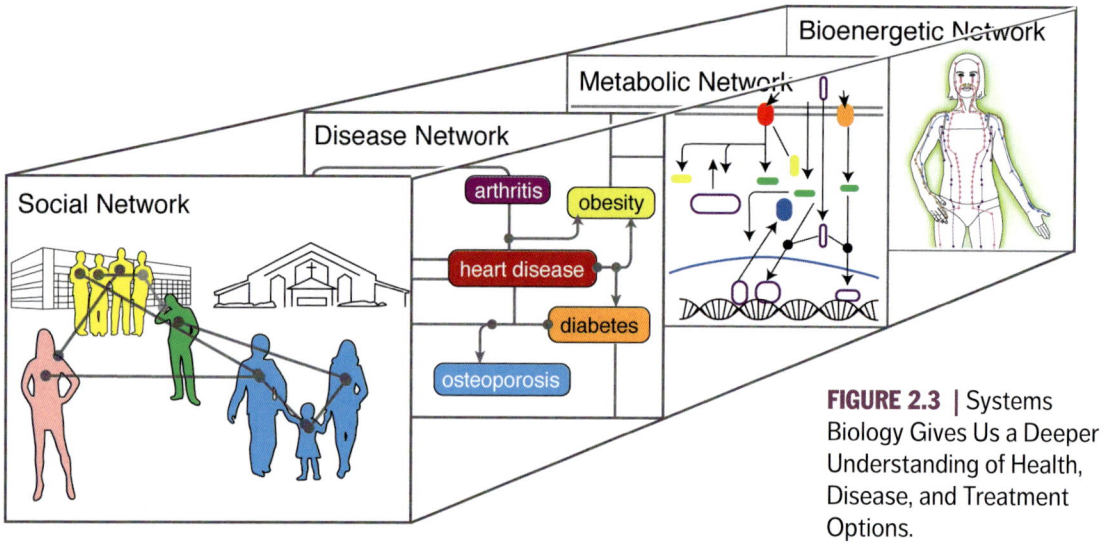

FIGURE 2.3 | Systems Biology Gives Us a Deeper Understanding of Health, Disease, and Treatment Options.

Systems Biology and **Your Health**

Today, new technologies such as genomics, information technology, nanotechnology, bioinformatics, network biology, and translational research have given us a dramatically improved understanding of how we become ill. This new way of looking at the complex interactions in the human body is called systems biology.

Systems biology allows us to see that several major factors can contribute to the development of a specific disease in any given individual.

Social networks affect disease. Studies have shown that people with better social connections and support handle life challenges better than those who are isolated and lonely. These social connections may include family, partners or spouses, friends, peers, religious communities, or social groups. In general, financial, emotional, and even physical stresses tend to be cushioned if someone has a good support system. This tells us we can't view a patient as an isolated disease. We also need to view the person in the context of a social network, as this will influence how that person will develop and express disease.

Diseases are linked to each other. Someone who is obese is more likely to develop heart disease, diabetes, and arthritis than someone who is not obese. These diseases are different, but they also tend to occur in conjunction with one another. In medicine, such diseases are called comorbidities. When a patient has comorbidities, we find it is usually because their diseases share similar metabolic underpinnings.

Different diseases may share similar metabolic pathways. The chemical pathways that influence one disease may be influencing another at the same time. A good example of this is inflammation. This low-grade fire in our bodies can simultaneously affect diseases such as coronary artery disease, arthritis, osteoporosis, Alzheimer's disease, and even cancer. The cells in our bodies constantly send chemical signals to each other. When we are inflamed, chemicals travel around our bodies, lighting fires in many areas. That is why one metabolic dysfunction can result in many diseases. But here lies an opportunity to treat many diseases by using one approach that deals with the underlying problem.

Our bioenergetic networks affect our health.
Traditional Chinese medicine has used the concept of bioenergetic networks for thousands of years. According to Chinese medicine, bioenergetic networks, also called meridian systems or biopsychotypes, affect the functioning of our metabolic pathways. By understanding the imbalances in these networks, it is possible to predict where disease will occur and simultaneously treat and prevent illness.

With a systems biology perspective, we can move away from the idea that disease will simply strike us as some misguided lightning bolt from the sky. We can look at the myriad interacting internal and external factors that create health or disease. And we can learn to start affecting these factors in many dimensions—not just to treat and prevent illness, but to promote health itself.

Functional Medicine

Functional medicine, a term coined by one of our mentors, Jeffrey Bland, PhD, FACN, CNS, explains how diseases are affected by multiple systems. It details how external factors—stress, our community support, environmental toxins, diet, lifestyle, and exercise—interact with internal factors in our bodies. These include factors related to our genetic makeup; our hormonal, immune, and neurotransmitter balance; inflammation; gut health; and musculoskeletal health. Functional medicine is a modern, scientifically based approach, but many of its

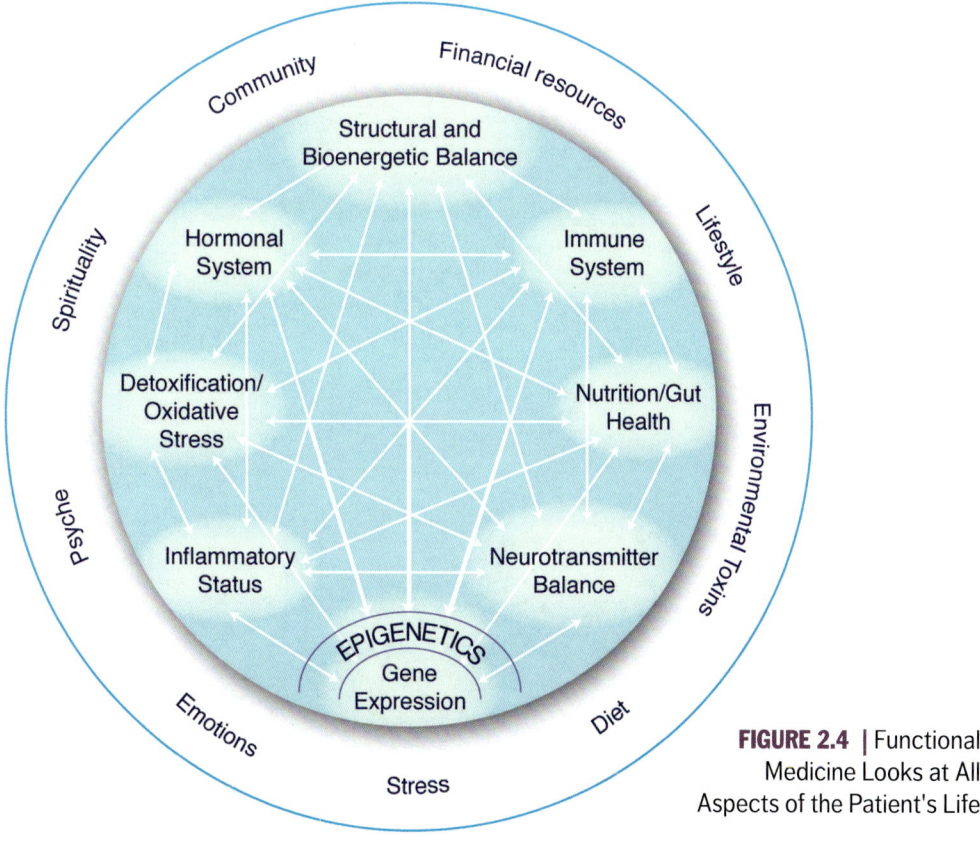

FIGURE 2.4 | Functional Medicine Looks at All Aspects of the Patient's Life

principles—especially the idea that we have multiple interacting and self-regulating systems—mirror the ideas of health and disease promoted by age-old principles of Chinese medicine and Ayurvedic (Indian) health-care philosophies.

By looking at the body as a complex web of these interacting systems, we can view health as a dynamic balance between internal and external factors. We can understand that each person is biochemically and psychologically unique, responding in different ways to the many influences each of us faces.

Changing the Way We Think about Medicine

People often seek out wellness by trying alternative therapies because of the focus these systems place on returning to an active state of wellbeing. In the old medical paradigm, physicians were resistant to alternative therapies, with the result being that patients either saw their conventional doctor or tried complementary or alternative therapies. The two approaches rarely coexisted—indeed, many patients never told their physicians about their use of complementary therapies. This has changed as the medical profession has become more accepting of integrative medicine.

It is our opinion that medicine will and should continue to change. New inventions, drugs, ideas, surgeries, and technologies will continue to advance the science of medicine. Genetic advances, biotechnology, and nanotechnology will be used to help our bodies heal in ways that we could never have imagined.

We also envision a new kind of medicine in which people will be asked to play a more active role in their own health care. What's more, we will be asked to recognize illness at a much earlier stage. As we each become more attuned to our health, we will be able to transform it.

What we have learned using this approach is that when we affect multiple systems at the same time, we can accomplish three things at once—reduce the symptoms of illness, prevent future illness, and promote a feeling of health and vitality. This is what we call Transformational Medicine.

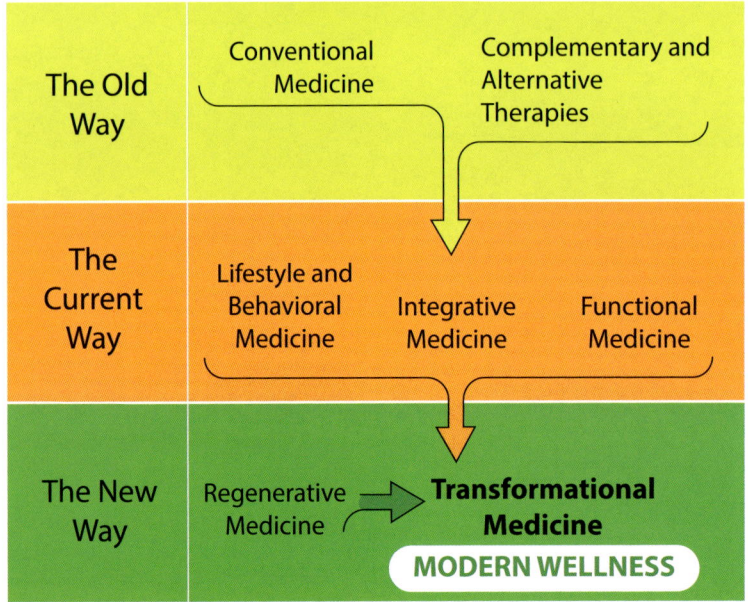

FIGURE 2.5 | The Development of Transformational Medicine

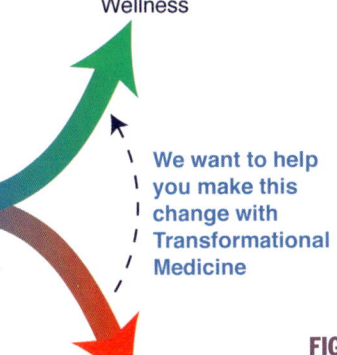

FIGURE 2.6 | Changing the Trajectory of Your Health

Transformational Medicine

In practicing both integrative medicine and functional medicine, we have learned to use the best of both complementary and conventional medicine to create a new state of vibrant health and wellbeing for our patients. We have come to realize that we all can move toward wellbeing by transforming our symptoms of dis-ease or dis-comfort into a new state of better health, and this is an approach we can each apply to our lives on a daily basis.

To transform your health, you need to see where you came from, assess where you are, and then make positive changes to influence where you are going.

Predisposition to illness. We all have a certain set of predispositions to illness. This may be due to our genes, a poor or toxic environment, emotional trauma, a dietary deficiency, or numerous other causes, alone or in combination. This sets us on a trajectory toward illness, whatever that illness may be.

Assessing your current health. To assess your current health, ask yourself if you have any symptoms of discomfort or disease. If you have a disease or health crisis, we would like you to see this as an opportunity for change, an inflection point.

Transforming your future health. We believe you can turn your trajectory away from illness and toward health and wellbeing.

What we have shown is that the principles of Transformational Medicine can reverse illness and slow the rate of aging. *Modern Wellness* will now include ways to reverse aging.

YOUR Transformational Medicine Wellness Plan

In Transformational Medicine, we think of your diagnosis as being made up of five main aspects. Together they help us understand the whole: the multifaceted, multidimensional being that is you, the person who wants to understand what is going on with your health.

The five aspects we use to evaluate a patient are:

1. Making an **expanded medical diagnosis**, then using the best of conventional medicine, including genomics, to evaluate treatment in the safest, most cost-effective way possible.
2. Evaluating and treating the **effects of stress** on the body.
3. Evaluating and treating imbalances in **nutrition**, **immune function**, **metabolism**, and **body chemistry**.
4. Evaluating and treating **hormonal imbalances**.
5. Evaluating and treating **pain imbalances** in body mechanics and bioenergy.

For those who choose to do this, Modern Wellness now includes options to help reverse aging.

We then develop your Transformational Wellness Plan. By combining your goals, your risk factors, and our cutting-edge assessment, we can address any reversible factors, rebuild your vitality, and reduce your pain—with the goal of helping you become healthier and more resilient at the end of the process than when you started.

Transformational Medicine is an applied primary care approach that can be used to resolve many common medical problems. It doesn't replace the need for a primary care doctor, nor does it replace the need for a specialist. It augments both.

> **In Transformational Medicine**, we spend time and effort on prevention and early intervention to reduce the burden of illness both now and in the future. Because our patients take a greater role in their own health care, they develop and expand a new sense of wellbeing. Our goal is for you to participate actively in your health care, to transform your health, treating illness if it exists, learning to heal your body, avoiding future illness before it happens, all the while promoting a sense of vitality and wellbeing!

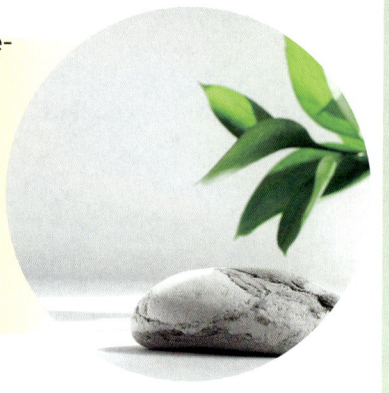

Modern Wellness

We're at the dawn of a new age, one where we're starting to turn back the clock. Some people are now aging backward. Yes, you read that correctly! The mind-blowing concept of getting biologically younger while getting chronologically older is now possible.

Although the science of longevity and immortality is still young, in the future we'll be able to reverse aging, reverse illness, rejuvenate our bodies, and rekindle our vitality. We will touch on this repeatedly throughout this book.

Companies like Google and Amazon are investing heavily in biotech companies researching the biology that controls aging and lifespan. In 2023, Bryan Johnson, a wealthy tech entrepreneur, made headlines when he announced the results of his $20 million-a-year program to change his mind and body. Blueprint, as he calls it, employs a group of physicians, nutritionists, and scientists to tightly control and monitor his life. (Complete details are at blueprint.bryanjohnson.com.) The program has made him "the most measured man in human history," tracking hundreds of biomarkers with the goal of attaining maximum health and youth. After two years on his program, he claims he slowed his pace of aging by the equivalent of 31 years and started aging slower than the average 10-year-old. His biomarkers normalized and began correlating with those of significantly younger men. For instance, his free testosterone index (FTI), one measure of biological age, was reduced by 20 years. His sleep and athletic performance were in the top 1 percent. He had an 80 percent reversal in gray hair. His brain white matter intensities—small imperfections we see on brain MRIs as we age—reduced by 20 years.

Bryan is being completely transparent about his progress in the hope that others can learn from his benefits and mistakes. Still, unless you are both extremely wealthy and extremely motivated, his results aren't something the typical person can duplicate. What can the average person do to change their rate of biological aging?

One step would be to determine your biological age with a DNA methylation test, such as the one from TruDiagnostic, that accurately predicts your true (real) biological age, as opposed to your chronological age, or age in years. The TruDiagnostic test can also be used to show if we're changing the rate at which we're aging—it detects if we are getting biologically younger.

Plastic surgeons have been making people look younger for decades. Newer techniques for cosmetic procedures, such as laser therapy, don't require surgery to make you look younger. Regenerative medicine using platelet rich plasma (PRP) and stem cells can help regenerate tendons, joints, and ligaments. Regenerative medicine can also help make the skin appear younger and can help regrow hair. Using newer and simpler techniques, we are now able to help people avoid some surgeries and return to more active lifestyles.

How long we can live an active life free of disability and disease isn't yet clear. It's possible that 120 years isn't unreasonable—and our potential lifespan may be much longer. At the beginning of this book, we talked about most people's reaction to this. Now, reimagine yourself living to a ripe old age filled with vigor, happiness, and fulfilment! What then?

A gym rat who works only on his upper body and arms will see bulging muscles in the mirror but won't see that the rest of his body is unbalanced. Someone who erases facial wrinkles with Botox and fillers may not see that the rest of their body is flabby. Trying to partially repair a crumbling building isn't a good approach to renovating it. To turn back the biological clock, you need to start with the basic principles we outline in Transformational Medicine. Then the rest is easy!

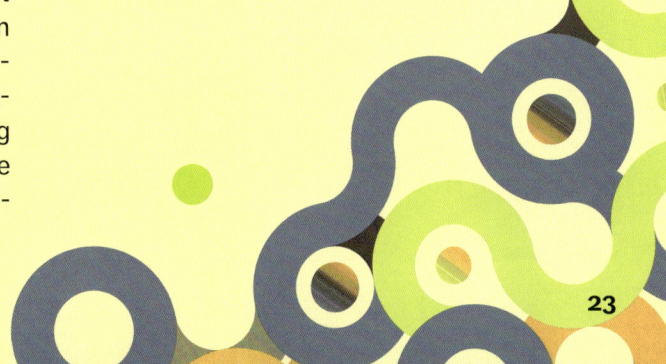

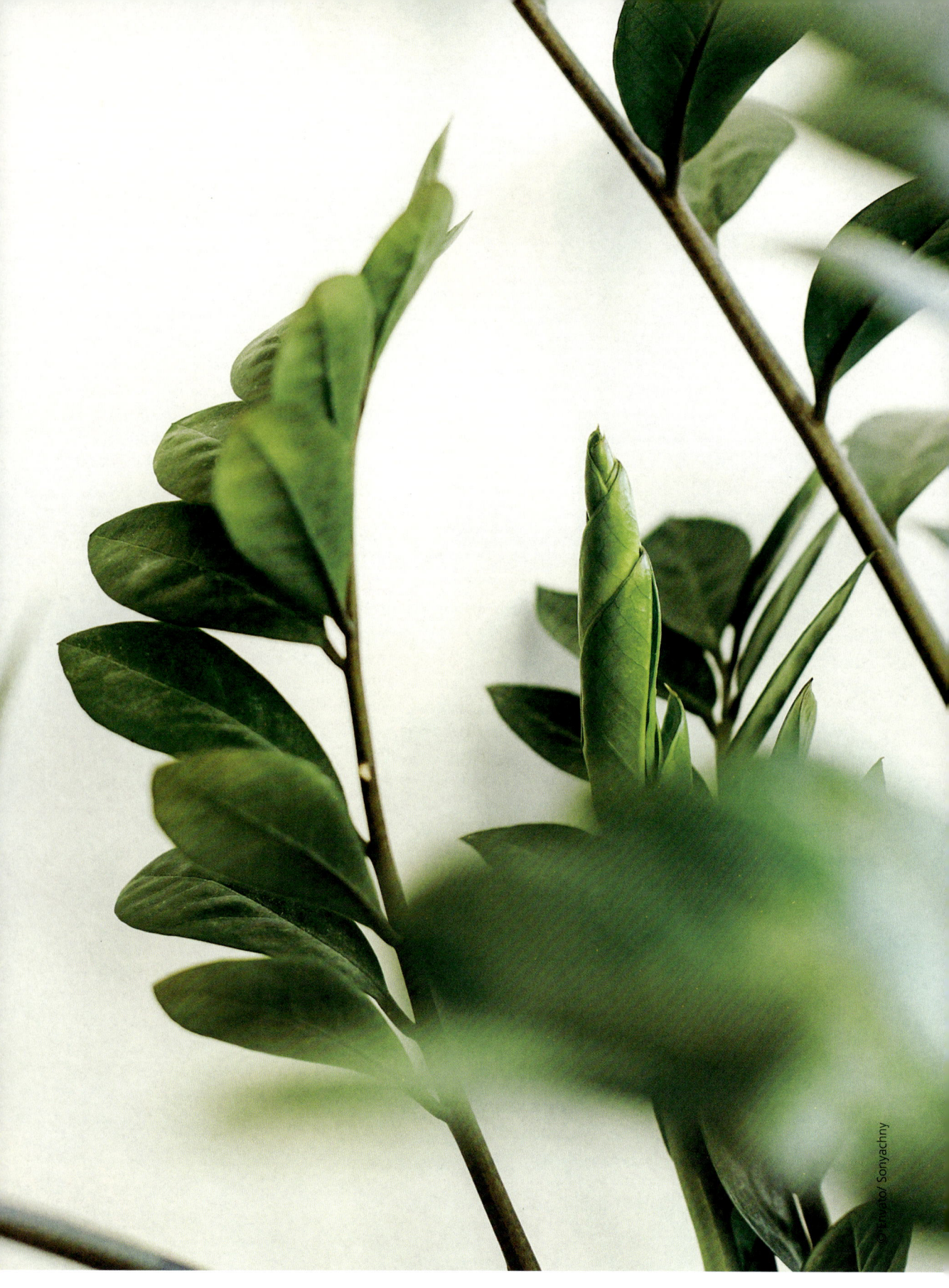

CHAPTER 3

Using Illness and Dis-ease as a Fulcrum to Transform Your Life

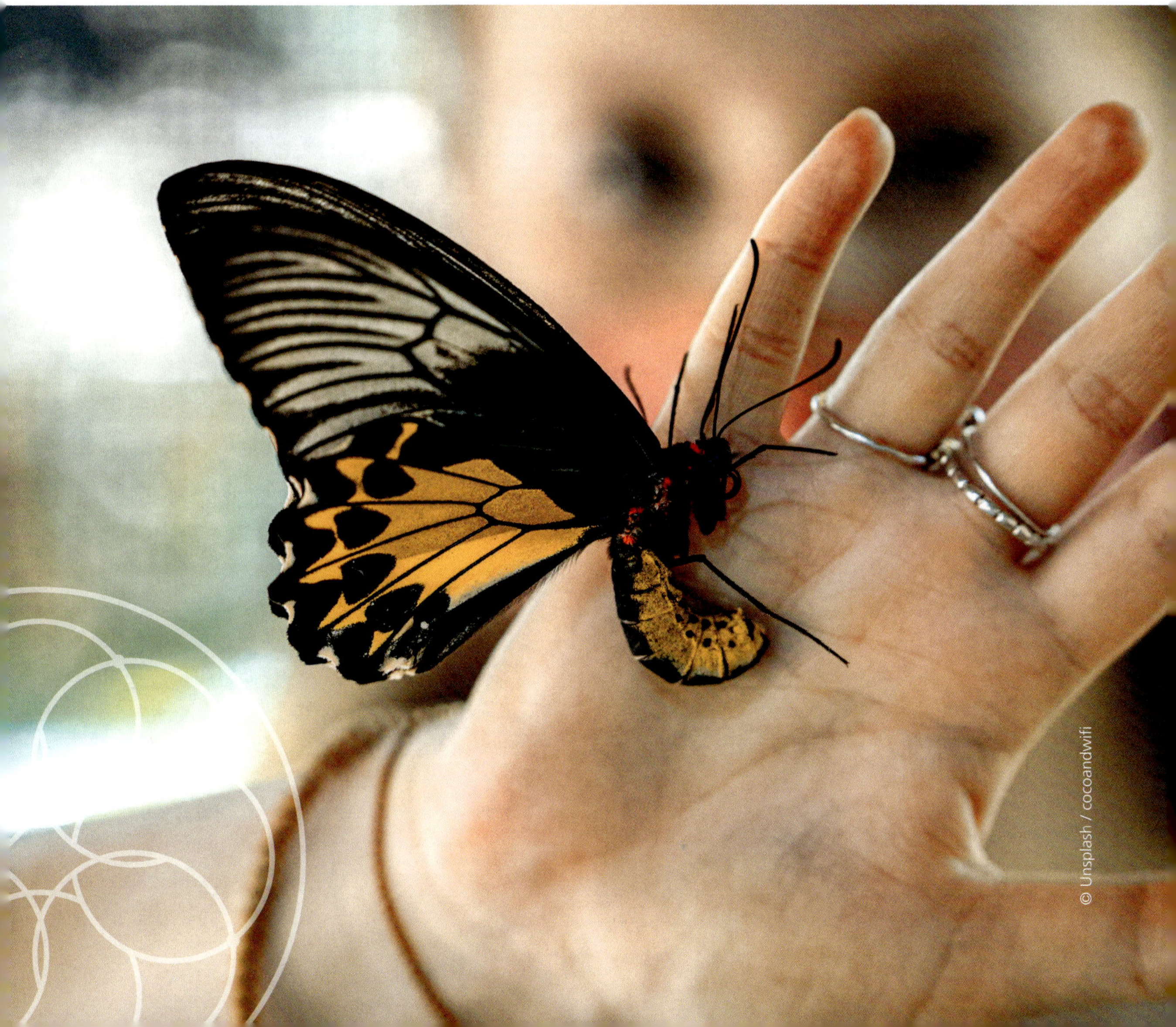

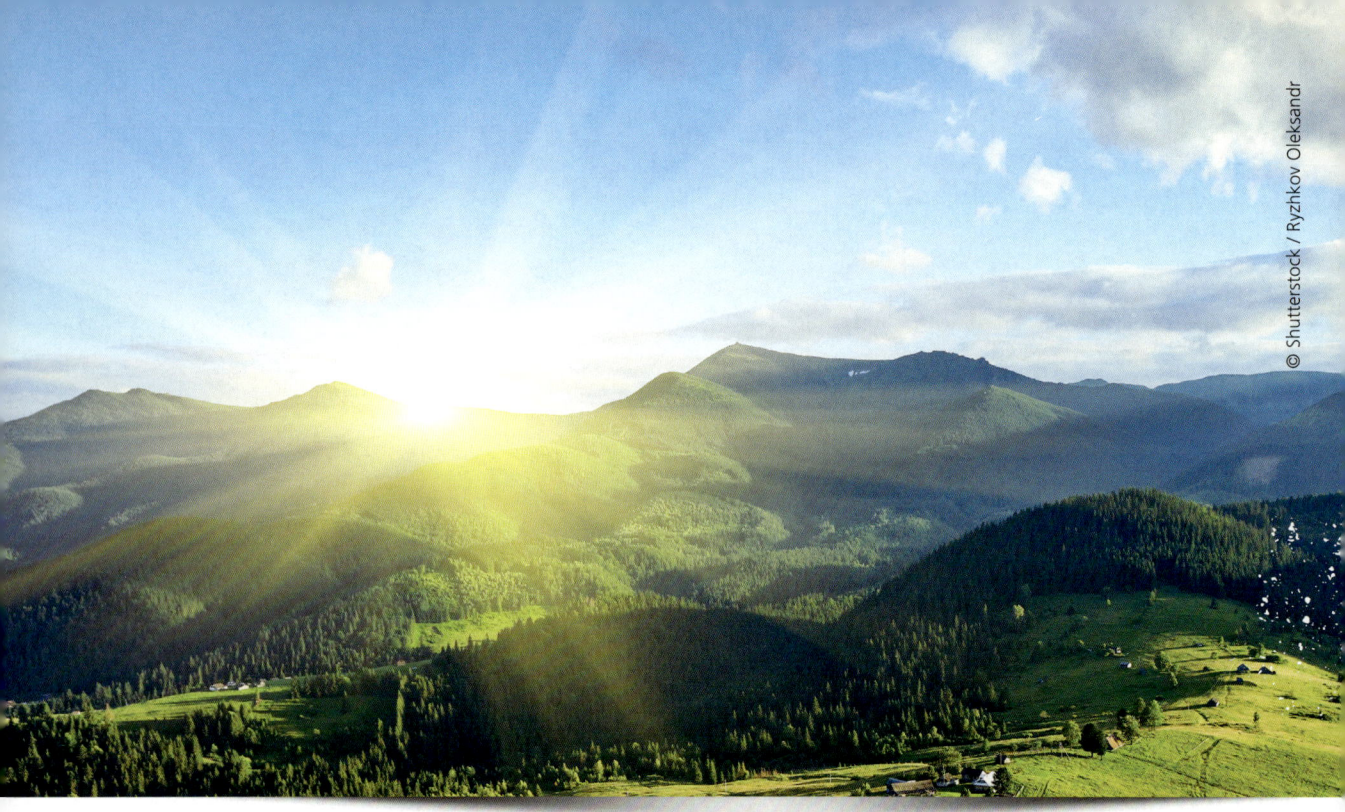

How a Journey into the Heart of Healing Led to a **New Vision of Health**

The word *heal* is derived from an Old English word that means "to make whole." This book offers insight into healing and tools you can use to move toward wholeness. We'll explore how you can use your symptoms or your current illness to create change in your life and help you on your journey toward health and wellbeing.

We are taught in medical school to stay impersonal as we interact with patients. Theoretically, this detachment helps us think through patients' problems clearly and unemotionally, but it actually may keep us from understanding our patients as more than just a medical problem to be solved. We have found that understanding our patients as individuals is crucial for providing compassionate care. It's what brought us to integrative medicine. We've found over the years that many doctors who ask us about practicing integrative medicine come to us after feeling burnt out with the failures of conventional medicine. Some have experienced illnesses that conventional medicine couldn't diagnose or treat very well.

We both know from personal experience and from treating thousands of patients that integrative therapies can be highly effective in ways conventional medicine can't. Chronic fatigue syndrome introduced Steve to integrative therapies, while Sandi used them with amazing results to recover from a severe head injury following a bike crash, and later, to recover from West Nile virus.

The path to healing often begins with a personal crisis, a disaster, or an illness. Although it is initially stressful, this time of introspection often leads to a journey of self-discovery.

More Questions Than Answers

When we met during medical school in Johannesburg, South Africa, we both realized that we shared a similar philosophy of openness to different treatment modalities, no matter what they were. As study partners, we would swap stories of our experiences treating patients. For example, some of our patients with back pain reported that they had seen a chiropractor as a last resort before surgery, only to have all their pain resolve permanently. We listened as patients told us how they had used alternative type therapies to recover from cancer, autoimmune diseases, chronic pain and even bizarre symptoms that never made sense to any conventional doctor. We were equally aware, however, of patients who had seen a traditional African healer and been given a concoction of herbs, only to develop kidney failure afterward. There was even the patient who was told by an alternative medicine practitioner not to worry about his heartburn, but then had a heart attack only a few weeks later.

For us, these stories pointed to the idea that a rational balance between conventional medicine and the safest, most effective alternative therapies could result in an economical, patient-oriented form of medicine. Deep down, this just made sense to both of us. Without realizing it, we were embarking on what would become a life's journey of learning to assess and integrate alternative therapies with conventional medicine. When we started in the late 1970s, all we knew was that we wanted to learn more. Years later, Andrew Weil, MD, would describe this as integrative medicine.

We wanted to know what made people get well. Why did they feel better? Was it the therapy or their belief in it? Why had some therapies persisted in cultures for generations?

We began seeking out anyone in the healing arts who was achieving superior results. We interviewed everyone with skeptical but open minds. We studied with the most highly skilled of these healers. For instance, once a week we spent a half-day with a well-known doctor trained in both osteopathy and naturopathy. He was highly respected for curing patients with complex conditions. We listened in amazement as patient after patient told us how he had resolved their problems. His methods were inexpensive, simple, safe, and effective. We realized that we needed to open our eyes to a new vision, to expand our paradigm beyond what we knew, in order to broaden the resources for healing in our medical practice.

We were also lucky to be able to spend time with a famous African traditional healer named Credo Mutwa, who helped us see disease from a different point of view. As physicians, we treat epileptic seizures with medication to stop and prevent them. Credo had a different perspective. He told us, "In our culture, having a seizure is called *tswala*, the calling to become a healer." He went on to explain how they felt the seizure opened up an area in the brain necessary to become a shaman. What a different way of viewing a disease! We certainly don't espouse this, but we marveled at how a different paradigm could give a whole new dimension to a health problem.

During our medical education, we decided that we wanted to travel around the world to meet healers from different cultures and healing traditions who were able to successfully

What Is Integrative Medicine?

Integrative medicine respects and treats the whole person—body, mind, and spirit. The integrative approach is grounded in modern scientific medicine but makes use of all effective therapies, both conventional and alternative. Integrative medicine emphasizes therapeutic partnerships for treating health problems and for promoting better health and the prevention of illness.

treat conditions considered incurable. We decided that if we couldn't explain how someone had gotten better, we would follow up on it. Almost as soon as we decided this, people came to us with stories of famous healers and miraculous cures around the world. For our purposes, we defined a "miraculous cure" as one that defied conventional medical outcomes. With this as our new agenda, we left South Africa in 1984 for a trip overseas that would last two years.

The Journey Begins

Our travels took us through Australia, the Philippines, Hong Kong, Taiwan, Japan, Hawaii, the United States, the United Kingdom, and Europe. Open to healers of all sorts and shapes, we met indigenous healers, psychic surgeons, acupuncturists, tai chi and qigong masters, faith healers, energy healers, homeopaths, and herbalists. Along the way, we encountered enlightened people and charlatans, masters and magicians. For us, certain questions remained: why were some of these people getting good clinical results and what could we learn from them? How could we tell the difference between a quack and a true master?

Consider our visit with an acupuncture expert in Australia, who took Sandi's hand and began taking her pulse (one of the traditional Chinese forms of medical diagnosis). He looked over at Steve, smiled, and said gently, "Your wife is ovulating today." I stood back, astounded, as he then turned to her and said, "Your sunny disposition belies a great sadness."

He was correct. Sandi's father had died suddenly a few years earlier, right in the middle of our final medical school examinations. Forced to continue with her exams to complete medical school, she had never adequately grieved his death. Later that day, the expert took us to his office for an acupuncture treatment. "You will feel good," he told Steve before his treatment, "but Sandi's sadness will need to come out." Sandi later described the feeling of a tap being turned on when he stuck a needle in her ear. The waves of tears and sadness continued to pour out for days after the treatment, only to be replaced by a sense of love and connectedness to her late father. We knew then that we wanted to learn how to do this. A short treatment had changed our lives forever!

We visited the Philippines, intent on getting closer to the truth about the healers known as psychic surgeons. Many were in an area close to the city of Baguio. Dismissed by many Western scientists as nothing more than charlatans and magicians, these psychic surgeons saw thousands of patients each day. Were they helping or were they simply a hoax? We wanted to see this phenomenon for ourselves.

We found ourselves journeying out of Baguio into the valley below on a bus filled with chickens, dogs, and a myriad of local Filipinos. Our goal was to visit a psychic surgeon known only as Rosa, who took no money and offered her treatment as a spiritual service. Sandi asked her if she would treat an unattractive, raised purple scar on her foot, which

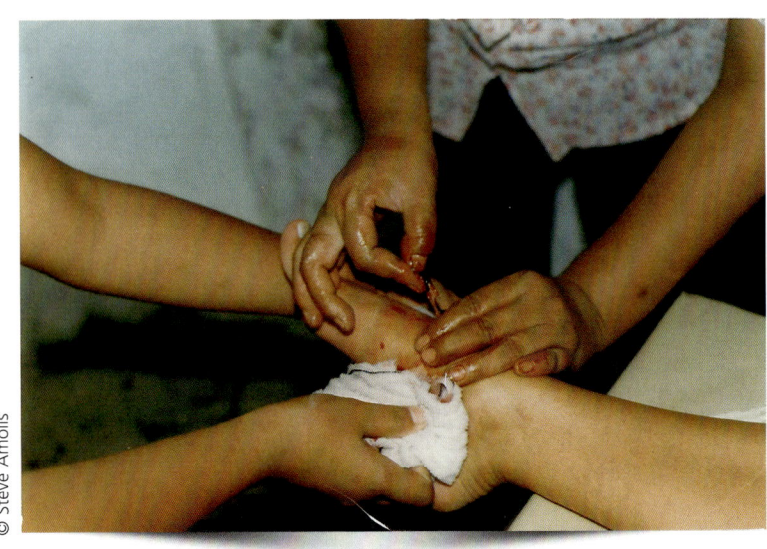

Filipino "psychic surgeon" removes flesh from Sandi's foot.

had not changed over the prior three years. Rosa answered that she could not take the scar away, but she could take away the infection underneath. Quickly, painlessly, and with a sleight-of-hand maneuver, she seemed to pull some flesh out of the scar. Interestingly, the scar—swollen and purple—shrank and turned pink overnight. It remains that way to this day.

We stayed for weeks, watching hundreds of patients receive this form of healing. One patient still sticks in our minds. He was a famous American actor who had gone to the Philippines hoping to heal his lung cancer, which had spread to his brain, paralyzing one side of his body. He initially made some startling improvements. One day after a treatment, he had a seizure. One hour later, he got up and began walking around. He was convinced he was cured. Unfortunately, despite the apparent improvement, he died two weeks later. Did the treatment really help him or prolong his life? To us, the answer was no.

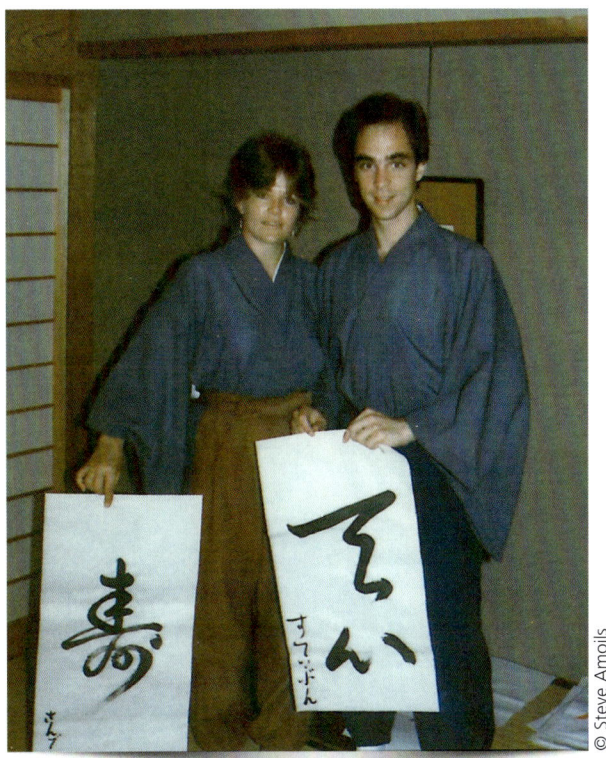
Studying calligraphy in Japan.

Traditional Studies in Japan

In Japan, we were fortunate to be chosen to participate in a seminar on traditional Japanese arts. We lived in a small traditional village near Kyoto, where we immersed ourselves in centuries-old Japanese culture. We wore traditional Japanese garb and studied various art forms such as the tea ceremony, calligraphy, flower arrangement, noh drama, and a martial art similar to aikido. Ultimately, through our contacts there, we met and studied with a true master of acupuncture, Mii Sensei.

Each day in his Osaka office, together with his seven students, Mii Sensei saw up to a hundred patients. Decades before there was research evidence to confirm acupuncture's effectiveness, we watched as Mii Sensei reversed asthma symptoms, removed pain, treated strokes, and seemingly fixed a whole host of other problems quite effortlessly. He was able to achieve these improvements in his patients simply by performing an acupuncture diagnosis and then inserting fine acupuncture needles at highly specific points on the body.

In Japanese, "sensei" means not

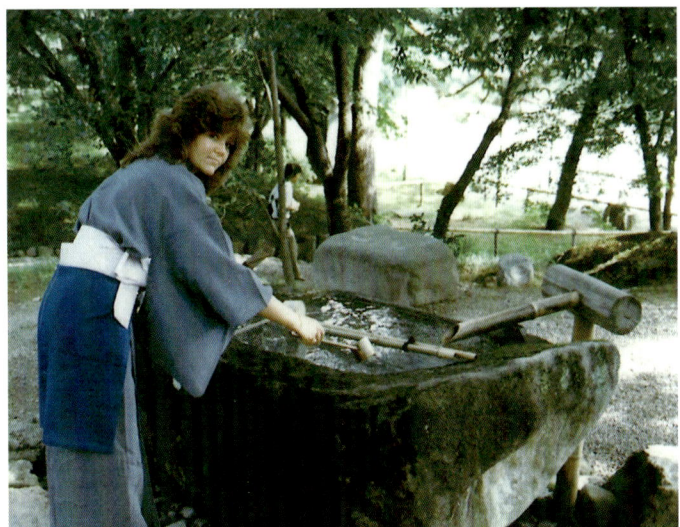
Mindfulness: Sandi preparing for a ceremony by washing her hands

just doctor or master but teacher as well. As a teacher, Mii Sensei had an innate sense of how his students were feeling. On days we were discouraged and down, he was nurturing and supportive. However, if he felt we were becoming overconfident, he would quickly bring us back to earth.

Mii Sensei taught us about the origins of Oriental medicine, as well as its focus on prevention and wellbeing. He often reminded us, "In ancient China, in every village it was the responsibility of the physician to keep the community well. The doctor was only paid if people were well. Once they got sick, he stopped getting paid. It was therefore the job of the physician to teach people to stay well and to stop disease before it arose."

Mii Sensei also taught us something that has become a guiding principle for us with every patient we see: "At each visit, you must treat the patient's current problem, heal the problems of the past, while simultaneously preventing future illness. You must do all three to practice good medicine." This became a foundational concept to our approach to medicine.

Celebrities from all over the world came to consult with Mii Sensei. Rock stars, wealthy businesspeople, members of the Japanese parliament, athletes, and ordinary people were all treated with the same dignity, compassion, and integrity. When Koji Gushiken, the "old man" of men's gymnastics at twenty-six years of age, returned to Japan with his Olympic gold medal, he brought it to Mii Sensei, attributing his health to the acupuncture master.

Our First Integrative Practice

We returned to South Africa in 1986 and began working in a large family practice in Johannesburg. During this time, we began to see the benefit of combining complementary therapies with conventional approaches. One day, a muscular metalworker came in to see Steve, bent over and moaning and groaning in pain from a sprained back. He was anxious to get back to work and implored Steve to do more than just give him painkillers or send him for physical therapy. Steve explained manipulative therapies and acupuncture to him. Not quite sure what to think, he nodded in agreement, desperate to get some relief. Thirty minutes later, after his treatment, he walked back into the waiting room, completely pain-free. He began to dance for the front office staff and the people in the waiting room, cavorting exuberantly.

Our integrative practice began right there. This case resulted in an onslaught of patients who began to come to us for many different pain conditions. Seeing how effectively—and quick-

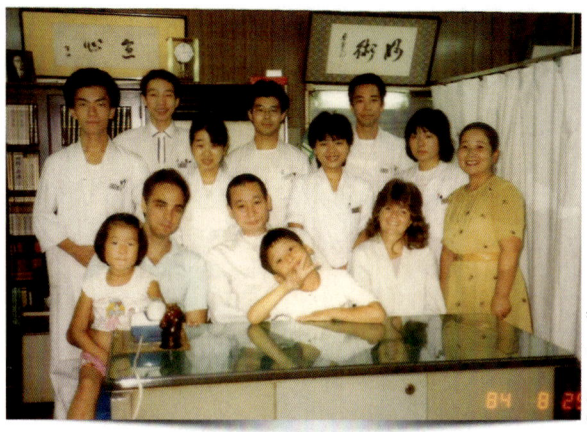

Mii Sensei and his students, children and wife complete the picture. Mii Sensei is seated in the middle front row, flanked by Sandi and Steve.

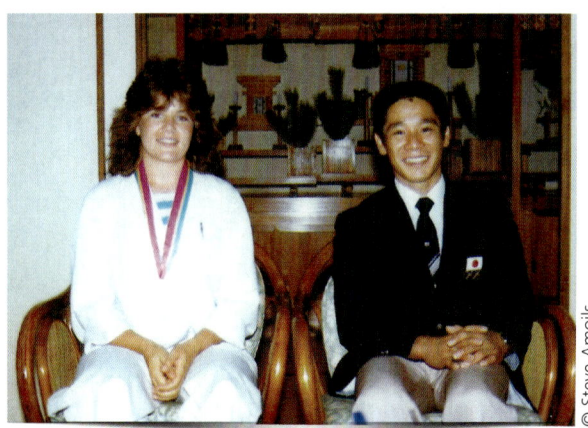

Koji Gushiken, winner of the men's gymnastic Gold Medal at the 1984 Olympics, attributed his good health to Mii Sensei's acupuncture treatments.

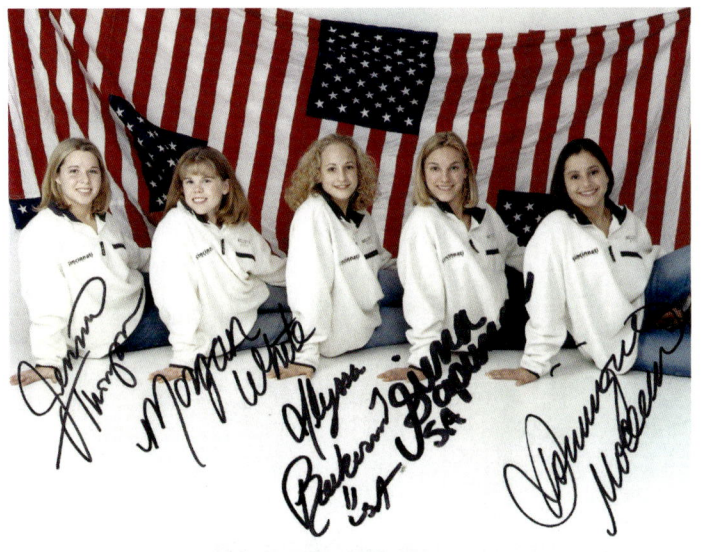

Photo given to us by members of the US Women's Gymnastics Team.

cacious combination. Because patients were doing so well, he gave us his full encouragement.

Since those early days, we have had the honor of treating hundreds of athletes, many of them world-class, including members of the US women's gymnastics team. We had come full circle from watching our acupuncture sensei in Japan treat an Olympic gymnast to treating Olympic athletes ourselves.

The Journey's Culmination

We immigrated to the United States in 1987. After completing our family medicine residencies at the University of Cincinnati, we worked with several family practice groups that ultimately merged into one. As board-certified primary care doctors, we began incorporating effective complementary therapies into our family practice. In 1999, at the request of the five-hospital group for which we worked, we opened the Alliance Institute for Integrative Medicine. In 2004, our center was chosen as one of the leading clinical centers of integrative medicine in the United States by the Bravewell Collaborative. As such, we worked in partnership with national leaders in the field of integrative medicine, doing research and learning where integrative medicine is working—and where it is not. We have developed substantial clinical experience in this area. Our center has averaged over thirty thousand visits a year for the last twenty years.

ly—these therapies worked to resolve our patients' health crises helped us realize that what we had learned around the world could be applied in a conventional medical clinical setting.

A few months later, a senior partner asked Steve what he was doing that was so successful. In just one day Steve had treated three celebrity athletes: a runner who was a world record holder in the 800-meter hurdles, a soccer goalkeeper with Manchester United, and a tennis player who had won the Wimbledon doubles title many times. Steve explained that people wanted a treatment that was effective, yet quicker, cheaper, and less invasive than the traditional methods they had come to expect. Acupuncture, manipulative therapies, massage, and energy healing were proving to be an effi-

Here are our **Research Results**

We have been fortunate to be part of the Bravewell Collaborative, and then to be part of the Bravenet PBRN (Practice-Based Research Network), a group of integrative medicine centers of excellence. While working with the Bravenet center, we participated in several collaborative research studies. The results have made valuable contributions to research on integrative medicine.

In one collaborative study, we looked at the reasons patients had for seeking integrative options for their care around the country. We surveyed 4,182 patients from nine different Bravenet integrative medicine centers.

The top reasons they gave for seeking care at an integrative medicine center were:

1. I want to improve my health and wellness now to prevent future problems.
2. I want to try new options for my healthcare.
3. I want to maximize my health regardless of whether or not my illness is curable.
4. I want to be in a place that acknowledges the connection between mind, body, spirit, and community.
5. I want to receive objective advice on nonconventional approaches.

In the SIMTAP Study (Study on Integrative Medicine Treatment Approaches for Pain), a prospective observational study, we looked at 409 patients who were treated for pain at nine Bravenet integrative medicine centers. In this study, we showed that an integrative approach to treating chronic pain had a significant impact on patients' pain as well as on associated symptoms and quality of life. This success was in the context of patients with long-standing chronic pain, with an average duration of greater than eight years. The trends on decreased pain, stress, depression, and fatigue, together with improvement in physical quality of life and overall wellbeing, were consistent over the 24-week period and point to the sustainable effects of integrative interventions.

The PRIMIER (Patients Receiving Integrative Medicine Effectiveness Registry) study in 2013 involved a network of fourteen clinical centers. They all collected patient-reported outcomes and extracted electronic health record data into a large national registry, with the goal of helping to improve the health and wellbeing of patients. Patients were monitored as they were treated with integrative medicine for over six months.

The study was published in the journal *BMC Complementary Medicine and Therapies* in 2016. It showed some interesting results:

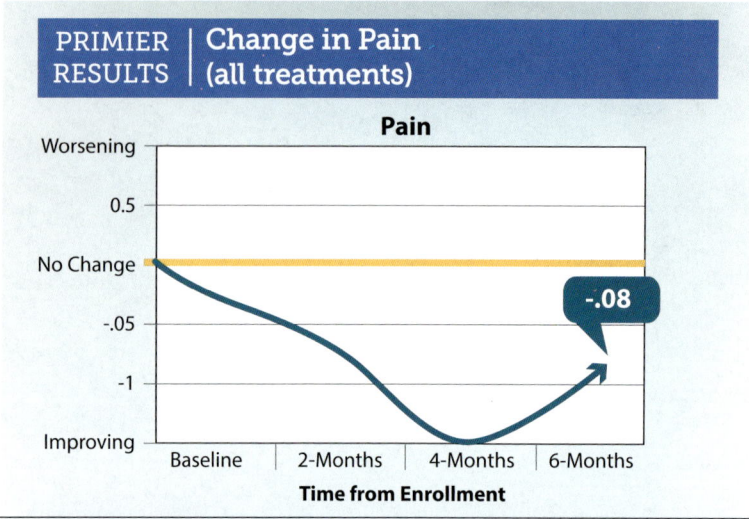

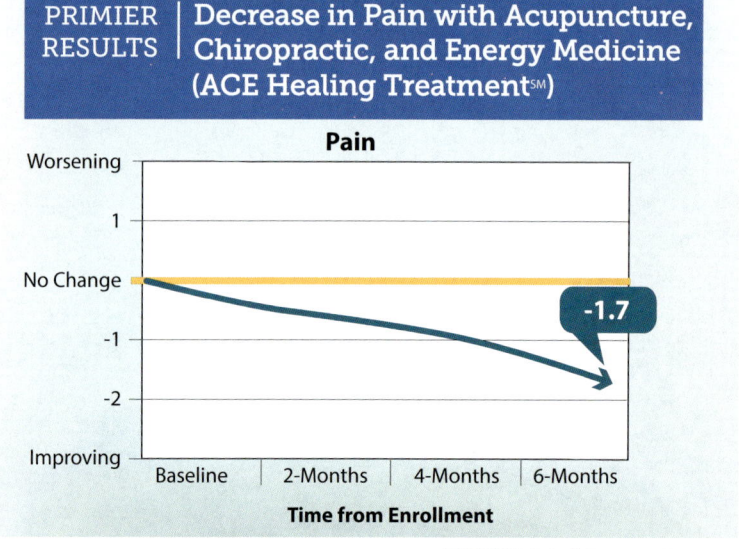

FIGURE 3.1 | Primier Results

1. We measured patient activation scores, or how patients transitioned from lower levels of knowledge, skill, and confidence in managing their health to higher levels of understanding the importance of taking a proactive role in managing their health and gaining the skills and confidence to maintain behavioral changes over time. We found that as patients remained in the study, there was a general trend to move toward higher patient activation scores. The higher scores correlated with improvements in clinical outcomes such as less pain, an increase in preventive screenings, and a reduction in ER visits.

2. Stress, depression, and pain all decreased over six months.

3. When patients were treated with multiple modalities at once, their pain decreased even further. This approach was based on the combined acupuncture, chiropractic, and energy healing (ACE) treatment protocols we use at AIM.

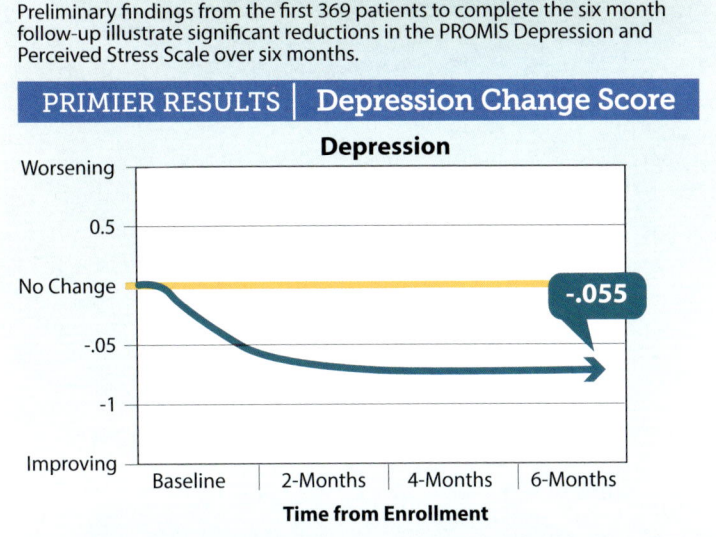

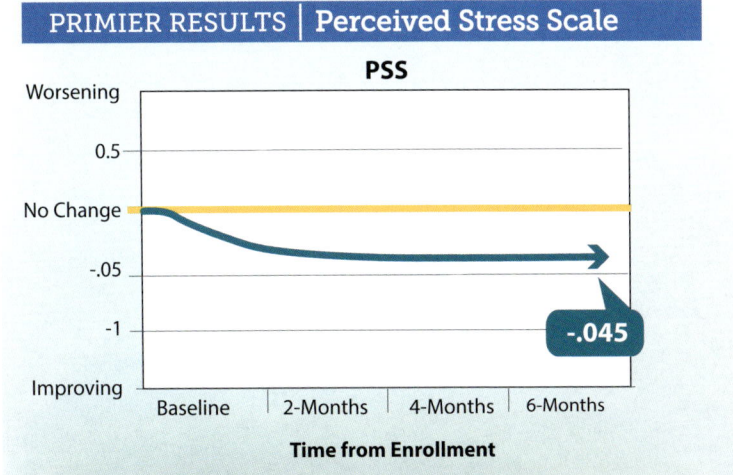

FIGURE 3.2 | Primier Results

Partners in Wellness

In 2022, we began a new endeavor. Our practice was absorbed by The Christ Hospital Health Network, a large private hospital system in Cincinnati. The Christ Hospital is nationally ranked in cardiology and highly ranked in multiple other specialties. While patients come in for treatment of specific health issues, The Christ Hospital has realized that most of them really want to focus on wellbeing and prevention. With this in mind, we plan to work together to develop:

- A first-in-kind, best-of-class, **wellness-oriented direct primary care program**
- **A unique pain and rejuvenation program**, incorporating multiple different modalities to help heal and then rejuvenate the body
- **Integrative medicine programs to reverse aging and illness**
- **Unique programs for:**
  - Allergies and sensitivities unresponsive to conventional approaches
  - Irritable bowel syndrome and other functional gut disorders
  - Weight loss and metabolic balancing
  - Hormonal optimization in menopause, andropause, or women with PCOS (estrogen or progesterone dominance)
  - Chronic fatigue syndrome (especially for post-Lyme disease, chronic mold exposure, long COVID syndrome, and similar syndromes)
  - Immunity boosting for people who keep getting sick
  - Adjunctive cancer care
  - Preventive Cardiology
  - And more . . .

> By working with a large, reputable hospital system, we feel we can leave a larger footprint on health care and set a record of accomplishment that other hospitals can follow. It has been our long-held belief that any terms we use for the medicine we practice will disappear as this type of medicine gets reabsorbed back into the mainstream and simply becomes **Good Medicine!** If we have our way, insurance companies will start paying for this type of approach.

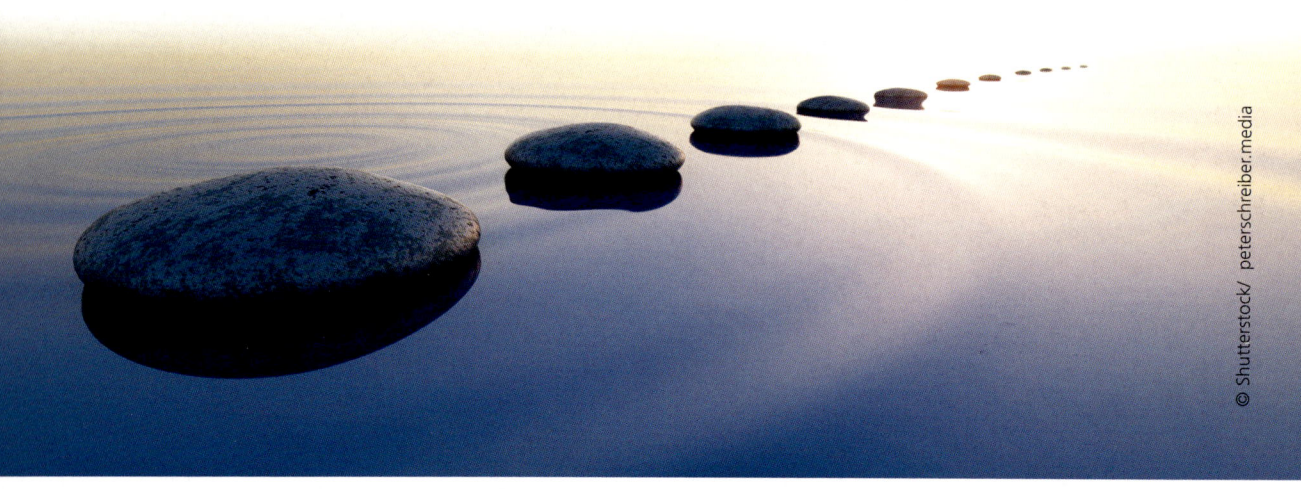

34 CHAPTER 3 | Using Illness and Dis-ease as a Fulcrum to Transform Your Life

CHAPTER 4
How to Approach an Illness

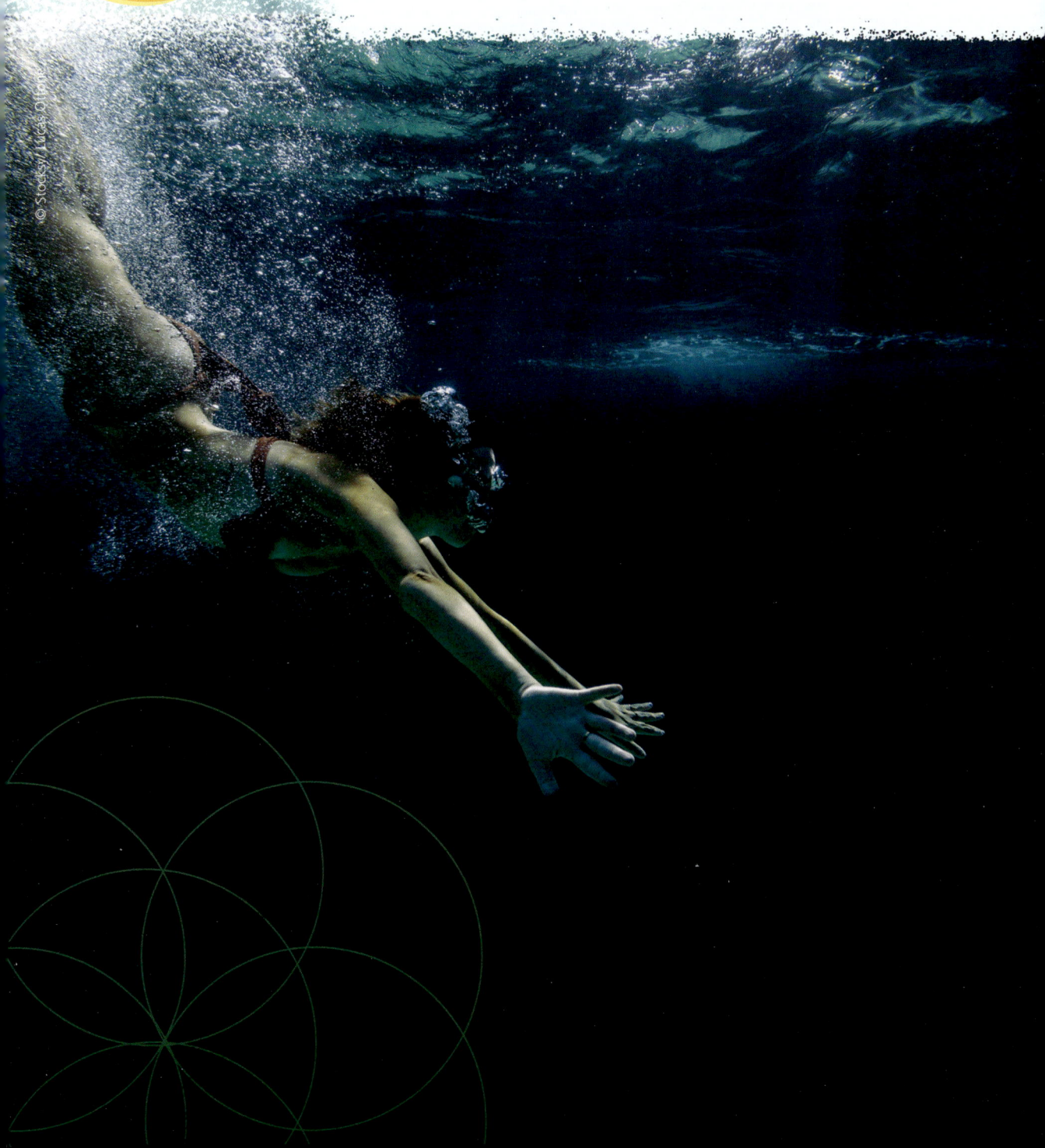

Patients often come to us with a new illness, feeling like they were struck by lightning, out of the blue. They may have recently had a full physical by a competent doctor and subsequently declared healthy. Then a few months later they have a full-blown illness. **How did this happen?**

Unfortunately, what this situation tells us is that their illness has escaped conventional and early detection techniques. More importantly, preventive measures have failed. In this chapter we will to show you what we see as the path from wellness to illness.

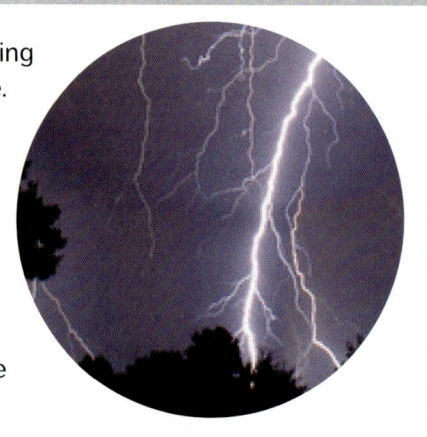

The Evolution of a Philosophy

Conventional medicine as it is practiced today is outstanding in many areas, yet quite archaic in others. One day we will likely look back at medicine as it is today and ask ourselves how we allowed patients to go through such barbaric practices. Why were we so ignorant? Change is happening very rapidly in medicine today. It's being disrupted, even revolutionized, by exponential growth in new sciences: genomics and gene splicing, metabolomics, proteomics, microbiomics, computing technology and mobile interconnectedness, nanotechnology, robotics, 3-D printing, stem cell technology, CRISPR gene editing, and artificial intelligence. Fields that were unimaginable just a decade ago now flourish—and fields we can't imagine now will develop in the near future. Nonmedical basic sciences will soon be just as likely to provide answers to medical dilemmas as medical science itself.

An Expanded Medical Diagnosis

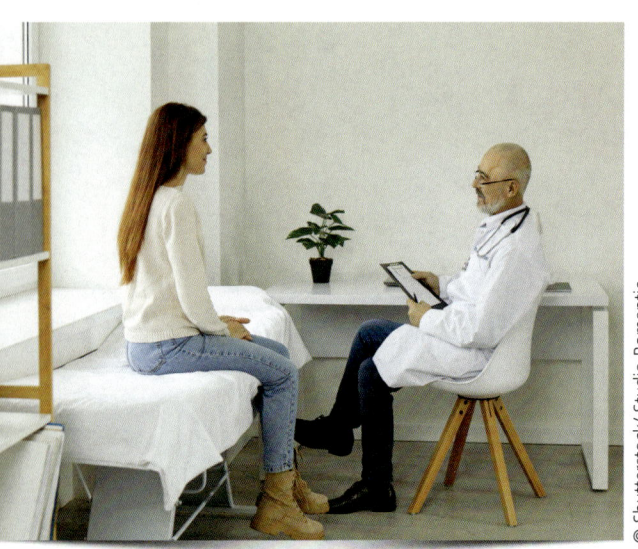

A full workup by a conventionally trained medical doctor remains the first and most important step in the diagnosis of medical problems. If you have a clear-cut issue that needs a specific test or treatment, we encourage you to see your primary care physician first. Your primary physician is the person who can take care of you or refer you to the right specialist or testing center.

But what if your chronic health problem doesn't improve, despite time and skillful standard treatment? This might be the time to seek out a physician who can delve further into the issue and help you resolve it. A slightly different approach to a health problem can lead you toward a profound transformation.

What about those of you who are healthy but want to maintain your health or go further to achieve peak performance?

We often say to patients, "We have yet to find someone who is completely normal or completely healthy—including ourselves." Everyone, once we start looking, has some kind of health issue. They may have minor aches and pains, gut disturbances, mood or sleep problems, skin eruptions, or some other minor concern. But when we view minor problems from the vantage point of looking for functional problems, we can see early fluctuations that are potential warnings of bigger issues down the line.

> It is health that is real wealth and not pieces of gold and silver.
>
> —Gandhi

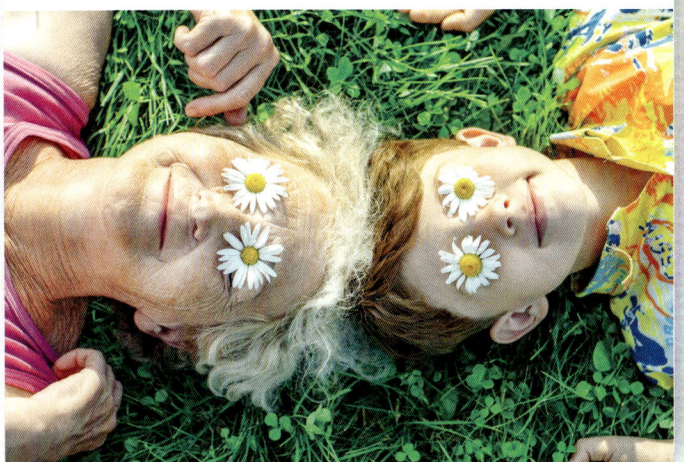

We outline the following steps to tweak your body, mind, or metabolism to **facilitate optimal health**.

Begin with a Conventional Medical Workup

One of the primary reasons to have a yearly physical is to check your conventional health markers. How is your blood pressure? Are your glucose and cholesterol levels normal? Is your stool clear of blood? Abnormal markers indicate that your body isn't fully functioning, even if you feel reasonably well. The goal is to identify malfunctions in your system so normal functioning can be restored before you get sick. In matters of health, sooner is always better than later. It is much easier to intervene early on than down the line when a disease has taken deeper root in your system.

Usually, when one of the health markers on your lab tests is abnormal, the problem isn't urgent—but it is important. Every time you restore balance to your body chemistry, you've lowered your risk of a more serious health problem. Sometimes, highly abnormal markers make further medical intervention or medication a necessary step. For instance, if you have very high triglycerides (tiny fat droplets in your blood), you're at an increased risk of an attack of pancreatitis. If your glucose levels are dangerously high, you're likely to have diabetes and need immediate treatment. Usually though, abnormal health markers simply tell us in which direction to point you in order to help you make a change. If you feel healthy but want to further optimize your health, we still recommend a conventional medical workup. Occasionally, this will uncover a medical issue, but in most cases your standard exam and lab work will all be normal. They give you the starting point for further steps that can enhance your health and wellbeing. If you strive for peak performance in your life, this approach will help you attain it through optimized health and an improved ability to handle stress.

Desperate for a Diagnosis

Medical science puts us on a quest to pinpoint a single cause for an illness. Because of this, we've come to think that having a diagnosis is a prerequisite for a cure. When there is no name for a set of symptoms, patients are concerned that they're not being taken seriously or that a treatable cause is being missed.

A diagnosis alone, however, is often not enough. It tells us nothing about the cause of a person's symptoms. When someone has a heart attack, for instance, we know what happened but not why. The underlying cause may be very high cholesterol levels, high levels of inflammation due to gum disease, cocaine abuse, or any number of other reasons.

As physicians, we strongly support using the best of scientific medicine to make a diagnosis. We will always do our best to find out what is happening by taking a thorough medical history, performing a physical examination, and using lab and radiological tests, and even invasive testing if necessary. However, there often comes a time when we realize that the best of medicine still can't explain what's going on.

This is especially common when patients have had multiple symptoms for prolonged periods of time. At that point, we start looking "under the hood" to see what systems are malfunctioning.

When the Tests Are Normal, But You Don't Feel Normal

At times, you may simply feel off or not yourself, yet you may not have a diagnosable illness. Often, your conventional lab markers are within the normal range, even though you don't feel well. Normal lab results don't necessarily mean good health. For instance, the common conventional blood tests for kidney function may not indicate a problem until your kidney function is 50 percent compromised. Similarly, conventional liver function tests, such as aspartate transaminase (AST) and alanine transaminase (ALT), may not indicate problems such as cirrhosis until liver disease is quite advanced.

If you don't feel well, we want to rule out a serious underlying condition, such as a tumor or a blocked artery. Most of the time, though, causes of common nonspecific medical complaints, such as fatigue, are difficult to pinpoint or treat.

One reason is that medical tests aren't always sensitive enough to pick up causes of common symptoms. Good examples here are migraines and irritable bowel syndrome. In these cases, the patient may be completely debilitated by pain, yet the results of conventional testing are normal.

These are good examples of what we call functional problems. The patient's normal function has been disturbed, but there is no evidence of an illness or organic pathology, such as a brain tumor or inflammatory bowel disease. A functional disturbance such as a migraine may not progress to anything dangerous or life-threatening, but it can severely impact a patient's daily life and wellbeing. On the other hand, it could be the start of a progressive path toward illness.

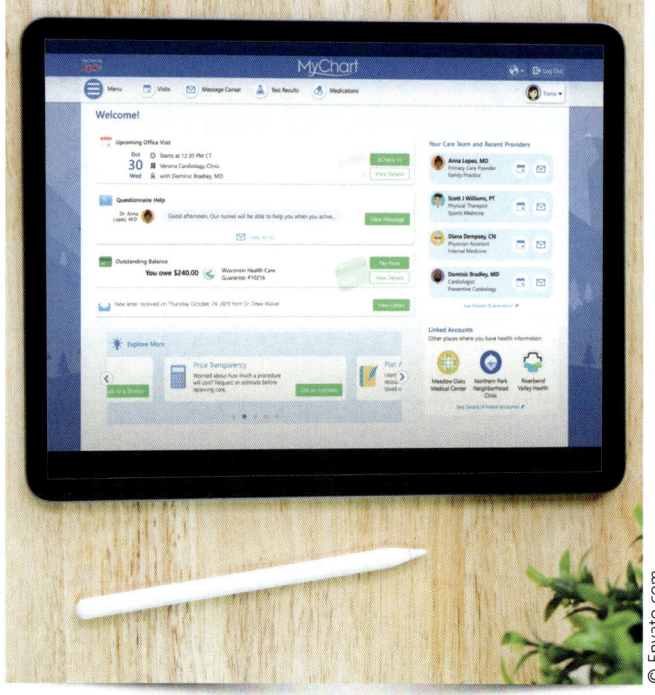

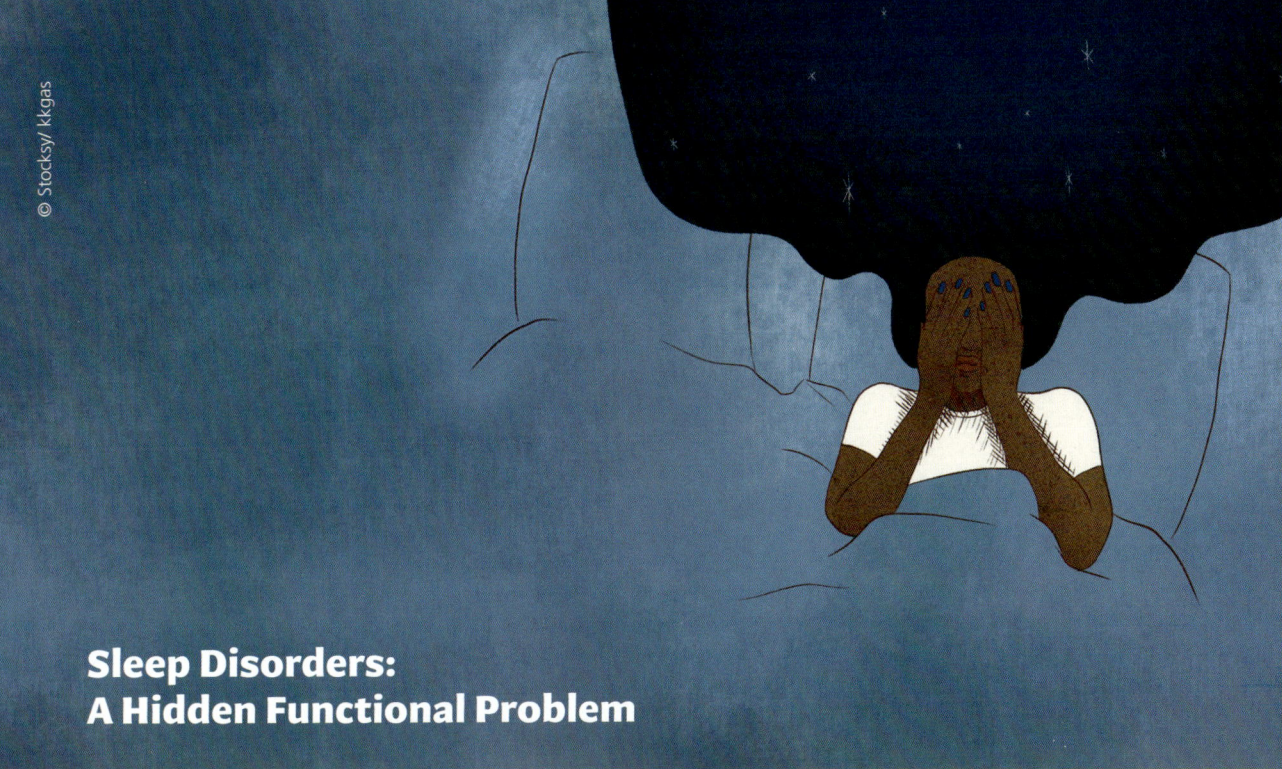

Sleep Disorders: A Hidden Functional Problem

Sleep is extremely important to help the body regenerate, yet too often we find that our patients, even young children, don't get enough sleep. The cause could simply be too much to do, too many distractions, or a poor sleep environment. It could also be that a sleep disorder is the problem.

Sleep disorders include:

- **Chronic insomnia**, where you have trouble more than a few times a week falling asleep or staying asleep more than a few times a week for three months or longer.
- **Teeth grinding or clenching** (bruxism), which can cause temporomandibular joint (TMJ) problems, headache, and tooth damage.
- **Sleep apnea**, or shallow start-and-stop breathing that causes loud snoring and frequent mini-awakenings from lack of oxygen throughout the night. The disrupted sleep causes daytime sleepiness, and long-term lack of oxygen may eventually lead to heart problems.
- **Restless legs syndrome**, which causes a crawling or "antsy" feeling in the legs and a powerful impulse to move the legs. This usually happens when the person is sitting or lying down and prevents restful sleep.
- **Narcolepsy**, a sleep disorder that causes trouble sleeping at night and sudden periods of extreme daytime sleepiness.

Daytime sleepiness is the most usual sign of poor sleep from a sleep disorder. It can cause memory and mood problems, irritability, and depression, and is a significant cause of work-related accidents and car crashes. Other indications of a sleep disorder include unexplained chest pain, palpitations, shortness of breath, and fibromyalgia-like muscle soreness. Lack of sleep also raises your level of the stress hormone cortisol—and high cortisol levels are associated with weight gain, insulin resistance, and type 2 diabetes.

A Progressive Disturbance: From Wellness to Illness

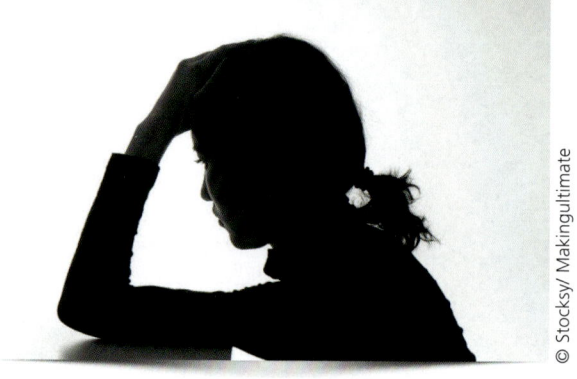

Many times, a patient comes to the doctor with a vague or ill-defined health complaint with no detectable cause. Some examples include:

- Fatigue
- Insomnia
- Moodiness, irritability, anxiety, and depression
- Lowered libido or impotence
- Headaches
- Frequent infections
- Indigestion, heartburn, bloating, diarrhea, or constipation
- Weight gain or weight loss

Doctors often dismiss these symptoms as minor problems that may be psychosomatic or related to depression. In most cases, the physical exam and lab work are normal. However, this is where we believe that viewing symptoms in a different light can help reverse the course of illness and even turn you toward wellbeing. Learning to understand a problem as a disturbance of function can dramatically alter the way you look at it. Treating a sleep disorder, for instance, can significantly improve a person's life. Learning that what doctors label as psychosomatic disorders are really functional disorders can offer new and exciting ways to treat them. Irritable bowel syndrome (IBS), for example, is often dismissed as psychosomatic, but when we treat it as a functional disorder of digestion, our patients improve.

When Do You Get Sick?

Getting sick is a process. Patients don't just suddenly develop chronic diseases such as type 2 diabetes. At first, they develop what we call functional imbalances. These are small changes that begin to occur long before the patient has all the signs and symptoms that define a particular disease. Increased inflammation, oxidative damage, and altered immune function can start long before blood sugar problems rise to the level of type 2 diabetes, for example. We feel it is important to recognize these imbalances when we first see them, take them seriously, and correct them. The earlier a condition is diagnosed, the greater the likelihood that it can be reversed, returning you to a healthy state.

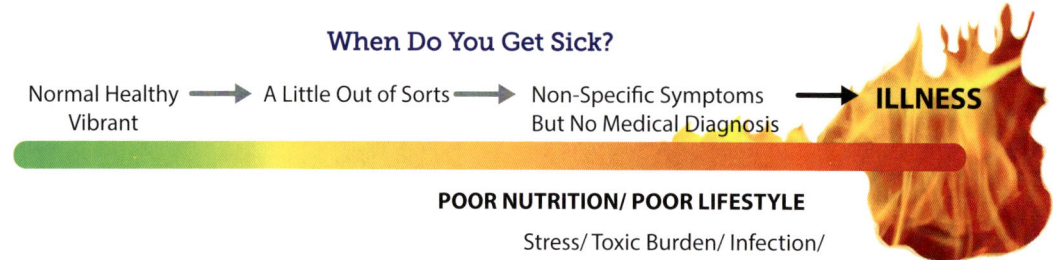

FIGURE 4.1 | When Do You Get Sick?

Identifying Your Genetic Risks

To understand how we progress on the path from illness to wellness, we need to understand genetic makeup as well as the factors that affect how genes are expressed. In medical school, we were taught to think of genes as fixed and immutable, conferring upon us some inevitable disease. This is not the case. About 70 percent of our genes can be up- or down-regulated. In simple terms, they can be turned on or off. This is called *altering gene expression*. It turns out that our environment, our lifestyle, our emotional traumas, our diets, and numerous other factors affect our genes. All these factors together are called **epigenetic factors**. Think of your genes as your hardware and your epigenetic factors as your software. You know that good apps can make your electronic devices work much better. Similarly, a glitch in your app can shut down your device. Your genes are not always your destiny—you do have some control over them.

Let's look at this example in real life. If many of your family members have type 2 diabetes, for instance, you're at greater risk for it as well. Why? Is it just your genes, or is it also the diet, lifestyle, and exercise habits you've learned from your family? You can't change your genes, but you can modify the environment they are exposed to—in other words, you can change your genetic expression. Modifiable risk factors mean you can lose weight, eat a better diet, and exercise more. Making such changes is no guarantee against getting the disease, but it can prevent or delay it and make it easier to manage if it does happen.

We can get a general idea of your risk of illness from your family history. This alerts us to your risk for conditions such as diabetes, heart disease, Alzheimer's disease, and various types of cancers. It is now possible to study the entire human genome and know all your approximately 22,000 genes. Each gene can have thousands of variations, however. The resultant permutations are diverse and make us all unique. Beyond this, our genes are constantly being influenced by our lifestyle, diet, and environment. No wonder it's sometimes difficult to figure out what's going on!

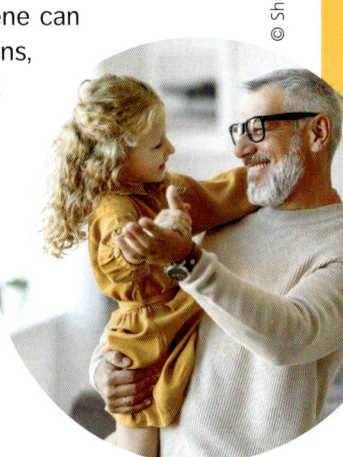

Understanding **Epigenetics**

You inherited your chromosomes, which contain your genes, from your parents. You have 23 chromosomes in total, inherited from your parents. Within your chromosomes are the 22,000 or so genes that produce the proteins encoded in your DNA that run your body and form the foundation of who you are as a unique individual.

As we stated above, you can't change your genes—but you can change the way they work. This is done through the epigene, which sits next to the gene and instructs the gene on how to express itself. Epigenetics is the study of how your behavior and your environment affect your epigene, and thus your genetic expression.

Your genes work by expressing proteins according to instructions encoded in your DNA. You can't really change those instructions, but you can turn genes on and off through epigenetic changes, such as what you eat or how much exercise you get.

Genes change very slowly through the process of evolution. Over many generations, genes that confer a survival advantage will tend to spread, while genes that are harmful will tend to die out. Our epigenetics, however, change all the time, depending on what we're eating and what we're doing. Genetic changes can't be reversed, but fortunately, epigenetic changes are reversible. In other words, you can't change your hardware—your DNA—but you can definitely upgrade your software.

Biological and Chronological Aging

Simply getting older is the biggest risk factor for both chronic illness and dying. If we compare the lifestyle risk factors associated with both death and illness, even the worst culprits, such as smoking, drug and alcohol abuse, pollution, and toxicity, pale in comparison to what age does. And as we get older, the effects of age keep getting worse. Genomic instability, telomere attrition, cellular senescence, altered intercellular communication, mitochondrial dysfunction, deregulated nutrient sensing, stem cell exhaustion, mitochondrial dysfunction, loss of proteostasis (protein stability), and epigenetic alterations are all scientifically recognized hallmarks of aging.

Aging is the one thing that remains assured for all of us, yet up to now there has been little we could do about it. We're now rethinking whether age and illness must always go together.

Most of us know precisely how old we are chronologically. Yet, if we just look around, we see that colleagues our own age are aging at vastly different rates. Some look years younger, while others look much older. In other words, their biological ages don't always match their chronological ages. Studies in twins show that epigenetic modifications are highly influential on the way they age. Epigenetics is the interface between the outside world and your genes. Outside influences such as diet and environmental toxins can turn genes on and off. The main way epigenetics affects our genes is through DNA methylation—an epigenetic mechanism that both affects gene expression and is affected by your environment. ==Methyl tags attach to your DNA and change gene expression by changing what areas of the DNA can be transcribed. A portion of DNA with a methyl tag can't be read, so in effect, methylation turns genes off. A methylation change that silences a gene will affect every other function in the body, since all other functions rely on instructions from the DNA to begin. Fortunately, DNA methylation can be changed, which means we may be able to reverse damage and improve outcomes.==

Up until quite recently, we weren't able to measure biological age accurately. This is rapidly changing. High-tech labs are now able to measure 900,000 (out of 26 million) methylation marks on the DNA of white blood cells. We were used to seeing lab results of up to 100 markers. Now we're using 900,000 markers, and that number will increase rapidly in coming years. Algorithms that use methylation patterns can detect the epigenetic effects of your environment and lifestyle dating back to childhood.

By examining methylation, we can get a detailed look at how your body is self-regulating and how well it's aging.

Methylation patterns seem to be able to predict chronic diseases such as Alzheimer's disease. And now, algorithms using methylation marks have created third-generation biological age clocks that can detect differing rates of aging in different organ systems. These clocks predict not only your actual biological age, but also your rate of aging. Chronologically, we age at the rate of one year per year, but biologically, aging rates vary considerably, confirming what we see when we look at our contemporaries. Some of us are aging excessively fast, while others are aging slowly, at say 0.7 years per year. This way of looking at aging gives us a radically different view of how to intervene.

Methylation patterns, for instance, can quickly tell us if some anti-aging approaches are actually helpful. Metformin, for instance, is a drug long touted as a way to slow aging. (It turns out that it doesn't seem to help.) Typically, to test this hypothesis, we would have to test two groups, an experimental group and a control group, and then wait until they died to see if an intervention worked. But because methylation patterns are affected quite quickly, if we want to try out a new intervention, whether it be a lifestyle or dietary change, a drug, or a supplement, we can know the answer in three months. We don't have to wait until the end of someone's lifespan to see if an intervention worked or not. This is called a N-of-1 study, and it may be the best way to do a controlled test on any patient.

This is both a watershed moment, and a confluence of medicine, science, and functional

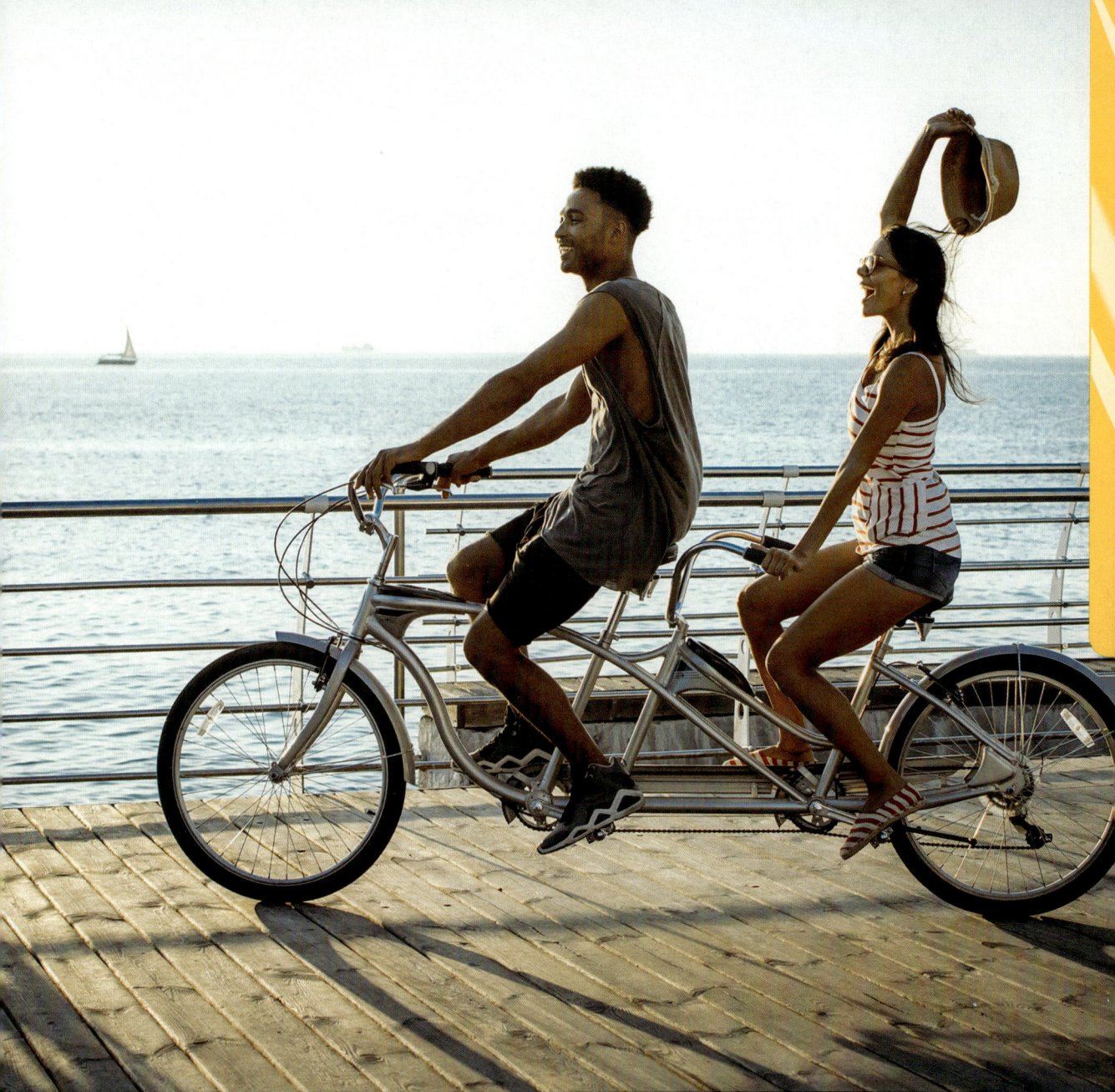

medicine. Since we now have a good marker for biological aging, and a way to measure if an intervention works, we should be able to see rapid strides in anti-aging in the coming years. No longer are we going to be stuck with someone's opinion. Now we can see real data.

We have begun using the TruDiagnostic epigenetic test to look for signs of accelerated aging in some of our patients. The test uses a powerful algorithm called DunedinPACE to show how fast you're currently aging—it's like a speedometer for aging. Many chronic illnesses that appear as we get older can be predicted—and possibly prevented—years in advance by tracking markers of accelerated aging. Using the TruDiagnostic test lets us show our patients what their future health may be. The results motivate our patients to take preventive measures, such as improving their diet and lifestyle, and lets them see within a few months how effective their steps have been.

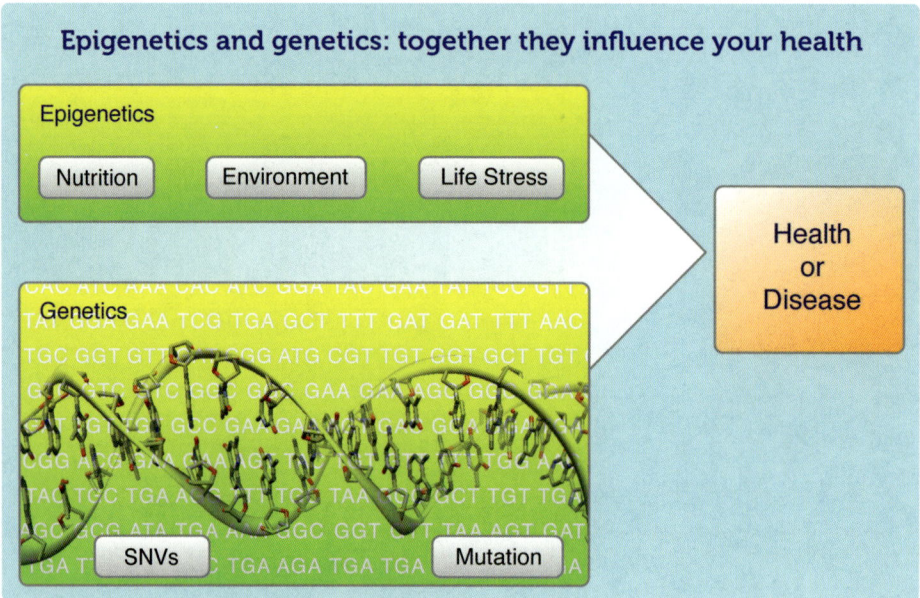

FIGURE 4.2 | Epigenetics and Genetics

Genomics and Multiomics:
The Future of Personalized Medicine

The International Human Genome Sequencing Consortium, part of the collaborative Human Genome Project (HGP), published the first draft of the human genome (the collection of all human genes) in the journal *Nature* in February 2001. More than 2,800 researchers took part in the consortium and shared authorship of the paper. The full sequence was completed and published in April 2003. The sequencing revealed that humans have between 20,000 and 25,000 genes. At the time, we stood in awe at the dawning of a new age; the HGP gave us the ability to read the complete genetic blueprint for building a human being. When we understand the code written in the book of life, we can better understand disease and aging.

Initially, we were excited about normal variants in genes called single nucleotide variants, or SNVs. These used to be called single nucleotide polymorphisms, or SNPs, but as science evolves, terminology often changes to reflect its development. We realized that SNVs influenced the variability we saw in our patients. SNVs explained, for example, why different patients metabolized drugs and nutrients differently, based on genetic differences in the way they manufactured and used proteins, the building blocks of the body.

The MTHFR (methyltetrahydrofolate reductase) SNV was given much press when it was discovered. The MTHFR gene helps activate the B vitamin folate into an active form called methyltetrahydrofolate (MTHF). Because MTHF is involved in a variety of processes, ranging from spina bifida in newborns to heart disease, strokes, depression, and arthritis in adults, we were very excited to learn about it. We thought the SNV that made this gene less effective at converting folate revealed a treatable root cause of many health issues. Alas, this was an oversimplification! It turns out there are multiple SNVs that metabolize folic acid. In addition, folic acid levels also depend on nutrient intake, as well as the health of the gut and the functions of the trillions of microbes living there.

Genomics today is still a work in progress. *We've come to realize that with very few exceptions, no single gene or gene variant is directly responsible for aspects of your health. Rather, many genes—sometimes thou-*

sands—work together to control how your body functions in both health and illness.

The amount of genetic data is immense. Analysis of genomic data is like looking at the stars at night. As you zoom in closer, each star opens into other universes, revealing even more data. Today, genomic analysis, although highly scientific, is still open to interpretation. The experts don't always agree about what they're seeing. An analogy would be describing clouds in the sky to friends— what you see may not be the same as what they see.

If millions of genetic variations combine to create what we see as human uniqueness, we must further understand that the variations interact with each person's own unique environmental stresses (microbiome, lifestyle, diet, emotional, and physical) to produce unique outcomes. Simple tests that we have used in medicine for decades simply aren't sensitive enough to give us an understanding of what is really happening. To do this we need to understand multiomics, the multiple data sets that interact in the body: the genome, proteome, transcriptome, epigenome, metabolome, and microbiome. Researchers can analyze this complex aggregate of data to find new biomarkers that can warn that disease is brewing, long before it becomes visible by conventional testing. Multiomic technology shows us that people at elevated genetic risk for a range of diseases have changes in their blood proteins and metabolite levels that can be detected long before disease symptoms appear.

The predictive power of big data, all analyzed by artificial intelligence and deep learning, will let us see disease coming long before it happens—and we will be

> ❝
> A long healthy life is no accident. It begins with good genes, but it also depends on good habits.
>
> —**Dan Buettner**

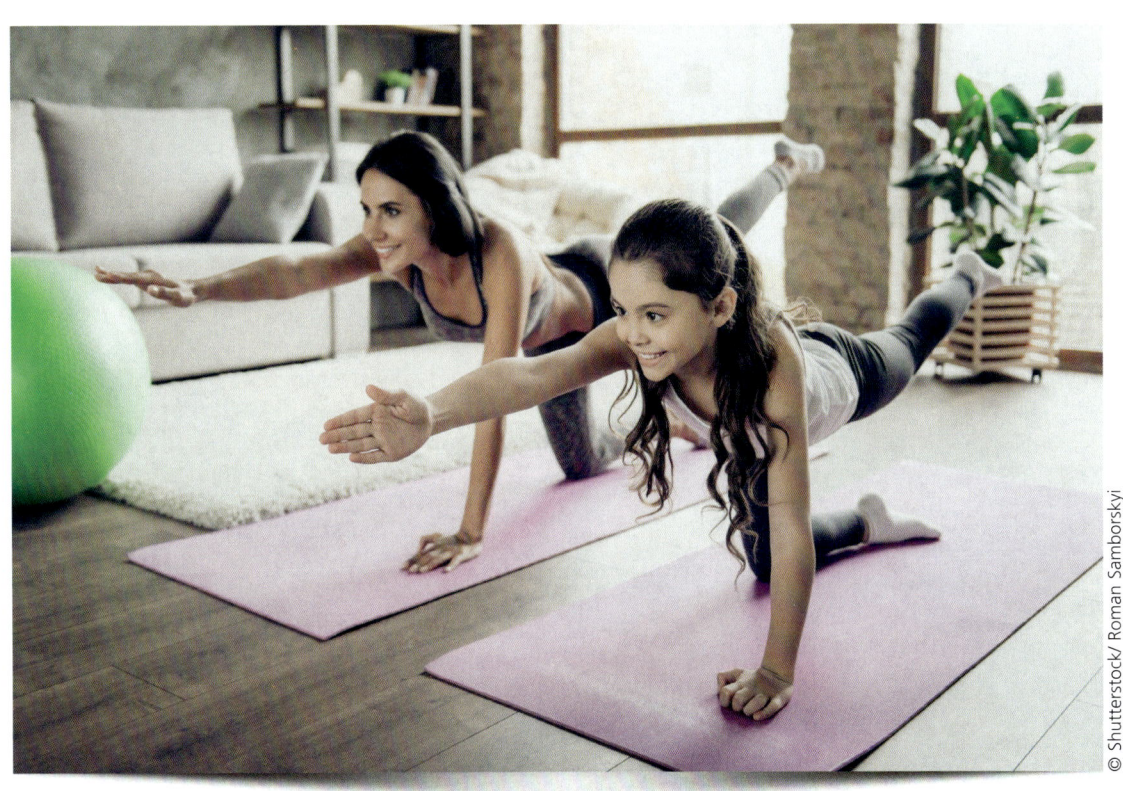

able to see in real time how effective preventive interventions for lowering risk are.

Epigenetics: How Diet, Lifestyle, and Environment Affect Our Genes

It's the old argument: nature versus nurture. Your genotype is your individual genetic makeup—your own personal instruction manual, or hardware, for your body. The genes you inherited are with you for your whole life, but they don't necessarily determine your health. Epigenetic factors can flip the genetic switch, either toward health or toward disease. You might have inherited the group of genes that predispose you to lung cancer, for example, but if you don't smoke, and you avoid the cigarette smoke of others, those genes are unlikely to be switched on.

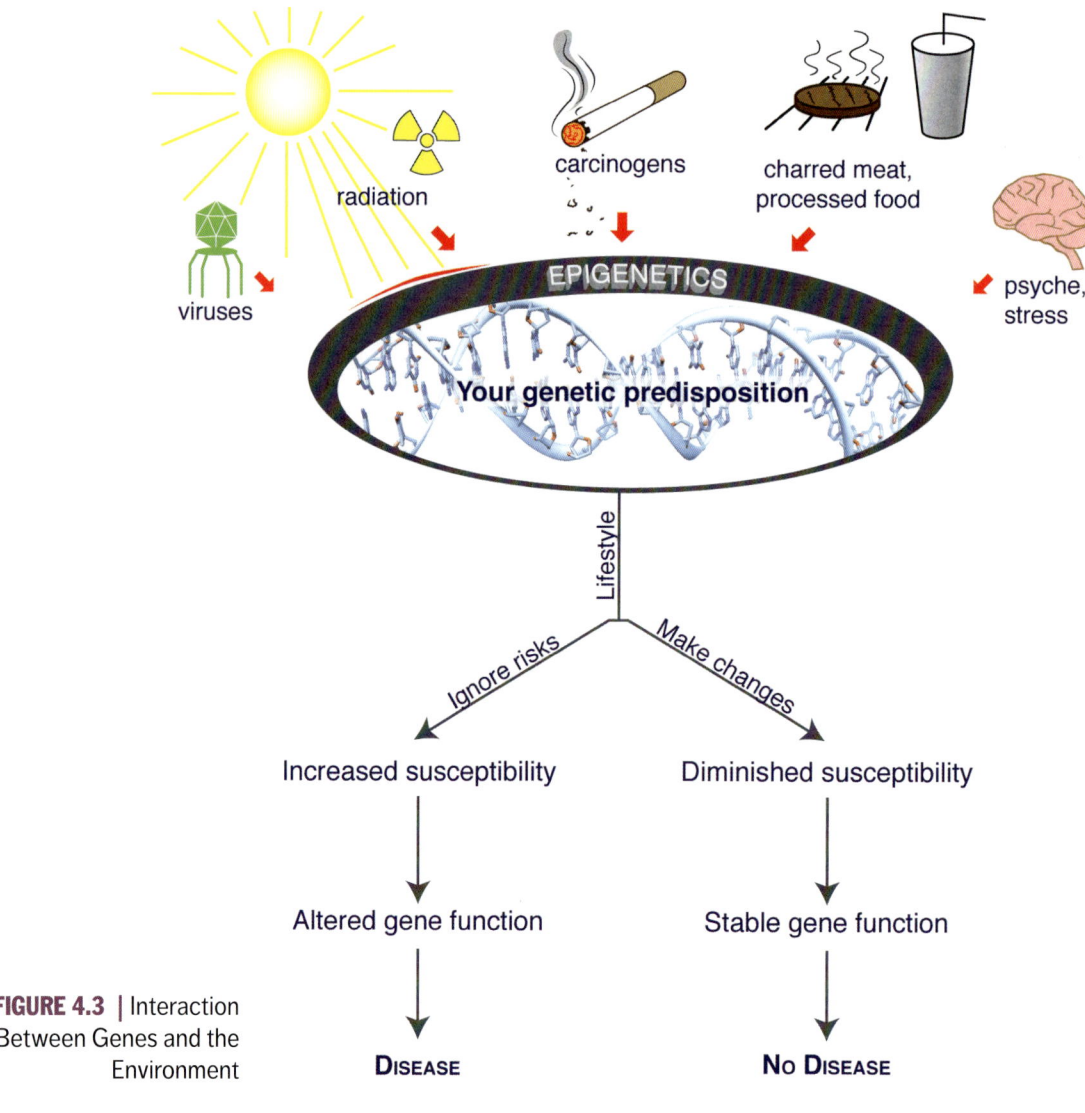

FIGURE 4.3 | Interaction Between Genes and the Environment

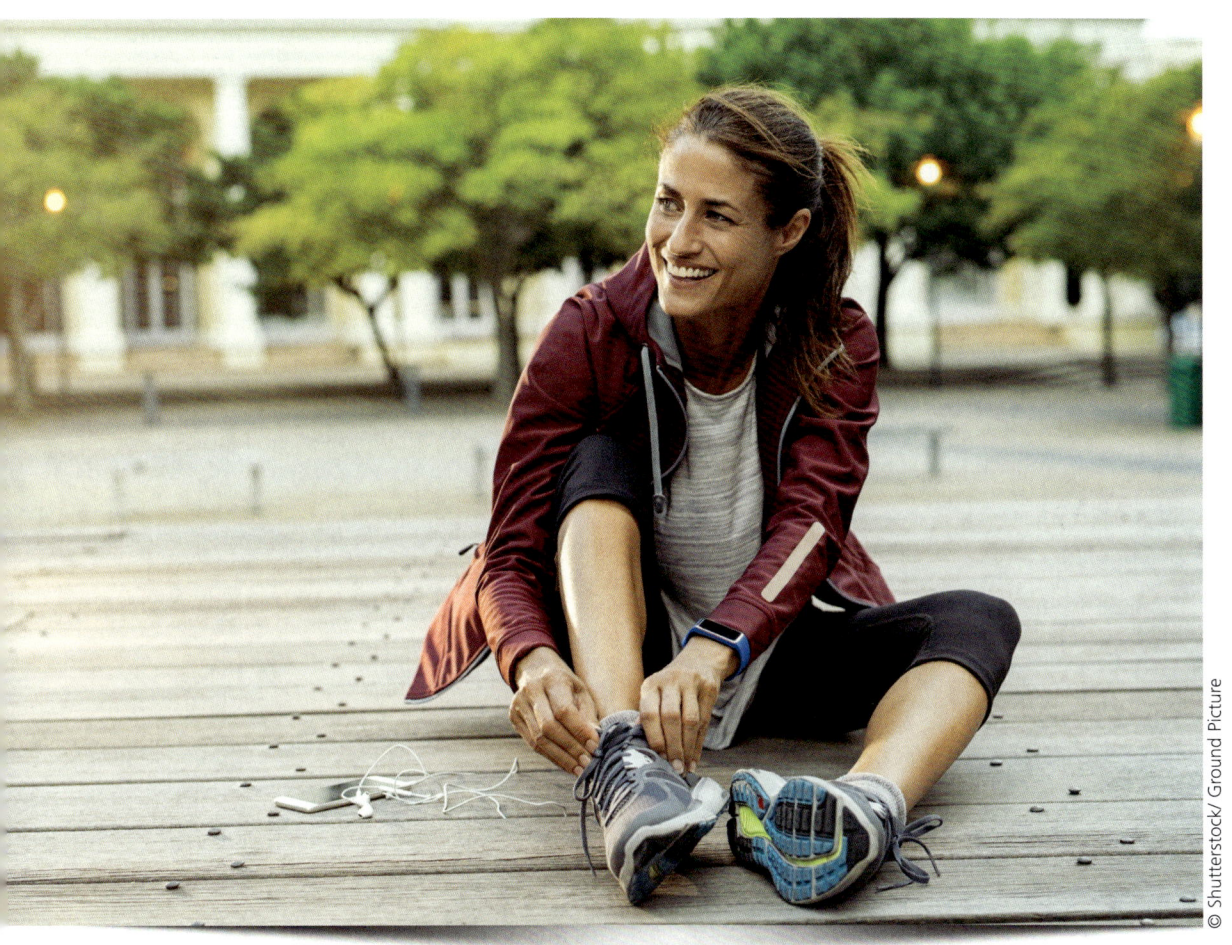

The Pima, Native Americans who live in the Sonora Desert of southern Arizona, are a classic example of the interaction between genetics and epigenetics. This nation has the highest rate of type 2 diabetes in the world—about 38 percent of the adult population.

Why are the Pima so susceptible to diabetes? For thousands of years, the Pima lived in an environment that sometimes provided plenty of food and sometimes provided very little. Their genes adapted by allowing them to store body fat very efficiently during the good times to prevent starvation during the inevitable lean times. This is sometimes referred to as the "thrifty gene."

The genetic heritage of the Pima hasn't changed over thousands of years, but their lifestyle has. For more than a century, the Pima have lived on reservations. Instead of the hunter-gatherer diet of game, fruit, berries, and other foods, they now have a Westernized diet much higher in fat, refined carbohydrates, and processed foods. In addition, they are far less active than their ancestors were. Their genes, which originally kept them alive by resisting starvation, now interact with their diet and lifestyle—their epigenetics—to produce a very high rate of obesity and diabetes. Pima Indians living in the very remote Sierra Madre region of Mexico share the same genetic heritage but have far lower rates of diabetes—only about 7 percent of adults. The difference is their environment. The Mexican Pima eat a more traditional diet and are much more physically active. The contrast between these two groups clearly shows how genetic tendencies toward a disease can often be countered by diet and lifestyle.

How the Diet of a Mother Affects Her Offspring

Agouti mice have a much higher incidence of obesity, diabetes, and cancer than other mice and are therefore frequently used as subjects in scientific studies. Typically, these mice are fat, with a pale-yellow coat. A famous study in 2003 compared the health of pregnant agouti mice fed two different diets. One group was fed a diet supplemented with folic acid, vitamin B12, choline, and betaine, all of which promote methylation, while the control group was fed a standard diet. Rather than being fat and yellow, the offspring of the mice on the supplemented diet were slender with brown coats and had a much lower incidence of obesity, diabetes, and cancer. What's more, this protective effect persisted into the second generation.

So, it seems that a diet high in B vitamins protected the next two generations of mice. However, when the supplemental diet was stopped with the next generation, the protective effect wore off. Isn't it interesting how a simple change in the environmental exposure of the agouti mice genes had such a profound impact on the health of the next generations?

Epigenetics in Action: The Agouti Mouse

Yellow agouti mice become obese and have a high risk of diabetes, cancer and shortened lifespan.

Brown agouti mice are thin, with a normal lifespan and reduced risk of diabetes and cancer.

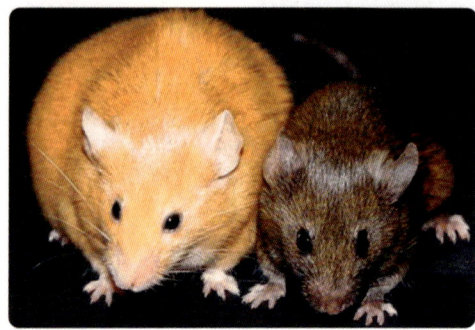

Photograph reproduced with permission from Environmental Health Perspectives: Weinhold B, Environ Health Perspect 114:4 (2006).

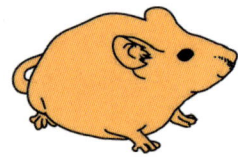

regular mouse food / mouse food fortified with methylating nutrients

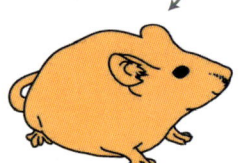 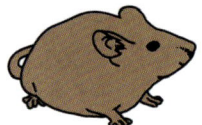

FIGURE 4.4 | Epigenetics in Action

Expanding Your Medical Options

If you have lingering health issues that have persisted for three or more months with no resolution with conventional medical care, this might be a time to reconsider your approach. You might even know that you have a genetic tendency toward a particular health problem. Alternatively, you may simply want to improve your health to head off illness later in life. In any of these circumstances, you might want to take proactive steps.

An Expanded History: The First Order of Personalized Medicine

You are not simply a "heart attack," a "back pain," or a "cancer." You are you, a unique individual, and you have a unique story your doctor needs to understand. The initial medical diagnosis is, in fact, only part of the story. *If we really want to find out what is going on, we need to get the whole story or, as we like to say, the story behind the story!*

To better understand how you got sick, we need to be able to personalize your story:

- We need to know your risk for illness—your family history and genetic predisposition as well as the current environmental and lifestyle factors that place you at risk.
- We want to know what your health was like before you got sick. Illness doesn't happen in a vacuum. It is part of a process.
- We want to know what the precipitating factor or triggering cause of the illness is. This is the tipping point to illness. Any of several factors can be the last straw that causes us to get sick. The tipping points can include infections caused by viruses, bacteria, or even parasites; an emotional crisis; physical trauma such as a car accident; or major physical stressors such as surgery.
- We want to know what the mediators of the illness are—chronic stress, for example, can predispose you to sickness. If we understand this, we can design treatments to antidote the illness.

Why We Need the Whole Story

We can easily go for the quick medical fix. In fact, in many cases, such as a severe infection, we should. This is why conventional diagnosis and treatment are so useful. However, if we miss the story behind the story, we lose the chance to harness the transformational opportunity of an illness. Every illness, no matter what it is, gives us a chance to reevaluate what we are doing and bring ourselves into balance in some way. If we simply go for the quick fix, we lose the chance to find and correct the underlying problems that left us vulnerable and continue to leave us vulnerable to recurrence. If we don't, the problems accumulate, becoming more and more likely to cause future problems. *In functional medicine, these factors are called antecedent factors—they set us up for future illness.* As doctors, we need to know about your stress level; your nutritional, metabolic, and immune risk factors; how your hormones are doing; and whether you have any pain in your body.

Every time we get sick, that is feedback from our bodies. Consider the type of illness that stops us in our tracks—when we get it, we're usually very run down or stressed out. So rather than viewing illness as a bother, consider it a message with valuable information to be used to help us get better.

An Expanded Medical Workup

In a medical workup, lab tests are an invaluable aid to letting us know how you are. Sometimes, a simple lab test may tell us all we need to know. If you're feeling fatigued and the lab test shows anemia, we can presume the anemia is associated with the fatigue, and then we start investigating the cause of the anemia and decide on the most appropriate treatment. However, there are many times when some-

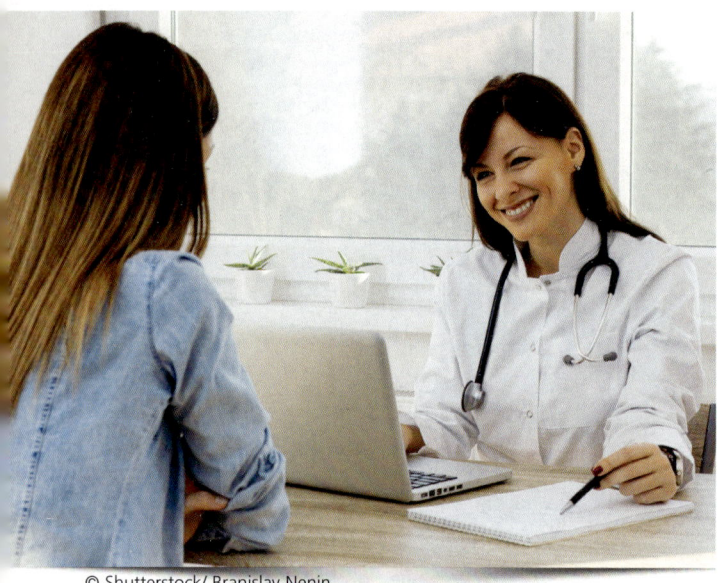
© Shutterstock/ Branislav Nenin

one may complain of fatigue yet have normal lab tests. This is where the systems approach we discussed previously can be so helpful. We can use functional lab tests to find out which system is malfunctioning.

Functional Lab Tests: Your Epigenetic Risk Factors

To discover what system or systems are malfunctioning, we can use conventional lab tests and order additional tests from laboratories that specialize in functional medicine evaluations. We do this testing because often the magical, clear-cut diagnosis you have been looking for may not exist. Instead, you may have a complex problem involving a malfunction in one or more systems in your body. To heal, it may be necessary to look at all of these systems and consider how to improve the balance within each one. A systems approach can be especially helpful with chronic illness. By improving the functioning and balance of the major systems of the body, many patients find that their symptoms just melt away!

If, for instance, we want to ascertain your nutritional status, we might order standard tests such as vitamin D, red cell magnesium, folic acid, and vitamin B12 levels. We can also use indirect tests such as homocysteine (which can indicate a need for vitamins B6, B12, or folic acid), or we can test for methylmalonic acid (to help us understand if your body needs more vitamin B12). We might order specific functional lab tests if we want to know if you're absorbing nutrients and have sufficient amino acids (protein building blocks) to help you repair your body. We can also test further to see if you have enough of the good anti-inflammatory fats called omega-3 fatty acids. If we want to check to see if you're inflamed, we might use a conventional test called high-sensitivity C-reactive protein (hs-CRP). Or we could check chemicals called cytokines, such as interleukin 6 (IL-6) or tumor necrosis factor alpha (TNF-a), or complement levels such as C4a, which further let us know about your inflammatory status. If we want to know if your body is dealing with oxidative stress (i.e., "rusting"), we could test markers that let us know about oxidative status.

Functional lab tests can be used to check stress-related problems, neurotransmitter imbalances, nutritional, metabolic, and immune problems, and subtle hormonal imbalances.

The list of these tests is extensive. As physicians, we need to constantly evaluate and balance the benefit of the information (including false-positive results) we will get from the results against the cost of the tests. This is similarly true if we decide to do further radiological testing, such as CT scans, MRIs, and ultrasounds.

Ultimately, we want to know where you are, what the causative factors are, and why you are in the situation you are in.

We call this a *systems approach* to lab testing. Using a systems approach, we are not trying to make a clinical diagnosis. We are looking for an imbalance in an underlying system, which we can then rectify. When we correct the imbalance, symptoms of illness often simply melt away.

Understanding a Diagnosis:
What It Means to Tease Out a Story

Let's start with a closer look at conventional Western medicine, which is highly effective in diagnosing and treating so many illnesses. We all want precision and accuracy, and that's what conventional medicine can usually deliver. Let's follow two stories that illustrate the ways acute illness is commonly approached by conventional medicine.

Sam awoke with a sore throat. Two hours later, he started shivering as his temperature rose to 102.5°F. Sam decided to go to work anyway, so he took two Tylenol tablets and headed out the door. At work, he began to feel even worse. By 5:00 p.m., he wasn't sure he even had enough strength to get home. At the urging of his wife, he called his family doctor, who fortunately had evening hours that day. Dr. Smith took a quick history from Sam and examined him, taking notice of his enlarged tonsils, which were coated with a thick, white discharge. A throat swab showed Sam was positive for strep throat. Dr. Smith gave Sam a prescription for penicillin. Less than 24 hours later, Sam was feeling much better, and two days after that, he hardly knew he had been ill.

Nila was playing soccer for her college team when she felt a snap in her knee. It happened just as she planted her foot and began to pivot toward the oncoming ball. Within seconds, she dropped to the ground in agony, hardly able to move. Her knee was swelling rapidly, and she struggled to stop her tears from flowing. Before she knew it, the team trainer had arranged for her to be taken to the local emergency room. An MRI revealed a ruptured ACL (anterior cruciate ligament) and torn cartilage (medial meniscus). The orthopedic surgeon on call, a well-known sports physician, confirmed the diagnosis and scheduled her for surgery, assuring her that after rehab she would be playing soccer again within a few months.

Ah, the miracle of modern medicine! These stories are the ones we love to hear. We go to the doctor, and they fix us. We feel better and go back to living our lives. But in the real world, these examples don't tell us the whole story.

Antecedent Factors

Let's take a closer look at Sam's situation. When Sam came down with strep throat, he had been under significant stress at work. Not only that, but his relationship with his wife was at an all-time low. She had been depressed since the birth of their second child, less than a year after the first baby. Sam and his family had been living on fast food and takeouts. Their children, both infants, were frequently ill due to infections they picked up at day care. Sam was at a breaking point from the combination of stress, lack of sleep, and poor nutrition. And that's when he got sick.

Let's also look more closely at Nila. At first glance, it might appear that Nila just suffered from a mechanical injury. Simply put, the forces applied to twist her knee were greater than the strength of her ligament or cartilage. The result was that her tissues snapped under the shear force. However, Nila, too, was at a crossroads in her life. She loved playing soccer and being slim and fit, but exercise had taken over her life, mainly because it kept her weight down. She also forced herself to run five miles every day and work out at the gym whenever she could while keeping up her schoolwork. Given her academic schedule, that level of exertion left her vulnerable to a stress injury. Secretly, Nila also suffered from an eating disorder. No one noticed her slipping away from soccer parties into a bathroom so she could purge her french fries into the toilet. Nila silently suffered from exercise anorexia and bulimia that had been going on since her high school days. High levels of exertion and poor nutrition left her vulnerable to a stress injury.

Stress and the Mind–Body Connection

Both Sam's and Nila's stories illustrate the influence of psychological factors on the development of illness. In Sam's case, stress played a role. And a thorough history would have turned up that Nila had been hiding a long history of eating disorders as a way to cope with the stresses of being a high-achieving student and athlete.

Immune Function

In Sam's case, it is important to find out more about his poor diet. We also need to know about his stress, his long work hours, and the infections his children were bringing home from day care. These factors all affected his immunity. With a healthy immune system, Sam would probably not have come down with strep. But because his system was so vulnerable, he became sick.

Nutritional Deficiencies

We can argue that no matter what Nila had done, the shear force applied to her knee would have snapped the ligament. This is possibly true. But let's consider another way to assess her susceptibility to injury. Nila's frequent purging resulted in a low level of nutrients, particularly two essential amino acids found in protein—glycine and proline—that are necessary to maintain healthy ligaments. Other nutrients that help build muscle and joint strength are the B vitamins and vitamin C, as well as a host of cofactors. Nila's habit of purging seriously depleted these nutrients, leaving her vulnerable to injury.

Injury and Imbalances in the Body

The body's muscles are in a dynamic state of push and pull, or tensegrity. In Nila's case, tight hamstrings and a weak vastus medialis obliquus muscle (VMO) on the upper inside of her knee could easily have contributed to her injury.

The Tipping Point

Unfortunately, since conventional medicine is so focused on finding a singular cause for illness, doctors sometimes get caught up looking for the one single thing, such as a virus or high cholesterol, that might have caused the illness. In reality, most illnesses are caused by a constellation of factors coming together.

After treating thousands of patients over more than forty years, one concept has solidified for us: when people lose control over their health, they lose their sense of control over their lives, and thus their destiny. Patients struggle with conventional medicine because these treatments aren't designed to restore control. They are simply given "this-for-that" solutions, a series of tradeoffs between benefits and side effects.

In explaining to patients how to deal with the stress of a newly diagnosed illness, we often use a metaphor: If you're in the sea when a huge wave comes for you, don't stiffen up because the wave will break you. Take a deep breath, relax, sink down, and let the wave pass. Another wave may come along, but soon you will learn to surf.

When life or disease throws you a huge wave, the biggest priority is to retain control over yourself. How?

- **Educate yourself** about the best options available through conventional medicine.
- **Use the concepts** of healing we outline in this book.
- **Surround yourself** with a community that reinforces and supports you.
- **Contemplate your life spiritually**. Does your life have purpose and meaning? What is the illness trying to teach you? Can you make changes that will allow you to feel more fulfilled as a human being?

This is the transformation we seek in **Transformational Medicine**. Remember that while curing isn't always possible, healing always is! **Illness is something that happens to us. Wellbeing is something WE CHOOSE TO MAKE HAPPEN!**

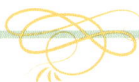

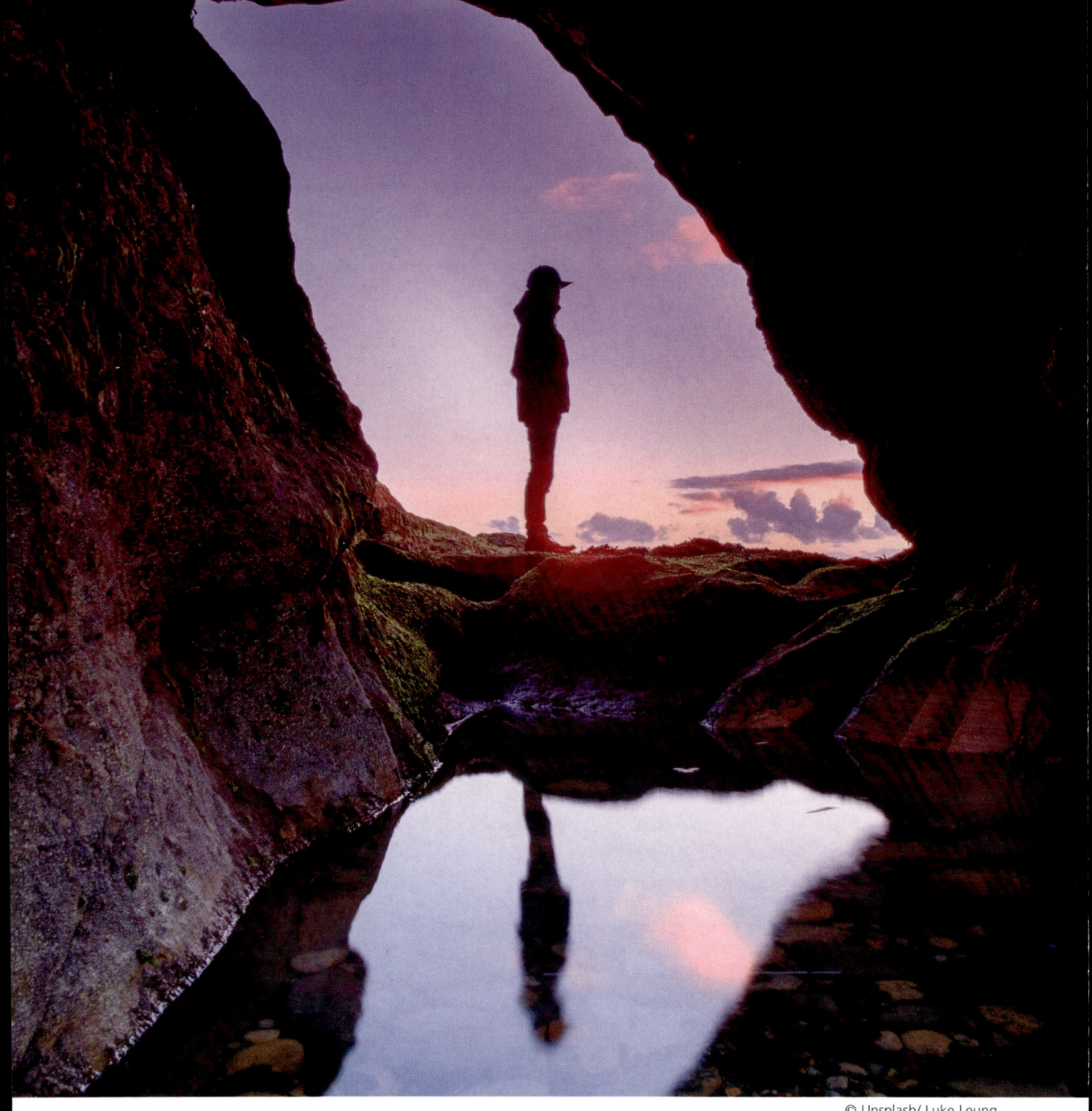

CHAPTER 5

Stress and The Road to Illness

Addressing the Trajectory Toward Chronic Illness

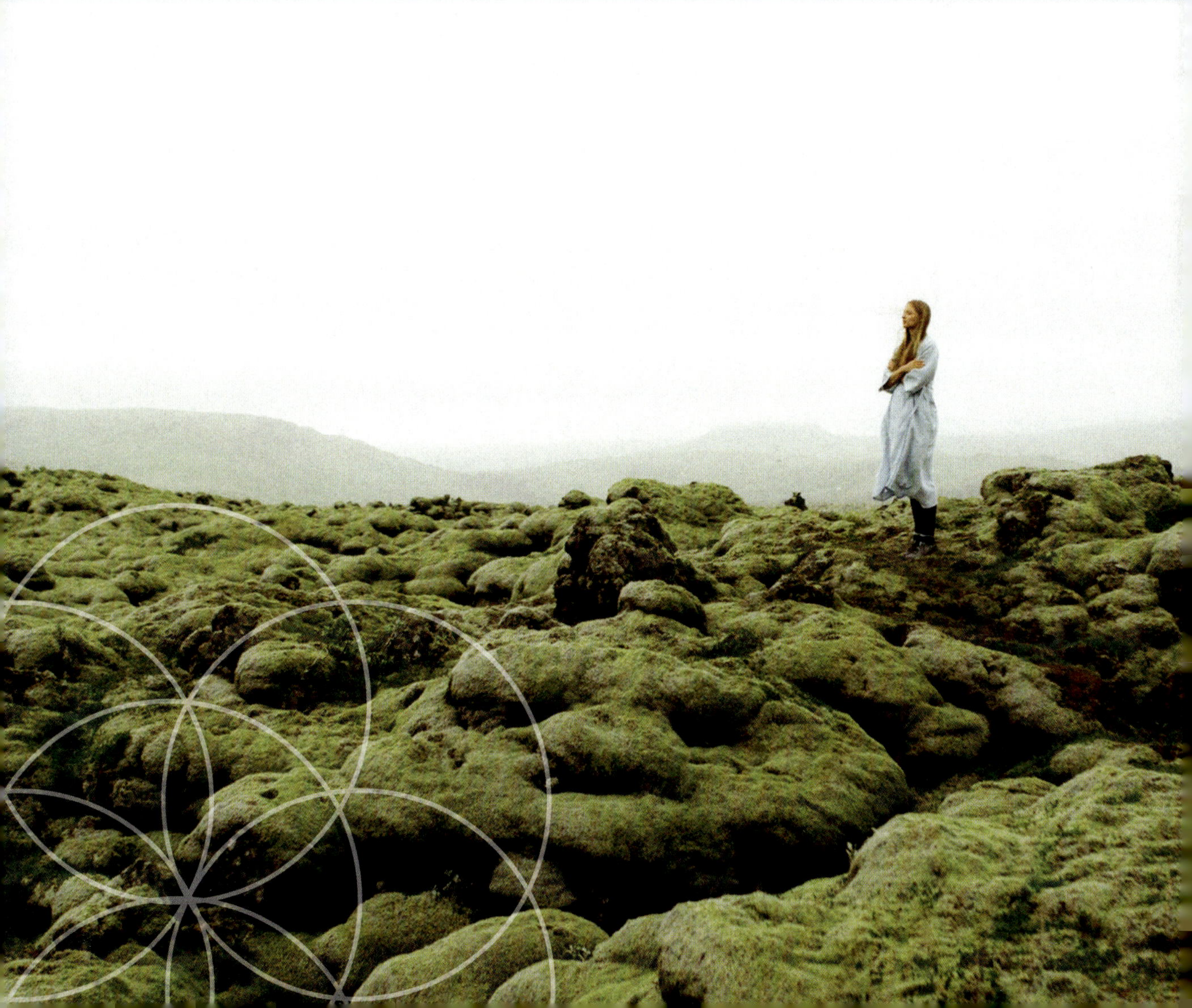

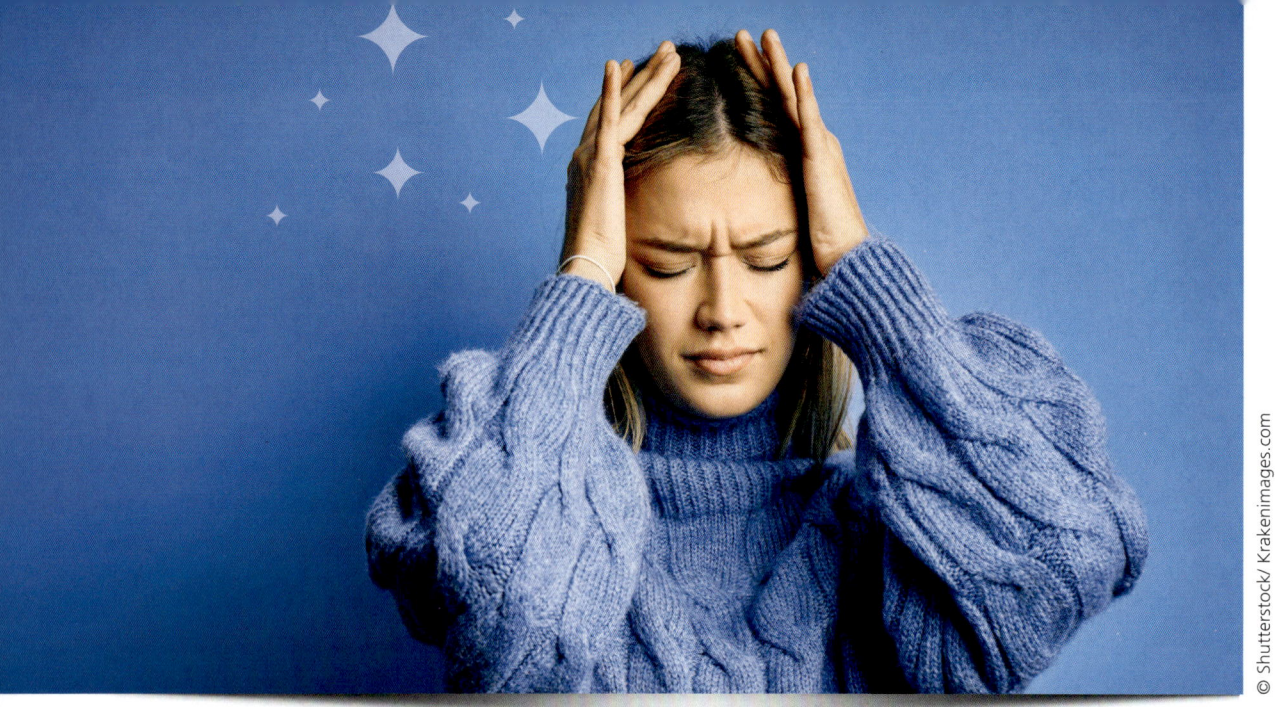

Most of our patients tell us the same story in different forms. It is the story of how they got sick, and it always involves both physical and emotional stress. If you or someone you love has chronic illness, you'll want to give some thought to the stresses that may have contributed to that illness. Getting sick is a process, and reducing stress is often the first step in preventing illness.

Stress and Illness

Stress is a term that gets used a lot, but what does it really mean? We define stress as the body's response to physical, emotional, or mental demands. Our bodies handle stress by producing hormones that help us cope. When we're faced with a sudden danger—a close call in traffic, for instance—our bodies respond by releasing the hormone adrenaline or epinephrine, which raises the heart rate and makes us more alert. Ordinarily, once the stressful situation is over, the body returns to normal. But what if the stress continues unabated? That's when stress can start to affect your health.

The Stress Curve

To understand how stress impacts your physical, emotional, and mental health, you need to know what a typical response to stress looks like. We call this the Stress Curve—check the diagram on page 58 to see what the curve looks like.

This pattern was first described in the work of the pioneering physician and researcher Hans Selye. In the late 1930s and early 1940s, Selye performed the initial studies on what he defined as the stress syndrome, then coined the term stress. His studies also looked at the effects of stress over time and at how we adapt to stress, described as the General Adaptation Syndrome.

Stress is a normal aspect of life. In short, controlled episodes, stress can be good for you. Selye called this *eustress*. Yet we now know that stress, left unmanaged, can lead to psychological and major physical problems, or what Selye called *distress*. Researchers have connected stress to almost every form of non-hereditary illness.

People respond to stress in unique ways. One person will thrive in a situation that causes another to crumble. However, we all have our breaking point. When we're overextended and overworked for too long, we inevitably suffer from extreme stress. Once stress becomes chronic and overwhelming, almost all of us tend to experience a similar pattern of physical and emotional responses that reflect profound changes in our body chemistry.

What's more, stress tends to become both invasive and pervasive. When stress is chronic, you may get so depleted from it that you feel you no longer have the physical and emotional stamina to change the pattern. In other words, try as you might, you can't just pull yourself together anymore.

Going NUTS

According to stress researcher Sonia Lupien, PhD, professor of psychiatry at the University of Montreal and the founder and director of the Centre for Studies on Human Stress in Canada, life events likely to be stressful are usually those that drive us "NUTS." That is, they are either new or novel (N), unpredictable (U), threatening to our personality (T), or induce a sense (S) of loss of control. Each time we get stressed, and, in a sense, go a little bit NUTS, our bodies react by releasing hormones and other chemicals, readying us for the "fight, flight, or freeze" response.

Initially, the elevated levels of stress hormones can be beneficial and even invigorating. However, over the long term, the effects of the pressure and strain tend to be debilitating, chronic, and cumulative.

In his book *Why Zebras Don't Get Ulcers*, neuroendocrinology researcher and Stanford professor Robert Sapolsky affirms that wild animals are less likely to experience the type of stress induced by the constant worry and anxiety that plagues humans. In the animal kingdom, when confronted with the threat of an attack by a predator, the stress response enables an animal to either fight or run for its life. Both scenarios require an intense physical effort. In terms of body chemistry and the nervous system, the physical exertion of running or fighting completes the stress response. When the danger has passed, the animal returns to a baseline state, free of ongoing worry (until the next predator comes along).

Like animals, humans are genetically hardwired for experiencing cycles of acute stress. When stress is followed by intense physical activity, we can return naturally to baseline and a calmer state of mind. This sort of stress doesn't give us ulcers.

Stress can be habit-forming and even addicting. The pulsating adrenaline high we feel when we deal with acute stress may make us want to go back for more. Think of a roller coaster ride. You may scream while you're on it, but as soon as you get off, you start thinking, "That was fun! Maybe I should do that again."

So, acute stress is fine as long as you can deal with it and then return to your baseline low-stress level. But what happens when we're exposed to stress day in, day out, with nothing to help antidote it?

Stuck in the Stress Response

Constant, escalating, never-ending stress can eventually make us sick. We can get stuck in the stress response and not be able to see a way out.

Let's presume for a moment that you have a manageable amount of stress in your life. We want to show here what happens when the demands of your life progressively increase your stress load, creating a scenario of chronic persistent stress that lasts for three months or more.

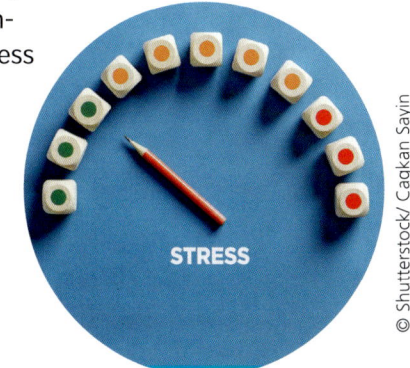

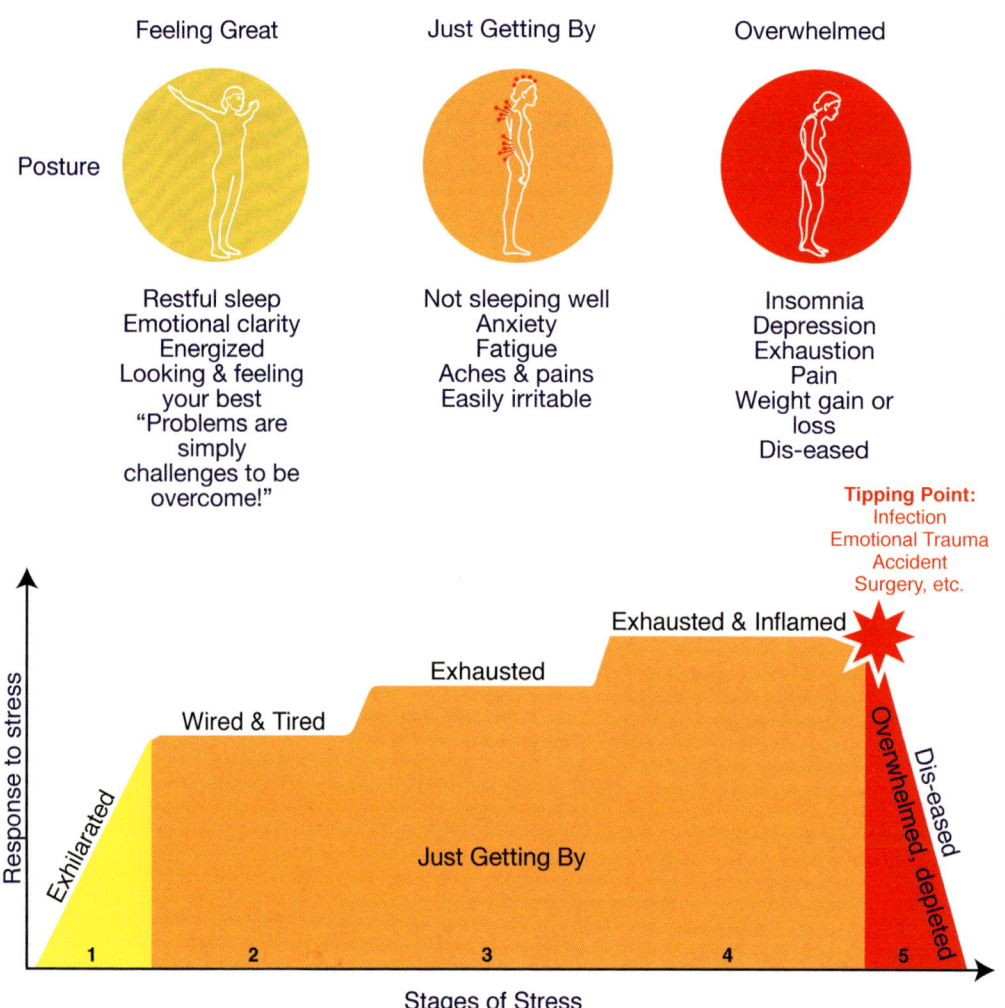

FIGURE 5.1 | The Stress Curve

When Stress Is Invigorating: The Exhilaration Aspect of the Stress Curve

Under initial mild or moderate stress, most of us typically respond well. If you're asked to complete a rush job with an urgent deadline, or you need to study for an exam, you can probably push yourself a little, respond to that stress, and meet the challenge. If it's an exciting opportunity, such as a new job, you'll probably even feel energized or exhilarated. At this early stage, problems are simply challenges to be overcome. This is the optimum response.

When You Max Out on Stress: The "Stressed-and-Just-Getting-By" Phase of the Stress Curve

The stressed-and-just-getting-by phase comprises three progressive levels:

- **Wired and Tired**
- **Exhausted**
- **Exhausted and Inflamed**

Behind the Scenes: Invigorating Stress

Neurotransmitters are the natural brain chemicals that underlie our moods, emotions, and energy level. They are the natural stimulants that drive us and play a major role in the stress response.

Some of the chemicals produced by our bodies serve as natural stimulants. That's how we're able to pull an all-nighter or get the driveway shoveled after the first big snow. When we feel invigorated, these natural stimulants have kicked in.

The chemicals in the brain that serve as accelerators to our mood and energy level are described as *excitatory neurotransmitters*. This chemistry—which includes epinephrine (also known as adrenaline) and norepinephrine (or noradrenaline)—comes into play when we're under stress and need to speed up our performance or respond to an emergency. Our bodies produce these natural stimulants to help us focus and give us the drive to respond to the task at hand. This same chemistry is present in all mammals and is evident whenever they are experiencing the fight, flight, or freeze response.

When stress becomes chronic, persistent high levels of excitatory neurotransmitters, unchecked by *inhibitory neurotransmitters* such as serotonin, stop being invigorating and start causing anxiety.

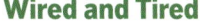
© Shutterstock/Lightspring

Wired and Tired

At what point does that sense of exhilaration become a drain? Let's say that the stress, pressure, long hours, and deadlines continue day in and day out. You may be an emergency room nurse, a single parent working two or three jobs, a student preparing for a big exam, someone grappling with an addiction, or a caregiver for a family member with cognitive degeneration. In these circumstances, you may be able to meet the demands of the tasks facing you, but eventually you will no longer respond as efficiently. Your ability to keep adapting to stress diminishes as your stress response changes. Your adrenaline remains high, making you feel wired, while your cortisol begins to drop, making you feel tired. The stress curve flattens out, producing the stage we call "wired and tired."

At this point in the stress curve, you might begin to experience unpleasant or unnerving physical symptoms:

Emotional Feeling	Possible Physical Symptom
Feeling stressed	Developing aches and pains
Hypersensitive	Hyperactive
Irritable	Racing heartbeat at times
Tense	Elevated blood pressure
Anxious	Hot flashes or clammy sweats
Fatigued	Restless sleep

Behind the Scenes: Wired and Tired

When we're wired and tired, our bodies are putting out too much of the stress hormone adrenaline—as well as neurotransmitters such as glutamate, epinephrine, and norepinephrine. This causes a racy, yet anxious, feeling. When we are healthy, the stress hormone cortisol is high in the morning and then drops progressively during the day. Typically, we should have lots of energy in the morning, then run out of it at night so we can sleep. In this phase of the stress response, however, cortisol drops during the day, but then rises at night. As a result, we feel tired during the day but more alert and awake at night.

Over time, stress wears away at metabolic reserves, depletes vital nutrients, and puts a strain on different systems throughout the body. Meanwhile, the body attempts to adapt. The mind tries to relax by secreting inhibitory or calming neurotransmitters such as GABA and serotonin—natural tranquilizers that act as brakes on a racing mind. The adrenals continue to make DHEA (the precursor for many stress and sex hormones) to try to protect the body, but despite this, blood pressure, cholesterol, blood sugar, and triglycerides may continue to climb.

Exhausted: Pushing Past Wired and Tired

What happens when you feel you must keep pushing despite the stress? What happens when you go past the wired and tired phase?

The body continues adapting to the chronic stress. It slows its metabolism, attempting to conserve energy. If you keep pressing on despite this, you move on to the next stage of stress. This stage is easy to recognize: **EXHAUSTION**.

As you become more depleted and move more deeply into the stress response, you become exhausted. Symptoms of exhaustion include:

- **Extreme fatigue and weakness**
- **A sense of constantly dragging**
- **Weight gain or difficulty losing weight**
- **Depression**
- **Decreased libido**
- **Cold hands and feet**
- **Menstrual irregularities**
- **Fertility issues** (both men and women)
- **Indigestion**
- **Recurrent infections**
- **Non-restorative, unrefreshing sleep** that does not improve fatigue.

Exhausted and Inflamed

We are genetically hardwired to adapt to increased stress by turning on inflammation. If we were cavemen, this inflammatory cascade would help us repair wounds more quickly and resist infection. However, inflammation in the face of chronic stress is different. When we reach the point of being exhausted and inflamed from chronic stress, health issues that are already present intensify. Asthma attacks become more frequent, migraines last a little longer, colitis may flare. Everything becomes a little worse as the body seems to catch on fire, figuratively speak-

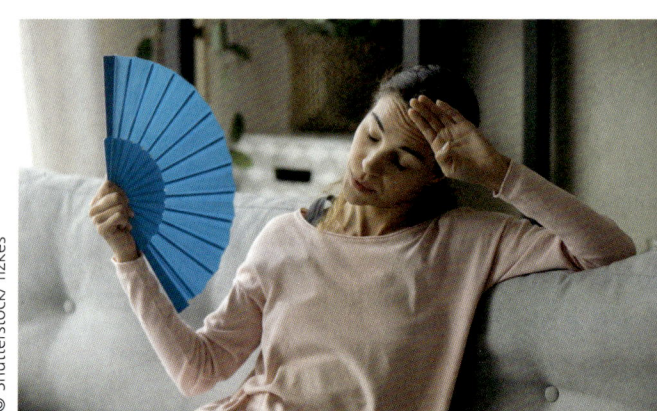

Behind the Scenes: Serotonin and Exhaustion

When continued lifestyle demands become too high for too long, our bodies can't keep up. Key stress hormones change. Adrenaline starts dropping, while cortisol levels fluctuate, tending to drop as you become more fatigued.

Unfortunately, at this point, the brain chemicals that would normally calm us, such as serotonin, also begin to drop. The result is that we feel depressed and anxious. Low serotonin levels can also be associated with other conditions such as PMS, irritable bowel syndrome, and fibromyalgia. Sadly, many people live in this state much of the time. This is why drugs such as selective serotonin reuptake inhibitors (SSRIs) are so popular. Medications like Prozac (fluoxetine), Paxil (paroxetine), Zoloft (sertraline), and Lexapro (escitalopram) normalize serotonin levels.

Your body's musculature also suffers in the face of chronic stress. Because the body is in catastrophe mode, it wants to protect itself by storing fat and breaking down muscle. Muscle tone is lost, and the body needs more time to recover from injuries. Even worse, your body can't fight off every infection or injury while in catastrophe mode. It simply doesn't have any energy to spare for repair.

---

ing. With chronic inflammation, the immune system is also overstressed, and as a result, we tend to get sick more often. We also have a sense of feeling progressively more out of sorts or that something is vaguely wrong.

Depletion, infections, and inflammation are common at this point. Low serotonin is associated with an overreactive immune system and higher levels of inflammation throughout the body. When serotonin drops, we tend to get sick more easily. Infections such as sinusitis may develop and then become chronic. The list of inflammatory conditions made worse by stress is seemingly endless: allergies; arthritis; asthma; autoimmune diseases; digestive disorders; eczema; hypertension; joint, shoulder, and back problems; and spikes in cholesterol levels. Furthermore, cuts, bruises, and other injuries tend to heal more slowly.

Whenever the immune system begins ramping up, inflammation levels increase throughout the body, which is just trying to defend itself—as if it were fighting infection. This can trigger flare-ups of conditions such as arthritis and colitis (and just about any disorder that ends with "-itis," meaning inflammation). Inflammation can affect any and all systems in the body. Increased inflammation is associated with:

- **Aching joints**
- **Plaque** and blockage inside arteries
- **High blood pressure**
- **Certain cardiomyopathies** (heart muscle problems)
- **Type 2 diabetes**
- **Diabetic complications**
- **Skin diseases,** such as psoriasis and eczema
- **Asthma**
- **Chronic obstructive pulmonary disease (COPD)**
- **Osteoporosis**
- **Allergy symptoms**
- **Heartburn or reflux (GERD)**
- **Colitis**
- **Cancer initiation** or promotion
- **Neurological diseases** such as Alzheimer's disease and Parkinson's disease

Mast Cell Activation Syndrome

When your stress reaches the exhausted and inflamed stage, your immune system can initiate a cascade known as mast cell activation. Mast cells are a type of white blood cell found throughout the body, especially in the skin, the intestinal lining, and the airways. These cells release a number of chemicals as part of the body's normal healing response to injury. These include histamines, which are well-known, as well as inflammatory chemicals called leukotrienes. In some people, histamines are also released as part of an allergic response—they're the chemicals that cause allergy symptoms such as itching and sneezing. We've learned that mast cells aren't only activated by injury or allergies.

High levels of stress, possibly along with exposure to environmental toxins, can lead to mast cell activation syndrome, the symptoms of which include:

- Hives, itching, and skin rashes
- Nausea/vomiting
- Diarrhea
- Wheezing and shortness of breath
- Headaches
- Depression and anxiety

We'll go into this in more detail on page 167. For now, we'll just say that mast cell activation syndrome is a diagnosis to consider if you are feeling unwell with a range of symptoms while also under a lot of stress.

Behind the Scenes: Exhausted and Inflamed

What happens to your body when chronic stress leaves you exhausted and inflamed?

Stress hormones: Your cortisol levels remain low, so little of this hormone is available to dampen the inflammatory response. DHEA also drops. (We discuss treatment of this on page 91.)

Inflammation: At this point, the ongoing stress sounds an alarm bell for your inflammatory system. This shift into a state of alarm is referred to as the *inflammatory cascade*. Your body alters the production of chemicals called cytokines. Most cytokines are the type called interleukins (because they're produced by leukocytes, or white blood cells). They're designated by the IL- prefix.

- *Pro-inflammatory cytokines*, as the name suggests, promote inflammation and tend to rise during the exhausted and inflamed phase. Pro-inflammatory interleukins include interleukin-1 beta (IL-1β), IL-2, IL-6, IL-8, IL-12, IL-17, interferon gamma (IFN-α), and tumor necrosis factor alpha (TNF-α).

- *Anti-inflammatory cytokines* tend to decrease during this phase. Anti-inflammatory interleukins include IL-4, IL-5, IL-10, IL-13, and transforming growth factor beta (TGF-β).

- *Chemokines* are additional messenger molecules that recruit and activate white cell subtypes in your immune system to make further cytokines. Chemokines include interleukin IL-8, monocyte chemotactic protein 1 (MCP-1), and macrophage inflammatory protein beta (MIP-1β).

Insulin resistance and the blood sugar blues: With increasing inflammation, the body becomes more insulin resistant. This means that the hormone insulin, which controls blood sugar, has trouble carrying blood sugar into the cells (we discuss this in more detail in chapter 15). This causes blood sugar highs and crashing lows. Often, we counter low energy with quick fixes—sugary snacks and junk food. Unfortunately, that just leads to more sugar highs and lows—more sugar cravings and more weight gain—and another vicious cycle.

The Tipping Point:
Total Exhaustion and the Final Straw

On the path to illness, exhaustion typically makes us more vulnerable. We may get sick more easily, have emotional crises and energy crashes, and be more susceptible to stress injuries and chronic health issues. When patients come to us with complex illnesses and a history of chronic stress and exhaustion, we trace back through their history to learn everything we can about the underlying cause(s) of their condition.

As physicians, we often find that after a long period of chronic stress, when yet another stressful event occurs in a patient's life, it becomes the final straw, pushing them over the edge of coping. They drop into the final phase of the stress response—they develop a disease. On the Stress Curve, we call this phase Overwhelmed and Depleted.

Patients often remark that they get sick just after the immediate stress abates. For example, they get a migraine on the weekend after a particularly intense work week. This isn't unusual. The body is designed to cope with acute stress. To use an extreme example, a person may get shot in the leg during a heated battle or injured in an important game. Because of the high circulating adrenaline, they might not feel pain until they get to the hospital and start calming down. When we see patients in the Overwhelmed and Depleted phase, they often ask us why they seemed to get sick just as life was getting easier. We tell them that they shouldn't worry about the war itself but the period after it!

Almost any kind of stressful event can become the final trigger for illness, particularly if it's intense enough. It could be a physical stress such as an accident, an infection, a surgery, or a toxic exposure in the workplace. It might be an emotional trauma, such as losing a job, a divorce, or the death of someone close. A person doesn't even need to be stressed beforehand if the acute stress itself is profound enough. However, most times the final straw is a single event for a system that is already exhausted—a system that has been overcompensating for far too long. It is after this tipping point or triggering factor that patients can develop serious illnesses. The time from the stressful event until the time of illness can range from a matter of days to eighteen months or even longer.

Unfortunately, society tends to misinterpret the cause of the disease. Health care providers tend to focus on the problem in front of them, viewing a single disorder as the cause and treating it alone. In reality, that particular illness or injury is simply the last straw. Our patients also tend to focus on one symptom or illness in their attempts to make sense of their lives. They may attribute their poor health to a viral infection that needs to be treated or midlife hormonal changes. Unfortunately, the problem usually goes much deeper.

==Such patients are suffering from a system-wide malfunction precipitated by a triggering event.== A virus may seem to be the cause, for example, but it's not the foundation of the problem. Often the deeper issue is severe depletion because of chronic stress that has developed over a period of months or years.

Sometimes the final stressful event seems insignificant. This is because we become psychologically primed by previous stressors. A loss early in our lives that is repeated later in some form can trigger intense emotional reactions. For example, your parents might have divorced when you were a child. You felt an intense sense of loss when your father moved out, but you got over it. Years later, though, when a beloved pet dies, that buried childhood sense of loss is triggered. You may seem to overreact emotionally and then become ill with something more serious within the next eighteen months. The death of a spouse or partner is so detrimental to the survivor's health that it's been called the widowhood effect. This is similar to what occurs in post-traumatic stress disorder (PTSD), when people cope with an enormously stressful event and then become highly sensitized to reminders of that experience. They may survive a wartime situation and later overreact to any sound that reminds them of gunfire, for example.

The Final Phase of Stress: Overwhelmed and Depleted

The name of this phase literally says it all. In this final phase of stress, you're depressed, apathetic, and dis-eased. At this point, disease literally sets in. Many of our chronically stressed patients are diagnosed with cancer or autoimmune disorders such as lupus, rheumatoid arthritis, or multiple sclerosis, or they struggle with emotional issues such as major depression. An experienced physician can diagnose any one of these illnesses without much trouble. However, many chronically stressed people develop complex symptoms that elude diagnosis.

Common symptoms in the Overwhelmed and Depleted state include:

- **Frequently feeling out of sorts** or ill at ease
- **Multiple symptoms** not associated with any disease
- **More than one disease**
- **Drastic weight gain or loss**
- **Depression, apathy, or hopelessness**
- **Feeling drained** or **emotionless**
- **Extreme difficulty in concentration**
- **Memory loss**
- **Dizziness, clammy sweats,** or **fever**
- **Rough skin and brittle nails**
- **Persistent fertility issues**
- **Edema (water retention)**
- **Lightheadedness**, especially when getting up or when exposed to increased heat, such as a sauna, a hot bath, or hot weather

Depletion: An Invisible Illness

If you're a patient whose system is overwhelmed or in a state of exhaustion, you may go to the doctor and be diagnosed with an illness or depression (or both). However, in our experience, most patients don't initially get any diagnosis at all. They may simply be told, "It's all in your head." Standard blood tests are usually normal, including a complete blood count (CBC), renal (kidney) profile, and liver function tests. Thyroid tests may be borderline or minimally abnormal, showing some thyroid sluggishness but nothing dramatic.

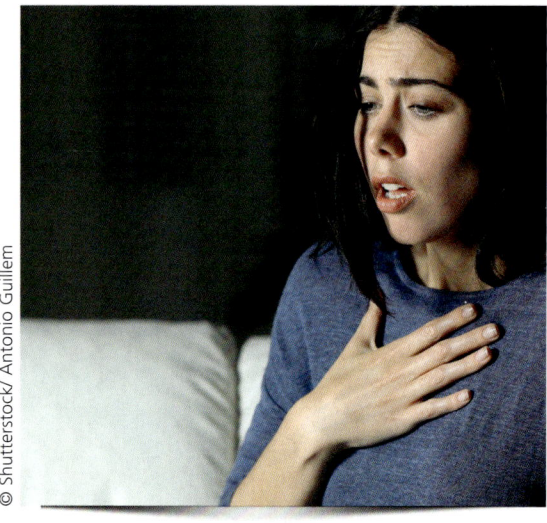

Behind the Scenes: The Depleted Phase: The Nervous System Out of Sync

Our autonomic nervous system is the part of our nervous system that runs our bodies on automatic pilot, regulating unconscious actions such as breathing and the beating of the heart—minute to minute, hour by hour, day in and day out. It consists of two parts: the sympathetic and parasympathetic nervous systems. The sympathetic nervous system controls our fight, flight, or freeze responses. Under stress, the sympathetic nervous system makes our muscles tense up; our heart races and our blood pressure rises. In contrast, the parasympathetic nervous system controls our rest and digest functions. Under the influence of the parasympathetic system, our heart rate slows, our blood pressure decreases, and digestion improves. These two systems are designed to be a check and balance against each other. However, when we are under prolonged stress, our sympathetic nervous system stays turned on, effectively pushing us further along the Stress Curve.

By the time a patient becomes depleted and exhausted, the autonomic nervous system may become dysfunctional, resulting in a condition described as dysautonomia. Two forms of dysautonomia are neurally mediated hypotension (NMH) and postural orthostatic tachycardia syndrome (POTS). In NMH, a patient's blood pressure is normal when tested in the office but often drops precipitously when the patient gets slightly overheated, such as after taking a hot bath or walking into a warm room while wearing a warm coat. The patient feels exhausted and sweaty and can often faint. POTS syndrome includes similar symptoms, along with a racing heart, even when sitting still or performing only mild activity.

Understanding Cortisol and Stress

In a healthy person with a normal circadian rhythm, cortisol rises in the early morning and gradually decreases during the day. Ideally, we should pop out of bed after a good night's sleep, full of energy, then gradually run out of energy at night, allowing us to fall asleep easily and peacefully.

In the Wired and Tired phase, though, cortisol is low in the morning and starts rising in the late afternoon or evening. After feeling exhausted during the day, a person in this phase will go to bed at night but find it difficult to unwind and fall asleep.

In the Exhausted phase, the cortisol levels dip even further, remaining low for most of the day, consistent with feelings of exhaustion. By the time we get to the Exhausted and Inflamed Stage, our low cortisol levels can no longer combat any inflammation.

In the Overwhelmed and Depleted phase, the adrenal glands are no longer responsive to stress and produce very little cortisol. The cortisol levels tend to remain low and flat throughout the day. Along with this scenario, neurotransmitters such as norepinephrine, epinephrine, and serotonin bottom out, leaving people feeling apathetic and overwhelmed. In these latter phases, we lose our resilience to stress and can no longer respond appropriately to life's ups and downs.

> "
> It is a lot harder to keep people well than it is to just get them over a sickness.
>
> – DeForest Clinton Jarvis

The Cortisol Awakening Response

One of the ways we assess resilience is to look at the cortisol awakening response (CAR). The steroid hormone cortisol is produced by your adrenal glands—two small, pyramid-shaped organs that sit on top of your kidneys. Cortisol is involved in many essential body functions, including regulating your metabolism, controlling inflammation, and regulating your immune response. All these roles are tightly linked to cortisol's other essential function: helping your body respond to stress.

We can measure how stress affects your cortisol by looking at your CAR. This is a measure of endocrine resilience and adrenal fatigue. Your body normally starts producing more cortisol shortly before you wake up. After you're awake, your cortisol keeps rising, usually by between 40 and 75 percent, in the next half hour. To measure your CAR, we use saliva testing done right after you wake up and again exactly 30 minutes later. The comparison should show a rise of at least 50 percent from the first measurement to the second. An increase of less than 50 percent indicates adrenal exhaustion. The smaller the increase, the more adrenally exhausted you are. We like this test because it gives us useful information while also being inexpensive, easy to do, and noninvasive.

You can see the impact of adrenal exhaustion in the diagram below, where the CAR response is an inverted V between morning and afternoon. A normal diurnal rhythm has a high peak in the morning then gradually tracks to a steady lower level. Ideally, your cortisol should peak closer to the tip of the V. If your CAR is flattened—that is, it doesn't peak as high as it should—that suggests your adrenal function is "normal" but waning. If your CAR is really flat, that suggests adrenal exhaustion. And what causes adrenal exhaustion? The unending demand for cortisol to help your body cope with constant stressors such as chronic pain, burnout, and chronic stress.

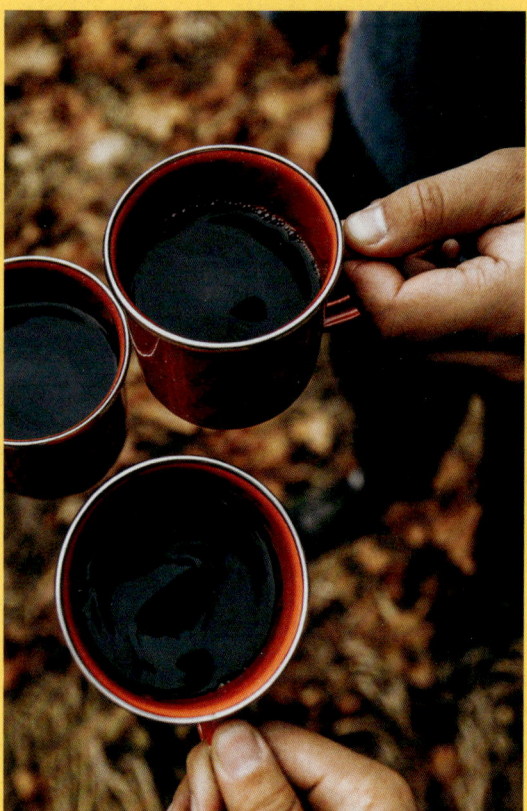
© Unsplash/ Nathan Dumlao

When patients tell us they are very fatigued all the time, we test the CAR. If it's low, we often say to patients "You've lost your morning kickstart." This helps them to realize that they're so accustomed to feeling tired all the time and self-medicating with coffee and other stimulants that they don't realize how fatigued they truly are.

How stress affects your adrenal glands

We measure how stress affects your adrenal glands by using Salivary Free Cortisol Testing. (Note: This is different from cortisol blood testing – as it measures free cortisol.)

Saliva samples are collected 5 times: upon awakening; 30 minutes later; 60 minutes later; mid-late afternoon; and at bedtime.

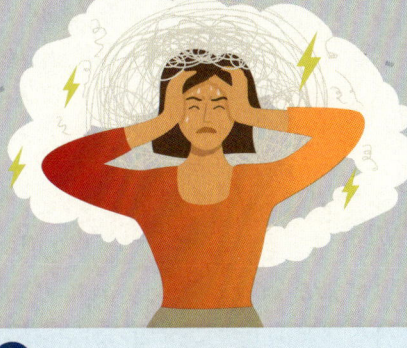

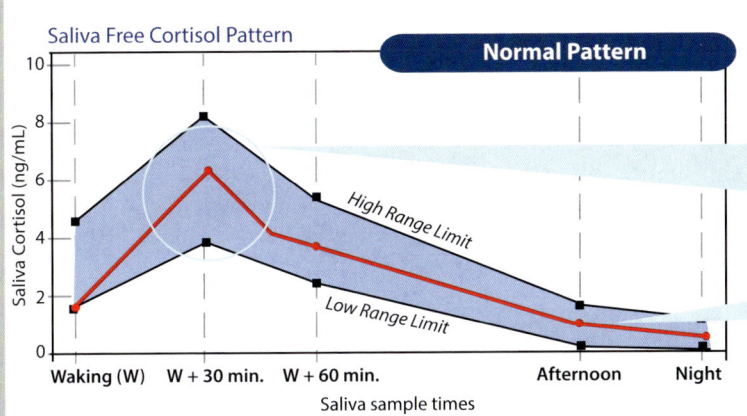

1 This inverted "V" pattern is called the cortisol awakening response and implies good adrenal reserves.

2 The normal cortisol curve shows a slow decline during the day. We should wake with energy then it should run out before we go to sleep.

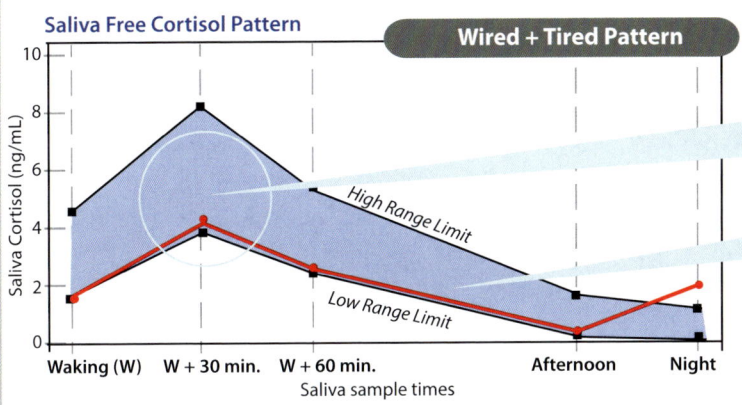

1 The cortisol awakening response (CAR) is still present although weakly so. This implies the adrenals still have reserve and can bounce back fairly easily.

2 The cortisol curve is low during the day ("tired") but shoots up at night ("wired").

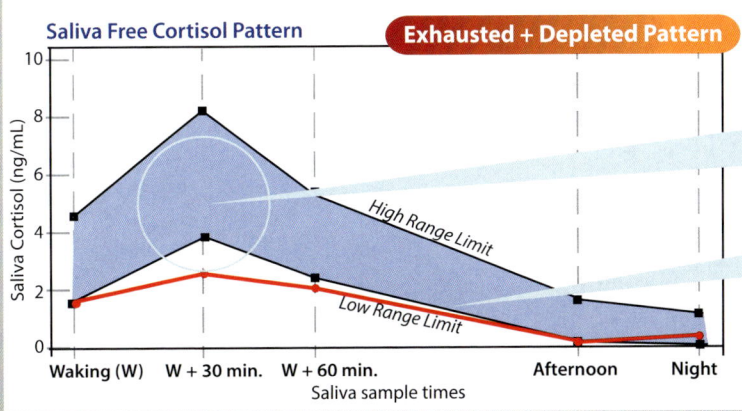

1 Absent Cortisol Awakening Response (CAR) indicates absent adrenal reserves.

2 A flattened cortisol curve is consistent with exhaustion.

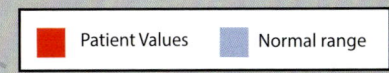

FIGURE 5.2 | How Stress Affects Your Adrenal Glands

Are You Depressed?

Many of our patients feel depressed but refuse help, saying they just need to "pull themselves together." They feel embarrassed to speak to anyone about their sense of feeling overwhelmed. We want to assure you that this is nothing to feel embarrassed about. It is a physical condition. When your neurotransmitters are depleted, you can't simply "pull yourself together."

The good news is that in most cases, depression can be easily treated.

According to the fifth edition of the *Diagnostic and Statistical Manual of Mental Disorders* (better known as the DSM-5), published by the American Psychiatric Association, a major depressive episode consists of at least two of the following symptoms:

- Depressed mood most of the day; feeling sad, empty, or tearful
- Significant loss of interest or pleasure in activities that used to be enjoyable
- Significant weight loss (when not dieting) or weight gain; a decrease or increase in appetite
- Difficulty sleeping or sleeping too much
- Agitation or slowing down of thoughts; a reduction of physical movements
- Fatigue or loss of energy
- Feelings of worthlessness or inappropriate guilt
- Poor concentration or having difficulty making decisions
- Thinking about death or suicide

The level of depression is considered significant if the symptoms have occurred nearly every day for at least two weeks. Some people struggle with depression for years before getting help. If you are suffering from any of these symptoms, don't feel embarrassed to talk to your physician about them.

Learning to Transform Stress

Understanding the road to illness can help you on your road to recovery and transformation. Understanding the Stress Curve gives you the ability to alter your trajectory away from illness and toward health. You have the power to alter that trajectory using a range of techniques that can help change your life by transforming stress into success.

This gives you a long-term view, but what about acute stress?

In Chinese calligraphy, the symbol for a "crisis" is made up of two different symbols, one meaning "danger," and the other meaning "opportunity." A health crisis is no different. We call this a Transformational Moment! Learn to look at acute stress differently – understanding both the danger, as well as the opportunity. Once you do this, you empower yourself to positively change both your health and your life!

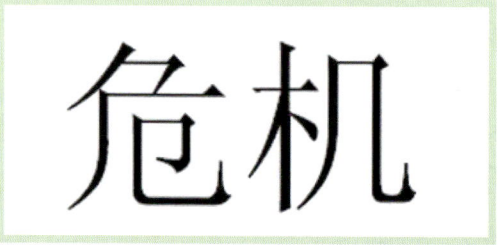

CHAPTER 6

The Persistent Effects of Trauma - A Sad Situation

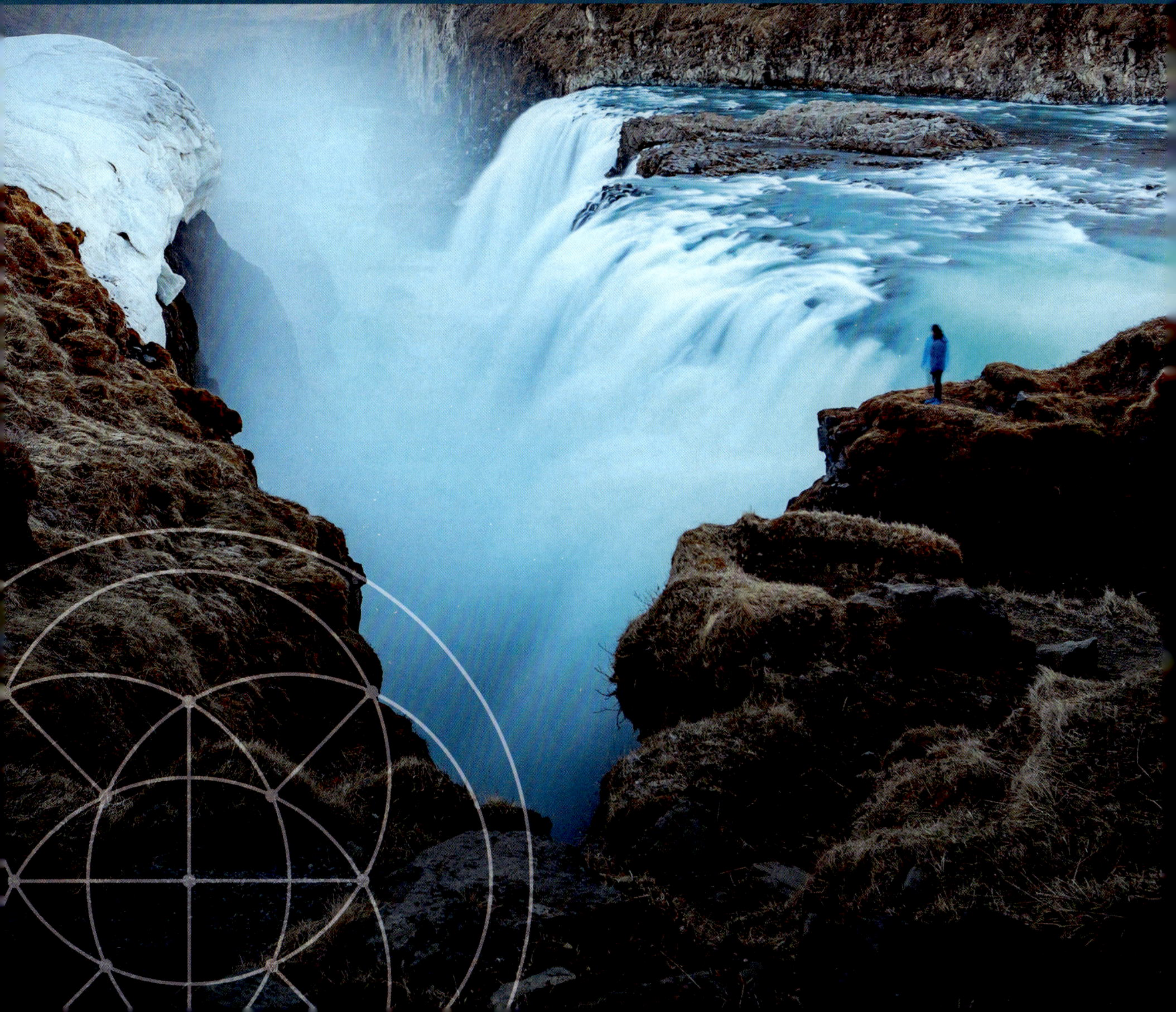

Trauma and mental illness are interconnected in several ways.

Trauma refers to an emotional response to a distressing or disturbing event, often involving intense fear, helplessness, or horror. The terms "Big T trauma" and "Little t trauma" are used to distinguish between different levels or types of traumatic experiences. Big T trauma typically refers to significant, life-threatening, or catastrophic events that result in severe emotional or psychological distress. Examples of Big T traumas include physical or sexual assault, natural disasters, war, loss of a loved one, serious accidents, or witnessing a violent crime. These events are often easily recognizable as highly traumatic and can have profound and immediate effects on a person's mental health. On the other hand, "Little t trauma" refers to less obvious or chronic events that can still have a lasting impact on an individual's well-being. These events are usually less severe and may not be immediately identifiable as traumatic. Examples of Little t traumas include ongoing bullying, emotional abuse, neglect, loss of a pet, parental divorce, or chronic stress. While the individual incidents may seem less significant, the cumulative effect and long-term consequences on mental health can be substantial. Unfortunately, social media has aggravated both Big T and Little t traumas. Rather than being a tool to unite people, social media has become a tool for bullying and polarization.

The categorization of trauma into Big T and Little t isn't meant to diminish the experiences of individuals who have gone through Little t traumas. Both types of trauma can have a significant impact on an individual's mental health and well-being. People who have experienced trauma may be at an increased risk of developing conditions such as post-traumatic stress disorder (PTSD), depression, anxiety disorders, or substance use disorders. Traumatic experiences can disrupt the normal functioning of the brain, affecting emotional regulation, memory processing, and stress responses. Trauma can lead to symptoms like intrusive memories, nightmares, hypervigilance, avoidance behaviors, mood disturbances, and difficulties in relationships.

Mental illness, including mood disorders, anxiety disorders, psychotic disorders, and others, can also occur independently of trauma. However, traumatic experiences can act as significant stressors and exacerbate existing mental health conditions.

Emotional trauma is also associated with chronic physical problems such as cardiovascular disease, hypertension, gastrointestinal problems, chronic pain syndromes, sleep problems, chronic headaches, dizziness and chronic fatigue. Because traumatized individuals are more prone to unhealthy coping mechanisms such as substance use, poor nutrition, and self-harming behaviors, they are also likely to have more secondary health issues.

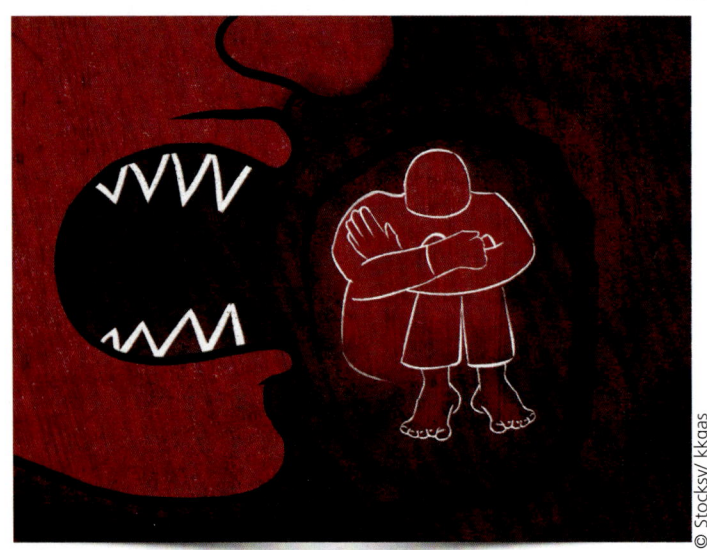

Trauma changes you. Healing is about creating a new version of yourself, the one that is stronger, wiser, and more compassionate.

– Michele Rosenthal

Trauma Is Common

Trauma is more common than we think it is. Adverse childhood experiences (ACEs), such as physical and emotional abuse, neglect, household dysfunction, racism, community violence, poverty, and lack of a supportive social structure, can cause toxic stress—stress that is prolonged, severe, or chronic.

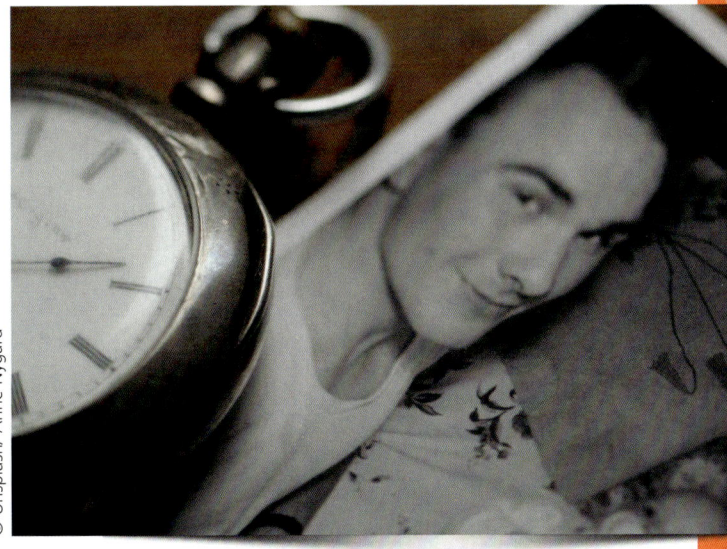

A powerful and persistent correlation exists between the degree of the ACEs and future violence, victimization, perpetration of crime and further abuse, and lifelong health and opportunity costs. People with a higher amount of adverse childhood experiences have a dramatically increased risk of heart disease, diabetes, obesity, depression, substance use, smoking, poor academic achievement, time out of work, and early death.

According to the CDC, adverse childhood experiences are common. About 64 percent of US adults have experienced at least one type of ACE before age 18, and nearly one in six (17.3 percent) report they experienced four or more types of ACEs.

Nature vs. Nurture: What Drives Mental and Physical Illness?

The debate over nature vs. nurture, or genetics vs. epigenetics, is complex.

Abused children often become abusive adults. Children who were sexually abused are filled with suppressed shame, guilt, and rage, often acting this out in antisocial or sociopathic behavior. Children raised by angry and violent parents are more likely to become angry and violent adults and to have trouble with addiction and trauma. Some become the next wave of young criminals, shooters, or rapists. Those who don't may externalize their emotions into misconduct or internalize them into physical problems and poor health. Is this learned or somehow passed on chemically?

We know that identical twins have similar inherited conditions. These include certain types of cancer, autoimmune disorders, body composition, metabolism, allergies and sensitivities, drug metabolism, sleep patterns, and even aging. However, if identical twins are reared apart, the impact of a different diet and lifestyle can play a large role in their health. The effect of epigenetics seems to be a major influence. Based on how they are brought up—the nurture they received and the diet and lifestyle they follow—they can develop completely different diseases and psychological patterns. For example, if both identical twins tend to high cholesterol, the twin who smokes and eats poorly may develop severe heart and lung disease, while the one with a healthier lifestyle might not. This is an example of how our own diet and lifestyle can affect us.

It's not just our own lifestyle that affects us—but also that of our parents and grandparents!

In the winter of 1944–45, the Nazis starved a portion of the population of the Netherlands, a time that came to be called the Hongerwinter. The children of women who were pregnant during this time and experienced malnutrition—in other words, children born near or soon after the end of the famine period—were thin and malnourished. When food became more plentiful, however, they gained weight and had normal development. These children were followed for years in the Dutch Famine Birth Cohort Study.

The results show that in adulthood these children were more susceptible to diabetes, lung problems, obesity, and other health problems—and had triple the risk of cardiovascular disease. Many developed depression in their 50s.

Studies of women who were pregnant during the 1998 Quebec ice storm, one of the worst natural disasters in Canada's history, showed that a mother's subjective distress during the ice storm predicted outcomes in their children, such as anxiety, depression, and aggression, IQ and language in childhood, obesity at age 5½, and insulin secretion at age 13. Genetic and epigenetic markers showed a tendency to higher inflammation, a tendency to develop type 1 diabetes, and an altered metabolic and immune response.

The babies of Tutsi women who were pregnant during the 1994 genocide in Rwanda show the epigenetic marks of the trauma their mothers experienced. Many of the affected genes are those associated with a higher risk for mental disorders such as PTSD and depression.

Pregnant women who use drugs, are abused or traumatized, or who have addictions or psychopathic behavior are more likely to have children with callous-unemotional traits. These children in turn may develop unstable or aggressive behavior. It is possible to identify these children using methylation marks.

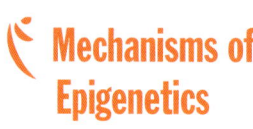

Mechanisms of Epigenetics

Trauma leaves a biochemical scar or "mark" on the nervous system. Studies on epigenetics show us that both physical and emotional abuse can be measured biochemically in our genes. Methylation marks, post-translational histone modifications, and post-transcriptional regulation by microRNAs are some of the ways abuse can be seen in the brain. These molecular events seem to play a big role in aggression and antisocial behavior. When a woman has epigenetic changes caused by trauma, she may pass those altered genes on to her offspring. She may also inherit altered genes from her own mother and in turn pass on those genes.

This is a big epiphany for those studying behavior. We have always thought that behavior was only learned from parents and those around us. Now we see that physical and emotional trauma can also leave a genetic mark that may alter the genes of the next generations, changing their behavior. This has deep societal implications for how we recognize mental illness and how we should respond to it, especially when it comes to criminality, addiction, and violence. Current measures to control these behaviors aren't working well by most measures.

To understand how to change behavior, we need to first see that there is a connection between genetics, epigenetics, neuroscience, ethics, philosophy, and law. This doesn't mean we can simply write off bad behavior as a software problem beyond our control. We need to learn more about how this affects us, and then what we can do to fix the problem.

Predicting Mental Illness

Can we now perhaps learn to predict who will develop mental illness?

We know that some soldiers who go to war are more likely than others to suffer from post-traumatic stress disorder (PTSD) from their experience. Why is this? Why do two soldiers who are in the same armored vehicle that endures a roadside bomb have quite different outcomes? One will walk away just with physical injuries, while the other will also have disabling, crippling emotional anxiety and panic attacks. Studies suggest that preceding emotional and physical abuse predisposes some people to PTSD.

Abuse survivors are more likely to have a

sense of hypervigilance, or sympathetic nervous system overactivation. This may lead to chronic pain, depression, and anxiety at much higher rates than other populations. Epigenetic studies show that hypervigilance affects glucocorticoid or stress receptors, serotonin pathways which then affect mood, and the oxytocin receptor. Oxytocin is a hormone secreted by nursing mothers and humans when they feel love and compassion. It is called the "social neuropeptide" because it promotes human attachment and social interaction. In the case of abuse survivors, the opposite happens. They feel isolated and unattached because the stress response to abuse reduces the number of oxytocin receptors in the central nervous system. As a result, they don't respond to oxytocin as well and tend to be depressed, anxious, and angry, a setup for future abuse.

It seems then that in the future we might be able to do a better job of measuring methylation marks and screening for previous abuse before sending someone to the frontlines of police or military duty. That way we might prevent problems before they start.

What Are Addictions?

People with addiction use substances or engage in behaviors that become compulsive and often continue despite harmful consequences. We generally think of addiction as a compulsion to act out in a self-destructive way. An addiction may be severe and life-threatening, such as an addiction to smoking, alcohol, or drugs. It may seem mild and innocuous, such as an addiction to shopping, or it may fall somewhere in between, as an addiction to sex, food, or gambling. Society has generally viewed addiction as a mental weakness and a moral failure. However, large studies show that trauma is involved in addictive behavior about 35 percent of the time.

Here are some common addictions:
- Substance addiction to drugs, alcohol, and nicotine
- Behaviors: compulsive patterns in gambling, gaming, shopping, and sex (porn)
- Food addictions: Sugar, salt, fat, and caffeine addictions lead the way to overeating and weight gain. On the other hand, consider orthorexia, where a person obsessively eats foods they believe are healthy.
- Work addiction: addiction to work or achieving professional success at the cost of personal relationships or wellbeing
- Internet addiction to social media, smartphones or online activities that can interfere with daily activities, social interactions, and sleep
- Exercise addiction, which can lead to excessive workouts, injuries, and isolation

Treatments for addiction are often only marginally successful. The person usually doesn't give up their tendency to be addicted, only what they are addicted to. Someone who gives up drinking may start or continue to smoke. Someone may give up smoking and start to overeat. The addicted mind doesn't change, only the addiction to a specific thing.

Addictions at their core are a deep psychic pull toward more self-love and away from deep traumas. Addicts are trying to restore an innate sense of happiness. Yet they can get a fleeting and temporary high as they fulfill their addiction, only to succumb to feelings of guilt, shame, and rage as it wears off. This creates the need for another fix. It's a terrible cycle to break. *The addicted brain doesn't want to stop.*

Past Trauma Begets Future Trauma

Trauma will reproduce itself, either as a learned behavior, or by epigenetic mechanisms, or both. If we do nothing to heal the trauma, we never really do anything more than cover up the symptoms. In other words, unless we can heal from the vicious cycle of trauma, we are destined to repeat it.

Although mice aren't humans, a study from 2014 is informative: male mice were traumatized by being made to stand on electrified plates and get shocked while they were exposed to the smell of cherries. Four generations later, the children of these rats still shivered and shook as if they were being shocked when exposed to the smell of cherries. Again, we can see this on their methylation marks.

The coping mechanisms we use to survive one trauma often become our next problem. For instance, someone sexually abused as a child may later develop chronic pain, anxiety, depression, and antisocial behavior. Physical diseases such as coronary artery disease, hypertension, autoimmune disease, and possibly even cancer may be affected by trauma. People who abuse alcohol may do so in part for epigenetic reasons, but alcohol abuse itself perpetuates further illness. The effects of alcohol stop the person from processing emotions correctly, making them more prone to depression, which in turn makes them more likely to drink. Alcohol abuse creates its own set of illnesses, including cirrhosis of the liver, heart disease, cancer, malnutrition, and many others.

Think of your genes as the hard drive of a computer and epigenetics as the software. Trauma seems to create a software glitch that causes people to act badly. As a society, we focus on the outcome of the glitch, rather than rewriting the software. We jail people who break laws and medicate those with depression. What if we could undo their methylation marks instead? Perhaps there is an out-of-the-box solution?

A SAD Situation

Humanity struggles with a deep-rooted core belief that we live in a zero-sum game. If I win, you lose. If you win, I lose. There can be no sense of mutual abundance. The result: a mutual sense of distrust, an automatic divisiveness. And if I want what you have, I get envious and greedy. Because I need to look after myself, I have no problem doing whatever I can to get what I want. I might dehumanize you in that quest. I may say I'm doing this for my family, my community, or my country. This is a type of tribal thinking that makes us want to band together. Like-minded cooperation allows us to thrive but can also serve to reinforce negative principles. We may form business alliances, armies, or even terrorist groups. We may pollute, rob, steal, or live in corruption. In our minds, we justify this as being OK, when in truth it is not. When we initially propose this concept to people, they deny that they do this, although they usually see it in others. Then they think about it and grudgingly admit that they, too, are colored by this same belief.

This isn't new. The biblical story of Cain and Abel, the sons of Adam and Eve, has been told for thousands of years. Cain was filled with jealousy and bitterness about the favor God showed to Abel, and thus felt justified in killing him. When the Lord God Almighty asked Cain if he had killed Abel, he lied, thus bringing down the wrath of God, who condemned Cain to a life of wandering.

We all want to go back to Adam and Eve's Garden of Eden, to live in abundance. And for the first time in history, it looks almost possible. Futurists talk about AI and newer technologies generating enough wealth that everyone might be paid for not working. All this might seem possible if we assume that people are inherently good. The problem is we are not. All of us are flawed, if not by something we have done, then perhaps by what our family, community, or country has done.

If we look back, it seems that much conflict is fueled by a history of emotional and physical trauma. This is often called karma. Karma is the philosophy: As you sow, so shall you reap. Good begets good, but, on the other hand, if you did something bad to me, I would do something bad to you to retaliate. This results in cross-generational hatred. Wars in the Middle East, Eastern Europe and Russia, Africa, and Northern Ireland are good examples. Less overt are the traumas sustained by ACEs (adverse childhood experiences), where a child who is raped or abused may become a rapist or criminal later. As we have discussed, trauma leaves methylation marks on our DNA that may last for generations. However, more common are the practices of destroying your enemy in business, on the sports field, on social media platforms or even in presumably sacrosanct marital or family relationships. When we do this, we feel somehow justified in bullying, or polluting, or continuing the cycle of abuse. Why?

For those who have been traumatized (and as we have discussed, that is most of us), we feel a sense of inadequacy or insecurity, a lack, a sense of brokenness in our lives. This is often the underlying feeling behind depression, anxiety, and PTSD, as well as generalized feelings of hopelessness, helplessness, and despair. This makes us more likely to try and appease these feelings with addictions, creating a never-ending cycle of pain, or aggression, or even self-righteousness. There are lots of ways to try to escape from our feelings of hurt. The point we want to make is that as humans, it is very difficult to overcome the pain of falling from grace, of being expelled from the Garden of Eden.

To add to this dysfunction, our societies are fed with constant misinformation and disinformation. Computer-generated AI will certainly add to this in the future. We are persistently led to falsely believe we live in a zero-sum world. Politically, this is creating a schism that is pushing people to extremes. This in turn appears to be fueled by social media algorithms that weigh hits, rather than truth, as being important. Yet, delving into societal dysfunction, the inherent message is often more insidious. Popular magazines and TV programs continually show us we need to be better looking, thinner, richer, younger, or something other than who we perceive ourselves to be. There is an inherent problem in this: If I win, you lose. Relationships aren't approached with a sense of balance. We are judged as having but never with equality. This further engenders a sense of anxiety, of lack, and of inadequacy.

In this scenario, people feel justified in dehumanizing others. And by stigmatizing and dehumanizing others, we are more able to justify malice. We may justify greed as a way of self-defense against a perceived sense of encroachment by others. Pollution in some form or other is often seen as a necessary byproduct to create wealth and power. If we then can't get what we want, we justify ways to achieve these goals. This is a setup for crime, war, food shortages, and famine. Climate change and pandemics, which threaten the survival of the human species, further aggravate this point of view and further divide people. We have come to see this as the norm, but it shouldn't be so.

And at the time, as we are traumatized, and continue to traumatize others, we leave *methylation marks*, visible scars, on the DNA of our nervous and immune systems. These are effectively software glitches that, up until now, have been self-perpetuating.

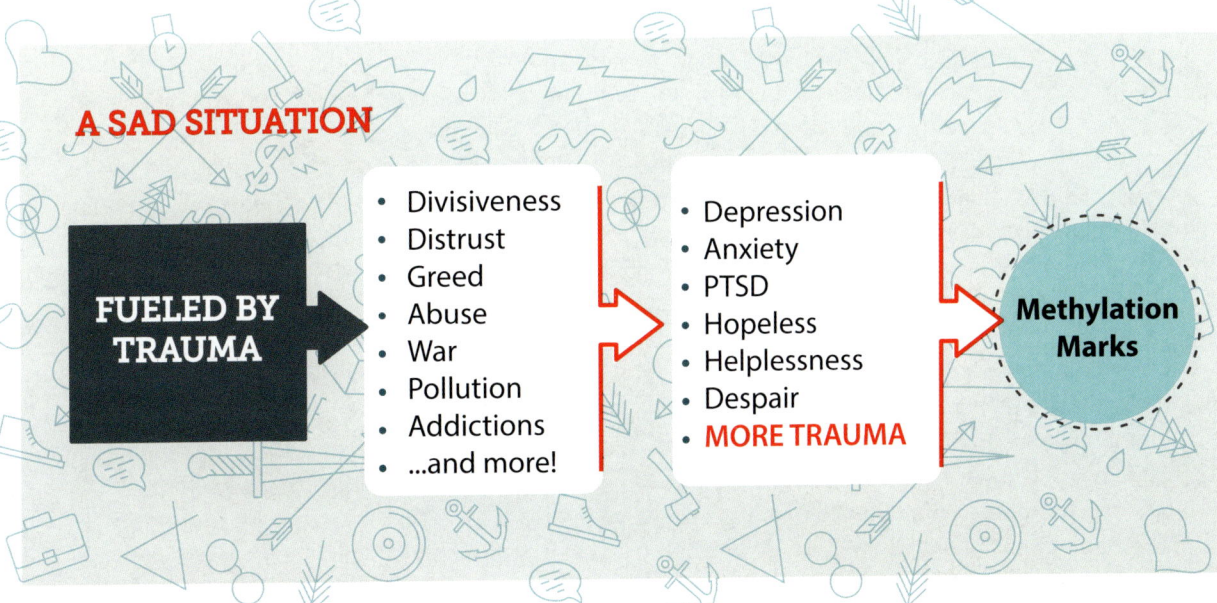

FIGURE 6.1 | A SAD Situation

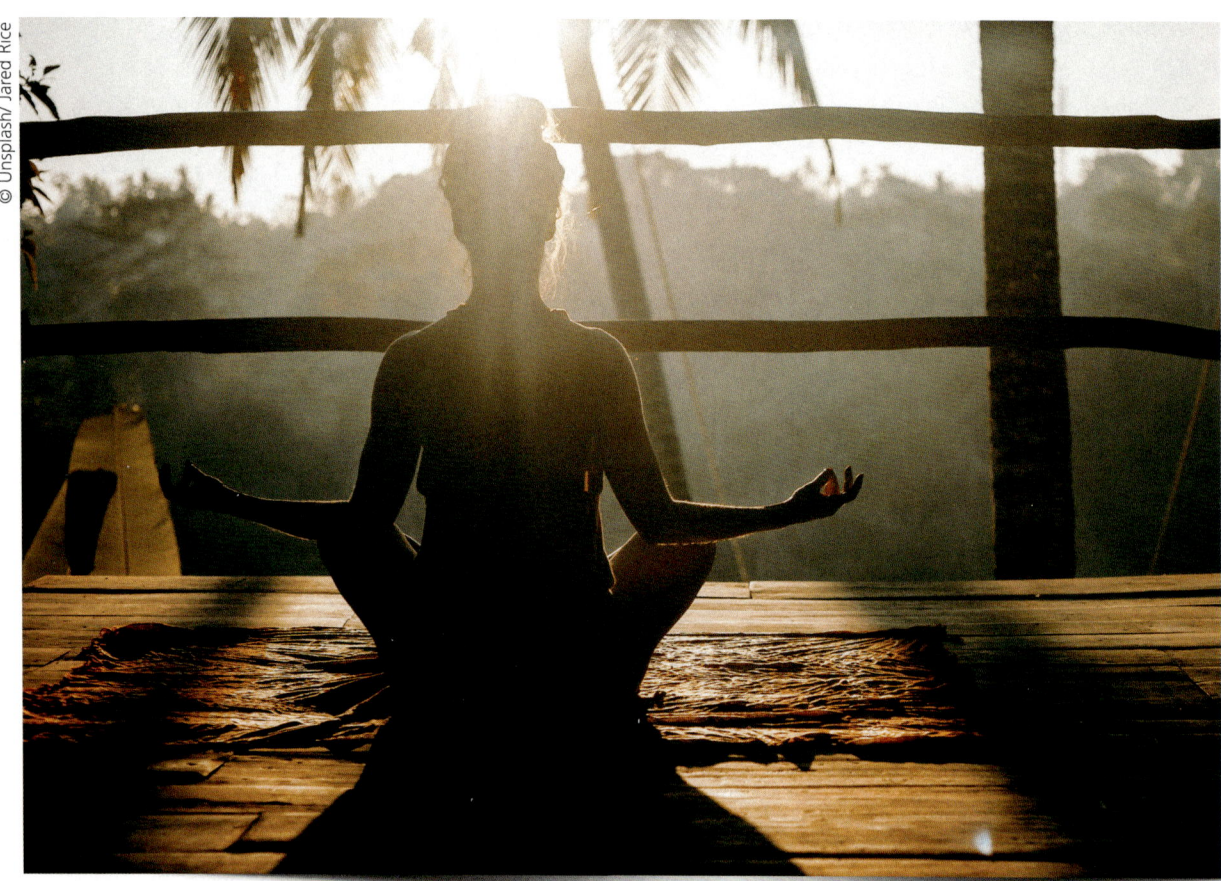

Healing from Trauma and Addiction

This book is about transformation! Throughout this book, we discuss physical transformation. We discuss tools for your toolbox: ways to get better. Because science and medicine have focused on physical mechanisms and antidotes, it's easy to understand physical ailments and potential magic bullets (drugs and surgery) as ways to get better. As wonderful as they may be, the expense is crippling our society. What's more, they can't fix everything.

Despite all this, we are hopeful that we can change at our very core. Studies suggest that the same genetic variants that put us at risk for bad behavior show plasticity. In other words, the brain is more sensitive to positive environmental inputs than it is to negative inputs, resulting in increased prosocial behavior. What this may mean is that the very people who get hit the hardest by trauma are the most likely to be able to be helped!

It is crucial to approach trauma and mental illness with empathy, understanding, and professional support. If you or someone you know is struggling with trauma or mental health challenges, we recommend seeking help from mental health professionals who can provide guidance, assessment, and appropriate interventions. A genuinely good therapist can help resolve old emotional traumas by gently guiding the person toward the time of the past abuse. If the person can lovingly and willingly experience the emotion present at the time of the trauma, they can often extinguish the emotional charge of the trauma, while retaining the memory. Ideally, they can then move toward forgiveness, self-acceptance, and self-love. It is important to retain the memory and not suppress it. It is only by doing so that we can stop someone from repeating the trauma. Without the emotional charge associated with the memory, they are able to live their life with a new-found sense of freedom.

If we have learned anything from systems biology, it is that there are always multiple ways to help. Treatment for trauma and mental illness often involves a combination of therapy, such as cognitive-behavioral therapy (CBT) or eye movement desensitization and reprocessing (EMDR), and medication, if necessary. Supportive interventions, self-care strategies, and building resilience are also essential components in the healing process. To fix the symptom, we often need to approach it in non-standard ways. Recent data shows that an enriched environment can reverse epigenetic marks. Talk therapy, meditation, massage, yoga, and tai chi can all bring about meaningful changes in physical and mental health. But we need to do more. Doing more of the same results in more of the same. We need something more effective and much faster.

The Promise of Psychedelic Drugs

Psychedelic drugs have been maligned as having no medical use and for being highly addictive with multiple toxic effects. All this turns out to be incorrect. New and exciting research in this field is yielding excellent results. The root of the word psychedelic comes from the Greek *psyche* (for mind or soul) and *delos* (to manifest or make clear). It turns out that, if wisely used in a medical setting, psychedelic drugs can help patients profoundly. For further information on this we suggest reading *How to Change your Mind* by Michael Pollan or streaming the content of the same name.

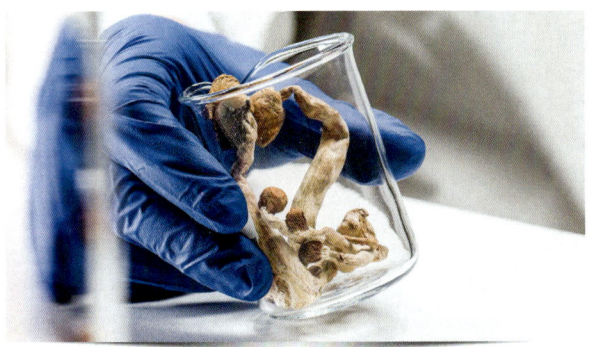

We have spoken with dozens of people who have used psychedelics for years, either illegally or as part of clinical studies. People using these medications often achieve an ineffable transcendent state, something that is so beautiful, so magnificent, so encompassing that it indelibly alters their life in a good way. While all report the same thing, "There are no words to adequately describe this," they all describe feeling the most incredible sense of LOVE! One person told us, "I felt as if all love in the universe originated from me, yet I was part of a universe of love. There was a complete sense of unity."

The result is a deep sense of spirituality, a profound sense of gratitude, and an intense humility and awe. What is more amazing is that, with increasing frequency, people who use psychedelics report that bad behaviors drop away. They report no longer even wanting to drink alcohol, smoke, or use drugs, even after only one treatment. They use fewer drugs, choose healthier foods, and improve their lifestyles. They are more loving to their spouses and partners and report a greater sense of purpose.

While taking psychedelic drugs, people often report reliving deep emotional traumas, often ones that they had completely suppressed. If they are not prepared for this possibility, the experience will be negative and upsetting, a so-called *bad trip*. Psychedelic drugs should be taken under the supervision of someone who can guide the person through the process. When this happens, some people report having "thirty years of therapy" in a session that lasted only a few hours. They leave with a sense that they are no longer encumbered by the traumas they have been carrying around forever. Life is good! Depression and anxiety melt way. They feel hopeful and loving. One person described it this way: *Looking back, my mind seemed to be like a ski-run with lots of moguls. I was filled with ruts that forced my thinking only to follow certain routes. Now, it feels as if my mental ski-run has been plowed, and filled with fresh beautiful snow. My mind enjoys a never before sensation of freedom, of lack of judgment of my self and others. I feel content. Happy and whole!*

Early studies seem to point to psychedelic medicines erasing the methylation marks. In other words, they are finally getting closer to erasing the traumas and halting the vicious cycles of mental illness and addiction.

Unlike antidepressants and similar medications, which need to be taken long term, psychedelics are used intermittently. The outcome, if used correctly, should be that people feel more love, more hope, less depression, and less anxiety. Traumas no longer hold any emotional charge. They are simply memories we recall in order never to repeat them.

This feeling of divine or universal love (also called "agape") seems to be the complete antidote for all emotional traumas. If you think about it, there is no opposite of love, only lack of it. It seems that when we restore it to humans, they thrive!

Psychedelics appear to offer a new, unique, and safe way to achieve better mental health. They remain mostly illegal, except under some medically supervised conditions. Our hope is that the research and development in these areas portends a better future for all our mental health.

> Love is patient, love is kind. It does not envy, it does not boast, it is not proud. It does not dishonor others, it is not self-seeking, it is not easily angered, it keeps no record of wrongs. Love does not delight in evil but rejoices with the truth. It always protects, always trusts, always hopes, always perseveres.
>
> Love never fails. But where there are prophecies, they will cease; where there are tongues, they will be stilled; where there is knowledge, it will pass away. For we know in part and we prophesy in part, [10] but when completeness comes, what is in part disappears. [11] When I was a child, I talked like a child, I thought like a child, I reasoned like a child. When I became a man, I put the ways of childhood behind me. [12] For now we see only a reflection as in a mirror; then we shall see face to face. Now I know in part; then I shall know fully, even as I am fully known.
>
> And now these three remain: faith, hope and love. But the greatest of these is love.
>
> —**Corinthians 13**

CHAPTER 7

How to Transform Stress into Success

Tools and Techniques to Help You Transform the Effects of Stress on Your Health and Your Life

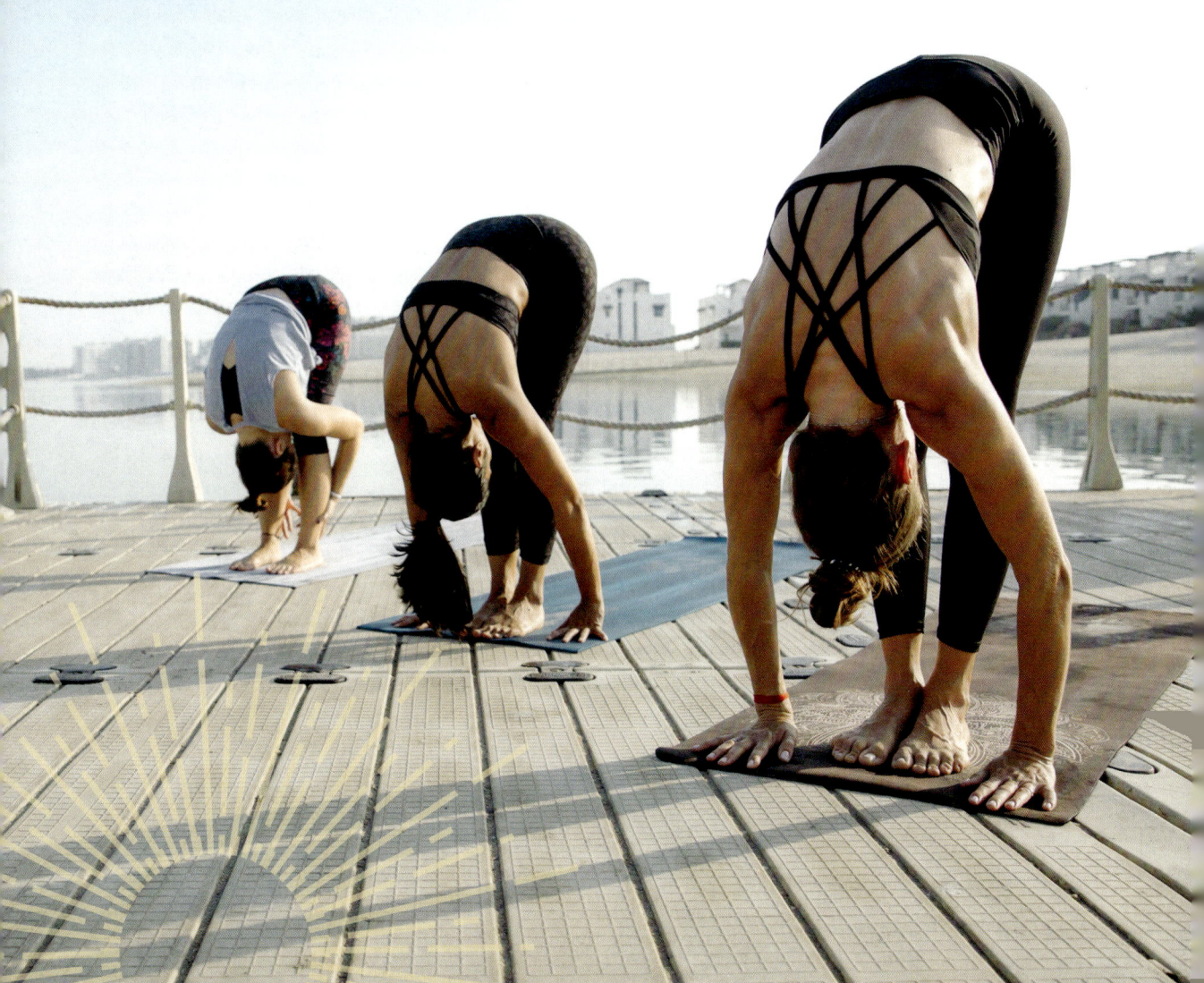

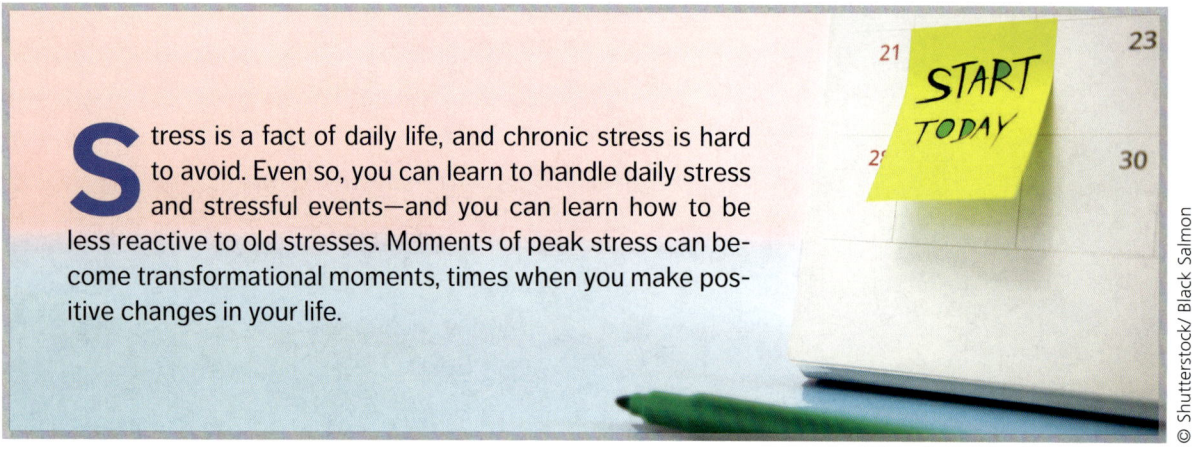

Stress is a fact of daily life, and chronic stress is hard to avoid. Even so, you can learn to handle daily stress and stressful events—and you can learn how to be less reactive to old stresses. Moments of peak stress can become transformational moments, times when you make positive changes in your life.

Dealing with Stress

Stress is a challenge to the body, emotions, and mind. Dealing with it takes a toll, but if you have a good understanding of how stress affects you, you are better able to handle it. Based on our experience with our patients, we've learned some important lessons for coping with stress. Here are some tips:

Aim for a healthy lifestyle. Stress, by its very nature, counteracts a healthy lifestyle. Stress will push you to eat junk food, lose sleep, and set up a cascading wave of chemical damage that will flow throughout your body. In earlier chapters, we outlined some healthy lifestyle approaches that can become a welcome refuge against stress. Here, we'll give specific suggestions on how to tailor your lifestyle to antidote stress.

Mend the mind to mind the body. The mind is a powerful tool, yet it can be both helpful and harmful to you. Learning how to develop a different outlook can powerfully reshape your life and literally reformat your body chemistry.

Restore the body to revitalize the mind. Body chemistry can affect how we look, feel, and think. Learn to treat your body with the respect it deserves. When your body feels vital and alive, so do you. In this chapter, we offer suggestions to help your body develop a profound sense of vigor that will help carry you through tougher times. We discuss the use of healing therapies, adaptogenic herbs, and even medications. Always work with a physician who understands the benefits and side effects of the medications you're being prescribed. When working with a practitioner who prescribes nutritional supplements, work with someone who also understands that "natural" doesn't always mean good or safe. Supplements may have interactions with medications and can cause harm. In addition, the quality of the supplements will affect the outcomes.

Techniques for Transforming Stress

Acute or sudden stress is different from chronic or long-term stress. We suggest you learn different ways to handle each of these.

Each episode of acute stress gives you an opportunity of choice. You can learn how to make decisions that will transform your health and your life.

To become whole again from chronic stress, you need to find ways to integrate deep rest and regeneration into your life. The goal is to move yourself back to the left side of the Stress Curve, returning to where you are Enthusiastic and Exhilarated once again.

Healthy Lifestyle Habits to Reduce Ongoing Stress

Simplify your life. Learn how to say stop, and learn how to say no. When you feel yourself getting overwhelmed, it is usually OK to stop. Learn to take breaks. Getting away for a while is a good thing. It gives you a needed sense of perspective.

Manage your time. Make a priority list of what is important to you. Don't overcommit. Learn to recognize when you are biting off more than you can chew.

Listen to your body. Your body will know that you are stressed before you do. Become skilled at recognizing your body's cues and become familiar with them. Irritability; tightness and tension in your head, jaws, or shoulders; or a gnawing feeling in the pit of your stomach may all be telling you that you are overdoing things.

Exercise. Make sure you exercise in a manner that is beneficial to you and be reasonable. Remember that running at midday in a high-traffic area may count as exercise, but it probably isn't improving your health.

Develop healthy ways to dissipate stress. Volunteer work, an avocation, or a hobby can be excellent ways to deal with stress. Whether you are helping to repair a hiking trail or tutoring shelter kids after school, using your gifts to serve others adds another dimension to your life.

Use social connections. If you enjoy socializing in groups, stay connected with ones you like, such as a religious organization, a self-help group, a support group, or a book club. Even online social groups or disease-specific support groups can give you a sense of social identity. On the other hand, if you're more energized by time spent one-on-one, tap those close relationships to sustain you.

Avoid stimulants and eat well. Reduce the use of stimulants such as caffeine and nicotine. Reduce alcohol. Minimize junk foods; go for a nutrient-rich diet.

Take time every day just for yourself. Consider a relaxation or meditation technique for 20 minutes once or twice daily. Even five or ten minutes a day is a good start toward this goal.

Mending the Mind and Minding the Body

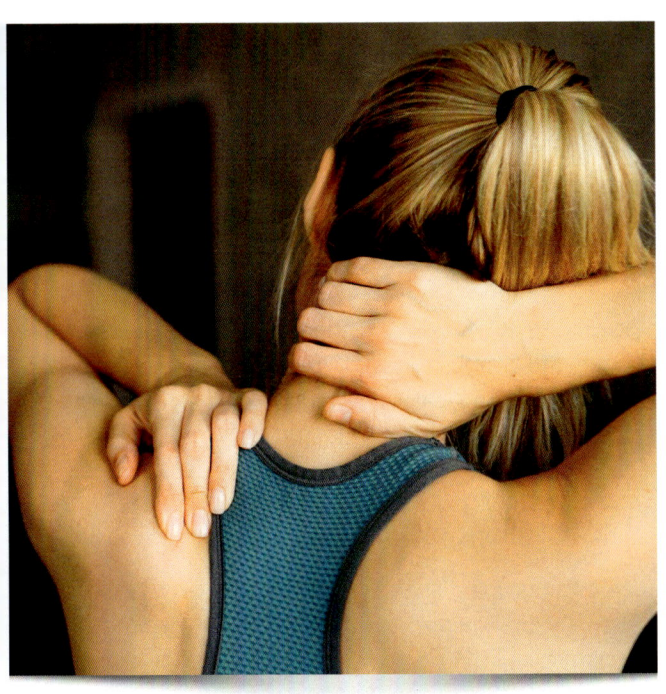

Researchers at Ohio State University have shown how powerfully psychological stress can affect the immune system. Janice Kiecolt-Glaser, PhD, is a professor of psychiatry and psychology at Ohio State University. Her husband, Ronald Glaser, PhD, was a professor of internal medicine, molecular virology, immunology and medical genetics, and head of Ohio State's Institute for Behavioral Medicine Research.

They compared the rate of wound healing after a skin punch biopsy (a small incision that removes some tissue from the skin) in two groups: a stressed group consisting of caregivers to a spouse or family member with advanced Alzheimer's disease, and an unstressed group. In the stressed group, wound healing took nine days longer on average. The study showed how much stress disrupts the immune system and makes us more vulnerable to infection and slower to heal. This finding has profound implications for medical care. If we can learn how to control or reduce stress, we can drastically affect how our bodies heal.

Mental Tips for Handling Stress

Stress has a major impact on emotions. As we feel more stressed, small things upset us more, and we feel more angry, anxious, or depressed. Fortunately, we have learned many mental tips from our patients that help them deal with their stress.

Journaling. Write down who or what is bothering you. Identify triggers: things that make you anxious, frustrated, or angry. As you do so, become aware of your own body's responses. Examining your physical reactions to thoughts and feelings that are stressful—rapid heartbeat, sweatiness, bowel habit changes—is part of this. Make notes on how you're dealing with stress. Eating more? Smoking? Ruminating or obsessing? Hoarding? Are these problematic behaviors? If so, develop a list of ways to address them in a healthy manner.

Develop self-compassion. Imagine a baby trying to walk. Each time she falls, you wouldn't deride her or tell her she's stupid. Learn to treat yourself with the same compassion with which you would treat a small child.

Be clear with other people. Make sure the people close to you understand your requests and intentions. We think that others understand what's going on inside our heads, but the truth is that often they don't.

Change your perspective. Speaking to others may help you get a different point of view. Whether it's through a friend, pastor, counselor, or therapist, learn to see problems from another's point of view.

Work on balancing your emotions. If anger is your issue, learn to deal with it. When you feel frustrated, go work out rather than taking it out on anyone. Count to ten before you say something in a negative manner. Practice forgiveness. Practice mindfulness.

Express yourself differently. Learn to give messages that begin with "I feel . . ." rather than "You are . . ." Learn to simply say, "I feel hurt when you . . ." or, "I feel angry when you . . ." This is a much better approach than cussing someone out, which is judgmental and tends to make people defensive.

Express yourself factually. So often, we don't tell people when they are hurting our feelings. This is usually with people we like, as we don't want to offend them. However, there is a way to do this. Tell them accurately and factually what you are feeling and when it is occurring.

Laugh. Can you find humor in a situation? You're in good company. Political journalist Norman Cousins once overcame a chronic illness by watching comedies daily. He wrote about his experience—and the healing power of laughter and humor—in his classic book *Anatomy of an Illness: As Perceived by the Patient*.

Develop resilience. Stress will always be part of our lives. Making ourselves more resilient to it is essential. Learn strategies to help you bounce back.

Try to find meaning in your life. Can you feel gratitude for the experience you are going through, despite its hardship? What do you think you are here for? What are you learning? Where are you going?

Forgive transgressions against you. Forgiveness does not mean you have to like someone. It means learning to bear no resentment. Remember, if you harbor anger or resentment, it is you that suffers, not the person you are angry with! Or, as the Chinese proverb goes, "If you seek revenge, you should dig two graves—one for yourself."

Remain hopeful. Trust that you will be okay. This too shall pass! Handling stress effectively is a learned behavior. Have faith in the process.

Accept what life throws at you. Remember the phrase, "Lovingly and willingly accept all things."

Psychological Transformation

Each one of us is physically unique. Similarly, we are all psychologically unique. Unfortunately, we may sense our uniqueness as a problem or an

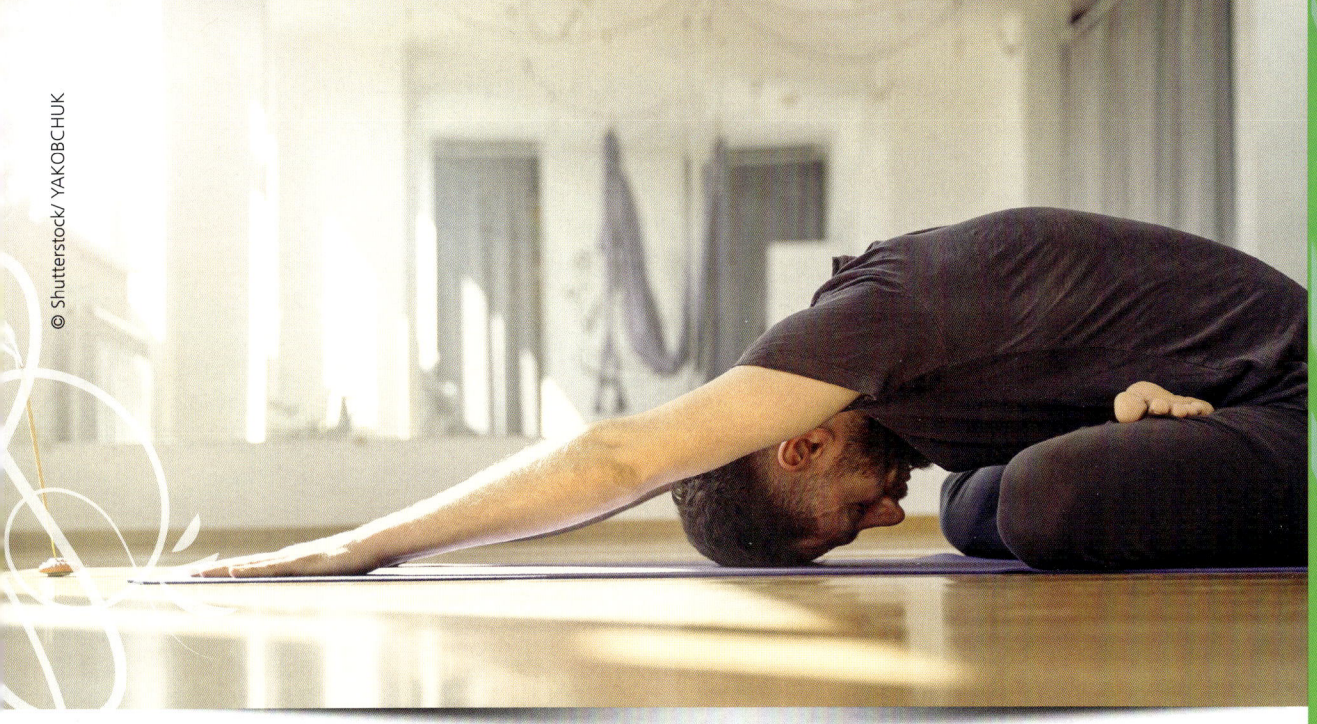

inadequacy—or even flip to the opposite side, where narcissistic qualities give us a false sense of greatness. Psychological transformation usually means discovering who you really are. It implies that you become more of your true self. Our true selves are usually stronger, kinder, and more loving than we believe. Yet our own psychological programming can hold us back from becoming our true selves.

You may have been brought up in a family where either over- or under-expressing yourself emotionally might be considered inappropriate. Patients tell us how they were forced to grow out of sync with their own personalities. A sensitive person may grow up in a macho family. An artist may grow up in a family, community, or time where their talents are undervalued. We are vulnerable to having alien attributes imposed on us by families, teachers, communities, and even advertising media. This leads to emotional miscues, or what we call mis-emotions.

An example of a mis-emotion is laughing if you are scared or crying if you are angry. Imagine you're the young child of an alcoholic, unhappy mother. One day you say to her, "Mommy, why are you so angry?" She glares at you, replying, "I'm not angry. Now go away." You decide that because she's an adult, she must be correct. She isn't angry. Therefore, as a child, you believe that your ability to sense anger must be wrong. You start misinterpreting emotions, but missing emotional cues leads to further emotional misunderstandings. This can lead to becoming self-destructive, critical of ourselves, and disparaging of others.

Physical disease and psychological pain can force us to examine these traits. The threat of divorce may bring a couple into counseling. Similarly, a heart attack may force a person to examine underlying anger, resentment, or other emotions and behaviors.

Transforming Toxic Emotions

To survive a bad situation, it is common to suppress a feeling or emotion. This feeling may resurface years later as a physical illness. By paying attention to your bodily sensations in times of stress, you can become aware of this link between suppressed emotional patterns and your physical reactions.

Psychologists know that if an illness serves as an unconscious strategy to cope with life, no amount of medicine alone is likely to heal the patient. Illness may reflect deep, secret anguish, grief, shame, thwarted goals, or some other form of human pain. Ignoring the underlying block is like ignoring a large splinter. Healing is difficult until the obstruction has been gently removed so the wound can heal. If you feel that your emotions are out of control, we suggest seeking a mental health practitioner for help.

However, most of us have emotional issues for which we don't see a therapist. In Chinese medicine, physical feelings encompass a full spectrum of emotion, spanning the mirror opposites, or the yin and yang aspects of that emotion. Have you ever seen a baby girl that has just been fed a new food? She will sometimes shake with ecstatic apprehension. From the outside, when we look at her tremulousness, we can't be sure if she's happy or anxious. Later, she will give the label "happy" to the emotion that goes with the feeling of blissful tremulousness. Similarly, a two-year-old boy having a temper tantrum may not understand what it means to be "angry." He simply feels out of control, needing to explode as tensions rise in his body. If we can help him understand how to better control his environment, and that he is experiencing an emotion of anger, we can help him control both his behavior and the physical consequences in his body—being tense and uptight. These unresolved primordial emotions continue to have power over our behaviors well into adulthood.

By learning to become fully aware of our physical feelings, we can often learn to transform our emotions, to flip from the negative side of the emotional spectrum to the more positive side. This technique implies an "emotional aikido" of sorts, using the power of a negative emotion on itself. We can turn anger into power, fear into courage, worry into selflessness, anxiety into tranquility, and sadness into transcendence. This way, we become more of our true selves.

Psychological transformation can therefore lead to new levels of psychological maturity with greater insight into and understanding of our own feelings and emotions. It calls for us to pay attention to our physical feelings.

We see patients transforming emotions every day. Here are a few epiphanies from some of our patients:

- "I realized that I am so busy worrying because deep down I feel like people are judging me. I thought that if everything was perfect, then people would see me in a better light. But the reality is that I can never be perfect, and people don't really care anyway. I am worrying all the time about myself. If I ignore the 'self' part of me, I stop worrying. I don't feel self-judged or self-pity. So now when I worry, I remind myself to be self-less, and then my worry-meter stops registering."

- "I sank into this sense of sadness, which I feel as a pressure over my lungs. As I did, heaviness seemed to lift off me. This was followed by a sense of calmness or peace, something like I had never felt before. I feel connected to everyone and everything. I never want to get rid of my tendency to sadness. It is my gateway to connecting to the universe!"

Transforming a Toxic Emotional Environment

We need to learn to deal with our emotions. We need to learn to see when our emotions and feelings are changing the way we see the world, just like tinted glasses. However, we also need to recognize when we are living in a toxic emotional situation. This may be an abusive spouse, a rage-aholic parent, an offensive boss, or cruel, or even bullying, friends.

==Dealing with a toxic emotional environment can mean moving on from it.== Leaving an

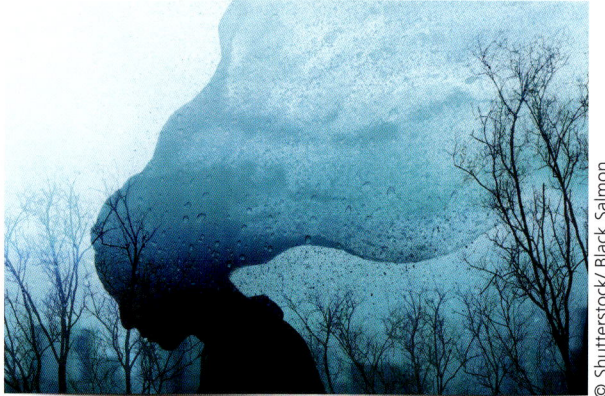

abusive partner is difficult—you may well need help from a therapist, a lawyer, and even the police. Learning to stand up for yourself is an important survival tool. If you are struggling with this, don't feel embarrassed about seeking help. It may be the most important thing you ever do.

Spiritual Transformation

The goals of transformational medicine are the optimization of physical health, psychological transformation, and spiritual growth. The last two goals can be differentiated. Psychological transformation implies that we change how we view just ourselves. In contrast, spiritual transformation implies a different way of viewing ourselves as part of the universe, of understanding how we fit into the universe. It is accompanied by greater love, more happiness, and less suffering.

In our quest to understand healing, we have had the privilege of treating or interviewing patients who have experienced what we consider miraculous healings. *(Our definition of a miracle is a patient's response to an illness that defies all conventional medical expectations of their disease.)* Many of these patients describe a profound connection with something greater than themselves. This may occur slowly or as a moment of clarity, in which a new insight or understanding is gained. These patients describe a sense of connectedness to their inner path that isn't dependent on physical or material comforts. It becomes a source of inspiration and orientation as they rededicate their lives to the spiritual and transcendent nature of the universe. There seems to be a spontaneous shift. They can see life in a completely different way, with changes in thoughts, emotions, and behavior. They feel less suffering.

In our experience, patients often have similar experiences after acupuncture or energy healing treatments. Following these profound insights, they tend to reassign their priorities, establish new ones, or simply experience an enhanced state of wellbeing, love, and connectedness. This often comes as an unanticipated but pleasant surprise. (For example, a patient may not be expecting this if they come in for treatment of their knee pain.)

Sometimes patients become acutely aware of an inner struggle. Traditional Chinese medicine describes this as a discrepancy between mind and spirit. The spirit may want something different than the mind thinks it needs. Your family may have expected you to be a physician or a lawyer, yet you may have had a profound need to become something else, such as an artist or a writer. In this manner of thinking, discord between your mind and spirit may lead to an illness. Healing then involves uncovering and resolving these areas of discordance, allowing insight into ourselves and our lives. As this new awareness develops, an apparent burden of stress is easily resolved.

Unfortunately, many of us will only take a spiritual leap when we are faced with insurmountable odds. This may come with personal misfortune or even the diagnosis of a terminal illness. No matter what, spiritual growth helps us learn how to cope and bounce back from a stressful situation. This enhances our resilience.

Personal Growth Is a Journey

Both psychological and spiritual transformation require constant work. We may grow in leaps and bounds at times or remain stagnant for prolonged periods. As with everything, we can choose how we want to work on ourselves.

Restoring the Body to **Revitalize the Mind**

All emotional and spiritual states have their physical counterparts. Functional MRIs of the brain show different areas lighting up with alterations in mood. Neurotransmitters in our brains relate to how we feel. Low serotonin levels, for example, result in anxiety and depression. Similarly, people in spiritual states of ecstasy, as well as drug-induced highs, have been shown to have huge outpourings of serotonin as well as another neurotransmitter called anandamide (N-arachidonoylethanolamine), or the "bliss chemical." Your physiology will mirror your psychological state. What if we help your physiology to feel better? We encourage you to learn how to help your body make more feel-good chemicals.

Medicines that Affect the Mind

Since the 1990s, the use of antidepressants has increased significantly. The development of selective serotonin reuptake inhibitors (SSRIs) created a relatively safe way to treat depression with fewer side effects than older classes of antidepressants. SSRIs such as fluoxetine (Prozac), sertraline (Zoloft), and escitalopram (Lexapro) mainly increase serotonin levels. These led the way to drugs such as venlafaxine (Effexor) and duloxetine (Cymbalta), which mainly increase serotonin and norepinephrine levels. Other drugs, such as bupropion (Wellbutrin), primarily affect dopamine levels.

Drugs can help people feel better. Certain drugs can also make patients feel worse. Beta blockers such as propranolol, acne drugs such as isotretinoin (Accutane), birth control pills, and even statin drugs can cause depression, for example. If you're feeling depressed, fatigued, achy, or anything unusual for you, ask your physician or your pharmacist if a prescription or nonprescription drug could be causing or aggravating your problem.

We are always amazed at how different doctors treat the same condition, depending on their viewpoints. A perimenopausal woman complaining of depression and hot flashes may receive estrogen from her gynecologist but antidepressants from her primary care doctor or psychiatrist. Both work. Why? Estrogen influences serotonin, and SSRI drugs influence both depression and hot flashes.

Drugs and psychotherapy are not the only way to help patients feel better. Besides teaching coping skills and lifestyle changing behaviors, we also find that correcting underlying functional imbalances can help overcome feelings of depression.

The Resurgent Use of Hallucinogenic Drugs

The use of hallucinogenic drugs in the 1960s was part of the countercultural revolution, justified as a way of expanding consciousness. While studies on LSD at major universities such as Stanford and Harvard showed promise, the government, the media, and the public's emotional tide turned against these drugs. They were ultimately criminalized.

The tide seems to have turned once more. This time, research is being done in a much more controlled and conservative fashion at many of the top institutions around the country. Multiple studies are showing significant benefits for people coping with high levels of stress, anxiety, and depression. Much of the research is being led by MAPS (the Multidisciplinary Association for Psychedelic Studies, maps.org). The studies have been very revealing.

> "
> Clouds come floating into my life, no longer to carry rain or usher storm, but to add color to my sunset sky.
>
> — Rabindranath Tagore

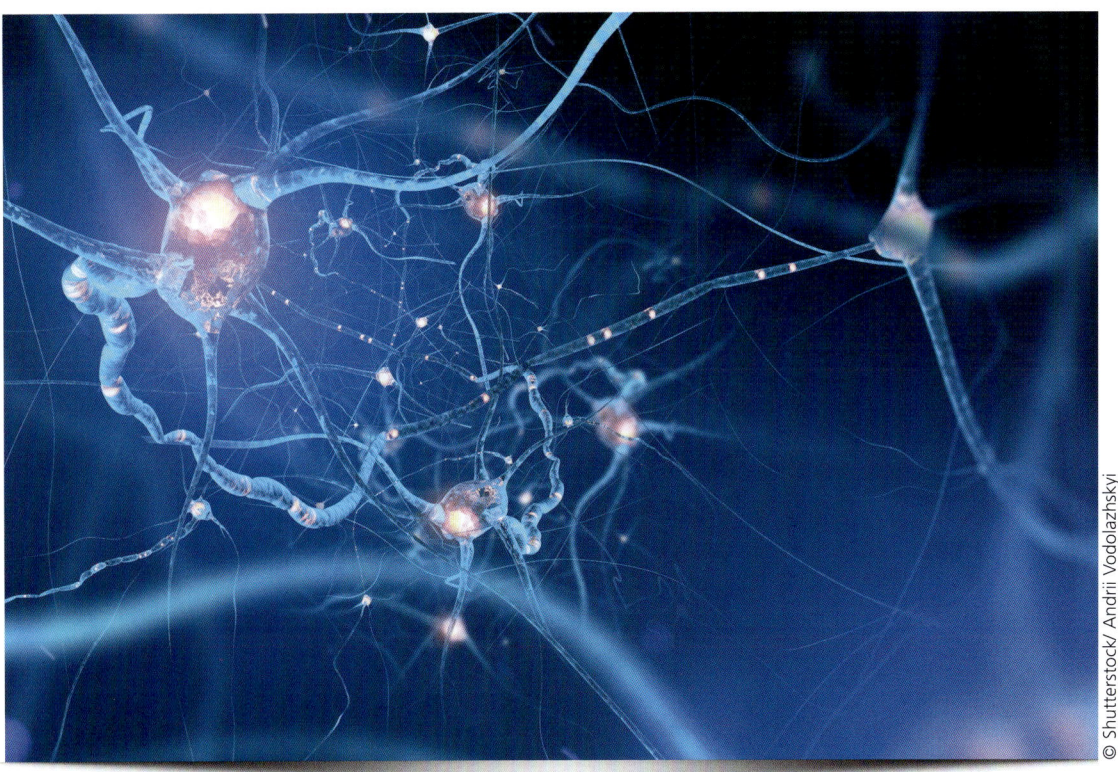

MDMA, commonly known as ecstasy or molly, is being studied as a breakthrough therapy for severe PTSD. Imagine how useful this is for highly traumatized people, such as combat veterans or rape victims, who have been unable to get help with any other therapy. In one study, 88 percent of patients with PTSD experienced a clinically significant reduction in PTSD diagnostic scores two months after their third session of MDMA-assisted therapy, compared to 60 percent of placebo participants. Additionally, 67 percent of participants in the MDMA group, compared to 32 percent of participants in the placebo group, no longer met the criteria for PTSD two months after the sessions.

Patients with end-stage cancer or other life-threatening illnesses often experience extreme anxiety, especially regarding dying. A study in Switzerland examined the effectiveness of LSD-assisted therapy for these people. Two months after treatment, participants showed a reduction in anxiety. No acute or chronic adverse events persisted beyond a day after treatment, and there were no treatment-related serious adverse events. Follow-up data at 12 months showed that the reduction in anxiety was still present.

Ketamine, a psychedelic drug that is FDA-approved for depression, can be used with or without antidepressants for treatment-resistant severe depression.

What is interesting about these and other psychedelic drugs, such as psilocybin or ibogaine, is that the real benefit appears to relate not so much to the specific drug but to its ability to induce what is called "ego dissolution," or the total loss of subjective self-identity. The patient experiences a transcendent state, a feeling of being at one with the universe. In most cases, the result is a positive change in outlook on life. The drug lowers anxiety and depression, removes or lessens obsessive-compulsive thoughts, and helps stop abuse of alcohol and tobacco. (Bill W., the founder of Alcoholics Anonymous, used LSD in the 1950s and was certain it would benefit people with alcohol abuse disorder. This horrified many AA followers and led to a backlash that meant LSD was never really studied for its value in substance abuse.)

In both studies and from anecdotal stories, it seems that the experience of the transcendent state is one of the critical factors in achieving a successful clinical outcome! In this way, these medicines are different from conventional drugs, in that this ego-less state is more than just an effect of the medicine itself. To cultivate the state, practitioners talk about the importance of *"Set"* (or the mindset with which you approach the experience,) the *Setting* in which you have your experience (it should be calm, nurturing, in or near nature), and the *Sitter*, or guide who is present helping you navigate the experience.

Microdosing is a term used for frequent small doses of usually either LSD or psilocybin. This has a different effect than the high doses typically used to create a psychedelic state. Since these drugs also work on serotonin, a feel-good neurotransmitter, people using low doses often report having a "very good day." They think better and feel more clear-headed and less moody. If antidepressants stop patients dropping into a negative mood state, these drugs push patients the other way, toward a positive mood state.

Microdoses of psychedelics have become topical in today's world. The initial research looks quite promising. Concerns about abuse and long-term effects remain, however. In addition, except for ketamine prescribed by a licensed healthcare provider, they remain illegal in the U.S. They should only be used under medically supervised conditions (which usually means being part of a study.)

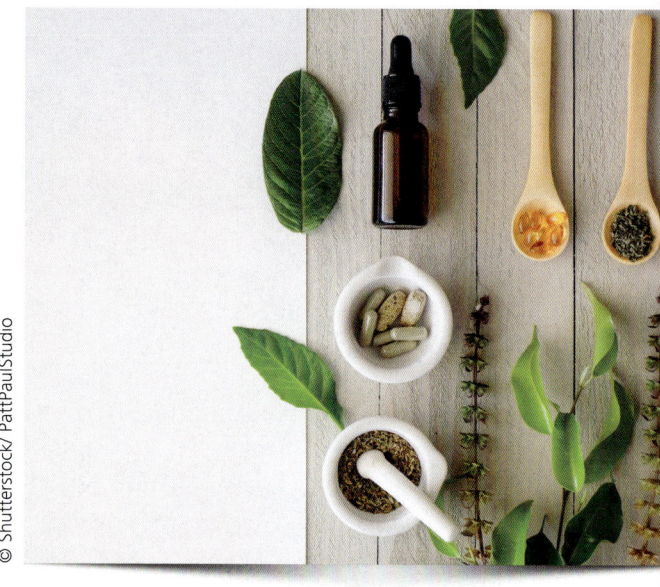

© Shutterstock/ PattPaulStudio

Supplements for Stress and Mood

In our experience, it is difficult to overcome chronic depression without supporting adrenal function and reducing inflammation.

Patients suffering from depression are often also chronically stressed. Simply put, their adrenal glands are shot. We can support the adrenals by using *adaptogenic herbs* to increase the body's resistance to stress and trauma, helping to balance the endocrine and immune systems and maintain a state of balance within the body. Adaptogenic herbs tend to tone down hyperfunctioning systems while improving systems that aren't functioning at an adequate level.

Adaptogenic herbs have been used safely for centuries in various cultures. They go by names such as restorative herbs, chi tonics, rasayanas, and rejuvenating herbs. Some examples of *adaptogenic* herbs are American ginseng (*Panax quinquefolium*), Siberian ginseng (*Eleutherococcus senticosus*), Asian ginseng (*Panax ginseng*), Indian ginseng or ashwagandha (*Withania somnifera*), and rhodiola (*Rhodiola rosea*).

Nutritional supplements can also be helpful for coping with stress. Nutritionists often advise taking more B vitamins during stress. Magnesium and zinc supplements are also often recommended.

Adrenal recovery can be supported with amino acids, such as L-methionine, L-histidine, and N-acetyl tyrosine. Neurotransmitter function also can be improved with nutritional supplements. Amino acids such as 5-hydroxytryptophan (5-HTP), L-theanine, and taurine all help increase serotonin levels. Levels of the neurotransmitter dopamine can be elevated with fava bean extract and N-acetylcysteine (NAC). NAC also increases glutathione, a strong antioxidant and main driver of the body's toxin-neutralizing system.

We suggest that you work with a qualified health practitioner who understands when and how to use herbal and nutritional products. These products are not regulated by the FDA, and their quality may vary. For one herb, one company may use the root, while another may use the bark or the flower. Some companies maintain pharmaceutical-like quality, while others have pills that don't degrade well or even contain contaminants. In addition, supplements and even vitamins may have drug interactions.

Treating the Body to Heal the Mind

Treating the body with integrative therapies is often an excellent way to help deal with stress. Numerous physical modalities, also known as bodywork, help both mind and body. These include acupuncture, massage therapy, energy healing techniques, the Feldenkrais method, the Alexander technique, Rolfing, yoga, and tai chi.

Practitioners of acupuncture have claimed for thousands of years that acupuncture needles affect both the mind and the body. Part of this is easy to explain. Acupuncture changes the blood flow in the brain. It also raises endorphins in the central nervous system, which makes us feel a little euphoric. This is what causes a runner's high, also called an endorphin rush. The philosophy of acupuncture goes deeper than endorphin changes, however. It connects the body and the emotions in a body-mind link we frequently see.

Transforming Chronic Stress

In this chapter, we want to help you learn how to transform chronic stress. First, you need to decide where you are on the Stress Curve. Check back to the diagram of the Stress Curve in the previous chapter. Your aim should be to get to the left side—the Exhilarated section—where stress is invigorating. Let's look at how you can do this.

Riding the Wave of Exhilarating Stress

In general, exhilarating or invigorating stress is the positive side of the stress response. We may have an exciting challenge in our lives—a new job, graduate school, or another child in the family. We are usually energized, motivated, and excited by these changes. At times like this, it's important not to neglect yourself. Recognize that you can only sustain this level of effort for so long before you move to the right on the curve. Maintain a sense of balance and control over your life. Develop a strategy for the long term.

Transforming the Wired and Tired Stage

You know you have pushed too hard when you find yourself on the Wired and Tired part of the curve. Fortunately, you can usually reverse these early changes quickly and easily.

We always suggest that you start by examining your life. We don't suggest making big changes—in fact, just the opposite. A much more effective approach is to make small but meaningful changes to address the major cause(s) of the stress. If tension or a toxic relationship is driving the stress, now is the time to deal with it. You want to address the cause of your stress before it results in burnout.

Lifestyle. Maintain a healthy lifestyle and keep your daily healthy lifestyle routine going. This is where exercise, especially aerobic exercise, can help burn off the extra adrenaline you are carrying around. Breath work will help you simultaneously revitalize and relax your body.

Body chemistry. Consider supplements and/or adaptogenic herbs to prevent depletion. We often use a blend of Chinese herbs. These include rehmannia root (*Rehmannia glutinosa*), schisandra fruit (*Schisandra chinensis*), jujube fruit (*Ziziphus spinosa*), dong quai root (*Angelica sinensis*), Chinese asparagus root (*Asparagus cochinchinensis*), scrophularia root (*Scrophularia ningpoensis*), Korean ginseng root (*Panax ginseng*), Chinese salvia root (*Salvia miltiorrhiza*), poria mushroom (*Wolfiporia cocos*), polygala root (*Polygala tenuifolia*), and platycodon root (*Platycodon grandiflorus*). Other options include American ginseng, Siberian ginseng, Indian ginseng, rhodiola, astragalus (*Astragalus membra-*

naceus), passionflower (*Passiflora incarnata*), valerian (*Valeriana officinalis*), skullcap (*Scutellaria lateriflora*), and magnolia (*Magnolia officinalis*).

Additional nutritional supplements. These include vitamin C, zinc, and B vitamins. If you are under a lot of stress, you may need up to 200 mg of vitamin B6 (pyridoxine) and 1500 mg of vitamin B5 (pantothenic acid) daily. These vitamins help you metabolize stress hormones. Phosphatidylserine, GABA, and L-theanine can also be helpful for reducing anxiety and helping you relax.

Healing therapies. Acupuncture, energy healing, and massage or other bodywork can be instrumental to help you reduce bodily tension and achieve restorative sleep. The effects of one session can last for several weeks. These therapies promote deep relaxation and counteract that sense of being wired by balancing stress hormones and calming your nervous system.

Transforming the Exhausted Stage

The sense of exhaustion we are referring to here isn't temporary fatigue. It is a state of profound depletion that occurs over a period of months or even years. Over the long term, it is usually not one single factor that wears us down and results in exhaustion. Ask yourself if the stress is occurring too often. Is it too much or lasting too long? You can tolerate high levels of stress for a time but consider setting a limit. Apply the same rule of thumb for psychological stress that you would for a physical health problem. Any condition that persists longer than three months is considered chronic. If the condition, whether physical or psychological, isn't improving, or if it keeps coming back, seek professional help.

Lifestyle. At this stage, you need to take more time for self-care, to look after yourself. To optimize your quality of life, despite the challenges you are facing, put yourself first. This is really a time to say "no" and "stop" to things that will deplete you. Take 10 to 20 minutes three to four times a day to meditate and relax. As for exercise, go gently; aim to do only about 50 percent of what you think you should do. If you feel tired when you exercise, cut down even further. This is also a good time to reduce stimulants, such as chocolate and caffeine, especially after noon. Avoid junk food and cut out alcohol. Find other ways to support your energy.

Body chemistry. To help your body cope, consider adaptogenic herbal supplements. We suggest slightly different ones to those when you are "wired and tired." American ginseng, Siberian ginseng, Indian ginseng, astragalus, schizandra, rhodiola, and licorice (*Glycyrrhiza glabra*) are helpful. (Licorice can raise blood pressure, so avoid it if you have hypertension.) We routinely suggest a combination of extracts of cordyceps mycelium (*Paecilomyces hepiali*), Korean ginseng root, and rhodiola root to our patients at this point.

Consider additional nutritional supplements. These are similar to when you are wired and tired, and include vitamin C, zinc, and B vitamins. You may need up to 200 mg of vitamin B6 (pyridoxine) daily and 1500 mg of vitamin B5 (pantothenic acid) daily. Phosphatidylserine, GABA, and L-theanine can also be helpful here.

Healing therapies. The healing therapies referenced in the Wired and Tired section—acupuncture, energy healing, and massage or other body work—can have a profound effect in transforming your health. We will discuss these in depth in later chapters.

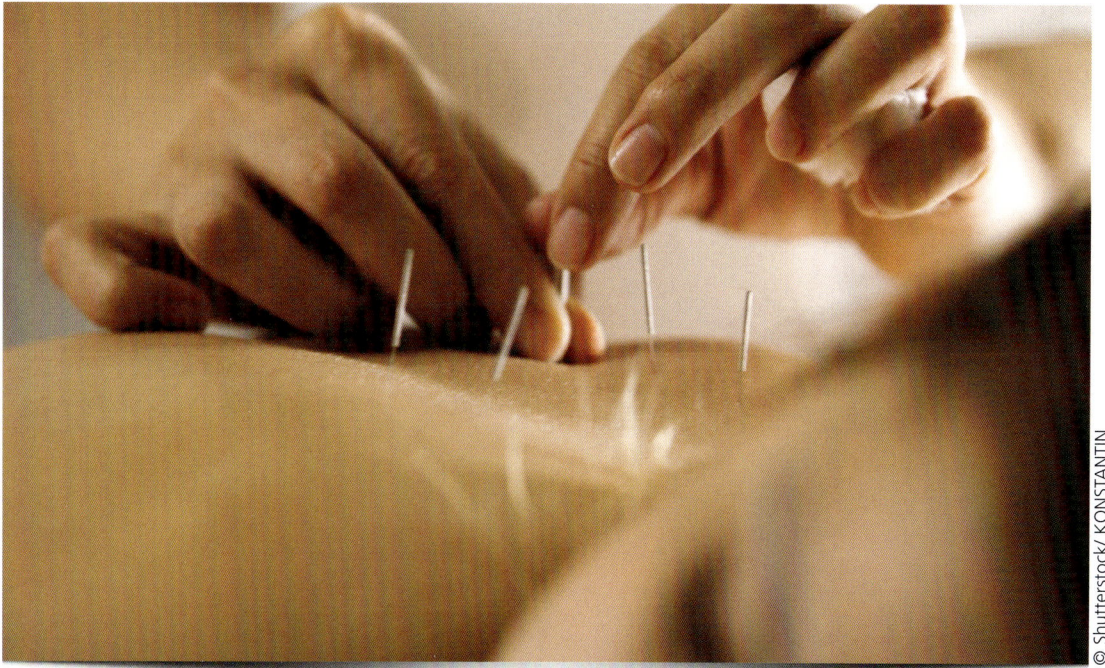

Transforming the Exhausted and Inflamed Stage

In the Exhausted and Inflamed Stage of the Stress Curve, your body is screaming at you. It's saying, "Help, I'm on fire!" Pay attention to your diet, mood, and lifestyle. At this point, we suggest following the same steps you would during the Exhausted phase. In addition, add in these steps:

Lifestyle. Make sure you are addressing insulin resistance, which can be caused by high cortisol levels. Ensure your diet is high in anti-inflammatory foods. Continue to exercise gently and aim for fifty percent of what you think you can do.

Mind-body techniques. At this point, mindfulness meditation once or twice a day for at least 10 minutes can be very helpful. Apps such as *Headspace*, *Calm*, or *Insight Timer* are good starting points.

Body chemistry. If you're depressed, consider an antidepressant or nutritional supplements such as 5-HTP to help increase serotonin. Higher levels of serotonin will also help reduce inflammation.

Nutritional anti-inflammatories. These include mercury-free fish oils, iso-alpha acids from hops (found in supplements like Kaprex by Metagenics, available through health care professionals), turmeric (*Curcuma longa*) or isolated curcumin with piperine (a black pepper extract) for improved absorption, bee propolis extracts with caffeic acid phenethyl ester (CAPE), and supplements containing boswellia (*Boswellia serrata*) resin extract. There are many other anti-inflammatory supplements. Work with an experienced nutritionist or integrative medicine physician to find the supplements that are best for you.

Anti-inflammatory medical foods. These are powders containing amino acids and supplements that can be used as a meal replacement. Examples are UltraInflamX PLUS 360 by Metagenics and AIMforwellbeing Inflammation Support by Ortho Molecular Products (both available only through health care professionals).

Healing therapies. Once again, the healing therapies referenced in the Wired and Tired section become an even more important part of your journey toward a return to health. These include acupuncture, energy healing, and massage or other body work.

Transforming Being Overwhelmed and Depleted

If you are overwhelmed and depleted because you're all the way at the right side of the Stress Curve, chances are good you're also ill. What can you do to speed your recovery?

Lifestyle. At this point, you need to be under the care of a physician. Everything we stated earlier about lifestyle becomes even more important. Once again, follow the steps outlined earlier in this chapter on how to deal with everyday stress. Only restorative exercise should be done at this phase. In other words, do not overexert yourself at the gym. You might think you need to get stronger to get past this phase, but what your body really needs is rest. Gentle yoga, tai chi, or qigong are all very helpful.

Body chemistry. If you are very depressed, you may need an antidepressant. You might also need testing and treatment for neurally mediated hypotension (NMH). Your thyroid may be sluggish. If this is the case, your TSH (thyroid-stimulating hormone) will be raised, but other thyroid hormones will be normal.

Nutritional supplements. Extract of rosemary leaf (*Rosmarinus officinalis*), selenium, zinc, bladder wrack or kelp (*Fucus vesiculosus*), and iodine can all help correct thyroid problems. To help with the fatigue, we use a combination of licorice root extract, ashwagandha, rehmannia, and Chinese yam (*Dioscorea polystachya*) extract. Licorice can make your blood pressure go up and should not be used if you already have high blood pressure. However, most people who are depleted and overwhelmed have low blood pressure.

Healing therapies. We have found that healing therapies have an irreplaceable role in your recovery. We have not found any conventional medical treatments that can do for you what integrative healing therapies offer. Therapies such ACE® (acupuncture, chiropractic, and energy healing) treatments and frequency specific microcurrent work well to restore normal function by restoring adrenal and thyroid function, balancing the autonomic and immune systems, and reducing inflammation.

Transformational Moments

Sometimes in life, we come to the proverbial crossroads, a place where we need to make a choice. We can go one way or the other, but we cannot stay the same. The problem needn't be one that concerns your health directly. It could be something that relates to work, relationships, finances, or some aspect of your life that suddenly careens out of control. We are suddenly faced with transformational moments.

Sometimes, transformational moments occur when we are listening to music, meditating, walking, or doing some activity when the thinking mind is essentially switched off. However, at other times, these moments occur when we feel overwhelmed.

A wonderful teacher once said to us, "Inherent in every problem is the solution. Inherent in every stressful situation is the energy required to overcome and transcend this same situation."

We don't choose transformational moments. Generally, they happen to us. They force us to think and look outside the box. There is no obvious solution, so we are forced to find a different way forward.

Seize the Transformational Moment

We have seen many patients harness the power of shock and stress and use it to recover and bounce back to a new and better level of being. Here are some tips for seizing your transformational moment:

1. **When you hit a transformational moment**, become aware of your emotions and feelings. Don't judge what you're feeling or try to label it.

2. **Pay attention to your senses.** A transformational moment can allow you to achieve a new state of being. Observe your sensations: your smells, tastes, sights, and sounds.

3. **Surrender to this feeling.** Learn to sink into it.

4. **Learn to transform the emotion.** Remember that e-motion = energy in motion. (Don't wallow in your emotion!)

5. **Allow yourself to transcend logic.** You may feel confused at first, but insight will develop.

6. **Consider adding acupuncture and energy healing.** These therapies can help you attain this new state of awareness.

7. **Lean on your faith and prayer if so moved.** They can be profoundly valuable for some in times of peak stress.

8. **Remember that a transformational moment is a process.** It is time-independent—it may occur in seconds, or it may take much longer.

9. **If you are having difficulty** coping, feeling out of control, or just plain not succeeding, seek professional help.

Get Well, Be Well and Stay Well!

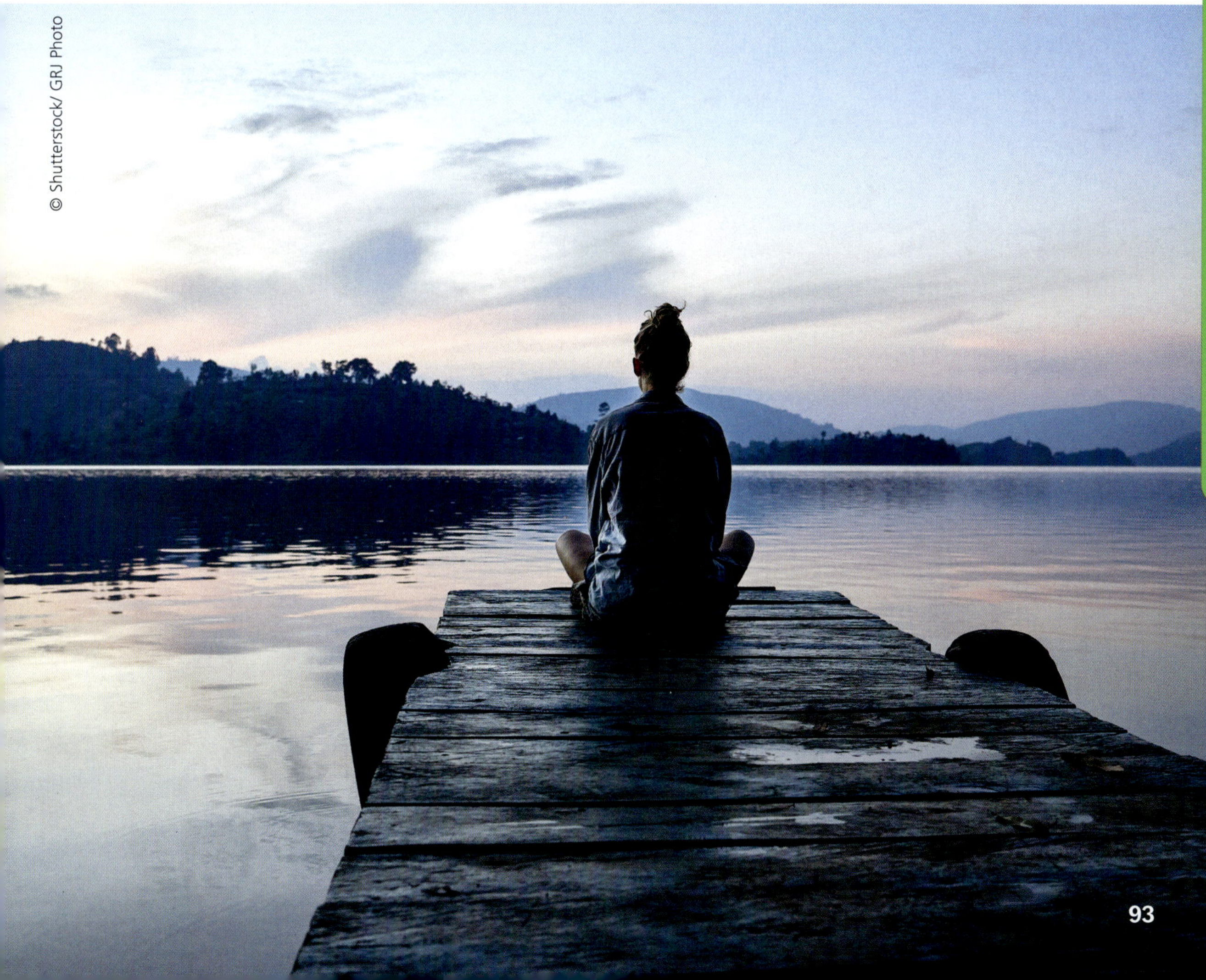

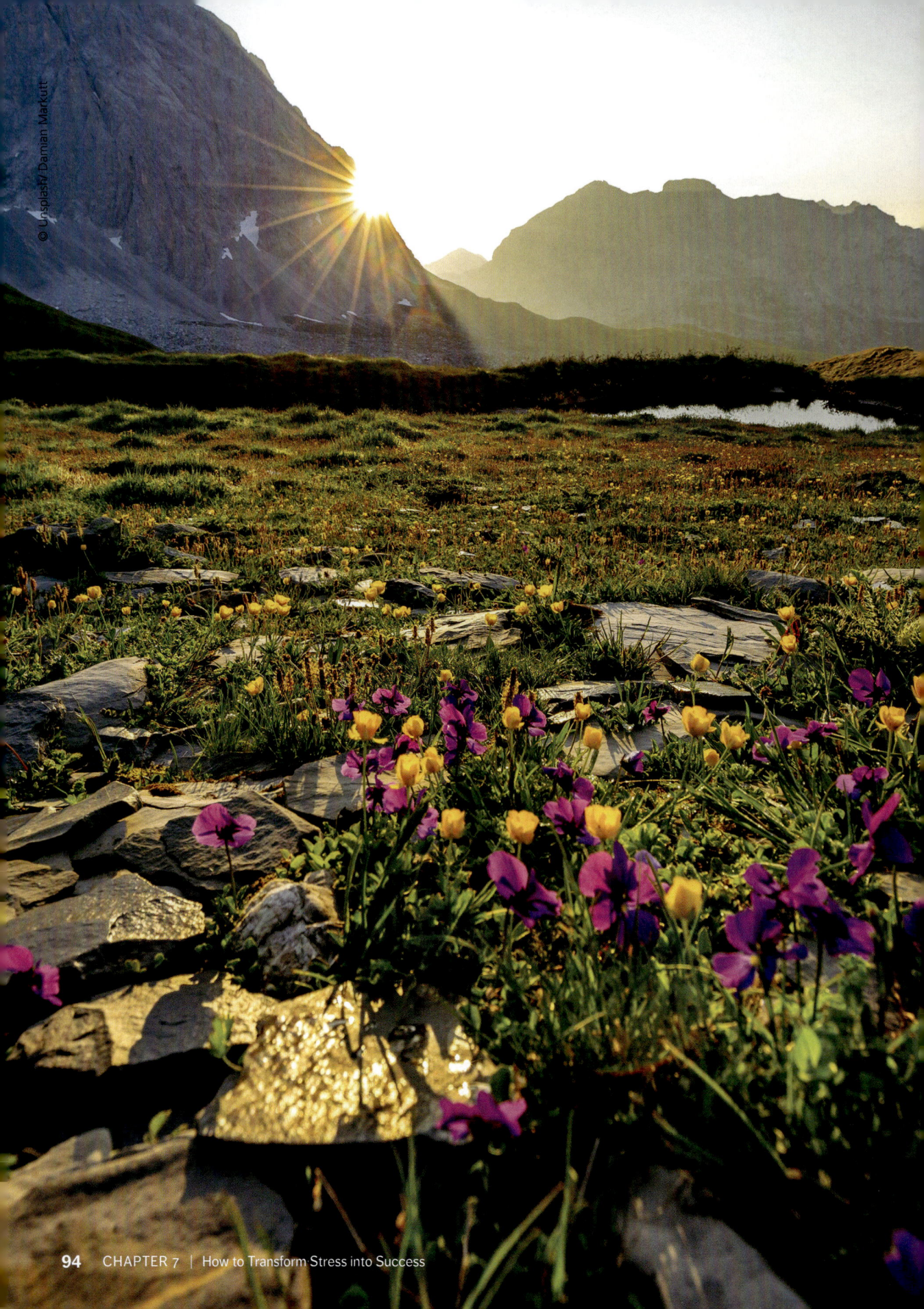

CHAPTER 8

Your Body on Fire

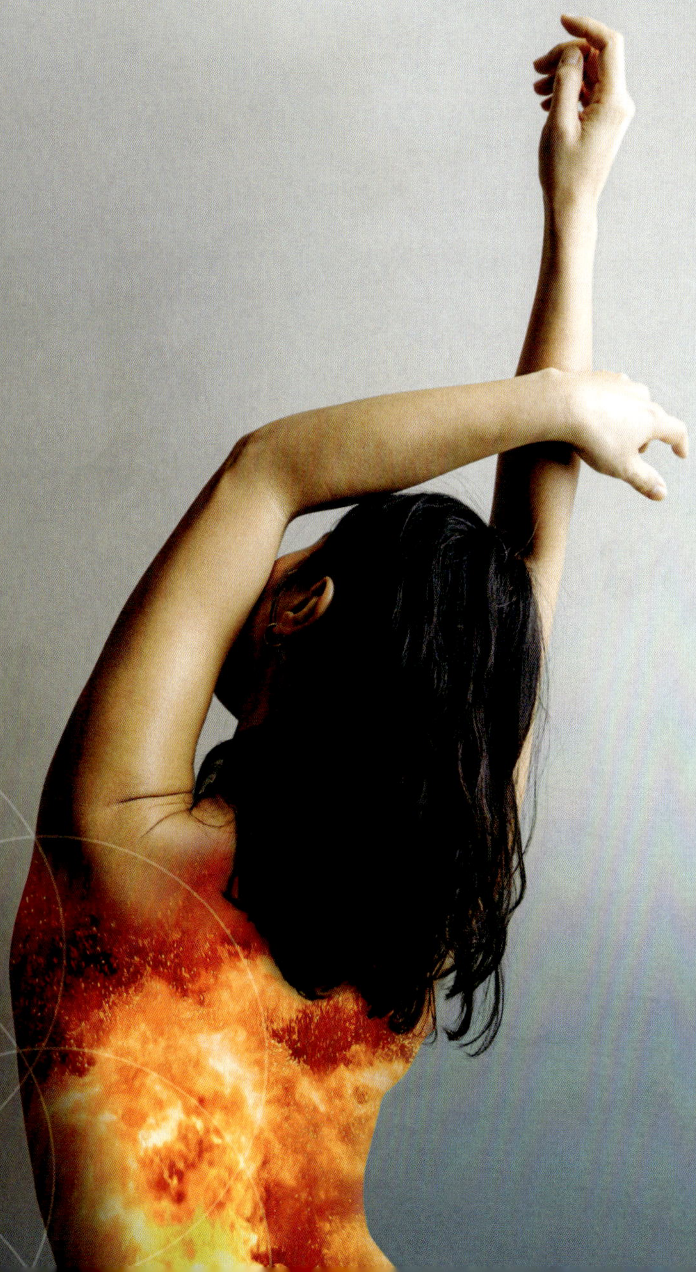

Metabolism and the Hidden Causes of Illness

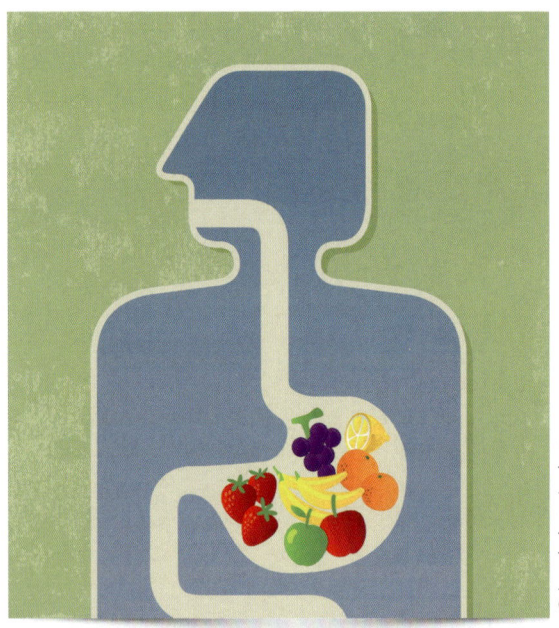

Your metabolism is the continuous sequence of chemical reactions that happens in your body to keep you alive. It's what keeps your heart beating, your lungs breathing, your brain thinking, and your body repair functions operating normally. These processes allow us to grow, mend injuries, and recover from illness. They essentially comprise every aspect of the body's function. This is the miracle of nourishment—the process by which what we eat becomes part of our cells and tissues. Metabolism provides the energy for our bodies. It is essential for every breath and every move we make.

We view metabolism as the leverage point for improving the health of our patients. The key is to identify imbalances in metabolism during the pre-illness phase, before the damage is done, because once the disease process deepens, it becomes much more difficult to reverse. Functional and conventional lab tests provide the lens through which we can see how the body is functioning; with them, we can monitor metabolism and body chemistry to determine which systems are out of balance. With this approach, we can devise a strategy to restore normal function at the earliest opportunity.

The Troublesome Triad of Inflammation, Oxidation, and Degeneration

Inflammation: The Body on Fire

To understand the ravages of aging and disease, let's look at the body's response to injury or infection. In both cases, the immune system responds by ramping up the process of inflammation. Signs of acute inflammation include redness, swelling, pain, and fever or heat. When you develop a fever during a viral or bacterial illness that affects your whole body, your body is turning on its defense mechanisms. That is also the case with the localized swelling, redness, pain, and warmth you experience when you sprain your ankle or cut yourself. In most cases, inflammation is a sign that the body's immune system is working efficiently to defend itself against foreign invaders.

When inflammation is chronic, however, it can be damaging to the body. This is because the inflammatory response releases many chemicals that affect the whole body. If you're getting over a cold, which most people do in a few days, the inflammatory response doesn't have much of a long-term impact. But if you have a chronic illness such as gum disease or diabetes, or are under chronic stress, your whole body is constantly exposed to these inflammatory substances. That's when painful chronic conditions such as arthritis, ulcers, colitis, asthma, and eczema can develop.

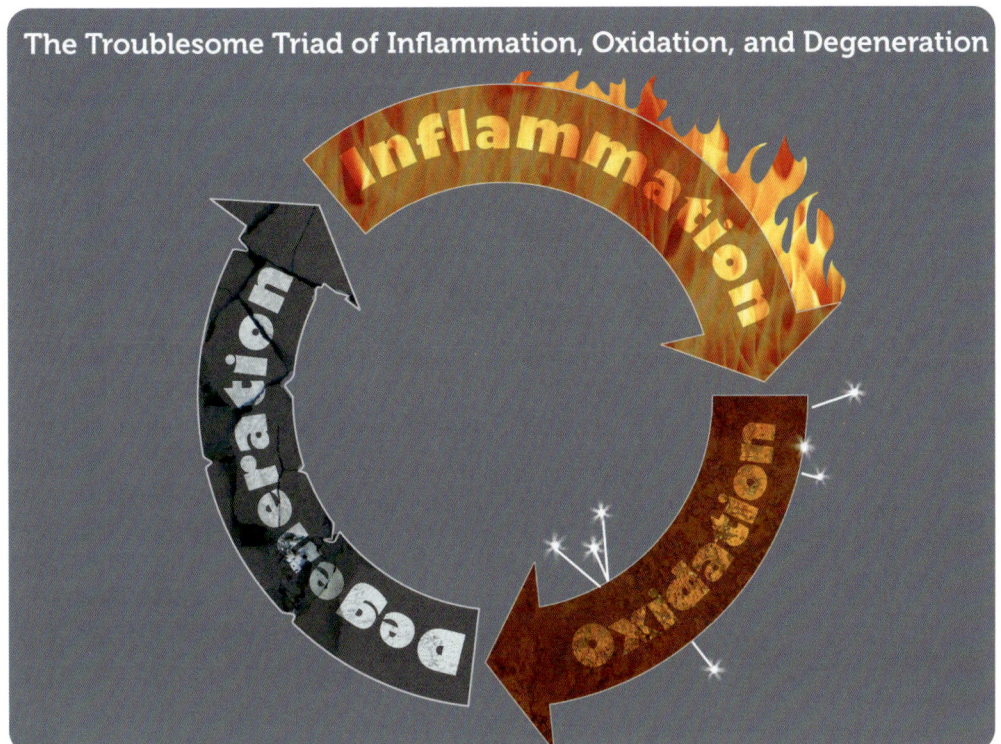

FIGURE 8.1 | Inflammation, Oxidation, and Degeneration

We now know that inflammation is also associated with many other major diseases, such as heart disease, cancer, and degenerative neurological disorders such as Alzheimer's disease.

Autoimmune conditions, such as multiple sclerosis and thyroid disease, are a different aspect of this process. With autoimmune illnesses, the immune function goes haywire, and the body seems to be raging out of control, attacking itself rather than the foreign molecules.

Inflammation and Infection: The Inflammatory Cascade

Acute inflammation is usually a good thing when it is associated with any type of injury or infection. Once the immune system recognizes an infection, the body begins producing chemicals called cytokines that signal a state of red alert. As the call goes out, these messenger chemicals course through the bloodstream, recruiting infection-fighting immune cells and launching an immune artillery. This shift to a state of emergency is referred to as the inflammatory cascade.

Our body always tries to maintain harmony. So, if there is an on switch for acute inflammation, there is also an off switch to put out the fire. This process is also performed by cytokines. Some cytokines drive (upregulate) inflammation; others switch off (downregulate) the inflammatory process, putting out the fire.

Lingering Inflammation

Chronic inflammation acts like a simmering fire that burns in our bodies, stimulating a cascade of chemical reactions that can destroy cells and compromise tissues over time. Inflammation can either occur locally or spread throughout the body. When inflammation occurs within a specific area or organ, it is described with a term ending in the Latin suffix "-itis." For instance, gastritis refers to inflamed gastric tissue in the stomach. Localized inflammation can lead to further disease. As an example, we know that at least 40 percent of stomach cancer is associated with the chronic inflammation caused by gastric ulcers.

Inflammation can also occur throughout the entire body. Systemic, low-grade inflammation can, over time, result in widespread disease. Coronary artery disease and strokes were once thought to be linked primarily to high cholesterol, but new studies show that inflammation within the arteries can be just as responsible for blocked arteries as elevated cholesterol. Chronic inflammation has also been associated with cancer, Alzheimer's disease and neurological disorders, insulin resistance and diabetes, and asthma and allergies.

When your cells are constantly exposed to inflammatory cytokines and other damaging natural chemicals, you can't switch off the inflammatory response. In the long run, these factors cause chronic diseases.

Dietary Causes of Chronic Inflammation

Because chronic inflammation can have a devastating effect on the body, it's important to understand what can trigger it.

Research over the past few decades has linked chronic inflammation to functional impairment of many metabolic processes, including digestion and detoxification. When these metabolic systems aren't working correctly, chronic inflammation can result.

When diagnosing an illness caused by chronic inflammation, we often start by looking at what the patient is eating. Unfortunately, the Standard American Diet is filled with foods that cause inflammation. Saturated fats, trans fats, and high sugar in the diet cause higher blood levels of an inflammatory chemical called arachidonic acid. (Many nonsteroidal anti-inflammatory drugs, such as aspirin and ibuprofen, work by counteracting this chemical.) Processed foods, junk foods, lunch meats, hot dogs, and sausages are filled with chemicals such as nitrates that promote chronic inflammation and disease. These foods are also largely lacking in fiber. In addition, many people have antibodies to certain foods that can aggravate a chronically inflamed state.

Good Fats, Bad Fats

We hear the low-fat message so often that we forget our bodies need dietary fat—the good kind, that is.

Good fats include omega-3 fatty acids from fish oil, flax seeds, and nuts, which tend to be anti-inflammatory. Other good fats include oleic acid, found in olive oil, and monounsaturated fats found in avocados.

Bad fats, on the other hand, are saturated fats (found in meat and dairy), and foods high in pro-inflammatory omega-6 fatty acids. Not surprisingly, fast food, junk food, and prepared foods such as frozen meals are high in omega-6 fatty acids. Heavily processed vegetable oils such as corn oil also contain high amounts of omega-6 fatty acids.

The ratio of omega-3 to omega-6 fats can play an important role in driving inflammation. Today, our diet tends to have a predominance of omega-6 fats. Thirty years ago, most eggs had a ratio of omega-3 to omega-6 of 1:6. Now that ratio is more like 1:15, or more! The same egg is more pro-inflammatory for a few reasons. The chicken's feed has changed (for the worse), and the chicken is stressed, cooped up in a cage with lights constantly turned on. Similarly, our highly processed diet can trigger chronic inflammation in our own bodies.

Inflammation and Weight Gain

Weight gain often plays a role in systemic inflammation, especially if it takes the form of fat around the belly, resulting in the so-called apple body shape. We tend to think of fat as inert tissue that just stores excess calories, but it is actually fairly active. Among other things, fat tissue produces inflammatory cytokines. This inflammatory effect tends to increase the propensity to gain weight, which then creates further inflammation. It's a vicious cycle that leads to many problems we see today that occur in clusters, such as type 2 diabetes and Alzheimer's disease (sometimes now even referred to as type 3 diabetes) or cholesterol problems and coronary artery disease.

Lab Tests for Inflammation

We can easily test your level of inflammation. One way to measure inflammation is to use conventional blood tests for a marker known as high-sensitivity C-reactive protein, or hs-CRP. This is a nonspecific test—it tells us that a patient is inflamed but not why. Other lab work can test for levels of immune system markers such as tumor necrosis factor alpha (TNF-α); interleukins such as IL-6, IL-16, and IL-β1, the complement component C4a; transforming growth factor beta (TGF-β) and many more. An indirect way to test for inflammation is to look at the patient's omega-3 index by testing the ratio of omega-3 to omega-6 fatty acids in the blood. Newer tests are becoming available to test for cytokine abnormalities. By measuring these, we can see which part of the immune system is being activated. Then we can work backward and figure out why. In our office, the doctors continue to explore the best options on how to understand inflammation—where it is coming from, and how to switch it off.

Oxidative Stress: The Body Rusting

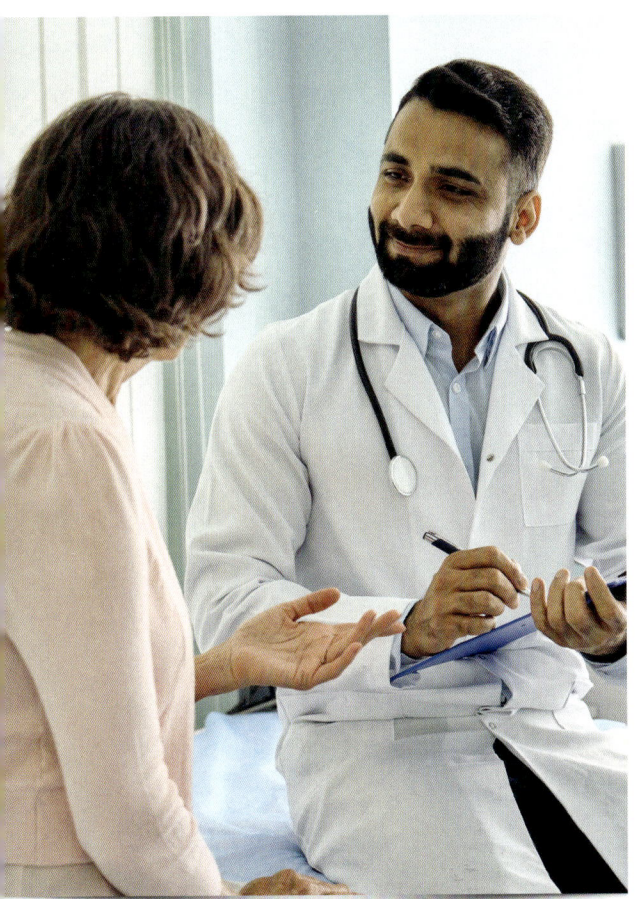

© Shutterstock / Ground Picture

Another primary contributor to aging and illness is oxidative stress, which might be described as the body "rusting." If you leave your car outside, unprotected and exposed to the elements, patches of rust can develop. Leave it out long enough, and the rust will eat into the structure and eventually corrode it. Similarly, our own bodies can rust from internal oxidation reactions. When cells burn glucose for fuel, or oxidize it, byproducts are produced, just as a car produces exhaust fumes from the gas it burns. In the human body, the exhaust fumes from oxidation are called free radicals. Free radicals act like chemical terrorists, making random attacks on cell membranes and other tissues, aging our bodies, and causing chronic illness and even cancer as they do so.

> He who takes medicine and neglects his diet wastes the skill of his doctors.
>
> **-- Chinese proverb**

Free radicals aren't just created when glucose gets oxidized. They are also natural byproducts of fighting infection or of chronic inflammation. They also occur with any kind of extreme exposure, such as overexposure to sunlight or ultraviolet rays or by the exertion of extreme sports, such as marathons and triathlons. Oxidative stress also results from exposure to chemicals, including food additives, pesticides, and preservatives, as well as organic and chemical toxins that have been found in the air and tap water of many major cities. In general, chronic stress increases oxidative stress on the body.

Fortunately, because free radicals are a normal part of metabolism, the body is well equipped to handle them. The human body has plenty of natural antioxidant chemicals, such as glutathione and vitamin C, that are designed to corral the free radicals and neutralize them before they can do much damage. At the same time, just as inflammation can be beneficial, so can oxidation, especially when the body is defending against bacteria, toxins, chemicals, or cancerous cells. For example, when fighting off viruses, the immune system uses oxygen as a form of chemical warfare to blow up these microbes.

Once again, the body has an elegant system of checks and balances. So, while oxidation can be useful to the body, there are times when the body's antioxidant mechanisms can't keep up with all the free radicals due to poor diet, illness, vitamin deficiencies, excess stress load, or other factors. It is during these times that oxidative stress is not held in check, and we can develop degeneration, cancer, and chronic illness.

Free radicals can't be easily measured directly. Instead, we can measure oxidative stress indirectly using functional lab tests.

Simply looking at a person can help you understand the level of oxidative stress they are under. We have all seen people who look years older than their biological age. This is often because their lifestyle has placed their bodies under high oxidative stress. Smoking, for example, ages the skin. Your body uses a lot of its vitamin C to counteract the toxins in cigarette smoke. That cuts back on the amount available to make collagen, the protein that supports your skin and keeps it flexible. The result is wrinkles.

Degeneration

Our own experience living in different cultures around the world has shown us that aging and degeneration don't have to go together. People who eat a traditional diet of mostly unprocessed foods, maintain low stress levels, and are physically active tend to age more slowly, retaining their youthful appearance and good joint health. They go gray later in life (sometimes decades later), and their skin retains its natural resilience. They also experience fewer degenerative diseases, such as heart attacks, strokes, and cancer, compared with their counterparts of a similar age and income level in industrial societies. This phenomenon is documented by author Dan Buettner in his book, *The Blue Zones*. Buettner studied places in the world where higher percentages of people enjoy remarkably long, full lives and tried to pin down what makes them different.

We all want to know how we can do this, too. How can we lower inflammation and oxidative stress? How can we learn to balance our metabolic processes so that we make ourselves more resilient to illness and more likely to age well? Let's look at some other parts of your metabolism.

Inflammation and Heart Disease

Chronic, low-grade inflammation contributes to heart disease by contributing to atherosclerosis—cholesterol-laden plaques that build up inside the arteries that nourish the heart. Plaques make the coronary arteries thicken and lose elasticity. Your immune system thinks the plaques are a foreign invader and responds with inflammation. In a complex process, immune cells are drawn to the plaques to remove the cholesterol and wall off the area of the artery wall. Sometimes, however, the walled-off area of plaque ruptures, spilling the contents into the artery, where they mix with blood and form a clot. Another name for a coronary artery blocked by a blood clot is heart attack. We'll go into this in more detail in chapter 17 on heart disease.

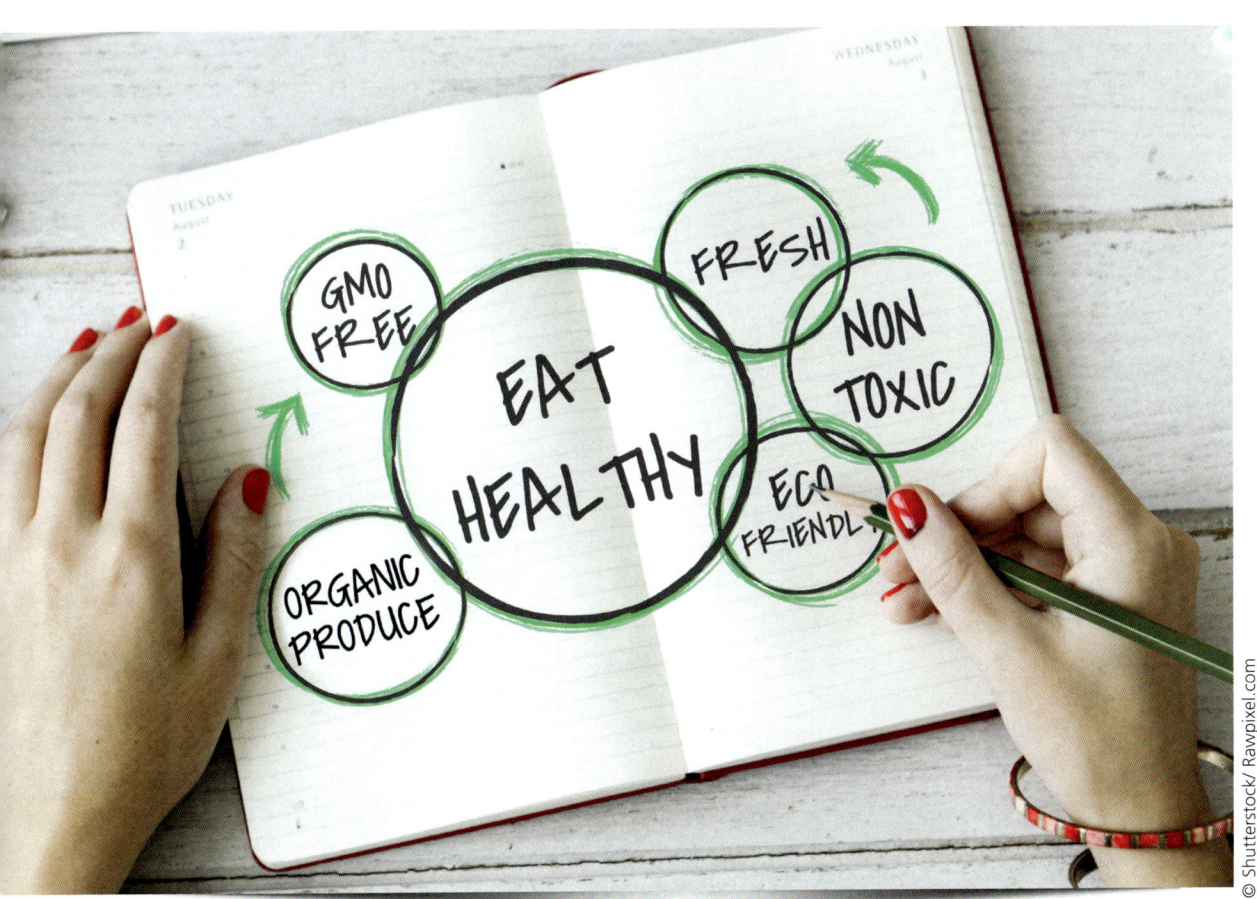

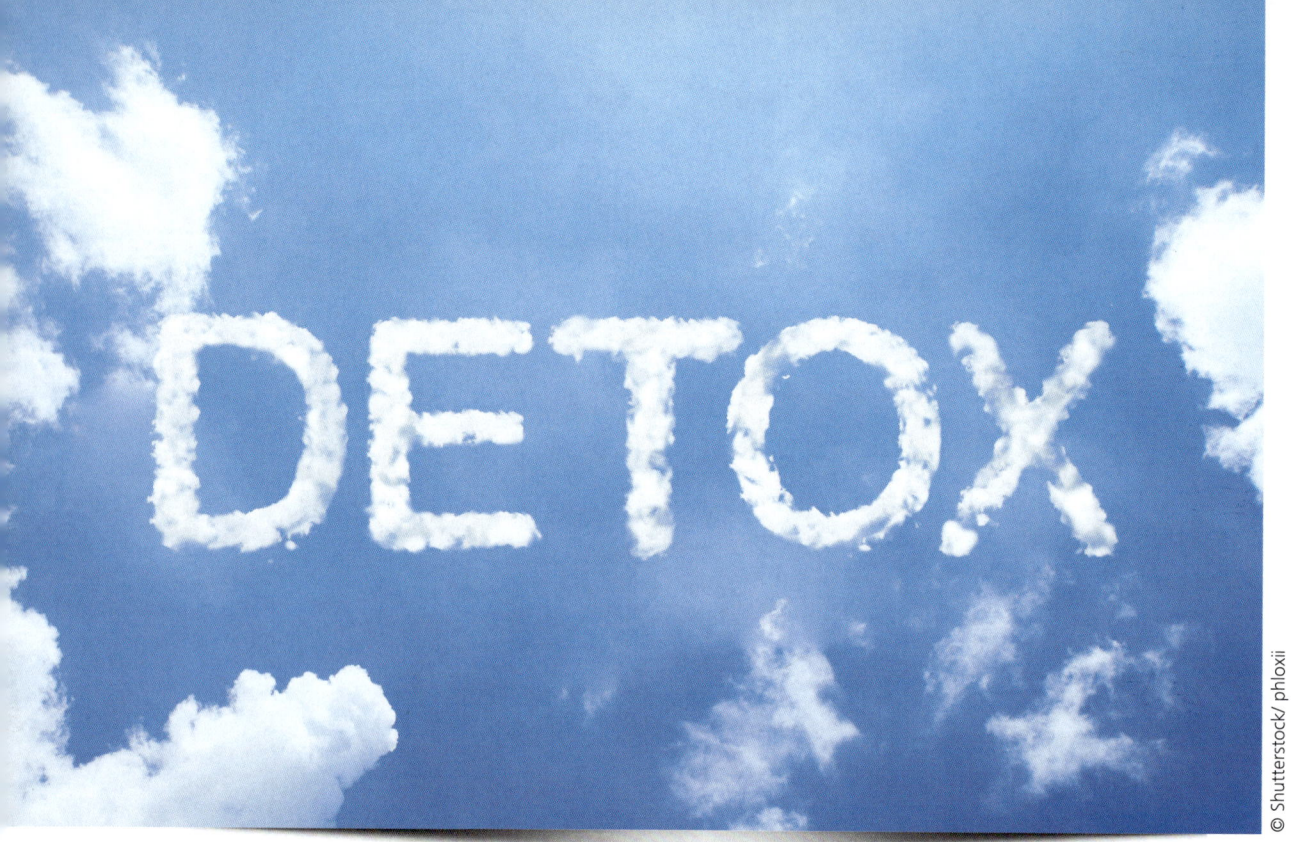

Detoxification:
The Body's Self-Purification

Your detoxification systems play an important role in your metabolism, reducing your risk of chronic illness by clearing your body of toxins.

Detoxification is another misunderstood aspect of health. Although toxins are removed from the body through the kidneys, colon, skin, and lungs, primary detoxification occurs in the liver, where toxins are broken down or degraded. When the liver's detoxification system is fully functional, it filters out many types of toxins recognized by the body as potentially harmful. This process disposes of toxins from our environment such as chemicals and drugs foreign to the body, which are known as xenobiotics. We are constantly exposed to toxins in tap water, pesticides, herbicides, food additives, vehicle and industrial emissions, environmental pollutants and prescription, non-prescription and recreational drugs, as well as through occupational exposures. Toxins also occur naturally within the body as byproducts of metabolism and include our own hormones, which also need to be detoxified and excreted.

Common Biotoxins

Exposure to biotoxins in the environment can cause cancer, autoimmune disease, and neurodegenerative disease.

- **Pesticides, herbicides** and **fertilizers**, including chemicals such as atrazine and glyphosate (Roundup®)
- **Solvents** and **VOCs** (volatile organic compounds), gases emitted from new carpets, paints, air fresheners, cleaning products and other sources
- **Heavy metals** such as mercury, lead, aluminum, and cadmium
- **Plastics** containing bisphenol A (BPA)

- **Molds** such as a*spergillus, penicillium, aflatoxin,* and *Cladosporium,* but especially black mold or *Stachybotrys chartarum*, also known as *Stachybotrys atra*
- **Biotoxins,** which can also come from infections, including from tick-borne diseases such as Lyme disease, babesiosis, ehrlichiosis, and from viruses such as Epstein-Barr, cytomegalovirus, and coxsackie virus

The list of biotoxins is quite extensive and unfortunately keeps getting longer! When working with a physician who can help with toxic overloads, it's important to try to narrow down this list by figuring out which are causing your problem(s), so you can receive more accurate treatment.

Symptoms of Impaired Detoxification

We may consume the best nutrition in the world, but if our body's self-cleaning detoxification systems aren't working, toxins can build up and put us at risk for illness. These symptoms of impaired detoxification are usually nonspecific but include the following:

- Exaggerated or altered response to medications
- Increasing sensitivity to medications or chemical exposure
- Increasing sensitivity to odors
- Multiple food sensitivities
- Chronic fatigue and muscle pain
- Impaired cognition, including memory problems and confusion
- Unusual tingling and numbness patterns
- A tendency to dysautonomia
- Recurrent ankle edema (swelling) for no obvious reason
- Hives; dry skin
- Recurrent illness
- A tendency to bloating and weight gain even though you watch your diet
- Dark circles under the eyes
- Canker sores
- Hormonal problems including PMS

If you're suffering from some of these symptoms, a history of exposure to potentially toxic chemicals at home or work may be a clue to investigate further. You might be suffering from an overload of toxins. These may include pesticides, herbicides, and many petrochemicals found in yard chemicals, dry cleaning agents, and car exhaust fumes. If you have a significant number of amalgam fillings or have had synthetic materials put in your body, such as implants or prosthetics, consider if your symptoms started within two years of having these procedures done. If you're on multiple medications, they may be interfering with your body's detoxification systems.

Detoxification Malfunction

Our detoxification processes are vulnerable to overload for a few reasons. Some of us have variants in our detoxification genes that simply make our detoxification processes slower than average. In our experience, patients may have variants that make them hypersensitive to alcohol, drugs, and chemicals. They simply take longer to metabolize them. They may feel woozy from a small amount of alcohol or develop side effects on a regular dose of medication.

Our detoxification systems may malfunction due to exposure to a wide range of chemicals in our environment and even our food. For example, certain drugs, herbicides, pesticides, and even charred meats can interfere with our ability to detoxify. When our detoxifying systems aren't working well, they create reactive intermediate products—byproducts of detoxification that are not fully broken down. They are highly toxic to our DNA, and may contribute to creating chronic disease, premature aging, and some forms of cancer.

Heavy metals such as mercury and lead can have a deleterious effect on detoxification systems, with an eventual impact on the health of cells and tissues. Although heavy metals aren't usually toxic when present in the body at low doses, the accumulation of multiple toxins in low doses can be harmful. Studies on rats showed a hundredfold increase in toxicity when mercury and lead in low doses were combined.

The same amplification of toxicity is likely to be true of exposure to multiple toxins from the environment. A low dose of a single toxin has little or no effect on most of us. It's the combination of multiple toxins in low doses that finally overwhelms our systems. Young children and the frail elderly generally have less resilience to the impact of multiple toxins. Children have immature detoxification systems, and the elderly may have systems that are compromised by the deterioration of aging and a lifetime of cumulative toxic exposure.

We may be exposed to heavy metals through eating fish tainted with mercury (usually bigger fish such as shark, swordfish, farm-raised salmon, tilefish, mackerel, grouper, sea bass, and tuna), mercury-containing products, mercury-emitting coal plants, and leaking amalgam dental fillings. Lead exposure may stem from lead paint used in houses built prior to 1977 or lead in water pipes. Many products imported from China have been tainted with lead or cadmium. Aluminum exposure may be due to aluminum-containing underarm deodorants, antacids, and pots and pans.

We're also now constantly exposed to microplastics—plastic debris less than five millimeters in length, or about the size of a sesame seed. Microplastics come from a variety of sources, including from larger plastic debris that degrades into smaller and smaller pieces and from microbeads, very tiny pieces of plastic added as exfoliants to health and beauty products, such as some cleansers and toothpastes. Tiny microplastic particles float in the air and easily pass through water filtration systems. They're now everywhere, which means we're exposed to them all the time, including in our food. The chemicals in microplastics are linked to a range of health issues, including reproductive problems, obesity, and developmental delays in children.

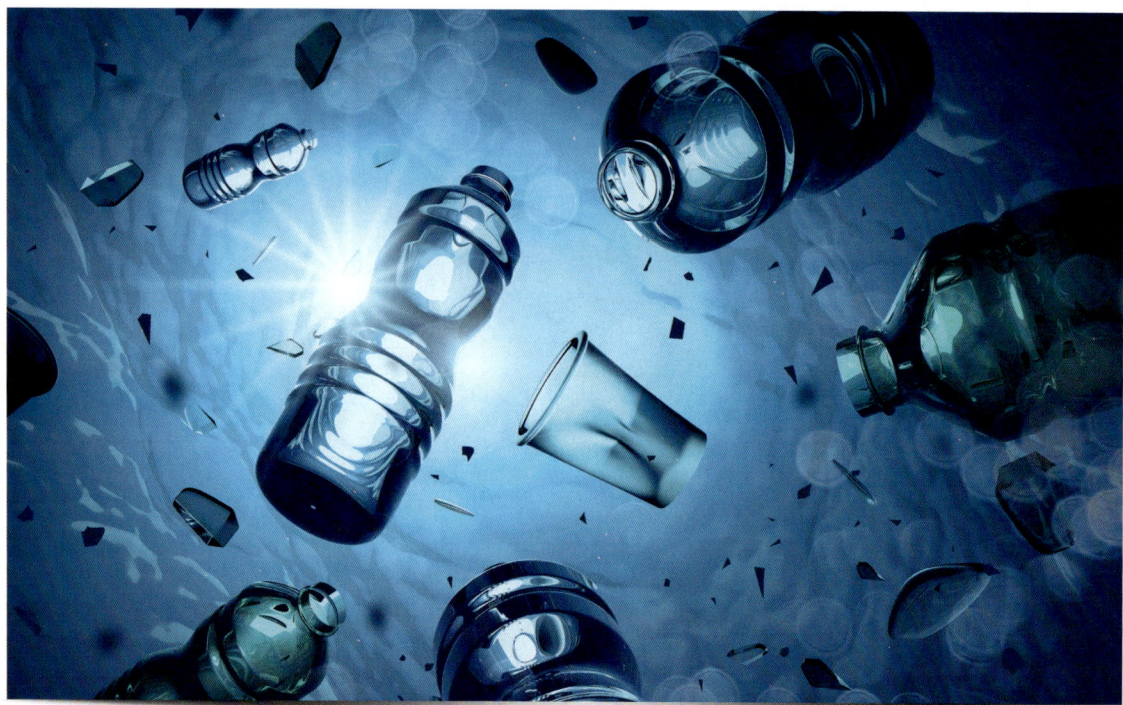

How Your Body Detoxifies

Phase I. Initial detoxification occurs in the liver, where environmental toxins, many drugs and even hormones go through the steps of a detoxification pathway referred to as phase I. The cytochrome P450 enzyme system in phase I is crucial for making the pathways work efficiently. After going through phase I, many toxins are neutralized and are then excreted through the gut into the feces. A positive balance of good bacteria in the gut makes this part of the detoxification process move smoothly. Other neutralized toxins are expelled through the kidneys into the urine. Toxins that can't be neutralized just by the phase I system pass through the phase II enzyme system and then pass out of the body through the feces or urine.

Phase I enzymes are supported by foods such as green tea, fresh coffee, and cruciferous vegetables (e.g., broccoli, cauliflower, brussels sprouts, kale, cabbage, and bok choy). Normal genetic variation in phase I enzymes can affect how well we detoxify.

Phase II. If a particular xenobiotic, metabolic byproduct, drug, or foreign chemical isn't adequately broken down by the phase I system, it becomes a reactive intermediary product, which can actually be more toxic than the original substance. Reactive intermediary products can cause DNA damage; over time, they may even cause cancer or chronic disease. Adequate levels of vitamin D and antioxidants can provide crucial protection against DNA damage from reactive intermediary products. But to remove the reactive intermediary products, your liver passes them through a second series of processes—the phase II enzyme system—to neutralize them and then excrete them through the gut or kidneys.

During phase II detoxification, enzyme systems can be supported by beneficial factors found in cruciferous vegetables, garlic, onions, artichokes, and whey. Once again, genetic variations may cause the system to detoxify at a faster or slower rate than normal. In fact, research has shown that the rate of detoxification can vary as much as thirty-five–fold from one person to the next.

Phase III. The next part of detoxification occurs via cell membranes all over the body. Although it is not officially called this, we refer to this aspect of detoxification as phase III. Cell membranes are composed of fats. An inadequate amount of healthy fats in the diet can result in brittle and inflexible cell membranes with limited capacity to take in nutrients or expel wastes. As a result, toxins may become trapped inside the body's cells. Poor cellular detoxification has been implicated in cancer and a myriad of other diseases—another reason good fats are so important in our diet.

Phase IV. In phase IV detoxification, neutralized toxins are excreted through the gut or the kidneys. In the GI tract, the disposal of toxins is facilitated by a positive balance of good bacteria. In the kidneys, the urine must be somewhat alkaline to be excreted optimally. Beneficial flora and a slightly alkaline balance in the body both have implications for the importance of diet in supporting healthy detoxification.

Eating to Detoxify

Many foods can help our detoxification processes. These are mainly vegetables and fruits (starting to sound familiar?). The best detoxifying foods are cruciferous vegetables such as broccoli (which is superb), cauliflower, broccoli rabe, brussels sprouts, kale, cabbage, collard greens, kohlrabi, mustard, rutabaga, turnips, arugula, radishes, wasabi, Chinese cabbage, bok choy, and watercress. Also helpful for detoxification are artichokes, onions, shallots, garlic, green tea, and fresh coffee. Most people don't eat enough of these foods, making them vulnerable to self-pollution.

We used to be skeptical about detox diets. Faddish detox diets, often endorsed by celebrities, are also often very unhealthy and ineffective. However, we've learned that following a detox diet for a short period does have some definite benefits. The goals of an ideal detox diet are:

- Stop input of all outside toxins as much as possible.
- Predominantly eat vegetables, with some fruit.
- Eat small amounts of clean protein if needed.
- Add herbs that encourage phase I and phase II detoxification.
- Add fish oil to help with what we call phase III detoxification.
- Drink lots of water to flush the kidneys, adding herbal support for this.
- Eat plenty of fiber from fresh fruits and vegetables to ensure regular bowel movements.
- Consider taking prebiotic and probiotic supplements.
- Ensure good skin elimination with sweating or far infrared saunas. (Far infrared saunas allow you to sweat out toxins without overheating your body, which may be problematic when you are fasting or on a restricted detox diet.)
- Ensure good fresh air for lung elimination.
- Ensure good sleep, as this is when the body detoxifies best.

Many years ago, we decided to test the concept of a detox diet by asking all our staff to join us on a three-week detox program. We monitored how everyone felt during this time.

We believed we already followed a pretty good diet so doing the detox program would be easy for us. But two days later, Sandi and I sat on the couch with severe headaches, feeling extremely lethargic. The caffeine withdrawal had really hit us! I remember saying, "There is no way I will ever ask another human being to do this." Then came the cravings for fast foods and sugar. Then, on the fourth day, a remarkable thing happened—our taste buds really kicked in. We began to crave and enjoy the natural flavors abundant in fresh veggies and fruit, shunning the taste of sweetened and artificial flavors. Sleep was a wondrous rejuvenating experience. We had vivid dreams and awoke feeling refreshed and vital. Our mental clarity improved. Our skin glowed!

Our colleagues had similar experiences. Their blood pressure and blood sugar also

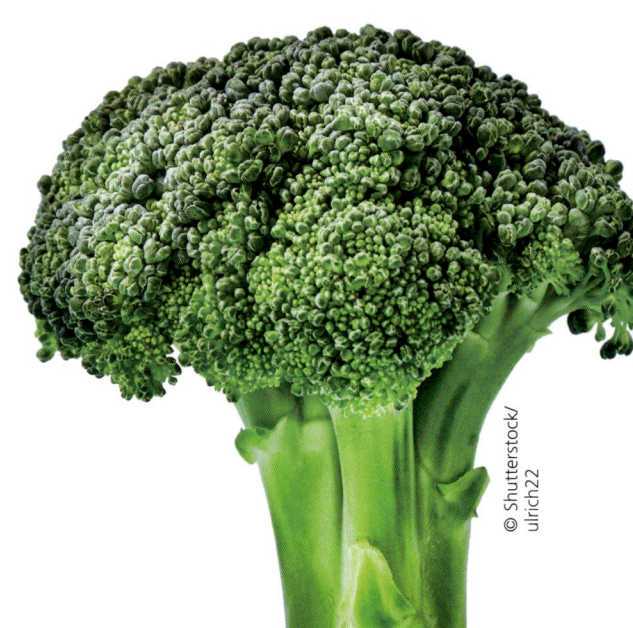

normalized. My LDL (bad cholesterol) dropped from 129 to 60 in three weeks. My HDL also dropped 20 percent, which is normal with detox diets.

We finished the detox diet with a radically new way of looking at the effect of food on our systems, promising ourselves we would never go back to the bad stuff. But alas, life happens. Birthdays, Thanksgiving, holiday parties—it's all too easy to fall back into your old, bad eating pattern. That's why we suggest doing a detox once or twice a year to reset your metabolism and your emotional and spiritual outlook.

Detox diets can be problematic, however. We have seen patients with chronic constipation get bowel obstruction. Some people feel so terrible in the first two days they can't continue. This is a common problem because your liver is dumping stored toxins. Fortunately, this phase usually passes quickly and most of our patients really enjoy the sensory awareness that reawakens during the next phase of the detox diet. The body starts to prefer natural tastes and odors, shunning those of fast foods and artificial chemicals. Sleep becomes more natural, and energy becomes more abundant. This is often interspersed with short periods of cravings as your body clears away old toxic loads.

Detoxing is a valuable process, but it can be challenging. We suggest you discuss detoxing with your doctor before continuing. For more information, see Chapter 9.

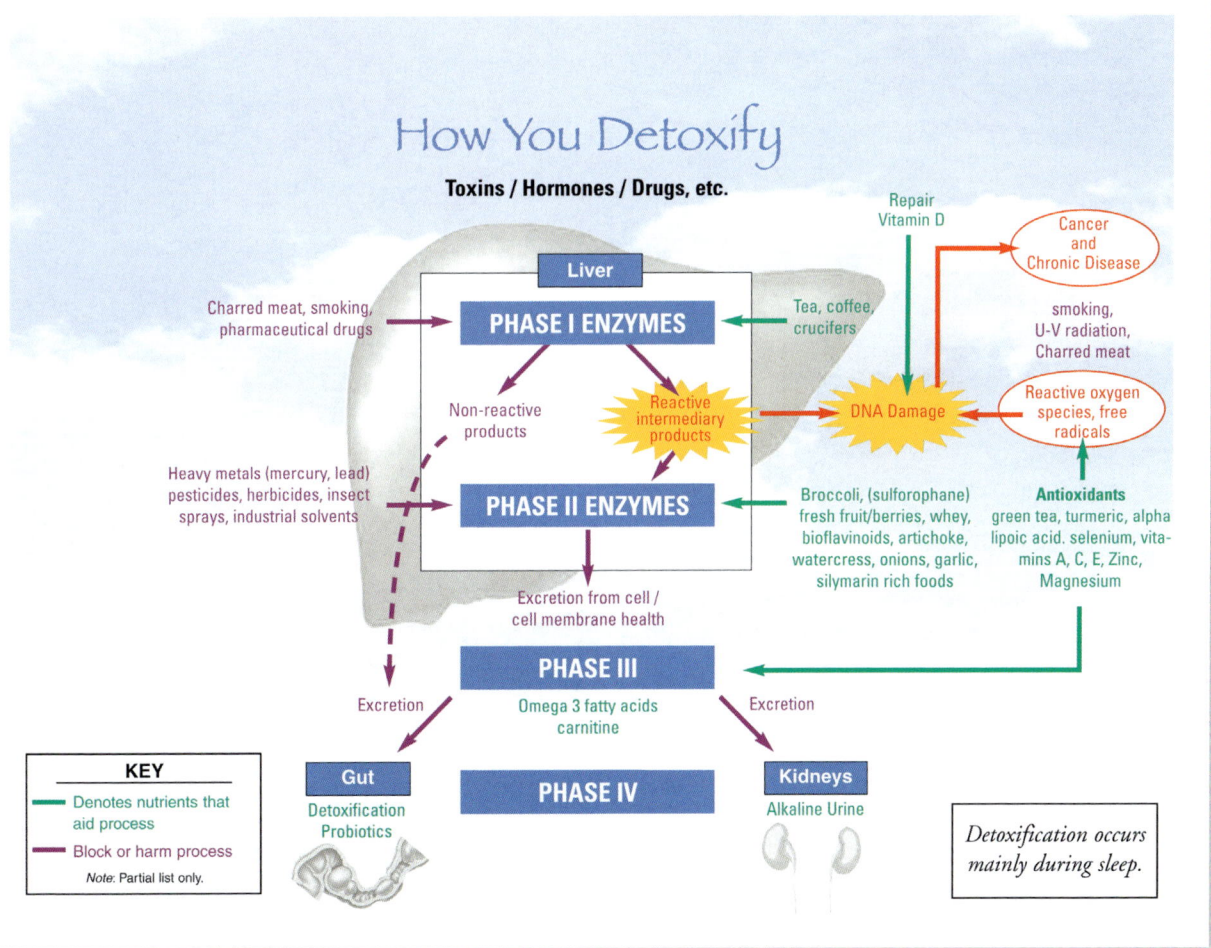

FIGURE 8.2 | How You Detoxify

Mitochondrial Dysfunction

Mitochondria are small organelles in every cell that create packets of ATP—the form of energy that fuels your body. When your mitochondria can't produce enough energy, it affects how your organs function and how you feel. Your batteries are literally flat. You feel exhausted and sick.

Mitochondria have their own DNA and genetic programming apart from the DNA in the nucleus of the cell. Some rare mitochondrial diseases are genetic in origin and are characterized by progressively worsening symptoms involving multiple organs or organ systems. These are sometimes fatal diseases with names like autosomal dominant optic atrophy, carnitine deficiency, complex I, II, III, IV, and V deficiency, Leigh syndrome, mitochondrial encephalopathy or myopathy, and others which usually need diagnosis and treatment at sophisticated medical centers dedicated to these diseases.

Mitochondrial dysfunction is different. It happens when the mitochondria don't work as well as they should due to another disease or condition. Mitochondrial dysfunction causes diffuse, widespread, and hard-to-diagnose problems. They can be incapacitating but don't necessarily lead to death. Whenever we have chronic disease, we have mitochondrial dysfunction. And vice versa—when we have mitochondrial dysfunction, we get chronic disease.

Mitochondrial dysfunction can result in fatigue, muscle weakness, cognitive issues, vision and hearing problems, acid reflux, diarrhea and constipation, breathing problems, and even seizures. Unfortunately, mitochondrial dysfunction is extremely difficult to correctly diagnose. Often we can diagnose it only by excluding other causes.

The mitochondria provide cellular energy, but they're also key players in thousands of reactions throughout the body. They're important in protein, carbohydrate, and fat metabolism; hormone, cholesterol, heme (blood), and neurotransmitter synthesis and metabolism; detoxification, especially of ammonia; and apoptosis. The mitochondria generate large quantities of free radicals, which need to be quenched by our antioxidant system. It is when the antioxidant system goes awry that we begin drowning in our own waste.

Mitochondrial dysfunction is a major underlying reason—though not the only one—for developing long COVID and myalgic encephalomyelitis/chronic fatigue syndrome (ME/CFS). We use antioxidant supplements to treat mitochondrial dysfunction, but we don't have a magic bullet for curing it. We do know that the best way to make healthy new mitochondria is to exercise, but people with severe mitochondrial dysfunction often can't do this. Exercise causes post-exertional malaise, which leaves them completely exhausted and feeling even worse. The next best way to start to heal your mitochondria is to lower your glucose intake. Once again, a good diet is the best solution! Lifestyle measures such as avoiding extreme heat or cold, ensuring adequate sleep, and alleviating stress can help.

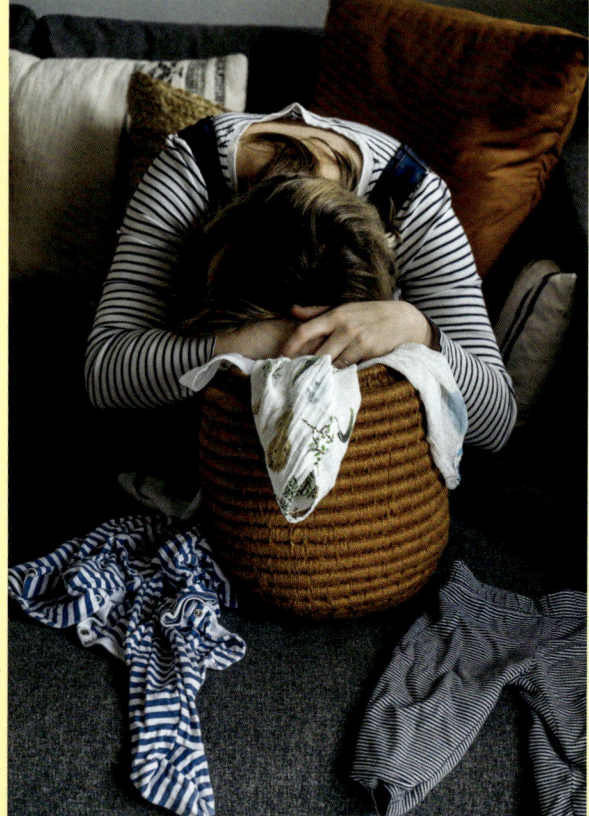

Unsplash/Monika Grabkowska

Cell Membrane Integrity

All cells in your body have a membrane that separates the interior of the cell from the outside environment. The cell membrane is semipermeable and regulates the transport of materials entering and exiting the cell.

When the cell membrane is damaged, the contents of the cell spill into the intercellular space and blood and cause havoc. A good example is the liver. Every day, some cells in the liver die; at the same time, the liver regenerates itself with new cells. This is a normal part of the liver's constant self-cleaning and renewal process. When the liver is working well, we see a normal range of the liver enzymes ALT (also called SGPT) and AST (also called SGOT) in the blood. If something goes wrong in the liver—it gets inflamed and causes hepatitis, for example—the cell membranes are damaged, more liver enzymes spill out, and the numbers for the enzymes in the blood skyrocket.

Cell membranes protect our cells and regulate how nutrients, hormones, and other cell signals get into the cell and how toxins get out. Maintaining the integrity of your cell membranes is important. The membranes are made of a lipid bilayer, sort of like a sandwich. Thin layers of lipids, or fats, form the "bread" of the sandwich, with a thin layer of protein between them as the "filling." Healthy cell membranes are strong but flexible and malleable. When cell membranes become dried out or inflexible, nutrients and cell signals can't get in properly, toxins can't get out, and ultimately the cells crack and explode, causing organ damage.

In general, polyunsaturated fats (good fats) are healing to the cell membrane, helping to keep it flexible and strong. Especially good are EPA and DHA, which we get from fish oil. Saturated fats, especially trans fats (now banned in many states) are toxic to cell membranes. Valuable as fish oil is, supplements may contain contaminants such as mercury and persistent organic pollutants. If you want to take a fish oil supplement, look for one that is highly purified. Your physician can check your omega-3 index with a blood test to know if you are getting enough EPA and DHA from your food and supplements.

Autophagy and Apoptosis

Autophagy, which literally means "self-eating," is the process your body uses to remove cells that aren't working well anymore because they contain old, worn-out, or damaged components or because they contain a virus or bacterium. These cells have become litter inside your body, slowing things up and keeping the cells from functioning properly. Autophagy is your body's cellular recycling system, a way of breaking down the old cells, reusing some components, and getting rid of leftover debris.

Efficient autophagy is key to good health. By quickly recognizing and getting rid of old cells that aren't working well anymore, autophagy makes space for new ones. Your autophagy ability is influenced by many factors, but particularly by your nutrition and your sleep. You need plenty of vitamin D, for example, to promote autophagy. Lowering your insulin level also promotes autophagy, as does increasing ketones. That's why intermittent fasting, which does both, can help prevent and heal illness and promotes longevity. Similarly, a deficiency of thiamine (vitamin B1) causes neurodegeneration, while thiamine supplements promote autophagy and help heal neurodegeneration.

A lot of autophagy occurs when you're asleep and your body can divert energy to cellular housekeeping. Getting enough quality sleep is important for autophagy throughout your body but particularly in your brain. When you're awake, your brain is highly active. When you sleep, it's less active and actually shrinks a bit. This allows cerebral spinal fluid to flow more easily throughout your brain and carry off both normal metabolic waste and the debris from old cells broken down by autophagy.

Apoptosis, also called programmed cell death, is the mechanism your body uses to get rid of cells that have been damaged beyond repair. The mechanism tells these cells to self-destruct. If apoptosis of a defective cell doesn't happen for some reason, this can lead to uncontrolled cell division– cancer.

Within your body, autophagy and apoptosis are in constant interplay to maintain homeostasis. Lifestyle, sleep, and nutrition are all vital elements for regulating the processes—more good reasons to focus on eating, living, and sleeping optimally to promote a good healthspan and a long lifespan.

You can Get Well, Be Well and Stay Well!

> " Wellness encompasses a healthy body, a sound mind, and a tranquil spirit. Enjoy the journey as you strive for wellness.
>
> **– Laurette Gagnon Beaulieu**

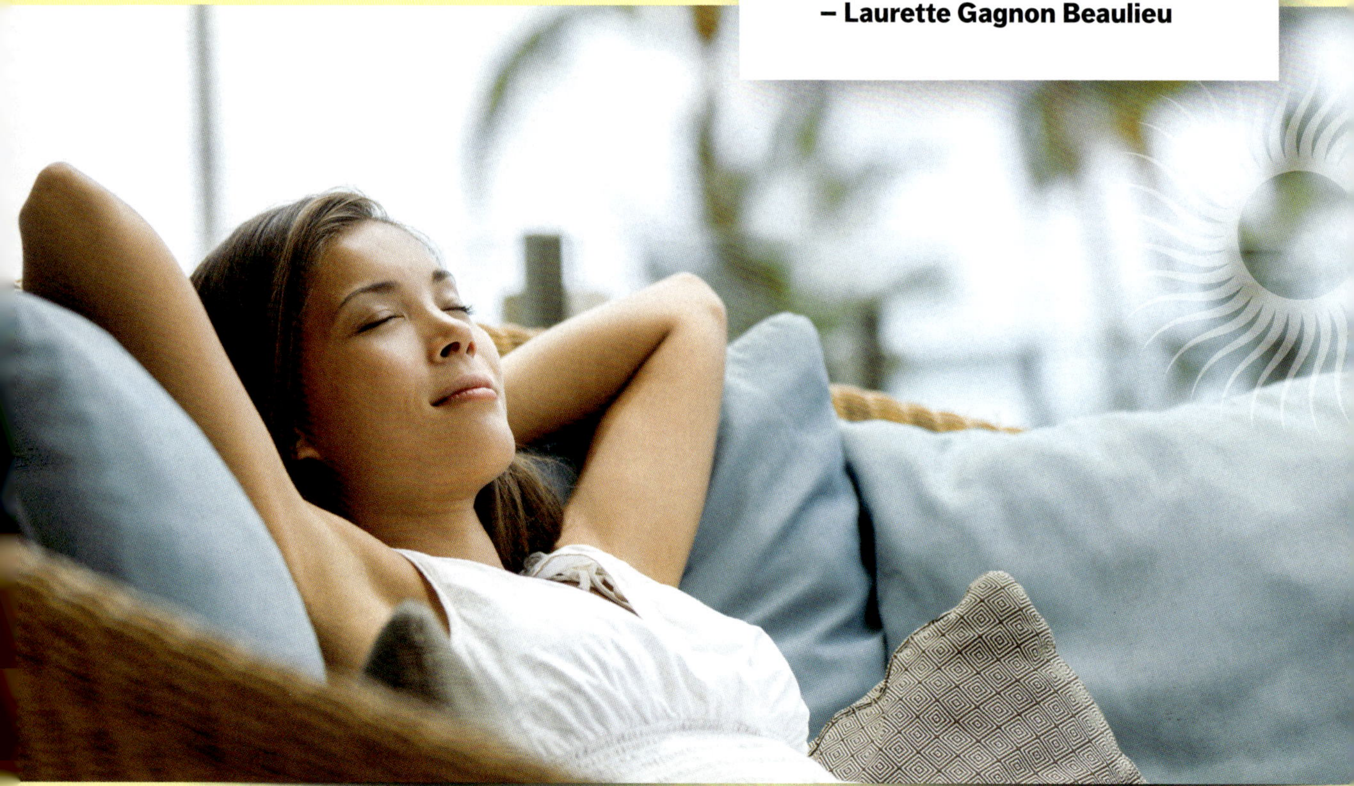

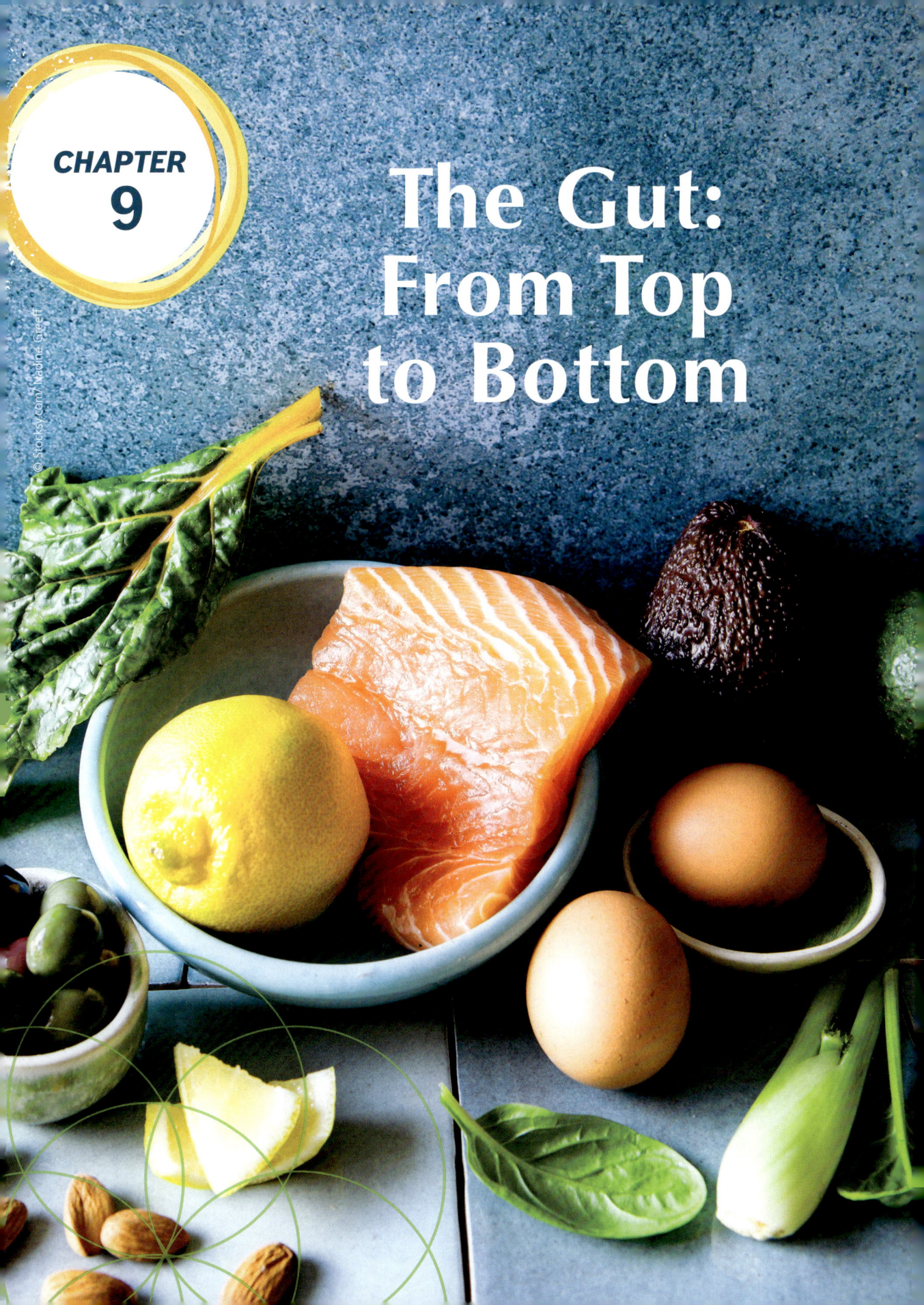

CHAPTER 9

The Gut: From Top to Bottom

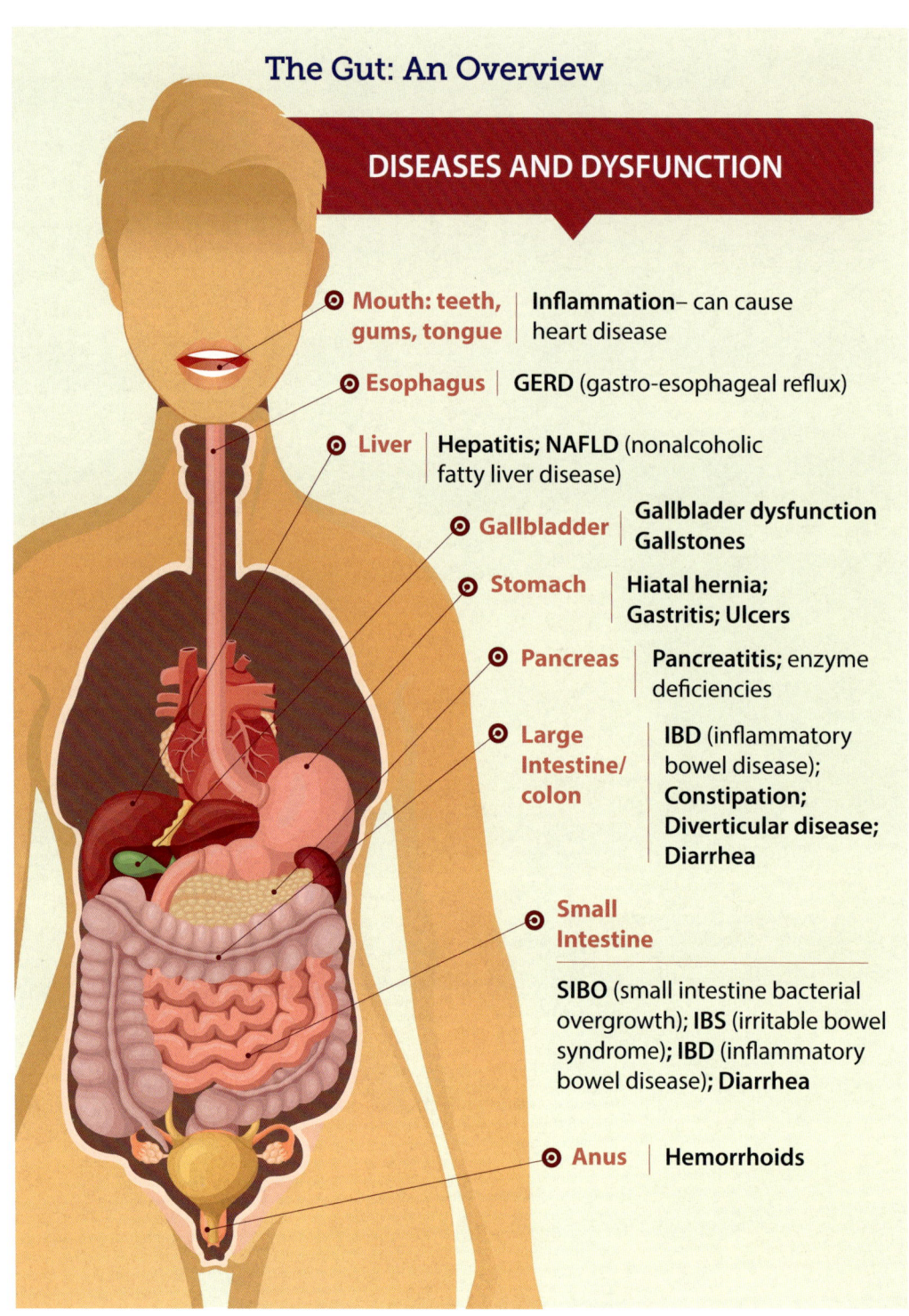

FIGURE 9.1 | The Gut: An Overview

Your genes, your food, and your lifestyle influence each other. Nutrition (what you eat), metabolism (how your body processes what you eat), and your immune system (how your body reacts to the environment) affect how your genes work, and vice versa. Knowing how well these processes are working, and making changes if needed, is important for your long-term wellbeing.

> Every time you eat or drink, you are either feeding disease or fighting it.
>
> —Heather Morgan, MS, NLC

The Gut, Digestive Function, and Elusive Illness

The health of the digestive system is one of the least-appreciated factors in our ability to repair and restore our bodies. The gastrointestinal (GI) tract serves as an assembly line that breaks down food, converts it into usable nutrients, and disposes of the spent food as waste. The digestive system is the source of all your nourishment and all the nutrients you have available for repair due to injury, illness, or aging. This miraculous system is also one of the major sources of your physical energy.

Your digestion starts with your mouth when you chew your food and mix it with saliva. Food then moves down your esophagus and into your stomach, where it mixes with stomach acid and digestive enzymes. From your stomach, partially digested food enters your small intestine; as it moves through, more digestive enzymes from your gallbladder and pancreas break food down even further. The digested food then moves on to your colon (large intestine), where water is absorbed from it and some dietary fiber is further digested. Finally, the remains of the digested food move out of your body.

Maldigestion and Malabsorption

To assimilate the necessary nutrients from our food, we first need to digest it (break it down into smaller parts) and then absorb it (pass it through the walls of the small intestine into the bloodstream). An inability to break food down well is called *maldigestion*. An inability to absorb it well is called *malabsorption*.

Maldigestion and malabsorption are quite common. Heartburn, for instance, is an occasional form of maldigestion that's usually mildly uncomfortable and goes away quickly on its own. But maldigestion can be more serious. Gastroesophageal reflux disease (GERD), for instance, is a severe form of frequent heartburn. Left untreated, it not only disrupts sleep but can lead to ulcers in the esophagus and even esophageal cancer. Malabsorption can range from simple diarrhea from a stomach flu to celiac disease and other serious conditions. Most digestive problems first appear as burping, heartburn, gas, and bloating. If left untreated, sometimes they progress to more serious symptoms. Ultimately, they can make us sick because they keep us from having the necessary nutrients to help us regenerate and heal. Let's look at this process in a little more depth.

Stomach Acid

Mundane, underappreciated, even maligned, the hydrochloric acid (HCl) produced in the stomach continues the digestive process for everything we eat once it travels from the mouth through the esophagus. Without sufficient HCl, we would have trouble digesting food properly.

==Although criticized as a cause of indigestion and heartburn, stomach acid is actually one of the secrets of good digestion.== Stomach acid is necessary to break down food to release its nutrients, particularly proteins essential for muscle repair and minerals essential for strong bones. This acid also destroys invading bacteria and other bad bugs.

Yet to watch the television ads, you might think that everyone in our society has an excess of stomach acid. We are implored to take various antacids or acid-blocking medications to stop heartburn, burping, and a host of related maladies. Although it's true that these medications have been effective at treating peptic ulcers and severe GERD, chronic overuse can cause medical complications.

In general, stomach acid should keep stomach pH low. When you don't have enough stomach acid, the pH rises, the stomach becomes less acidic, and bacteria such as *H. pylori* (the culprit behind many stomach ulcers), aren't killed or kept in check. Instead, they're able to grow and can cause damage to the stomach lining, leading to inflammation. When the protective mucosal lining of the stomach is damaged, it's exposed to stomach acid, which results in pain and can cause an ulcer. Heartburn—a burning sensation in the upper abdomen and chest—happens when stomach acid regurgitates, or refluxes, up into the esophagus, producing a burning pain behind the breastbone. If reflux becomes severe enough, it can even send stomach acid up into the throat, causing a sore throat and inflammation. If the reflux is severe and frequent, you have GERD. In extreme cases, the acid can spill into the voice box or larynx, causing hoarseness. It can even spill into the lungs, causing coughing and wheezing and making asthma worse. This is why drugs that switch off stomach acid are so effective in relieving these types of symptoms. Remember, however, that if you have an ulcer from *H. pylori*, relieving these symptoms will not treat the underlying cause. That usually needs to be addressed with antibiotics and acid-inhibiting drugs.

Paradoxically, it is often just as important to address the underlying issue of insufficient stomach acid, which may result in indigestion. Without sufficient stomach acid, food isn't digested fully, creating a sense of fullness after a meal that won't go away. Many of our patients come to us believing they have excess stomach acid, when in fact they have too little. They try antacids to no effect. In these cases, a single capsule of betaine HCl from the health-food store can alleviate all the patient's symptoms of burping and belching.

Ultimately, we must address the stomach lining if it is damaged. We'll explain how later in this chapter.

Digestive Enzymes

Enzymes are another underappreciated aspect of the body's digestive capabilities. Basically, they are catalysts—chemicals that make things happen faster. Digestive enzymes are necessary to digest foods as they pass from the stomach into the small intestine. These enzymes include proteases, which digest protein; carbohydrases such as amylase, which digest starches; and lipase, which digests fat. Your body produces most of its digestive enzymes in the liver and the pancreas. Enzymes produced by the liver are generally stored in the gallbladder until needed; they then flow through the bile duct into the small intestine to assist in digestion. The pancreas, meanwhile, produces its own enzymes that flow into the small intestine.

Low digestive enzyme levels typically cause symptoms of bloating and gas. When lipases are deficient, fats don't digest well. This can cause extremely foul-smelling stools that float and are difficult to flush. Sometimes a lack of digestive enzymes can be the result of significant digestive illness, such as a pancreatic disorder. However, in most cases, it's simply due to a deficiency of zinc, a mineral that is necessary

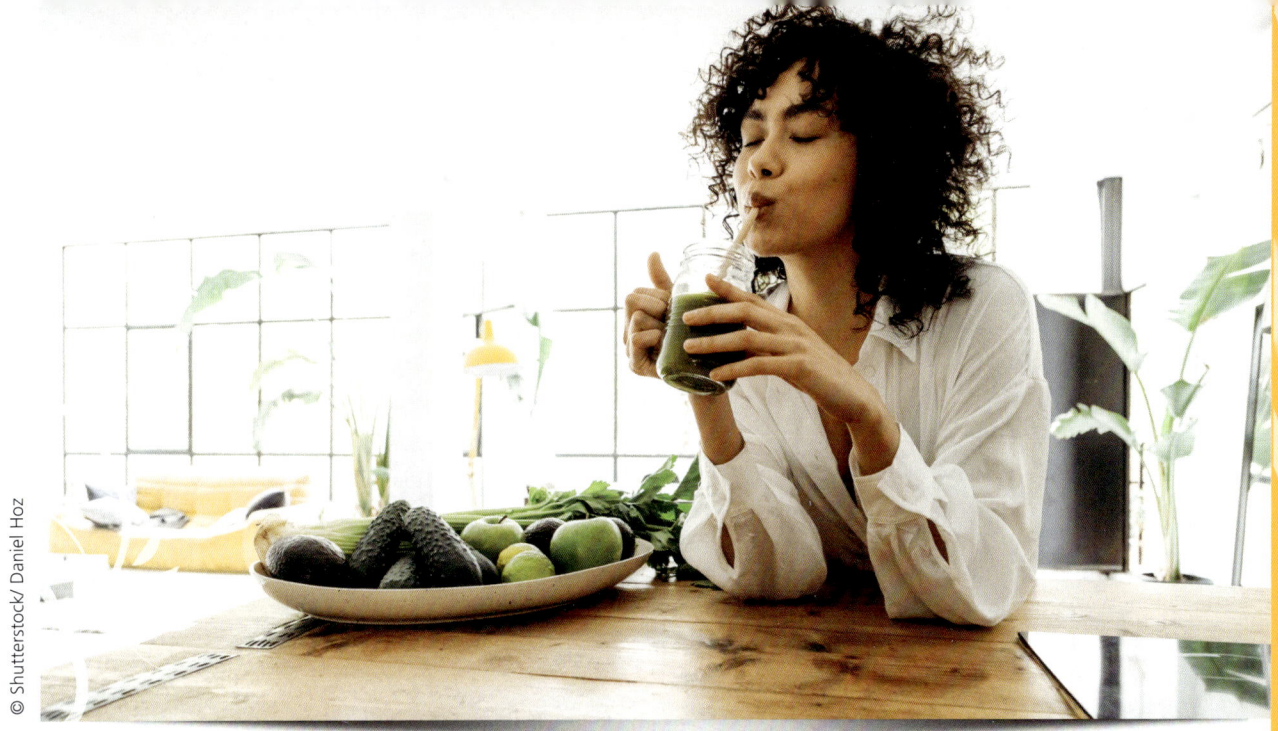

to help the microvilli (tiny projecting "fingers" in the small intestine) regenerate. Digestive enzymes are found on the microvilli, so sometimes zinc replenishment can have a profoundly beneficial effect on maldigestion.

Testing for maldigestion and malabsorption from a lack of digestive enzymes is often cumbersome and difficult. It is often simpler to try a digestive enzyme supplement to see if this helps. However, if the supplement works, it is still important to find out why the enzymes are low.

Malabsorption and Amino Acid Imbalances

Amino acids are the building blocks of protein—and your body needs plenty of them to build the many thousands of proteins that are hormones, neurotransmitters, enzymes, and other crucial body chemicals. Amino acids are also necessary for building tissues and making repairs. We have found that a surprising number of people have amino acid imbalances or deficiencies. When the missing nutrients are provided, the body can rebalance, and symptoms usually resolve naturally.

Testing for amino acid imbalances can be done with simple blood or urine tests at laboratories that specialize in functional testing.

Vitamin and Mineral Deficiencies

Vitamin deficiencies can be caused by insufficient intake, decreased absorption, or in some cases an overgrowth of bowel bacteria in the small intestine. If a deficiency is severe, you might have an illness such as pellagra, caused by a deficiency of the B vitamin niacin. In our overfed society, true deficiency diseases such as pellagra or scurvy (vitamin C deficiency) are rare, but minor deficiencies may cause nonspecific symptoms such as mental fogginess, irritability, skin rashes, and fatigue. Since minor deficiencies can be difficult to diagnose, we call this subclinical dysfunction.

In Africa, we unfortunately saw vitamin deficiencies such as pellagra and beriberi (from severe B vitamin deficiencies) and rickets (from severe vitamin D deficiency). In Western society, we sometimes see a form of dementia in older people caused by vitamin B12 deficiency; we also see anemias caused by deficiencies of vitamin B6 or B12. But we're more likely to see subclinical deficiencies—aches and pains or seasonal affective disorder—that may relate to vitamin D deficiency.

Mineral deficiencies can also have a profound impact on our health. Magnesium deficiency can cause muscle spasms and neurological symptoms, aggravate insulin resistance, and even increase the risk of irregular heart rhythm or heart failure. Zinc deficiency can cause hair loss and skin, immune, and digestive problems. It is also associated with loss of smell, taste, eyesight, and memory.

Testing for Vitamin and Mineral Deficiencies

In our experience, we have found the best way to test for vitamin and mineral deficiencies is with a combination of conventional and functional lab tests. If you are interested in this type of testing, we recommend you see someone who has expertise in this area. We can easily measure some vitamin deficiencies, such as vitamin D or vitamin B6, with simple blood tests.

Many functional medicine practitioners use organic acid testing (OAT), which is more detailed. This test looks at metabolic compounds in your urine and can help identify subtle imbalances and nutrient deficiencies before they show up on more standard tests. We use it to help us know how to optimize the body's chemical functions.

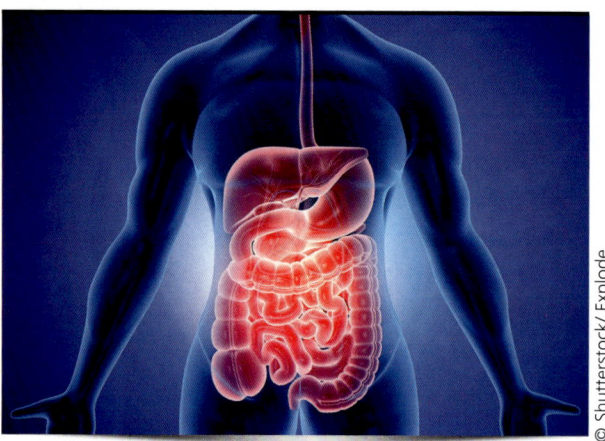

Friendly Flora—Your Inner Garden

The world inside your digestive tract is like an inner garden. From your mouth to the end of your colon, your digestive tract is home to trillions of bacteria, collectively called your gut microbiome. There are actually more bacterial cells in your intestines than you have human cells in your body. Most of the gut microbiome lives in your colon, where it plays several important roles in your digestion and overall health. The bacteria in your colon break down and digest dietary fiber, the cellulose and other complex sugars that are found in the cell walls of plant foods. These bacteria convert some of the fiber into butyrate and other short-chain fatty acids that are fuel for the cells that make up the lining of the colon. The bacteria also produce a range of metabolic byproducts that are important for your health, including vitamin K and some B vitamins.

Our internal flora is an entire ecosystem within the body, with the potential to be a thriving garden or a toxic wasteland. The gut microbiome is made up of thousands of different types of bacteria, including many that are beneficial and some that are harmful. When the good guys are in control, they keep down the bad guys and we thrive. Consequently, our immune system functions efficiently, we don't have severe allergies, and we digest and eliminate our food smoothly.

But when the harmful bacteria get out of balance and take over the beneficial bacteria, we begin to develop problems.

Dysbiosis

The gut microbiome is dynamic—the types and number of bacteria are constantly changing in response to your diet, your exercise level, the drugs you take (antibiotics, for instance), and your environment (exposure to toxins, for instance). Your gut microbiome is also very individual—as unique as a fingerprint. Only about 30 percent of all beneficial bacteria types are found in just about everybody. Even twins will have different microbiomes.

Overall, the beneficial or neutral bacteria in your gut outnumber the unfriendly bacteria. The bad guys are still there, but they're far outnumbered by the others, to the point where they generally can't do any harm. Sometimes, however, the balance of good and bad bacteria gets thrown off, a condition called *dysbiosis*. In the most obvious example, taking an antibiotic kills both good and bad gut bacteria, giving the bad guys a chance to grab hold. Less obviously but much more commonly, a diet high in processed and refined foods and low in natural fiber from fruits, vegetables, and whole grains creates the right conditions for dysbiosis. So do alcohol, stress, a sedentary lifestyle, and insufficient sleep.

In dysbiosis, the ratio of harmful bacteria to beneficial bacteria may be too high, or you may not have enough diversity among the different types of beneficial bacteria.

When you have dysbiosis, you may have symptoms such as bloating, indigestion, diarrhea, constipation, and sometimes malabsorption. Dysbiosis also plays a role in allergies, ulcers, autoimmune reactions, and illnesses such as irritable bowel syndrome (IBS).

Dysbiosis also has a negative effect on your immune system. To keep your immune system from being set off by all the bacteria in your gut, its activation is tightly regulated. Beneficial bacteria in the gut send signals to the large amount of immune tissue that surrounds the small intestine, telling it to stay calm. When dangerous viruses or bacteria take hold, the beneficial bacteria send signals telling the immune system to get busy. But when the balance between the beneficial and harmful bacteria is disrupted, your immune system is constantly activated. If the activation goes on long enough, you develop chronic inflammation—and the effects of that can go beyond the gut to impact other parts of your body, such as your joints and your heart.

Microbiome Malfunction

Children in less-developed countries tend to have a much lower incidence of allergies and autoimmune disease (see Hygiene hypothesis in Chapter 10). Researchers now believe that this may be because they are exposed to many pathogens early in life, which trains their immune systems to recognize bad bacteria for what they are and respond appropriately. At the same time, the immune system learns to be "tolerant" of the host, so that it is less likely to start an autoimmune reaction against the body. Another reason for this healthy immune reaction is related to the better health of the bacteria in their GI tracts. Studies show that these children have a more diverse microbiome—with 30 percent more bacteria species—because they eat a great deal more bacteria-supporting fiber than children in Western society.

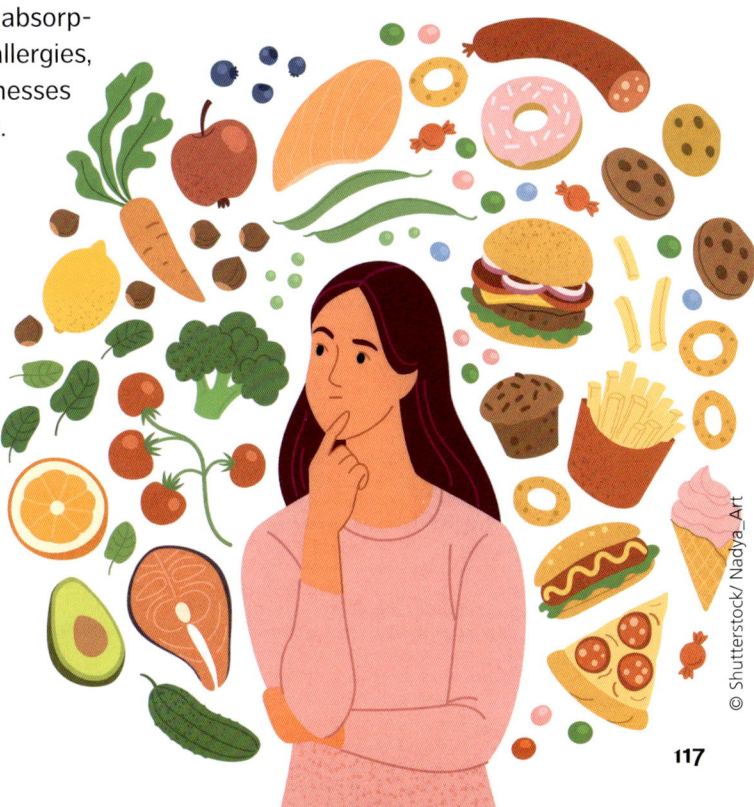

In adults, poor diet, antibiotic overuse, medications such as anti-inflammatories and birth control pills, and excessive alcohol use can all adversely affect the ratio of good bacteria to bad bacteria in our intestines, often with excessive yeast overgrowth as well. The resultant dysbiosis can lead to a breakdown in tolerance, allowing the immune system to inappropriately cause inflammation in the body.

Antidoting Dysbiosis

Americans have become more attuned to their intestinal flora, and, like many Europeans, now consume a range of sophisticated live-culture yogurts, kefirs, and other fermented foods, such as sauerkraut and kimchi, that naturally contain good bacteria. They also take probiotics—supplements that contain good bacteria. Probiotic foods and supplements are the perfect example of a functional approach to metabolism.

Improving your diet and adding probiotic foods and supplements is a good start for treating dysbiosis, but it's a bit like throwing grass seed on bare ground and expecting a good outcome without understanding when to water, when to apply weed killer (medications or supplements to kill the bad bacteria), and when to apply fertilizers. For your gut, the fertilizer is prebiotics—foods and supplements that contain complex sugars called fructo-oligosaccharides (FOS), which help the good bacteria grow.

Addressing dysbiosis can be a complex issue. It is important to work with a healthcare practitioner who is well versed in this subject.

SIBO

Small intestinal bacterial overgrowth (SIBO) occurs when there is an abnormal increase in the overall bacterial population in the small intestine.

The far end of your small intestine (the ileum) joins your colon at the ileocecal valve in the lower right quadrant of your abdomen. As an ordinary part of your digestion, the ring-shaped valve opens briefly to let digested food enter your colon, then closes again. Sometimes, the valve doesn't close quickly enough and bacteria from the colon backwash into the ileum. If enough bacteria end up on the wrong side of the valve, they can start to grow there. That can cause abdominal pain, diarrhea, gas, bloating, and cramps. In severe cases, the bacteria absorb so many nutrients that you become malnourished. SIBO can also cause leaky gut syndrome and inflammation. It's an often-overlooked cause of digestive problems and inflammation.

People with celiac disease, inflammatory bowel disease (IBD), low stomach acid, or irritable bowel syndrome (IBS) are more likely to get SIBO, but often it's caused by a bad bout of enteritis from an intestinal virus or food poisoning.

To treat SIBO, we first need to diagnose it, which can be done with a simple breath test. Then, we deal with the bacterial overgrowth with antibiotics. After that, dietary changes, along with prebiotics and probiotics, often help. If there's an underlying problem, such as irritable bowel syndrome, treating that will help prevent a recurrence. Because SIBO involves dysbiosis, it can also be a precursor of developing immune problems.

What should you do if you have persistent bloating but your SIBO test is negative?

If this happens, you may have a malabsorption problem. Typically, this may be from the sugars: lactose (found in dairy); fructose (especially the fructose in fruit juice and high fructose corn syrup), and sucrose (in table sugar.)

It is possible to test for malabsorption due to enzyme deficiency, but this can be expensive. Sometimes it is worth challenging yourself with high amounts of these sugars but do this at separate times. If you feel bloated, you have your answer!

If you have a problem, exclude these from your diet, or find an enzyme that will help you digest the sugars.

The Gut and the Immune System

Your small intestine is where most of your digestion and absorption occurs. As your food travels through the 20 or so feet of your small intestine, powerful digestive enzymes break it down into tiny particles that can be absorbed through the intestinal walls and into your bloodstream. The walls of your small intestine are only about the thickness of a paper towel. The interior wall of the small intestine is tightly wrinkled into many circular folds. Each fold has thousands of finger-like projections called *villi*. One square inch of the small intestine has about 20,000 villi—and each villus in turn has thousands of tinier microvilli. All those folds, villi, and microvilli are there to increase the surface area of the small intestine and let you absorb nutrients efficiently. The villi are coated with a mucosal membrane that helps keep unwanted molecules from being absorbed through the walls. Think of the small intestine as a sensor that can probe all incoming food to sort out the pure from the impure, the nourishing nutrients from potentially lethal toxins. On the tip of the microvilli exists another important barrier, the mucinous *Intestinal Epithelial Glycocalyx* ("glycocalyx" literally means "sugar coating"). The glycocalyx acts as the initial defense against bacteria and toxins and helps produce digestive enzymes and vitamins. It develops in infancy, aided by human breast milk and non-digestible fibers, another reason these factors are so important for us!

These cells, laid out end to end, are one cell layer thick, equivalent in size to a layer of plastic wrap laid over half a badminton court. The cells that line the wall of the small intestine are ordinarily held together very tightly at their junctions—they resemble tiles on a wall. To absorb nutrients, the junctions open up just enough to let small digested molecules into your bloodstream through a dense network of tiny capillaries. Once in the bloodstream, the particles are transported via the portal vein to the liver for further processing before they are finally sent out to the cells of your body to be used as fuel.

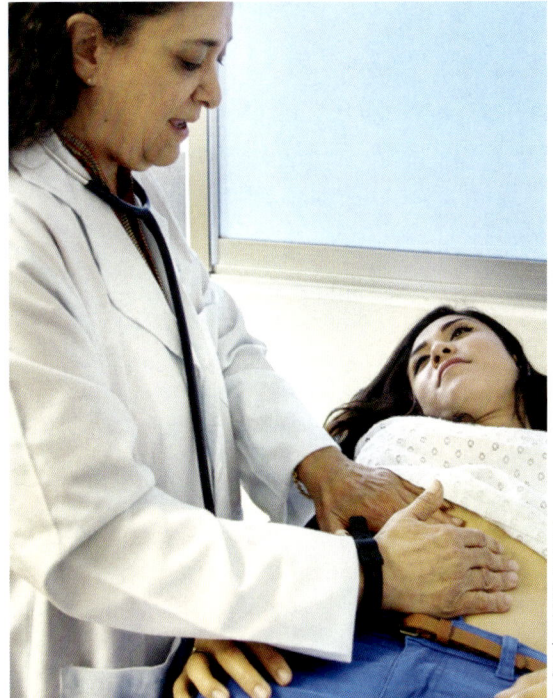

© Stocksy/ PER Images

Your small intestine is tightly linked to your immune system. Within the wall of the small intestine, you have between 30 and 40 areas of lymphatic tissue called *Peyer's patches*. These areas are part of your immune surveillance system, an early warning system for your body. Their primary function is to detect pathogens and initiate the immune response to attack them.

Lying just between the wall of the small intestine and the capillaries is a layer of lymphatic tissue that is the home for about 80 percent of your immune system cells. Called the gut-associated lymphoid tissue (GALT), this tissue is poised to pounce on dangerous bacteria, viruses, and toxins that escape the small intestine and try to enter the bloodstream. Because our modern life continuously stresses the small intestine with environmental toxins, a poor diet, drugs, and other substances, the chances of something bad escaping are high—and that can make your immune system go awry and turn on your own body.

Leaky Gut Syndrome

The delicate wall of the small intestine can be damaged by a poor diet, alcohol, pathogens, illness, stress, and a range of other factors. When that happens, the intestinal wall can become permeable: the tight junctions open too widely, allowing larger molecules that haven't been completely broken down to pass through and enter the bloodstream.

When the junctions in the lining of the GI tract open too wide for whatever reason, the result is called altered intestinal permeability, gut hyperpermeability, or, most commonly, leaky gut syndrome. This process can be compared to the way the pores in your skin expand and open wider when you take a hot shower.

In the gut, open pores are a bit of a disaster. When leaky gut syndrome happens, large molecules of undigested food are released directly into the bloodstream. The digestive tract's immune system quickly responds to these oversized molecules. The immune system reacts as if these foods were invaders, or antigens, and may launch an attack—even if the molecules are just food (or innocent bystanders, so to speak). In other words, the immune system falsely assumes that the foods are molecules that are making the body sick. It subsequently pours out antibodies, creating an immune and inflammatory response.

Leaky gut syndrome symptoms include gas, bloating, indigestion, diarrhea, constipation, fatigue, headaches, and brain fog. Inflammation from a leaky gut may be the hidden culprit behind some chronic digestive illnesses, such as irritable bowel syndrome. It may also be a factor in autoimmune illnesses such as chronic fatigue syndrome, and it may trigger food allergies and sensitivities. The inflammation caused by a leaky gut is often an underlying or contributing cause of aching joints and muscles, frequent minor illnesses, and a range of other symptoms, including sinus problems and skin rashes. We've come to realize that leaky gut syndrome is a common problem for many of our patients.

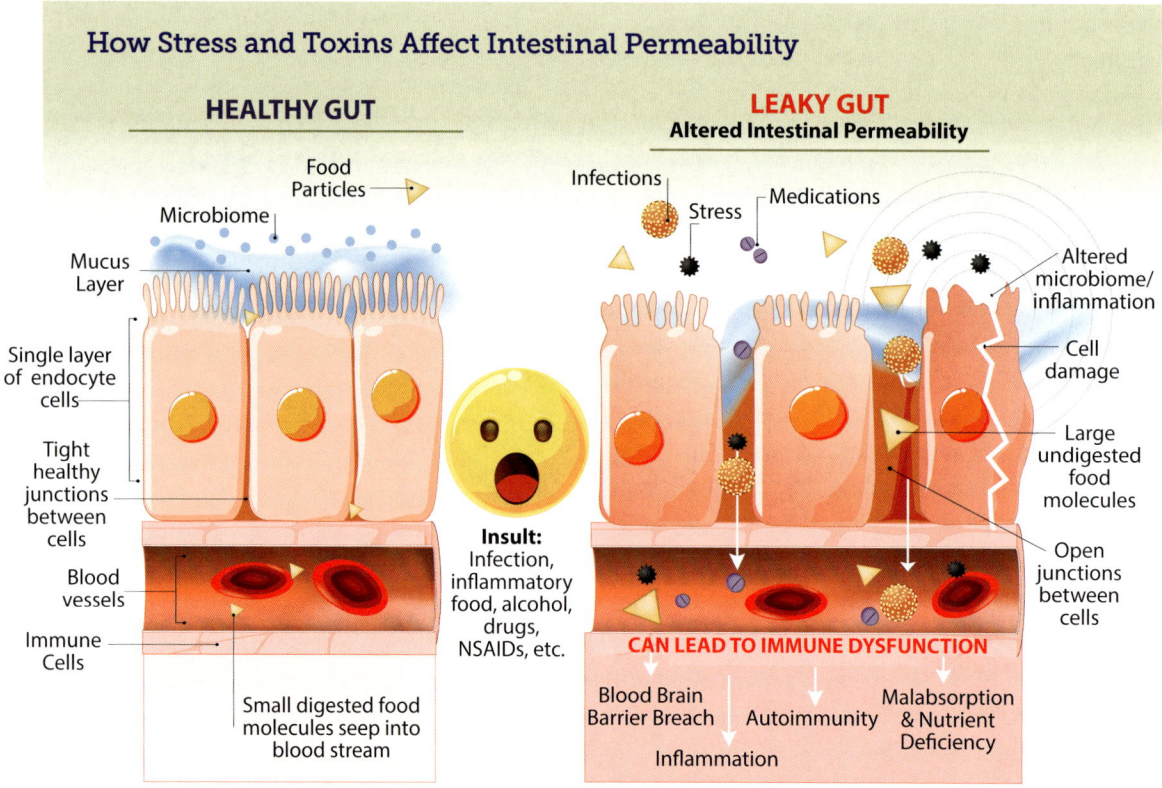

FIGURE 9.2 | How Stress and Toxins Affect Intestinal Permeability

Repairing a Leaky Gut

Fixing a leaky gut takes time but often leads to improvement of symptoms of food sensitivities and allergies. We work with our patients to follow the 5R model for improving gut health. It's a five-step process that works like this:

Step 1: Remove common food triggers such as gluten, dairy, corn, eggs, and sugar, which all can increase inflammation in the gut. Also remove any known allergens and food sensitivities.

Step 2: Replace essential digestive elements that have been depleted, such as digestive enzymes and hydrochloric acid.

Step 3: **Reinoculate** the gut with a healthy balance of good bacteria using prebiotic supplements and high-dose, broad-spectrum probiotics.

Step 4: Repair the leaky gut lining with amino acids like L-glutamine and herbal supplements like aloe vera, berberine, and marshmallow root.

Step 5: Rebalance the body to support gut health. Now that you've gone through the previous steps, you want to maintain the improvement. This is the time to address stress management, better sleep, and more exercise.

Although the concepts of 5R are simple, we recommend working closely with a functional medicine doctor to determine your personalized treatment plan.

As the gut lining heals, healthy foods that were removed can slowly be added back (except for known allergens). Going back to a diet full of junk and processed foods is likely to start the leaky gut problem all over again, however. It's important to move on to a better diet and stay with it—we'll explain the basics of a healthy, gut-friendly diet in the next chapter.

Is It Food Sensitivities or Food Allergies?

Leaky gut syndrome can cause food sensitivity and is also caused by reactions to food. Once you're sensitized to certain foods, you'll release antibodies every time you eat them. Removing the offending foods may help reduce symptoms, but you won't get better until you do something to heal the altered intestinal permeability.

It is very important to differentiate between food allergies and food sensitivities. An example of a food allergy is when someone eats an oyster or other shellfish then almost immediately starts struggling to breathe as their throat swells. Food allergies occur quickly, usually within minutes of eating the food. Food sensitivities are slow-motion reactions that usually occur hours to days after eating a food and usually aren't as dramatic. This is because they have different mechanisms. Food allergies are the result of IgE antibodies (think "E" for emergency) interacting with a protein in the food, while food sensitivities are usually the result of IgG (think "G" for gradual) antibodies reacting with food. In addition, IgA antibodies (think "A" for ate it) are often elevated in leaky gut. High levels of IgG and IgA antibodies usually imply a reaction that is happening on the surface of the mucus layer that lines the small intestine.

Symptoms of Gut Hyperpermeability, or Leaky Gut Syndrome

Gut hyperpermeability, or leaky gut syndrome, can lead to exaggerated antibody reactions to certain foods, also called food sensitivity. This altered immune response can be a contributing factor to a broad range of apparently unrelated conditions:

- Arthritis, autoimmune problems and fibromyalgia
- Chronic fatigue syndrome and multiple chemical sensitivities
- Cognitive malfunction, from brain fog to exacerbation of attention deficit disorder and autism
- Digestive disorders, such as inflammatory bowel disease (IBD), irritable bowel syndrome (IBS), malnutrition, and compromised liver function
- Food allergies and sensitivities
- Skin conditions, including acne, dermatitis, eczema, psoriasis, and urticaria (hives)

Food Sensitivity Symptoms

Unlike true food allergies, which can be immediate and life-threatening, food sensitivities are less immediate and less dangerous. Food sensitivities are usually the result of IgG antibodies reacting with food. Food intolerances are usually because the food irritates your digestive tract, or you lack the necessary enzymes to digest it properly.

A food sensitivity response can be delayed as much as twenty-four or even thirty-six hours, so we may feel ill and not know why. Moreover, food sensitivity symptoms are often not confined to the GI tract, making tracing symptoms to their original cause difficult. For instance, if we develop a headache on a Wednesday, we may not connect our throbbing head with the wheat in the sandwich we ate for lunch on Monday. The reaction usually involves gastrointestinal symptoms, such as cramps and diarrhea, but symptoms from food sensitivity can take other forms as well, such as headaches, runny nose, rashes, fatigue, joint pain, and difficulty losing weight. Food sensitivities have also been linked to many other conditions, including allergies, asthma, bedwetting, canker sores, constipation, chronic bladder infections, eczema, psoriasis, urticaria, IBD, migraines, heart palpitations, spontaneous bruising, ulcers, and serous otitis media (fluid in the middle ear).

You can develop a sensitivity to almost any food, sometimes after years of eating it without any problem. Because the symptoms are varied and don't happen right away, tracking down food sensitivities can be difficult—you don't always associate the food you ate one day with the diarrhea and headache you suffer twenty-four hours later.

Many different food components can trigger sensitivity or intolerance. Some common ones to look out for include:

- **Chemicals.** Examples include monosodium glutamate (MSG, a flavor enhancer), dyes and food colorings, and sulfites (preservatives found in wine and dried fruit).
- **Lactose.** Intolerance to lactose, or the sugar in milk, is related to a deficiency in the enzyme lactase. Without lactase, lactose can't be digested properly. This can result in abdominal pain, bloating, and gas when dairy products such as milk or ice cream are consumed. It is prudent to note that lactose is also used as a filler in many processed foods.
- **Fructose.** A person may have sensitivity or difficulty absorbing fructose, a sugar found

in fruit and high-fructose corn syrup. The symptoms are similar to those of IBS and lactose intolerance.

- **Fruits and vegetables in the nightshade family.** These include tomatoes, eggplants, bell peppers, chili peppers, potatoes, goji berries, and tamarillos. Eating these foods can cause a flare of arthritic symptoms in certain people.
- **Wheat.** Intolerance to wheat is not the same as wheat allergy or celiac disease. Wheat sensitivity can result in any of the symptoms we have discussed in this section.

The Gut as the Second Brain

You have at least 200 million neurons in the enteric nervous system (ENS) that automatically controls your gut—so many that the ENS is often called the "second brain." Just as your brain produces neurotransmitter chemicals to pass signals from neuron to neuron, so does your ENS. Your gut produces the neurotransmitters serotonin, dopamine, norepinephrine, epinephrine, and others. In addition, hormones such as estrogen are metabolized in the gut. Your ENS and your brain use these neurotransmitters and hormones to communicate with each other and coordinate your digestion with other parts of your body, like your immune systems.

In your gut, neurotransmitters function differently than they do in your brain. About 90 percent of the serotonin in your body is in your gut, for example. In the brain, serotonin plays an important role in keeping your mood stable; an imbalance in brain serotonin is associated with depression. But in the gut, serotonin's main role is to control motility. Serotonin production in the gut is a complex process that begins with your gut bacteria stimulating specialized cells in the intestines to produce it. Some of that gut serotonin ends up in the circulation and reaches the brain. This is how gut malfunction that affects the gut bacteria can in turn affect serotonin and other neurotransmitters and then cause brain malfunction. Inflammation in the gut, for example, changes how serotonin is metabolized, shunting it into a pathway called the kynurenine pathway. Remember how depressed you got when you had the flu? This was because the inflammation caused the same activation of the kynurenine pathway. Imagine if an inflamed gut was making you feel like that all the time!

It's not uncommon for patients with SIBO to suffer from anxiety and depression. It also appears that patients with anxiety are more likely to have IBS. So, which comes first? It's a chicken-and-egg problem. We know there is a bidirectional influence. Diet, exercise, overall health, gender, stress, and mood all affect the microbiome in the gut, and the microbiome in turn can affect how you feel.

Many neurological disorders are associated with gut dysbiosis. These include Alzheimer disease, Parkinson disease, autism spectrum disorder, attention deficit hyperactivity disorder (ADHD), multiple sclerosis (MS), and possibly some forms of epilepsy.

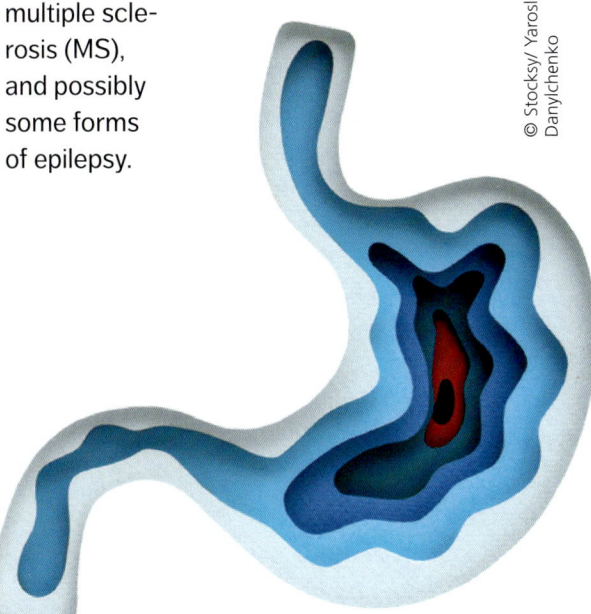

© Stocksy/ Yaroslav Danylchenko

In a stressful situation, your brain affects your gut by releasing a surge of the stress hormone cortisol. That diverts blood away from your digestion, which makes your intestinal muscles contract. You end up feeling "butterflies" in your stomach—or even throwing up or needing to dash to the bathroom.

Your gut makes its own hormones as well. These influence your appetite and how you digest your food—and your overall metabolism as well. For example, the hormone glucagon-like peptide 1 (GLP-1) suppresses your appetite and also has a powerful impact on how much insulin you produce and how well you use it. (We'll talk more about the value of hormones for weight control and blood sugar in Chapter 13.)

A change in one person's mood can affect others close to them. When someone in a household is given a course of antibiotics, which usually alters their microbiome, it also affects the microbiome of others in the same household. So, could it be that the mood change is partially due to microbiome change? Honestly, we don't know. But it's interesting to think about the wide range of effects the microbiome has.

Inflammation in the gut can cause a rise in the amount of lipopolysaccharide endotoxins, or LPS, in the circulation. LPS is released from the cell membranes of Gram-negative bacteria in the gut when they die (as they do all the time). In a healthy gut, the LPS stays in the intestines, where it is neutralized by an enzyme and then passes out of the body. When the gut is inflamed and leaky, LPS enters the circulation. Among other problems this can cause, high levels of LPS-stimulated inflammation are associated with major depressive disorder.

Changes in the microbiome that lead to a better balance of good bacteria can improve satiety and also reduce triglycerides (tiny fat droplets in the blood). In a recent study, supplementation with a spore-based probiotic appeared to help people feel full after eating and lower their triglycerides.

Because the bacteria in your gut produce neurotransmitters that can affect a wide range of functions, some probiotic supplements use specific bacteria strains that are thought to help improve production of specific neurotransmitters. Some are marketed as ways to improve mood, sleep, stress, and more. Do they work? The gut-brain axis is very complex, and it's unclear if it's that easy to manipulate it simply by taking some probiotic capsules.

We're often told by patients, "I'm taking a probiotic!" as if all probiotic supplements are equivalent. This could not be further from the truth. It's like saying, "I'm taking a vitamin," or even, "I'm taking a medication." Quality matters. Most probiotic supplements contain at least five billion (yes, billion with a b) CFUs per capsule at the time of manufacture. The bacteria species in supplements are predominantly Lactobacillus and Bifidobacterium because these are the most common bacteria found in the gut. Other species that are found in most probiotic supplements include Enterococcus, Saccharomyces, Streptococcus, Escherichia, and Bacillus. Look for products that contain spore-based bacteria. These bacteria are dormant and are more likely to survive the trip through your digestive tract and arrive in your colon ready to reproduce. To determine the best probiotic supplement for you, discuss your needs with your doctor or nutritionist.

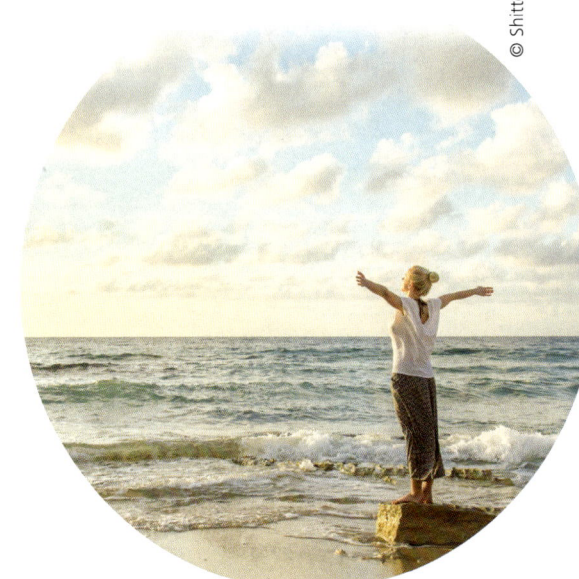

© Shitterstock/ Matej Kastelic

Food is Medicine; Food as Medicine

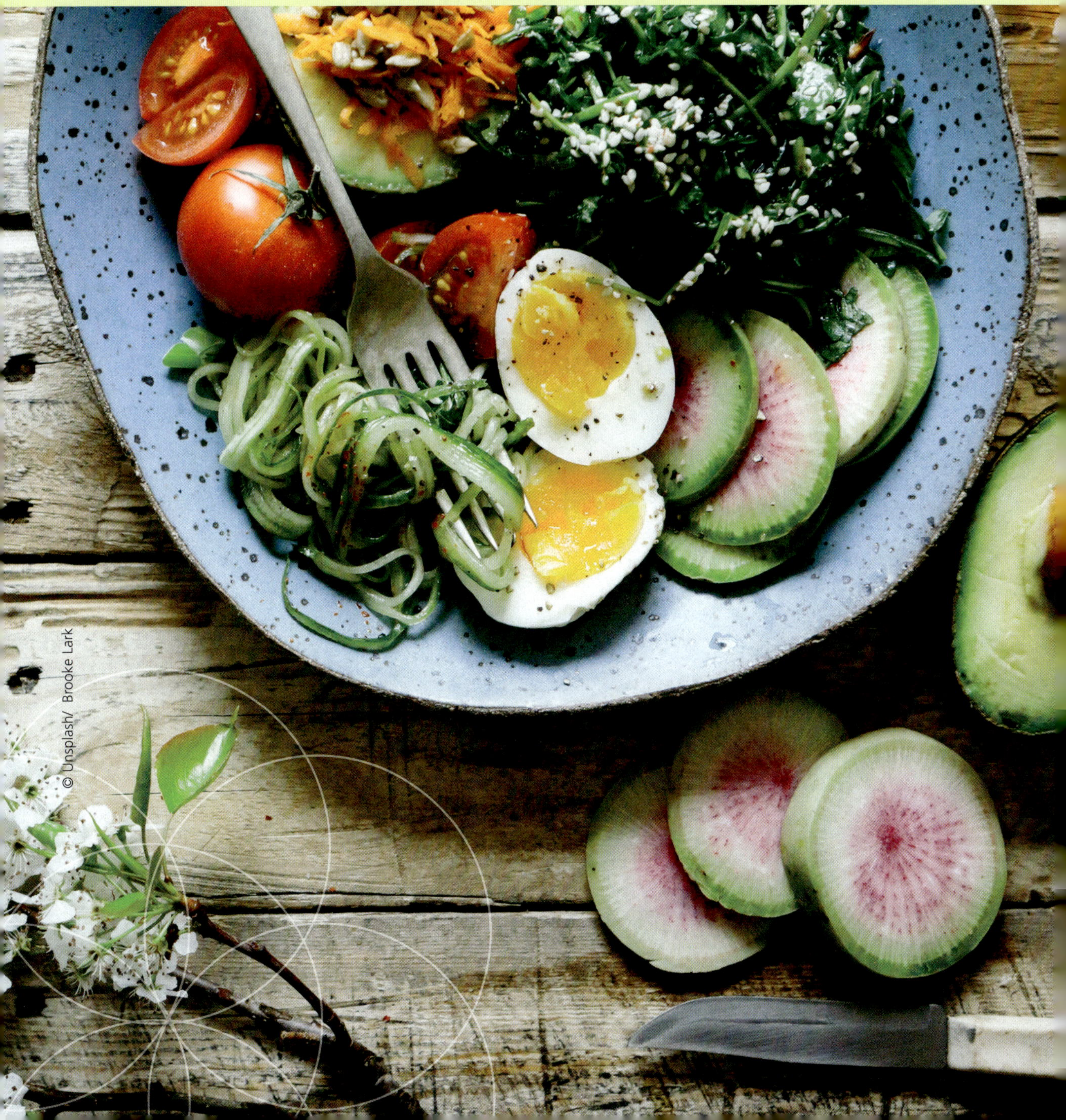

CHAPTER 10

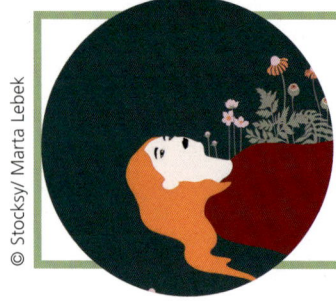

Did you ever think that changing your diet might save your life? You might be nodding your head if you thought about someone who was starving or someone living completely on fast food. But what about you? You may say, "I already eat a good diet!" But what if you changed your diet? Would it make a difference?

Growing Healthier with Every Bite

In one paradigm-shifting study published in 2001, patients who had experienced a heart attack were put on either a low-fat diet recommended by the American Heart Association (AHA) or a Mediterranean diet. The AHA diet at that time was essentially standard American fare but with the total fat intake lowered to 30 percent or less of calories. By contrast, the typical Mediterranean diet emphasizes fresh vegetables and fruits and includes whole grains, beans, and lentils, with olive oil, fish, and red meat in moderation. The researchers found that patients on the Mediterranean diet did so much better than those on the AHA diet (a 50 to 70 percent lower risk of recurrent heart disease) that they stopped the study early, feeling it was unethical to deprive half the subjects of the more efficacious diet. The study was eye-opening for many of us interested in nutrition.

It Doesn't Matter When You Start

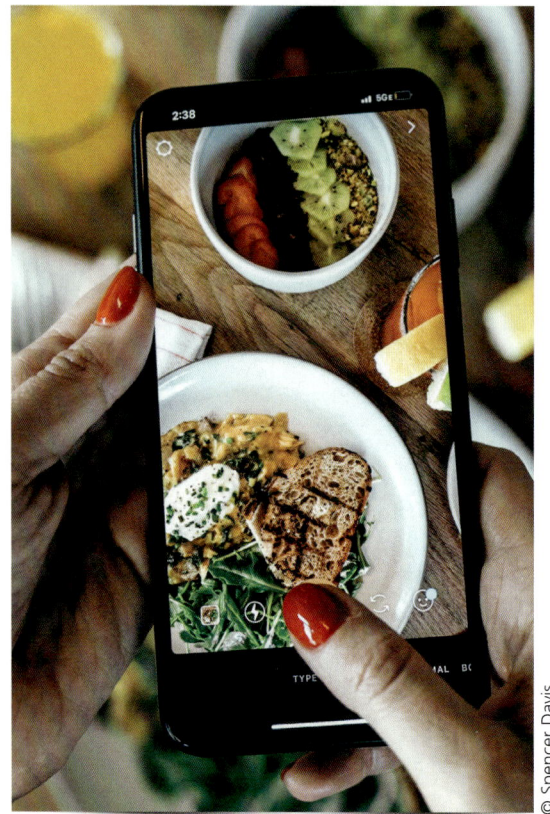

Improving your diet at any age can help. Another important study in 2004 found that introducing a Mediterranean diet to seniors between the ages of 70 and 77 resulted in a 50 percent reduction in disease risk, including heart disease, along with a significant reduction in arthritis and other health problems. Since then, multiple studies have corroborated this.

If you could take a pill to reduce your risk of degenerative disease by 50 percent, wouldn't you be rushing to get it? You might even be willing to pay an exorbitant amount of money for it. So why not make basic, inexpensive changes in your diet to achieve this type of result?

The first step is changing your concept of food. When you eat, you're marinating your cells in nutrients and sending messages throughout your body. Your choice of nutrients has a profound effect on your body chemistry, often within minutes. Long-term consumption of the wrong foods can result in inflammation, oxidation, and degeneration—the terrible trio we talked about earlier.

Eating **Mindfully**

Food companies know exactly how much our food intake can be manipulated by labels, smells, environment, textures (such as crunchiness), and a host of other factors. We get supersized, indulged, and overstuffed by food engineering that exploits our basic desire for sweet, salty, and fatty foods. As much as we like to think of ourselves as being conscious of our food intake, most of us rarely are.

Eating while you drive, watch television, or read removes awareness of the act of eating. Interestingly, it is your brain that sets the digestive machinery in process. This happens in response to the look, smell, and texture of foods, which then triggers a cascade of acids, enzymes, and digestive processes that help you assimilate food.

It's important to become aware of how you eat as much as how much you eat. Immerse yourself in the moment as you savor each bite. Really take notice of what your food looks like—as well as the aroma, flavor, and texture.

Slow down. In our fast-paced world, it's easy to overlook the importance of the ritual and pleasure of mindful eating. One way to slow down is by eating about 80 percent of the food on your plate, then pausing for 5 to 10 minutes. That short break can help you realize that you're already satisfied and don't really want to polish off your plate. That realization can also help you choose smaller portions going forward.

Diet and Lifestyle **Go Together**

In *Thrive: Find Happiness the Blue Zones Way*, Dan Buettner describes areas of the world where people commonly live active lives past the age of 100. He calls these Blue Zones. The areas he studied were Sardinia, Italy; the islands of Okinawa, Japan; Loma Linda, California (a Seventh Day Adventist community); the Nicoya Peninsula in Costa Rica; and the island of Ikaria in Greece. On Ikaria, almost a third of the population lives into their 90s. According to Buettner, Ikarians have about a 20 percent lower rate of cancer and a 50 percent lower rate of heart disease than people in industrial countries. Ikarians also experience almost no dementia. Buettner discusses the nine common features he found in the Blue Zones. They are:

- Moving naturally through frequent, moderate activity
- Developing a sense of life purpose
- Reducing stress
- Following the 80 percent rule: stop eating when you're 80 percent full
- Eating a plant-based diet derived mainly from fresh vegetables and legumes
- Drinking moderate amounts of alcohol (1 to 2 drinks daily) with family, friends, and food
- Belonging to a faith-based community
- Putting loved ones first; having a commitment to family

When all aspects Buettner identifies are combined for a healthy lifestyle, their power becomes evident.

>
>
> Wellness is not a 'medical fix' but a way of living – a lifestyle sensitive and responsive to all the dimensions of body, mind, and spirit, an approach to life we each design to achieve our highest potential for well-being now and forever.
>
> **– Greg Anderson**

Finding the **Right Diet**

Based on the diet of long-lived people in the Blue Zones, we believe a healthy diet has these attributes:

- Is plant-based, with plenty of vegetables, beans, fruits, and whole grains.
- Has limited dairy foods, preferably in the form of unprocessed cheese and live-culture yogurt.
- Limits red meat, poultry, and fish and has eggs in moderation. Red meat should be grass-fed. Poultry and eggs should be organic and pasture-raised. Fish should be wild caught.
- Uses plant-based unrefined oils such as olive oil (in fact, the more uncooked olive oil, the better) and avocado oil.
- Uses saturated fats from animal foods sparingly and avoids refined and processed plant oils.
- Limits sugar consumption.
- Avoids refined grains, processed and manufactured foods, and food with added chemicals.
- Avoids additives such as food dyes, flavorings, and preservatives.

In general, look for foods that are minimally processed, high in nutrients, and low in added sugar and salt. Beyond those basic principles, however, your healthy diet has the potential for a huge amount of variety, as we'll explain throughout this chapter.

A Nutritionally Dense Diet

A nutritionally dense diet is one based on foods that have nourished populations for centuries and provides food in their most unprocessed forms. Sometimes referred to as *ancestral foods*, these foods provided lean proteins, healthy fats, vitamins, minerals, and enough fiber-containing carbohydrates to allow hunter-gatherer societies to thrive. These ancestral food choices contrast sharply with our typical modern diet. The foods we eat now are highly refined and processed. They can be consumed rapidly and dissolve in our mouths with little need for chewing. These foods are depleted of important nutrients and are very low in fiber but are very high in added sugar, salt, and artificial flavorings.

We strongly recommend returning to a more ancestral way of eating by reducing the amount of processed food in your diet and increasing the amounts of whole grains, nuts, fruit, and vegetables. You can add nutrient density by making simple substitutions, such as:

- 100 percent whole wheat bread for white bread
- Oatmeal for sugary breakfast cereals
- Oven-fried sweet potatoes for french fries
- Fresh or frozen broccoli sauteed with olive oil and garlic for processed broccoli and cheese
- Fresh or frozen berries with yogurt for ice cream
- An apple or orange for cookies
- Lightly salted peanuts for potato chips

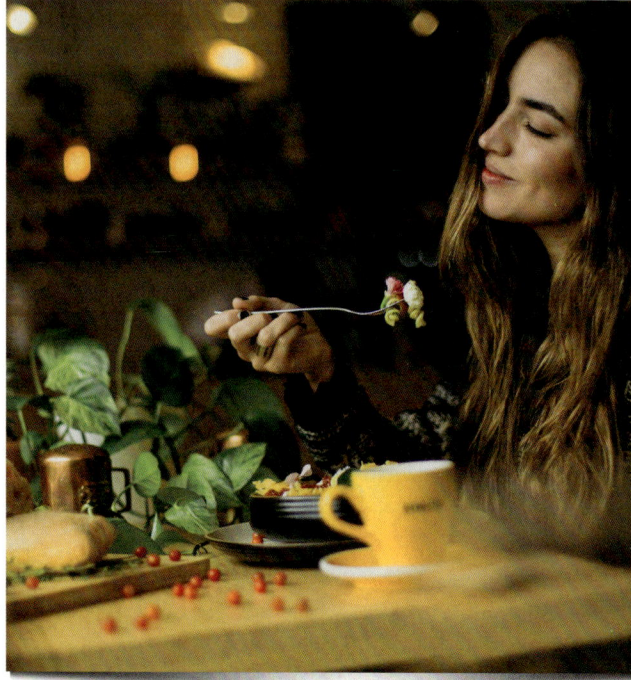
© Unsplash/ Pablo Merchán

Eat Your Broccoli!

Vegetables in the cruciferous family, which includes broccoli, cabbage, kale, and brussels sprouts, contain natural cancer-fighting compounds, along with plenty of folate, vitamin C, vitamin E, and fiber. Broccoli is particularly rich in an anticancer compound called *sulforaphane*. The broccoli plant produces sulforaphane to keep away insects that want to eat it—that's why broccoli has a slightly bitter taste. All cruciferous vegetables are also good sources of *indoles*, which seem to have anticancer action. The same compounds that protect these plants against insects seem to protect against cancer in humans by suppressing genes that promote tumor growth.

These cancer fighters become most available to our bodies when broccoli and similar vegetables are steamed or blanched for just one to two minutes.

Good and Bad Foods

Foods high in omega-6 fatty acids, such as soybean oil and corn oil, tend to be pro-inflammatory. The typical Western diet is filled with highly refined foods that are high in omega-6 fatty acids, often called the "bad" fats. The agricultural shift from grass-fed to grain-fed meats is a factor in the dramatic increase of omega-6 fatty acids in the American diet. So is the shift to fried foods, prepared/processed foods, and junk food, which contain a lot of cheap, processed vegetable oils that are high in omega-6 and low in omega-3 fatty acids (the good fats).

You can ensure that you're getting the essential good fats you need by eating foods rich in anti-inflammatory fatty acids. Foods rich in omega-3 fatty acids include fatty fish (e.g., wild salmon, sardines, and herring), and flax seeds and flax seed oil. Meanwhile, omega-9 monounsaturated fatty acids, another type of good fat, can be found in olive oil, avocados, and nuts.

Prebiotic and Probiotic Foods

A healthy balance of good bacteria in our gut plays a major role in our health. Prebiotic foods provide the dietary fiber your gut bacteria need to thrive. Think of them as fertilizer for your gut. Good sources of prebiotic fiber include apples, asparagus, bananas, barley, Jerusalem artichokes, flaxseeds, garlic, leeks, oats, and onions. Supplements containing inulin, the fiber that's found in most good prebiotic foods, can be used as well.

Probiotic foods are those that contain beneficial bacteria because they are fermented. Good probiotic foods include live-culture yogurt, kefir, sauerkraut, kombucha, lacto-fermented pickles and vegetables, aged cheeses, miso, tempeh, and kimchi.

Healthy Herbs and Spices

The distinctive flavors of herbs and spices come from the many polyphenols (complex natural chemicals) they contain. Polyphenols give these foods their healthful, antioxidant, anti-inflammatory, and anticancer effects. Turmeric (and the curcumin it contains) is well known for all these effects. Cinnamon helps to lower blood sugar. Garlic has antibiotic, anti-inflammatory, anti-nausea, and pro-detoxification properties. Rosemary, thyme, oregano, and hundreds of other herbs and spices used in foods abound with beneficial effects.

Nutrition Basics

To create your personalized nutrition program, start with the basics. In terms of pure simplicity, we like to quote author Michael Pollan, who states in *Food Rules* that we should eat:

1. Real food.
2. Mostly vegetables.
3. Not too much.

Real food. Real food is food your great-grandmother would recognize. Anything that has ingredients on the label you don't recognize or understand or has chemicals you can't pronounce, does not count as real food. Shop the produce section and the outer aisles of a supermarket, where the less processed products are, rather than the center aisles, where the boxes and bags of processed foods are kept. Even better than shopping in the supermarket is to get fresh produce from your local farmers' market. Eat seasonal, local, fresh, organic food whenever possible.

Mostly vegetables. Enough said.

Not too much. Learn to eat mindfully by taking the time to listen to your body. Whenever possible, try to eat without distraction. Set your phone and your work aside. Stop eating before you are full—the satiety center in your brain is about twenty minutes behind what you put into your mouth. Meals that include lots of fiber such as large salads and generous servings of fresh vegetables will help you feel full for longer while nourishing your body with important nutrients.

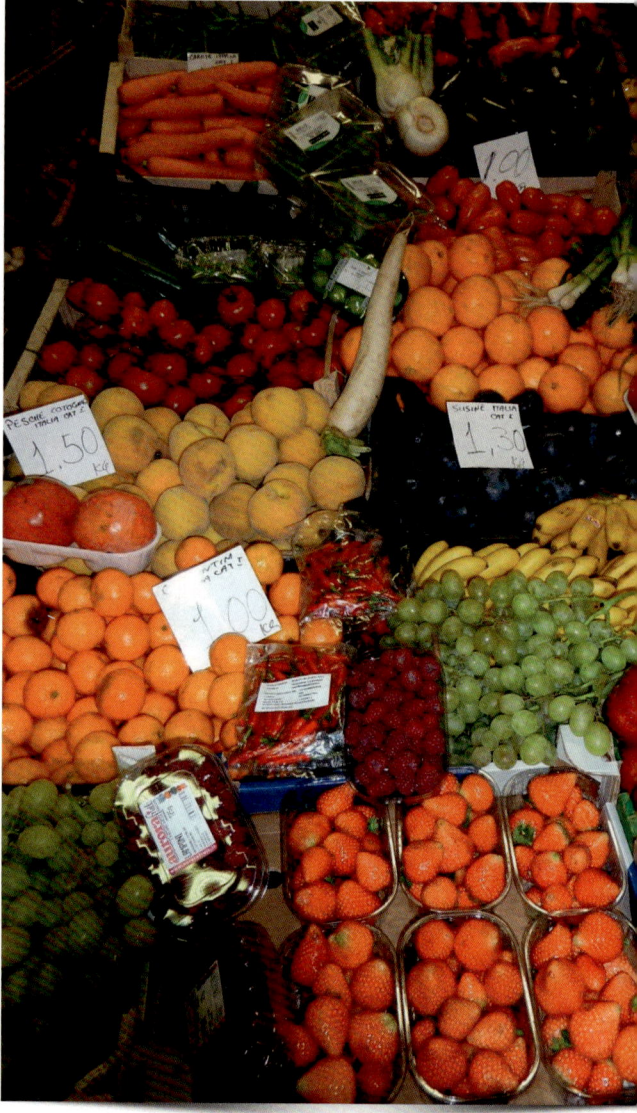

© Steve Amolis

> "
> Go vegetable heavy. Reverse the psychology of your plate by making meat the side dish and vegetables the main course.
>
> **—Bobby Flay**

Creating a Nutrient-Rich Diet

- **Eat lots of plants!** Aim to eat at least 5 servings of a variety of vegetables and fruits a day, but preferably 7-8. Aim for 42 servings/week. This may sound like a lot, but a serving is only half a cup. Eat at least twice as many vegetables as fruit. A Supernutrition Smoothie (see below) can help you achieve this in an easy way. Try to eat the colors of the rainbow to enhance the variety of produce you consume. Choose mainly less starchy vegetables, such as zucchini, peppers, tomatoes, broccoli, sweet potatoes, and greens.

- **Eat seasonal, local, and organic produce wherever possible.** Refer to the Dirty Dozen and Clean Fifteen below to save money and choose food wisely.

- **Eat plenty of fiber.** Benefits of fiber include stabilizing blood sugar, lowering cholesterol, and reducing the risk of type 2 diabetes and colon cancer. Fiber comes in two forms: *soluble*, which dissolves in water; and *insoluble*, which doesn't. Don't worry about the difference. Aim for eating 35 grams of fiber daily, which is easy to achieve with five servings of whole grains, fruits, and vegetables.

- **Eat red meat sparingly**. If you can, choose organic meat that has been regeneratively raised, grass-fed and finished (rather than corn-fed or finished).

- **Rotate your foods.** You are more likely to get food sensitivities if you eat the same food every day. Your body needs a variety of nutrients; your gut thrives on diversity. Broadening your diet will help you get the nutrients you need.

- **Eat a variety of whole grains (not whole grain flours), and avoid gluten if you can.** Try some new grains, such as amaranth, farro, einkorn, barley, buckwheat, millet, oats, quinoa, and black rice.

- **Avoid or eat less dairy.** Although they often don't know it, many people are lactose intolerant and can't digest dairy foods well. Choose grass-fed, organic milk, butter, yoghurt, kefir, and cheese in small quantities if you can tolerate it.

- **Eat more good fats.** Use first-pressed or cold-pressed extra-virgin olive oil as your primary source of dietary fat (at low or no heat), avocado oil (for higher heat cooking), and organic virgin coconut oil. Nuts and seeds, or oils and butters made from them, are excellent sources of nourishing fat.

- **Increase the omega-3s in your diet by eating fish such as wild salmon, herring, mackerel, and sardines two to three times a week.** You may also consider a mercury-free fish oil supplement. If you don't eat fish or don't like it, consider alternative sources of omega-3s, such as flaxseed oil, hemp oil, or a small amount of evening primrose or black currant oil. You can use these directly—a drizzle of nutty-tasting flaxseed oil on vegetables is a good

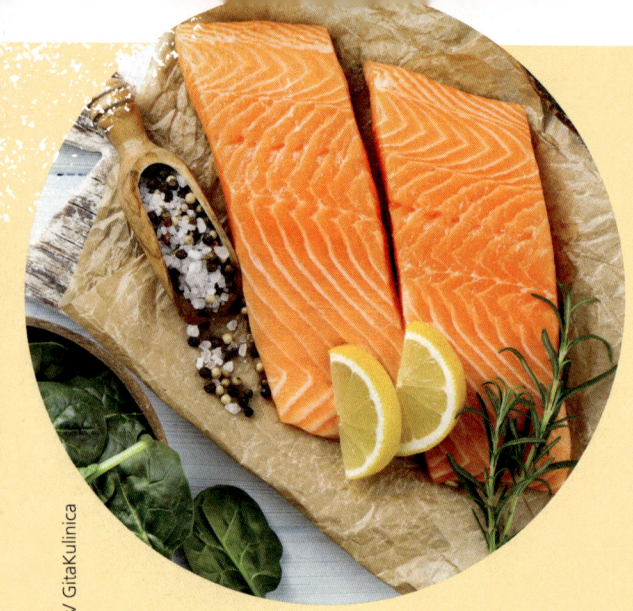

alternative to butter—or take them as supplements.

- **Eat pasture-raised organic eggs.** Pastured organic eggs are higher in omega-3 fatty acids and are more humane.
- **Drink filtered water.** Regrettably, it is almost impossible to measure the many chemicals that abound in our environment and can get into our water supply. An activated carbon charcoal filter on a tap or in a pitcher will remove most toxins. Reverse osmosis filtration and distillation are better ways of filtering your water but may also remove trace minerals that are healthy for you. Skip bottled water. Drink filtered water from your sink instead—it's free, it's environmentally friendly, and it doesn't use fossil fuel in the form of plastic bottles and truck fuel.
- **Spice up your diet.** Herbs and spices are healthful and make food taste fantastic, so use them with wild abandon! Many herbs and spices have proven anticancer and anti-inflammatory benefits. Dried herbs are as valuable as fresh ones. Examples include turmeric, cinnamon, oregano, and ginger.
- **Omit or drink alcohol in moderation.** One (for women) to two (for men) glasses of red wine per day are acceptable. Skip this if you are concerned about alcohol use or take drugs that interact with alcohol.
- **Add cultured and fermented foods.** Fermented and cultured products can encourage the growth of beneficial bacteria in your gut.

The Dirty Dozen and the Clean Fifteen

The nonprofit organization Environmental Working Group (ewg.org) releases an annual list of fruits and vegetables that are highest and lowest in pesticides and other agricultural chemicals. The foods on the Dirty Dozen list are high in chemicals, so it's probably better to purchase these only if they have been organically grown. The Clean Fifteen list is lowest in chemical residue; these foods are safe to eat even if they are not organically grown. The list may change a bit from year to year, but these foods typically appear:

The Dirty Dozen
Strawberries, spinach, kale, collard greens, mustard greens, nectarines, apples, grapes, cherries, peaches, pears, bell and hot peppers, celery, tomatoes. (Incidentally, raisins aren't considered fresh produce, but even most organic brands are high in pesticide residues.)

The Clean Fifteen
Avocados, corn, pineapple, onions, papaya, frozen peas, eggplant, asparagus, broccoli, cabbage, kiwi, cauliflower, mushrooms, honeydew, cantaloupe.

What to Avoid

- **Avoid processed and refined foods, which are low in nutrients but high in calories.** They are also often high in added sugars, salt, and fat. In particular, decrease your intake of refined carbohydrates such as enriched white flour and sweeteners such as sugar and high-fructose corn syrup.
- **Avoid charred meat and other foods.** The charred part of food can contain carcinogenic substances.
- **Avoid trans fats.** These fats are associated with an increased risk of oxidative stress and diabetes. Read food labels carefully: food manufacturers are allowed to list any food with less than half a gram of trans fats per serving as having zero trans fats.
- **Avoid genetically modified (GM or GMO) foods where possible.** USDA regulations say that food products must indicate the presence of GMO ingredients with a round green label on the package that says "bioengineered" or "derived from bioengineering." Alternatively, manufacturers are allowed to list a phone number to call or text for more information, or a QR code that takes you to an online disclosure. We are concerned about the effects of GM foods and believe it is better to avoid them when possible.
- **Avoid artificial food colorings and additives.** Many common food additives have been shown to interfere with normal vitamin and enzyme function. For example, yellow dye #5 can interfere with the action of vitamin B6.
- **Avoid processed meats.** These foods are full of fat, salt, and chemical additives. Stay away from bacon, ham, hot dogs, sausage, jerky, and smoked meats.
- **Avoid artificial sweeteners.** These register in your brain as sugar, making you crave sweet food and raising insulin. They also interfere with your gut microbiome.
- **Avoid fruit juices.** This includes all-natural ones with no added sugar. These drinks have little to no fiber, so they can cause a rapid rise in blood sugar. Should you choose to drink these, select freshly made, cold-pressed juices made mostly from vegetables with little or no added sugar.

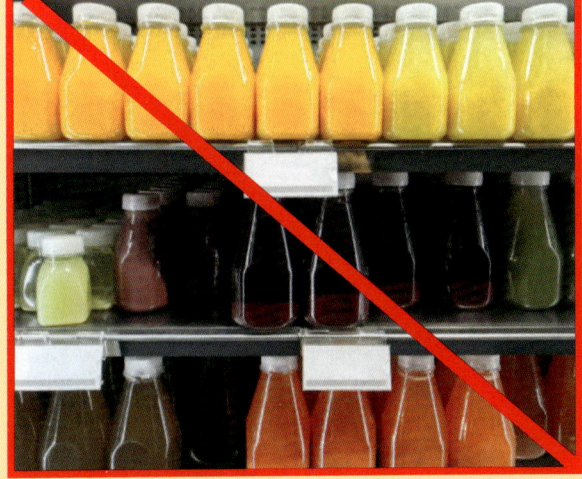

Tips on Decoding Food Labels

Making better food choices requires that we pay attention to what we are eating. A crucial first step is learning to read the ingredient list on the food label.

1. Look at the list of ingredients:

- Ingredients are listed by quantity, so the most abundant ingredients are listed first. If any of the first three ingredients are a form of sugar, think twice about the product. High-fructose corn syrup is just another way of saying sugar. So are pure cane syrup, beet sugar, brown rice syrup, dextrose, fruit juice concentrate, malt, and maltose. Be wary of fructose, or simple fruit sugar! When consumed as a fruit, the fiber in the fruit binds to the fructose, effectively negating its bad impact. However, if consumed as fruit juice or a fructose additive, it is highly toxic and addictive and even worse for you than glucose.
- Avoid all artificial sweeteners such as Splenda (sucralose), Sweet'N Low (saccharin), Equal (aspartame) and agave, which is high in fructose.
- Avoid products with more than seven ingredients unless you recognize all of them.
- Avoid products with artificial and hydrogenated ingredients.
- Avoid products that are enriched or fortified. These are indications that the food is chemically manipulated, rather than derived from nature.
- Also avoid products that claim to be low-fat, light, low-sodium, diet, healthy, or any other marketing term meant to fool you into thinking the product is somehow more healthful. The same can be said for "natural" products—sometimes these products aren't actually "natural" at all and require a closer look.

2. Look at the breakdown of servings, calories, fiber, fat, carbs, added sugar, and protein.

- Look carefully at the number of servings per container. The label gives the number of servings in the container and the number of calories per serving. Often a container includes several servings. If you eat the whole thing in one sitting, you could be getting a lot more calories than you realize.
- Serving sizes are not a recommendation of how much you should eat or drink: they are standardized in order to compare different foods. It's important to pay attention to serving sizes to understand how much of a certain nutrient you are consuming, but serving sizes are not meant to dictate your intake.
- The higher the fiber content, the better.
- Look at the fat content. Avoid saturated and trans fats (partially hydrogenated fats are trans fats). If the product has less than 0.5 grams of trans fat per serv-

Nutrition Facts

Serving Size 1 cup (228g)
Servings Per Container about 2

Amount Per Serving	
Calories 250	Calories from Fat 110
	% Daily Value*
Total Fat 12g	18%
Saturated Fat 3g	15%
Trans Fat 3g	
Cholesterol 30mg	10%
Sodium 470mg	20%
Total Carbohydrate 31g	10%
Dietary Fiber 0g	0%
Sugars 5g	
Proteins 5g	

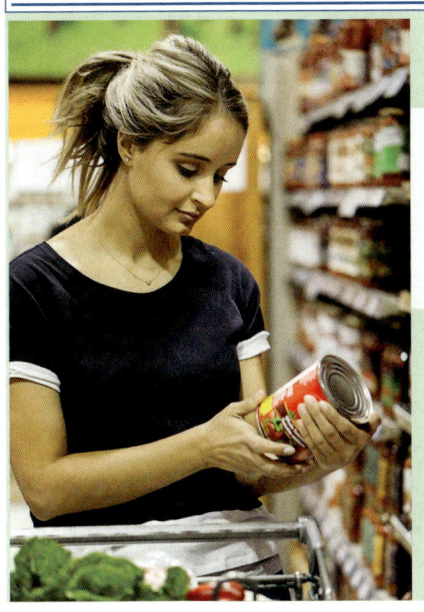

ing, the amount doesn't need to be listed. If you add up all the different fats, the sum should equal the total fat content. If not, hidden trans fats may be present.

- Avoid anything that has more than 10g sugar in a serving. Keep sugar to under 25 grams a day (about 6 teaspoons).
- Remember, the daily value amounts are approximate guidelines only.

Appropriate Portions

Several well-designed, carefully controlled studies have compared different dietary approaches and found that they're all about equally effective for weight loss, mostly because they all reduce calories. In the studies that went on for more than a year, the participants who lost weight almost always gained most of it back, no matter which diet they followed.

What the studies show is that what and when you eat matters, but so does how much you eat. To give you an easy way to choose your foods and control your portions, we like to use the fist method.

For a bigger meal, one plate equals about four fist sizes.

For a snack, you don't need much. Consider half a fist or two thumb sizes.

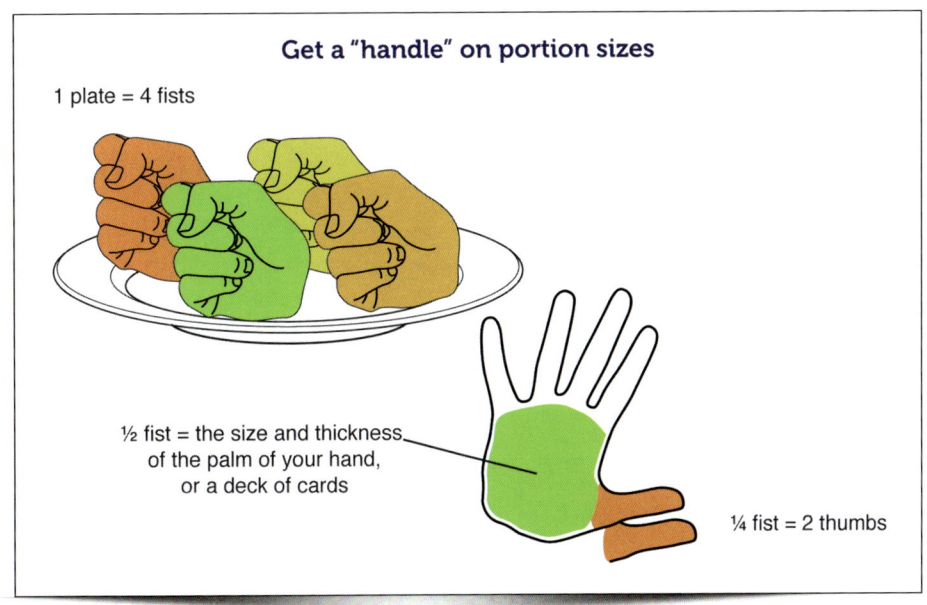

FIGURE 10.1 | Portion Sizes

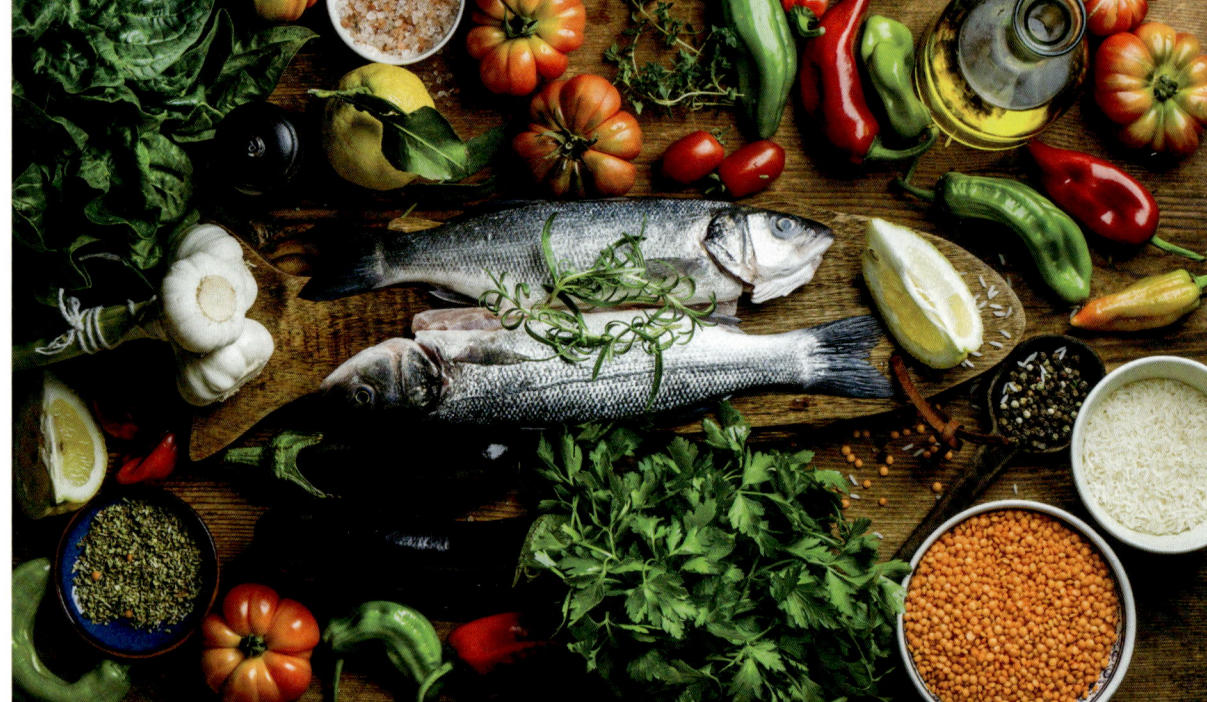

The Mediterranean Diet

The simplest and most delicious way to shift your diet away from processed foods and toward whole foods is to follow the Mediterranean diet. This eating pattern prioritizes whole grains, fresh fruits and vegetables, good fats, and lean protein. It's supported by a lot of excellent research showing that it helps prevent heart disease, stroke, diabetes, inflammation, impaired cognition, and other chronic conditions. This is the eating pattern followed by the long-lived and healthy residents of Ikarios we mentioned above.

The Mediterranean diet is a way of eating based on the traditional diets of people in countries near the Mediterranean Sea, including France, Greece, Italy, Israel, and Morocco. On the Mediterranean diet, meals contain minimally processed foods and are built mostly around plant-based foods.

The building blocks of the Mediterranean diet include:
- Plant foods such as fruits, vegetables, bread, whole grains, beans, nuts and seeds.
- Low to moderate consumption of dairy products, eggs, fish, and poultry; little to no red meat.
- Olive oil as the primary fat.
- Limited consumption of sweets, sugar-sweetened beverages, and white flour.
- Optional low to moderate consumption of wine (one serving per day for women and two servings per day for men), along with a meal.

The DASH (Dietary Approaches to Stop Hypertension) diet is based on research studies sponsored by the National Heart, Lung, and Blood Institute (NHLBI). It is very similar to the Mediterranean diet. The DASH diet has been shown to help lower high blood pressure and improve cholesterol levels, which reduce your risk of heart attack and stroke. The MIND (Mediterranean–DASH Intervention for Neurodegenerative Delay) incorporates the DASH diet, which means it's basically the Mediterranean diet with the addition of at least two servings a week of berries and a daily glass of wine. The MIND diet has been shown to help reduce the risk of cognitive impairment and dementia as we age.

What your main meal looks like on a Modified Mediterranean Diet

VEGETABLES: fresh, raw, stir-fried, lightly steamed, or blanched for 2 minutes: asparagus, broccoli, brussels sprouts, carrots, cauliflower, celery, dark green leafy vegetables (kale, spinach, swiss chard, etc), eggplant, garlic, mushrooms, onion, peppers, sprouts (all kinds), sweet potato/yam, tomato

WHOLE GRAINS AND LEGUMES: amaranth, barley, beans (black, kidney, lima, mung, pinto, soy/edamame), black-eyed peas, brown or wild rice, chick peas, couscous, cracked wheat, hummus, lentils, plain oatmeal, quinoa, split peas, sugar snap peas, whole grain or rye bread, whole wheat pasta

GOOD (UN-SATURATED) FATS: cold pressed vegetable oil/dressing, cold pressed extra virgin olive oil, nuts and nut butter (almond, cashew, peanut, walnut), olives, seeds (flax, salba, sesame/tahini, sunflower)

PROTEIN: chicken, edamame, eggs/egg whites from omega-3 enriched free-range eggs, fish, lean grass-fed beef, low-fat cheese and yogurt, turkey, tofu

- 2 FISTS VEGETABLES
- 1 FIST WHOLE GRAINS AND LEGUMES
- ½ FIST LEAN PROTEIN
- ½ FIST GOOD (UNSATURATED) FATS

HERBS: basil, bay leaf, chervil, chives, cilantro (fresh coriander), dill, marjoram, mint, oregano, parsley, rosemary, sage, tarragon, thyme, wild fennel

SPICES: allspice, anise seeds, caraway seeds, cardamom, cinnamon, coriander, cumin, fennel, fenugreek, ginger, hot pepper, mustard, nutmeg, paprika, saffron, turmeric

FIGURE 10.2 | Modified Mediterranean Diet

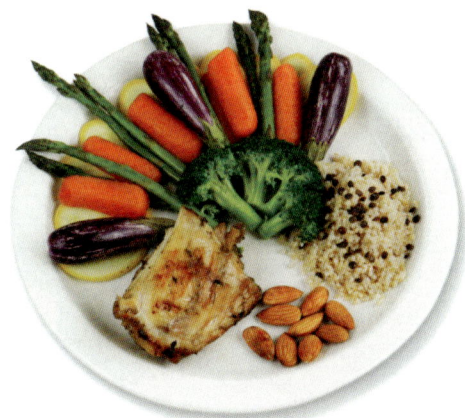

A modified Mediterranean diet plate example:

½ fist lean protein (e.g., grilled chicken)
½ fist good fats (e.g., almonds plus olive oil dressing)
1 fist whole grains and legumes
(e.g., brown rice and lentils)
2 fists low-glycemic vegetables

How Much Protein Do You Need?

When we suggest to patients that cutting back on animal foods might help their health, they often worry that they won't get enough protein. That's a good point. The body needs protein for normal growth and maintenance, but your needs vary depending on your health, your age, and your activity level. The current recommended adult daily intake of protein is 50 grams, based on a 2,000-calorie diet. It's less if you normally eat fewer calories; it's more if you're an athlete, pregnant, recovering from a serious illness or surgery, or are over the age of 65. If you have a chronic health condition, your protein needs may also deviate from this standard recommendation.

One egg contains about six grams of protein, an ounce of cheese has about seven grams, a quarter-pound burger has about 14 grams, a can of tuna has about 20 grams, and a baked chicken leg gives you about 30 grams. It's easy to see how most of us get far more than 50 grams of protein a day just from our regular diets—and it's equally easy to see that you could cut back on the animal foods in your diet quite a bit and still get plenty of protein. For example, a cup of cooked beans has on average about 15 grams of protein; a cup of cooked quinoa has about 8 grams; an ounce of almonds has about 6 grams. If you cut back on or even eliminate animal foods, you can still easily meet your protein needs.

Other **Healthy Diets**

Valuable as the Mediterranean diet and similar approaches are, they're not for everyone. Some other popular dietary patterns are both healthy and sustainable.

The Low-Carbohydrate Approach

The low-carbohydrate approach was originally popularized by Robert Atkins, MD, in the 1970s. On a low-carbohydrate diet, calories are less important than carbohydrate grams. The diet limits daily carbohydrate intake to under 100 grams (preferably under 50) or no more than 30 percent of your daily calories. You aim for 30 percent of your other calories from fat and 40 percent from protein. On a low-carb diet, you eat lots of non-starchy vegetables, limit fruit, and get your protein from meat, fish, poultry, eggs, nuts, and dairy products.

The Paleo Approach

High-protein diets such as the Paleo diet are based mostly on animal foods, with smaller portions of vegetables, fruits, and nuts. The idea is to mimic the supposed diet of our Paleolithic-era ancestors, who hunted and foraged for their food. We don't know exactly what they ate (probably whatever they could catch or find, including insects), but we do know their diets didn't include almost all the foods we eat today, such as sugar, dairy foods, coffee, and many others. Compared to our modern diet full of processed foods and additives, the Paleo diet is healthier. It is also low in carbohydrates, which can help with blood sugar stability. However, the emphasis on meat and the very restricted choices of other foods make it hard to follow for long.

What your main meal looks like on a Low-Carb Diet

VEGETABLES: *fresh, raw, stir-fried, lightly steamed, or blanched for 2 minutes:* asparagus, broccoli, brussels sprouts, carrots, cauliflower, celery, dark green leafy vegetables (kale, spinach, swiss chard, etc), eggplant, garlic, mushrooms, onion, peppers, sprouts (all kinds), sweet potato/yam, tomato

WHOLE GRAINS AND LEGUMES: amaranth, barley, beans (black, kidney, lima, mung, pinto, soy/edamame), black-eyed peas, brown or wild rice, chick peas, couscous, cracked wheat, hummus, lentils, plain oatmeal, quinoa, split peas, sugar snap peas, whole grain or rye bread, whole wheat pasta.

½ FIST WHOLE GRAINS AND LEGUMES

GOOD FATS ½ FIST

2 FISTS VEGETABLES

1 FIST LEAN OR VEGETARIAN PROTEIN

GOOD (UN-SATU-RATED) FATS: cold pressed vegetable oil/dressing, cold pressed extra virgin olive oil, nuts and nut butter (almond, cashew, peanut, walnut), olives, seeds (flax, salba, sesame/tahini, sunflower)

PROTEIN: chicken, edamame, eggs/egg whites from omega-3 enriched free-range eggs, fish, lean graass-fed beef, low-fat cheese and yogurt, turkey, tofu

HERBS: basil, bay leaf, chervil, chives, cilantro (fresh coriander), dill, marjoram, mint, oregano, parsley, rosemary, sage, tarragon, thyme, wild fennel

SPICES: allspice, anise seeds, caraway seeds, cardamom, cinnamon, coriander, cumin, fennel, fenugreek, ginger, hot pepper, mustard, nutmeg, paprika, saffron, turmeric

FIGURE 10.3 | Low-Fat Diet

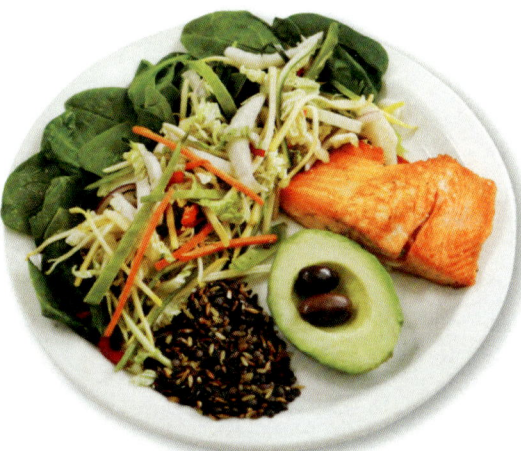

© Daniel J. Segal

A low carb diet plate example:

1 fist lean protein (e.g., grilled salmon)
½ fist good fats (e.g., avocado and olives)
½ fist whole grains (e.g., wild rice)
2 fists low-glycemic vegetables

The Low-Protein Approach

What about low-protein diets? There's some evidence that a low-protein diet may be helpful for improving longevity. Even so, while we feel most adults eat too much protein, we feel the low-protein approach is too limited, especially for very active adults and people over 65. Maintaining muscle mass is one of the most important parts of healthy aging. Some *sarcopenia*, or loss of muscle mass, is an inevitable part of growing older, but we can fight back and slow the loss significantly with regular exercise and a diet with enough protein. A low-protein diet may not be protective enough against sarcopenia.

The Protein Quandary

Valter Longo, PhD, a longevity expert, studied a group of patients in Ecuador with Laron syndrome, a hereditary disorder that involves a lack of receptors for growth hormone. People with Laron syndrome are extremely short. They tend to be long-lived and very rarely get cancer or type 2 diabetes, despite smoking, having poor dietary habits, and drinking a lot of alcohol. Dr. Longo concludes that their inability to respond to growth hormone is related to their longevity and good health despite poor lifestyle habits. Extrapolating from that, he feels we shouldn't stimulate our production of growth hormone—and one way to do that is to limit dietary protein. This is similar to the conclusion of T. Colin Campbell in his book, *The China Study*.

We're not sure about this, because a high-protein diet may help with maintaining muscle mass by stimulating the production of growth hormone and making your body more receptive to it. We know that having a 30-gram protein snack about two hours after working out helps maintain and even build muscles.

Is there a middle road? We think so, and the answer lies in looking at early humans. When game animals were scarce or hunters were unsuccessful, their diet was low in protein and they survived on foods they could gather, such as berries, tubers, nuts, frogs, small mammals, and fish. When game was more abundant or hunters were luckier, a period of high-intensity exercise would be followed by a period of feasting on protein. So perhaps the answer to high protein vs. low protein isn't binary. We're adapted to alternating periods of eating both. Overall, it's probably better to keep our protein intake within the recommended amounts as we age and exceed it only after exercising hard.

The Ketogenic or Keto Diet

The ketogenic diet can be very helpful for managing weight loss, prediabetes, and diabetes. However, it's not the right choice for everyone—and not always healthy when followed long-term. Discuss following this diet with your doctor or nutritionist before trying it. We've found that it is very helpful for our patients who are severely insulin resistant. We've also found that it can improve metabolic flexibility, letting you change your metabolism easily in response to exercise or diet.

To clear up some confusion about the ketogenic diet, let's start with an accurate definition. *Ketosis* is the normal metabolic state of elevated ketone bodies (such as acetone and butyrate) in the blood or urine. Ketone bodies are a normal energy source for the body when blood glucose levels are low. Ketosis often happens, for example, in the morning after fasting overnight. In ketosis, blood ketones are elevated, but the body's acid-base balance remains normal. It's important to understand that ketosis isn't the same as *ketoacidosis*, when very

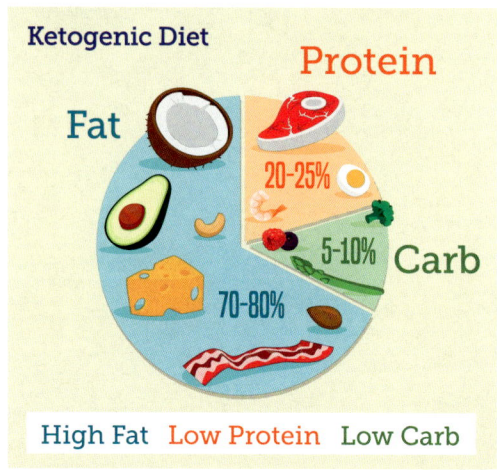

FIGURE 10.4 | Ketogenic Diet

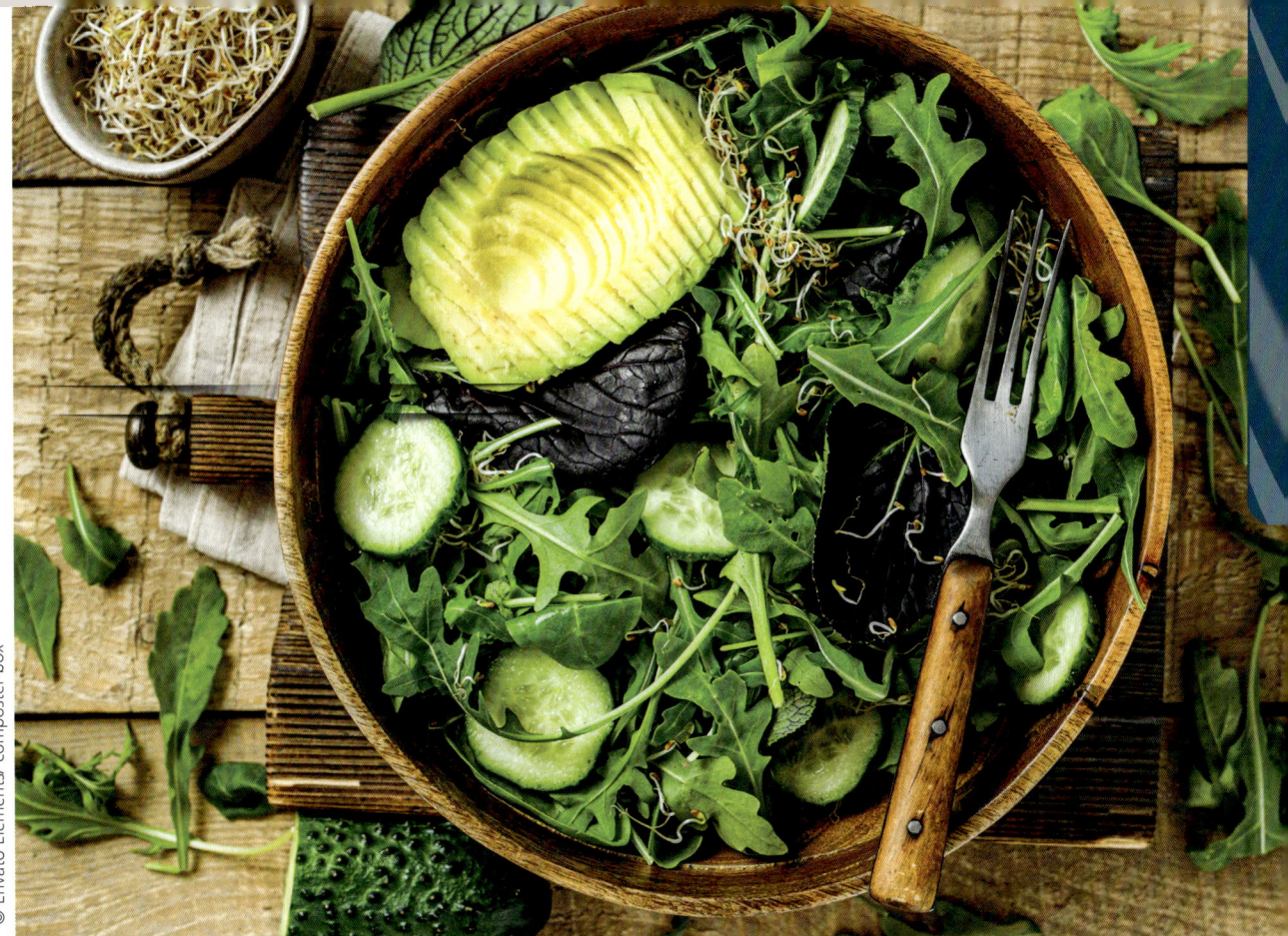

high ketone levels cause the blood to become dangerously acidic. This is usually seen in patients with type 1 diabetes who have very low or no insulin.

Your body goes into the metabolic state of ketosis when your daily carbohydrate consumption is below 50 grams. The body turns to fat as its primary fuel; instead of metabolizing glucose for energy, the body shifts its metabolism to break down your stored fat into ketones, which it then uses for energy.

The ketogenic diet is designed to put the body into a state of steady ketosis by limiting carbohydrates and increasing fat consumption. Because the ketogenic diet is rich in fat and low in carbohydrates, your liver shifts from producing glucose to using fatty acids to generate ketone bodies as fuel for the body and the brain. The ketogenic diet can be helpful for weight loss and for getting blood sugar under control by improving insulin resistance. Some studies report that people with Type 2 diabetes who follow the ketogenic diet can cut back on insulin and other medications or even stop using them.

On the ketogenic diet, 70 percent of your daily calories comes from good fats, 25 percent from protein, and only 5 percent from carbohydrates. By contrast, the Standard American Diet (truly "SAD") consists of 50 percent carbohydrates, 35 percent fats, and 15 percent proteins. As you can see, adopting a ketogenic diet means a big change in what you eat—your diet is a lot more restricted, though it's still healthy.

As mentioned, daily carbohydrate consumption on the ketogenic diet works out to 50 grams a day or less. On other low-carbohydrate diets, such as the Atkins diet, the Paleo diet, and the low-carb Mediterranean diet, daily carbohydrate consumption is generally in the 100-to-150-gram range. These diets don't limit carbohydrates enough to put the body into steady ketosis. We recommend that you get your carbohydrates mostly from non-starchy,

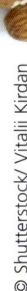

low-glycemic vegetables such as broccoli, spinach, kale, and zucchini. These foods are very low in carbs, so you can eat large servings—a cup of cooked broccoli has only 4 carb grams. By contrast, one medium baked potato has about 35 carb grams. The vegetables also give you plenty of phytonutrients and fiber.

The ketogenic diet is far more effective and easier to stick with if "clean keto" principles are followed. Clean keto means focusing on high-quality, nutrient-dense foods with minimal or no processing and no added sugar, chemical additives, antibiotics, or hormones. Look for grass-fed, pasture-raised, or regenerative meats and pasture-raised organic poultry and eggs. Fish should be wild caught. Vegetables should be organically grown; buy locally grown produce whenever possible.

Good low-carb vegetable choices include asparagus, broccoli, brussels sprouts, cabbage, celery, green beans, kale, peppers, summer squash, and zucchini. Berries such as strawberries, blueberries, and blackberries can be eaten in limited amounts; avoid other fruits.

Good fat sources are avocados, avocado oil, grass-fed organic butter, ghee, coconut oil, medium-chain triglyceride (MCT) oil, extra-virgin olive oil, flaxseed oil, sesame oil, and walnut oil.

Nuts, nut butters, and seeds are also encouraged on the keto diet. Good nut choices are almonds, almond butter, hazelnuts, hazelnut butter, pecans, and walnuts. Seed choices include chia, hemp, flax, pumpkin, and sunflower.

If you're a coffee drinker, you'll be glad to know that caffeine can significantly stimulate ketone production in a dose-dependent manner.

Switching over to a ketogenic diet probably will involve a big change from your usual diet. Many people experience a few days of mildly unpleasant symptoms, known as the "keto flu." Symptoms include headache, achy muscles, feeling foggy or irritable, fatigue, nausea, and constipation. Although you might feel sick, you aren't really—it's just your body adapting. You can help the symptoms pass faster by drinking lots of plain water, eating often, eating plenty of colorful low-carbohydrate vegetables, and taking it easy for a few days if necessary.

Suggested Meals

Nutrition is complicated. To make your food choices a bit simpler, we give you some ideas for meals and snacks based on the Mediterranean approach.

Breakfast

If you are following a low-carbohydrate or Mediterranean diet, aim for a breakfast that contains protein, healthy fats, and optional high-fiber carbohydrates. Here are some breakfast categories to choose from:

- Eggs
- Nuts, seeds, and grains: grain-free granola, nut butter and fruit, superfood trail mix, rolled or steel-cut oats
- Meatless option: potato-vegetable hash with tofu
- Yogurt: fat-free, live-culture milk yogurt, low sugar kefir, low-sugar nut yogurt
- Protein smoothies and shakes

Lunch and Dinner

The illustrations earlier in this chapter are examples of the fist method showing what your meal would look like on a Mediterranean diet and a low-carb diet. These are maximum portion sizes for your main meal. No matter what size your plate is, try to keep the proportions the same as those shown.

Fasting and Time-Restricted Eating

Fasting has a long history in religious and spiritual practice—and in medicine, dating back to Hippocrates. Today, we realize that fasting is a way to hit the reset button on your health. We like to think of it this way: You can't repair a road while heavy traffic is on it. You need to stop the traffic. Fasting involves the same idea. It allows the body time for self-repair and rejuvenation.

Work by the longevity researcher Valter Longo, PhD makes a good case for doing a very low calorie five-day fast every 6 months or so, mostly to prevent diabetes, heart disease, cancer, and neurodegenerative disease. A fast of this length stimulates your body to break down and recycle the components of old and damaged cells, a process known as *autophagy*. Fasting also activates stem cells, which have the potential to develop into many different types of cells in the body. Stimulating their production can help rejuvenate you.

A short, water-only fast of just 24 hours is enough to leave many people feeling depleted, not rejuvenated, and fasting longer than that on just water can cause health problems, like electrolyte imbalances and loss of lean muscle mass. Fortunately, based on his research, Dr. Longo has found a way to make a five-day fast safe and relatively easy to do.

Dr. Longo developed a fasting-mimicking diet (FMD) that provides the benefits of a long fast without the problems water fasting alone can have. To get around the health risks and reduce how hungry you feel, the fasting-mimicking diet (FMD) tricks your body into thinking you're not eating at all. Your body goes into energy-conserving starvation mode, begins autophagy, and produces more stem cells.

It works because the FMD provides 400 to 500 calories a day from plant-based complex carbohydrates, 400 to 500 calories from healthy fats, 25 grams of plant-based protein, and supplements for vitamins, minerals, and omega-3 fatty acids.

While we think the FMD has value for our patients, especially those who are at risk of diabetes, it's not for every patient. People who are pregnant, over the age of 70, have liver or kidney disease, or have a serious chronic condition shouldn't do it. The FMD also isn't something you should do on your own. We strongly recommend following the FMD only while working with your doctor or an experienced dietitian to make sure the diet is right for you and to help you get the best results safely. Instead of trying to reproduce Dr. Longo's fasting foods, we recommend using his convenient ProLon® diet kit for your fast.

Juice Fasting

Juice fasting is a popular wellness trend, but we don't recommend it. The idea is that the juice provides nutrients while promoting detoxification. The problem is that many juice drinks used during a juice fast are made palatable with the addition of fruits to sweeten them. The high sugar content may counteract many of the benefits of the fast. In addition, such juices usually lack fiber, which is important for restoring and maintaining the gut microbiome.

Supernutrition Smoothie

Most of us struggle to get necessary nutrients without a lot of extra calories. One easy way to achieve this is with what we call a Supernutrition Smoothie. This makes a great breakfast.

Here's the basic recipe:
- **Start with 1 cup filtered water** or ice cubes in a blender container.
- **Add protein.** Options are 2 tablespoons of organic tofu or a powdered protein such as a whey, rice or pea protein or spirulina-based powder.

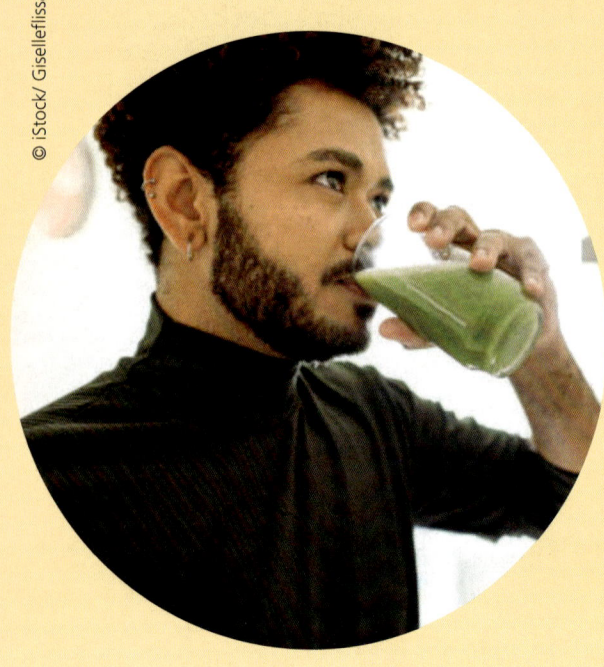

- **Add vegetables.** You can do this by adding 2 cups of leafy green vegetables such as spinach, kale, parsley, and others to taste. Alternatively, use an organic vegetable-based powder available from your health-food store. Look for one that contains cruciferous vegetables, such as kale and brussels sprouts, as well as flax seeds.
- **Add fruit, only if needed– but not too much.** Berries are always a good choice; a banana will give the smoothie a creamier texture.
- **Add good fats.** Try freshly ground flax seeds or 1/2 tablespoon of flax seed oil, or 1 tablespoon of chia seeds. (If you don't like the taste of these, take 1000 to 2000 mg omega-3 mercury-free fish oil capsules as a separate supplement.) You can also add half an avocado for silky texture.
- **Add 1 tablespoon fiber.** We suggest unflavored psyllium husk or inulin fiber.
- **Add flavorings or powders to taste.** Some ideas are 1/4-inch ginger root, peeled and grated; cinnamon or nutmeg; 1/4 to 1/2 teaspoon powdered green tea; 1 to 2 teaspoons nut butter; 2 tablespoons yogurt or probiotic powder; powders such as unsweetened cocoa, maca, reishi or pomegranate.

Blend together and enjoy!

Intermittent Fasting and Time-Restricted Eating

There are two ways you can get the benefits of fasting without doing a prolonged fast. One way is intermittent fasting, where you eat your usual meals five out of seven days a week. You choose to fast or eat very lightly on the fasting days. The idea is to give your body regular, shorter chances to clear out dead and damaged cells and produce extra stem cells.

Another viable approach is time-restricted eating. We're very accustomed to eating three meals a day, with plenty of snacks in between. Most of us start eating with breakfast in the early morning and don't stop for more than a few hours at a time until we go to bed. In fact, most Americans get over half their daily calories in the evening, when they eat dinner and then consume a lot of snack foods before bedtime. Along with the reality that about 70 percent of the typical diet comes from processed foods, this eating pattern may help explain why so many Americans are overweight.

We recommend a different eating pattern, where you eat your normal dietbut consume it only during a daily 12-hour window. So, if you have breakfast at 7 a.m., your last meal of the day should be at 7 p.m. Don't eat again until 12 hours later. You're still eating your usual (preferably healthy) diet and taking in the same amount of food, but you're consuming it in a more compressed time frame. This does two important things for your health. First, it reduces the number of low-quality calories you take in over the course of an evening. Second and more important, by going 12 hours without eating, your body must use the calories you took in during the day to fuel you through the evening and overnight. You burn more calories and store fewer as fat —in fact, your body might even dip into your fat reserves before you eat again.

Time-restricted eating, as this eating pattern is known, can be very helpful for people with metabolic syndrome, prediabetes, and diabetes. It improves insulin resistance, brings down cholesterol, helps reduce inflammation, and is an effective weight-loss tool, particularly if you stick with it for more than a few months.

You can take time-restricted eating up a notch by going longer from the time of your last evening meal until your first meal of the next day. Examples are a 14:10 or 16:8 pattern, where all your calories are taken in during an eight-hour window. Our patients who want to lose weight find this approach very effective if they eat their usual amount at meals and stick to low-calorie snacks. We don't suggest doing this for prolonged periods.

An additional benefit of time restricted eating is that it has positive effects on the microbiome. The "good" or beneficial bacteria divide more slowly, so they tend to survive, while the non-beneficial or "bad" bacteria, which divide rapidly, suffer from starvation and tend to die out.

Detoxification: The Body's Self-Purification

In Chapter 7, we discussed detoxification. In this chapter we discuss the basic approaches to "Detox Diets."

Eating to Detoxify

Detox diets are similar to fasting, but with significant differences and some drawbacks. The concept of regular detoxing comes predominantly from American naturopathic physicians. Leaving aside the many fad approaches to detoxing, the general principles of a detox diet are:

- Stop input of all external toxins, such as alcohol and caffeine, as much as possible. Avoid refined food, preservatives, colorings and flavorings.
- Eat predominantly vegetables, with some fruit.
- Eat small amounts of clean protein (wild or sustainably caught fish, organic egg, organic chicken, organic grass-fed beef, live-culture Greek yogurt, lentils, quinoa, tempeh).
- Add herbs that upgrade liver Phase 1 and Phase II detoxification, such as milk thistle, dandelion, ginger, and turmeric.
- Add fish oil to help with what we call Phase III detoxification.
- Drink lots of filtered water to flush the kidneys.
- Ensure good elimination with ensuring regular bowel movements through adequate fiber, prebiotics, and probiotics.
- Ensure good skin elimination with sweating, far infrared saunas, or dry brushing

the skin. (Far infrared saunas allow you to sweat out toxins without overheating your body.)
- Ensure good fresh air for lung elimination; practice deep breathing several times a day.
- Ensure good sleep, as this is when the body detoxifies best.

Supplements for Better Metabolism

Do we really need dietary supplements? You may have heard that all supplements do is make expensive urine, or that you just need a one-a-day multivitamin with minerals. These statements are both incorrect. Supplements can dramatically improve health. Yet on the other hand, they may not always be good for you. They can fuel various diseases and interact with certain drugs.

Let's look at some factors to consider:

Supplements for Nutritional Deficiencies

As medical students in South Africa, we watched a young woman enter the hospital in heart failure. She struggled to breathe as her heart beat rapidly. Her swollen legs and altered mental status were a clue to the cause of her illness—chronic vitamin B_1 (thiamine) deficiency, resulting in a disease known as beri-beri. An intravenous infusion of thiamine resulted in an astounding recovery. She was better within hours, an example of how vitamins can make a difference. Does that mean we should give thiamine to everyone with heart failure? The answer is clearly no. Understanding nutritional deficiencies helps us use the correct nutrient for the correct problem.

Vitamin D is another good example. In general, excessive sun exposure can lead to an increased risk of skin cancer. In attempting to

Fasting and Eating Disorders

We don't recommend fasting or time-restricted eating for anyone struggling with disordered eating. Someone with anorexia who severely restricts their food intake might find fasting an easy way to disguise their illness. Fasting can also be a way to disguise orthorexia, which is an unhealthy focus on eating in a healthy way. Fasting can sometimes be a slippery slope into disordered eating tendencies, especially if you have a history of disordered eating, find yourself obsessing over food and nutrition, or prioritize changing your physical appearance over your physical and mental health. If you or someone you know is struggling with an eating disorder, we urge you to ask for help.

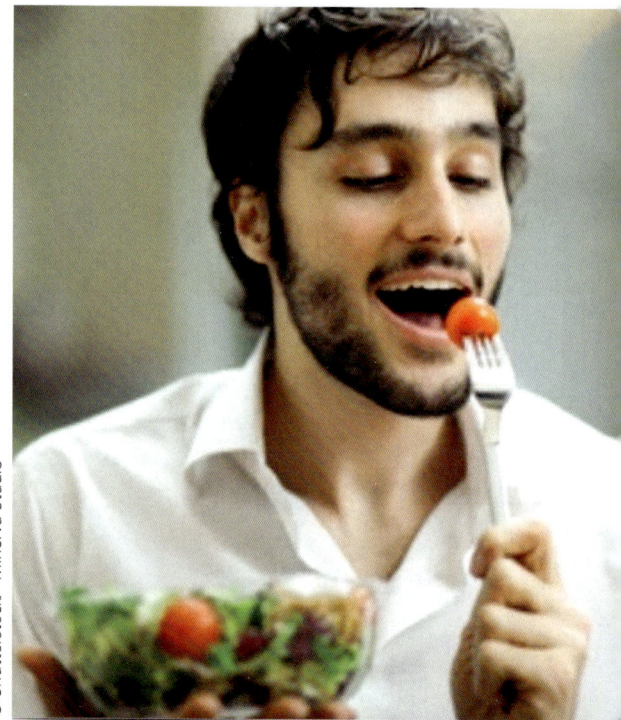

© Shutterstock/ Minerva Studio

avoid this risk by using sunscreen and protective clothing, many people have become deficient in this important vitamin, which is derived from adequate sun exposure on your skin. Checking your vitamin D level with a blood test is a good idea. If it is low, supplementing with vitamin D3, or cholecalciferol, can help prevent or improve many conditions including hypertension, depression, osteoporosis, and autoimmune diseases, as well as seasonal affective disorder (SAD). People with SAD get cabin fever or depression in the winter months and crave warm, sunny climates. Vitamin D supplementation may be a much less expensive alternative!

Supplements for Better Metabolism

We can use nutritional supplements to take a functional approach to helping the body detoxify, lower oxidative stress, reduce inflammation, improve methylation at the correct time, improve digestive function, improve probiotic balance, and maintain equilibrium of the immune system. This only helps, however, if the correct high-quality supplements are used.

Realize that no one supplement will be the ultimate solution to preventing illness. The diets we have outlined above will help promote normal function of your body systems. However, if clinical evaluation and functional lab testing still point to an imbalance, supplements can be added to promote ideal functioning. The advantage here is that dietary supplements tend to have multiple benefits. For example, good antioxidants will usually help detoxification and lower inflammation.

Supplements for Improving Detoxification

Numerous supplements can help improve your detoxification. N-acetylcysteine (NAC) has been used in emergency rooms for decades to treat acetaminophen (Tylenol) overdoses, protecting the liver from damaging free radicals as it helps excrete the drug. Doses of 500 mg to 1000 mg twice daily can help the liver with its detoxification functions.

NAC also helps increase levels of glutathione, a major antioxidant. It also appears to help an agitated mood. Supplements with ellagic acid, watercress (*Nasturtium officinale*), artichoke leaf (*Cynara scolymus*), juniper berry (*Juniperus communis*), red clover (*Trifolium pratense*), stoneroot (*Collinsonia canadensis*), fenugreek (*Trigonella foenum-graecum*), and milk thistle (*Silybum marianum*) can also all help improve detoxification. Glutathione itself should only be used if in a liposomal or other highly absorbable form.

Antioxidant Supplements

The classic antioxidant supplements are vitamins A, C, and E, and the minerals zinc and selenium. These are often touted as the solution to many degenerative diseases, such as macular degeneration. However, studies on these supplements have not always been positive. For example, one study concluded that smokers who take vitamin A have higher lung cancer rates. Vitamin C, when injected in extremely high doses, appears to help reverse early atherosclerotic disease. However, oral doses don't seem to do the same. Men with higher blood levels of vitamin E tend to have lower levels of prostate cancer, but studies on supplementation with synthetic vitamin E showed that this could increase prostate cancer rates. Another confounding variable is that a substance that appears to be an antioxidant in the lab may turn into a pro-oxidant in the body.

A green tea extract known as EGCG is

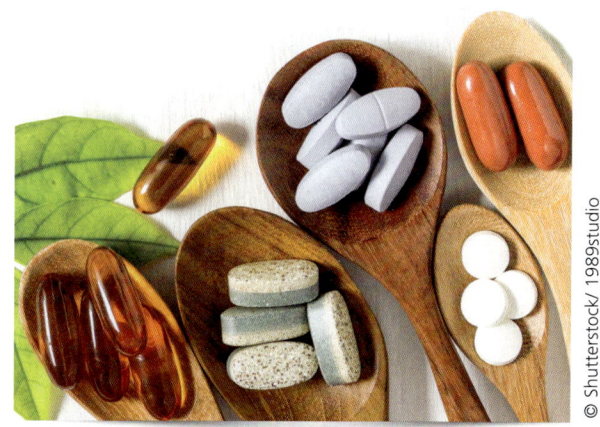

A Question of Quality

The quality of dietary supplements is extremely important, but the supplement industry isn't as carefully regulated as the pharmaceutical industry. Consumers are pretty much on their own when it comes to finding top-quality products. Look for products that reputable manufacturers make using pharmaceutical grade ingredients. The manufacturer should also guarantee the potency levels on the label and state that good manufacturing practices (GMPs) were followed, at a minimum! A supplement should be safe and effective as proven in clinical trials, case control reports, and other clinical documentation.

The products you purchase should be batch-tested to ensure a scientific evaluation of ingredients. They should be free of heavy metals, pesticides, and contamination by fungus, bacteria, or toxins. (Unregulated supplements from China and some other countries may be tainted with drugs, heavy metals, and other toxins.) Herbal supplements should come from organically grown plants. The products should meet the quality and purity standards set by the United States Pharmacopeia (USP or USP-NF), NSF International, and the Natural Products Association. The most effective products are manufactured by companies with scientific knowledge about the products they sell. Finally, look for companies that employ fair trade practices and that are concerned about sustaining the environment.

---

believed to be one hundred times more potent as an antioxidant than vitamin C and at least twenty-five times more potent than vitamin E. Even more impressive are resveratrol and pycnogenol—the antioxidants found in red wine—and Enzogenol, an antioxidant derived from New Zealand pine bark. These products appear to mimic the benefits of a calorie-restricted diet without the food restriction. Resveratrol, found in the skin of red grapes and in red wine, appears to regulate the sirtuin family of our aging genes. Resveratrol's actions may help explain the so-called French Paradox—why the French can smoke, eat a high-fat diet, never go to the gym, and yet have a lower heart attack rate than Americans. It's possible the resveratrol they get from regularly drinking red wine with meals may help, although it's more likely that their largely Mediterranean-style diet plays a role. Products with resveratrol derivatives are being studied for their impact on aging and illness and for their value in maintaining bone health in older adults.

Enzogenol fed to mice in a study helped them live longer, healthier lives. It also appears to help regulate brain function, prevent migraines, and regulate eye disease, heart disease, and even attention deficit hyperactivity disorder (ADHD). However, effective doses of these supplements have yet to be determined. Antioxidants appear to work better when multiple supplements are used in combination with one another. So while they are promising, we suggest you review antioxidants with someone familiar with current research data on nutritional supplements before taking them.

Supplements for Lowering Inflammation

Curcumin, an active compound in turmeric, has great anti-inflammatory benefits when tested in the lab. However, in humans, study outcomes are variable. This may be because curcumin is absorbed 2,000 percent more effectively if it is taken with pepper or a pepper extract (as it might be, for instance, in an East Indian diet). Curcumin also has an anti-inflammatory effect on the gut and the gut microbiome. EPA, a fatty acid found in fish oil, has anti-inflammatory benefits, as do the botanicals boswellia (*Boswellia serrata*), devil's claw (*Harpagophytum procumbens*), cat's claw (*Uncaria* spp.), willow bark (*Salix* spp.), and ginger (*Zingiber officinale*).

Supplements for Maintaining Immune, Metabolic and Endocrine Balance

Supplements can be used to support immune function while simultaneously dealing with stress. Examples here are astragalus, Siberian ginseng, ashwagandha or Indian ginseng, and rehmannia. Mushroom extracts and echinacea can help prevent colds. Plant sterols and sterolins can help regulate T-cell immune function, ameliorating chronic fatigue, allergies and boosting immunity.

We list only a few supplements to help you understand how to think about them. There is a broad array available. Find a health care practitioner who is knowledgeable in this area and can help you understand which is the best one to take.

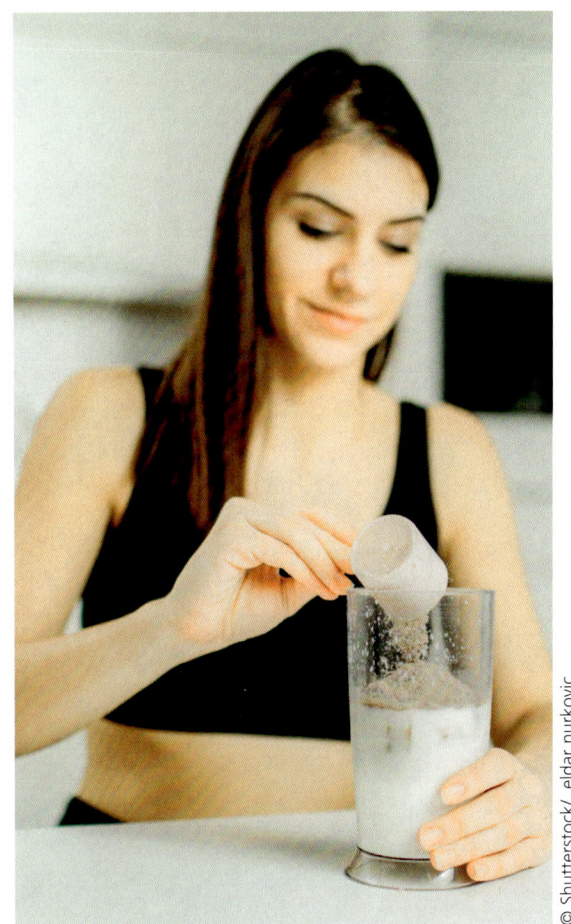

© Shutterstock/ eldar nurkovic

Food or Drug?

One of the big differences between food supplements and drugs is that drugs in general are new-to-nature molecules. In other words, we may not have detoxification pathways to adequately deal with the metabolic byproducts of drugs. In addition, drugs tend to have side effects and interactions, especially when you start taking more than one. Sometimes we only find out years later what these interactions are.

Food supplements in general are much less likely to have side effects and interactions. In general, Mother Nature has helped us decide which foods humans have tolerated over thousands of years.

Food supplements are often, but not always, better tolerated than drugs. While a drug may have one or two benefits, it may also have multiple side effects, which can lead to needing more drugs to control them. One food supplement, on the other hand, is likely to have multiple benefits. Vitamin D, for instance, may benefit osteoporosis and depression, may decrease pain, may reduce autoimmune disorders, and may even lower hypertension. Fish oil supplements may help heart disease, arthritis, osteoporosis, depression, and a host of other problems. The body is used to foods in combination. This is not true with drugs.

Synergistic Nutritional Benefits

The more drugs we take, the more likely we are to suffer from drug interactions and side effects. Nutritional substances are different. In nature, foods have multiple elements all working together to benefit us. Functional medicine providers are trained on how to combine supplements for optimal benefit. By understanding the various systems of the body, we can learn to analyze this and design specific programs that affect multiple systems.

You may need some nutritional supplements to antidote a subclinical nutritional deficiency, others to speed up detoxification, and still others to act as antioxidants or anti-inflammatories. We can use them even more to balance or modulate the immune system. Finally, we can use these in addition to medications if necessary.

When we analyze and understand the body from a functional medicine standpoint, we learn that the treatment that reverses illness is often the same treatment that promotes health. What's more, the same process appears to help multiple disease processes at the same time. This is the essence of Transformational Medicine. We use one program to transform your illness process into a wellness process.

A Transformational Supplement Program

A transformational supplement program can include vitamins, minerals, amino acids, enzymes, herbs, probiotics, and medications. It should ensure that hormones and mood are balanced. Your program should be selected in conjunction with a comprehensive lifestyle approach. We strongly recommend working with a doctor who understands functional medicine.

If you are taking any sort of dietary supplement, always tell your doctor. Supplement-medication interactions may create unexpected side effects.

You will know that your transformational supplement program is working when:

1. You feel better.
2. Your lab markers change.
3. Your health begins to improve.
4. You develop a sense of resilience—the ability to bounce back.
5. You develop a new, positive sense of vitality.

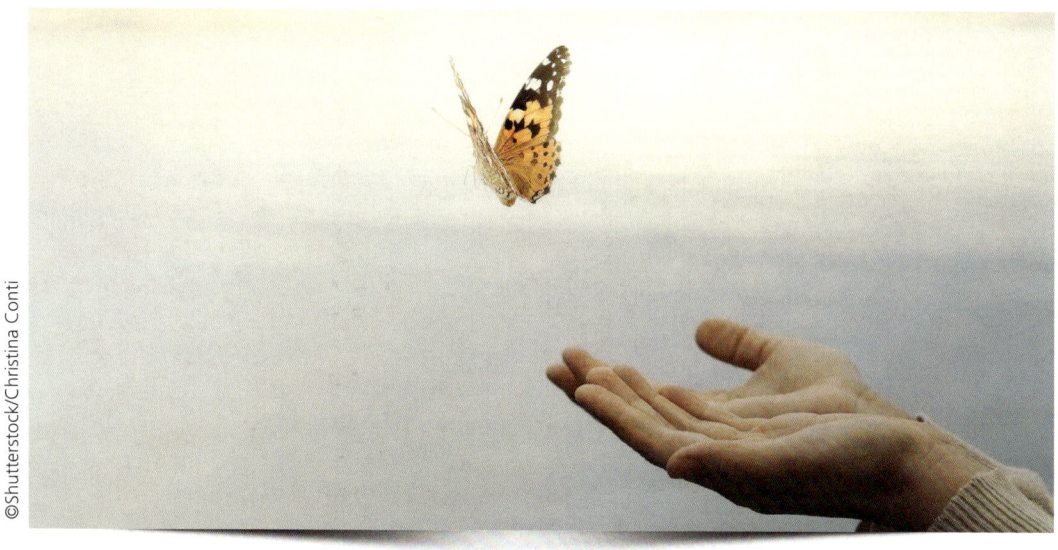

Don't be confused by labels

Labels are often inaccurate and misleading. Here's what they say and what they mean.

CHICKENS AND EGGS

Our ancestors ate eggs that had a balanced ratio of omega-3 (anti-inflammatory) and omega-6 fatty acids (pro-inflammatory) of about 1 to 5, respectively. Currently, conventionally raised eggs have an omega-3 to omega-6 ratio of about 1 to 45, leading to greater inflammatory impacts in the body. The nutritional decline of conventional eggs is physically evident in more brittle shells and dull-colored yolks. Grading (AA, A, or B) is based on freshness, shell characteristics, and defects, not nutrition.

Conventionally raised hens, or "battery caged" hens live in cages that provide less space than a standard sheet of paper and are stimulated with light, hormones, and other techniques to make them large quickly. Most cannot stretch their wings and do not see the outdoors. They are provided feed and drugs that rapidly increase their weight in a short period. These poor conditions result in poorer hen health and less nutrient density in eggs.

Raising claims describe a hen's living environment.

- The term **"natural"** is virtually useless as all eggs meet this standard, which is that nothing was added to them.

- **"Cage-free"** *implies that hens are allowed to roam in an indoor space that allows for wings expansion and dust bathing.* However, they are often denied access to the outdoors. This indoor living space may be overcrowded and unhealthy for their living conditions. This has no real benefit to the nutrient value.

- **"Free-range"** hens must be given access to outdoor space and may be offered the availability of wild food such as plants and insects. However, the length of outdoor time, the number of outdoor access points in the henhouse, and the outdoor conditions are not defined. The term free-range makes us think of a chicken roaming free on the range. However, as you read above, you see that this is not true. This has little benefit to nutrient value.

- **"Organic"** eggs come from uncaged hens that are free to roam indoors and have access to the outdoors. They are fed an organic diet without conventional pesticides or fertilizers. This is a good starting point when choosing eggs but does not specify all necessary living conditions. While we agree with feeding chickens an organic diet, this will not necessarily make the inflammatory value of the chicken or egg any better.

- **"Pasture-raised"** chickens and eggs imply hens are provided and encouraged to utilize full outdoor access spent roaming pasture grasses to gather food and exhibit their natural behaviors during day. At nighttime, hens are safely in the henhouse, allowing a more natural wild habitat. This is the type of chicken your great-grandparents would have eaten. While "pasture-raised" eggs have no legal definition or third-party verification, this term is often used by small farmers who raise their chickens similarly to that in nature. Pasture-raised hens yield eggs with rich yolk colors that are a result of the naturally pigmented carotenoids found in wild plants and insects. Shell color varies depending on the hen's breed. The best source of pasture-raised eggs is from a local farmer, where you can ask questions about the raising environment, feed, and time spent outdoors. Farmers often want to show how well they treat their animals and will be transparent when disclosing information. Choose pasture-raised eggs that are clean and crack-free. They may vary in size which is okay.

PREFERRED

- **Organic, pasture-raised eggs and chickens** are the gold standard when choosing poultry. Some local farmers may be too small to be USDA-certified organic; this is okay if they are using organic feed, as long as it is not corn-based.

FISH

Fishing and aquaculture have a significant environmental impact on our oceans and seafood supply. According to the Monterey Bay Aquarium Seafood Watch Program (https://www.seafoodwatch.org), one-third of fish populations are over-fished and over half are fully fished, leading to a decline in wild fish populations. Fish farming, also known as aquaculture, farms fish in a range of contained environments from natural ponds to high-tech tank systems. Overcrowded farms limit how much fish can swim, leading to their health decline and sometimes causing disease to spread. Between the cramped living conditions and unnatural diets, farmed fish generally do not thrive. Commercially raised farmed fish are often fed grain- and seed-derived pellets (like from soybean and canola) and less fish oil, which is their naturally preferred source of food. This has led to a decrease in omega-3 content in farmed salmon. The decline in natural carotenoids (the chemicals which give the fish the pink color) in the fish feed results in less vibrant pink flesh, which in commercially raised fish is sometimes hidden by the addition of pink and red dye.

It is important to know optimal sourcing and the preferred raising and catching practices for fish and seafood when seeking optimal health and environmental impacts. The Seafood Watch Program has excellent, thorough online resources including a fish search engine that generates information such as type, method, and location and a Seafood Calculator that provides recommendations based on age, gender, and weight. While wild-caught fish is generally thought to be the gold standard, there is more being sold than available. A study from the National University of Ireland in Galway found 73 percent of 233 deep-sea fish collected from the North Atlantic Ocean contained plastic bits. Educate yourself on best practices to avoid toxic exposure and seafood extinction.

PREFERRED

A highlight on salmon: Wild-caught salmon from Washington (Pacific Ocean) that is caught via lift nets are considered the best choice option. These populations are generally healthy and any non-salmon fish that are caught are returned to the water alive. When choosing farmed salmon, indoor recirculating tanks offer less sewage discharge into surrounding rivers and seas, less disease, and less impact on other aquaculture systems. However farmed salmon are less likely to have the high fatty content found in open-water fish. Currently, 84 percent of Coho salmon (and only 0.01 percent of farmed Atlantic salmon) are produced by this method; they are labeled as "land-based" or "tank-based."

BEEF

Beef and dairy production requires large amounts of pesticides, chemical fertilizers, fuel, feed, and water which is affecting our health, the environment, the climate, and animal welfare.

- Don't you love the flavor of a good steak? Prime beef's enticing flavor qualities are thought to come from the fat content paired with a savory, umami taste finished off with a seared browning of protein and carbohydrate (called the Maillard reaction) once cooked. These are very stimulating sensations to our pallets, likely leading to beef being a preferred protein source. The Maillard reaction and the type of marbled or "prime-beef" fat are primarily responsible for the inflammatory nature of beef.

- Fat content (and subsequent tender mouthfeel once cooked) varies greatly depending on the choice of cut and is shown by white cobbling. To achieve greater cobbing, meaning the fat that makes beef taste good, farmers feed conventionally raised beef with a high corn diet. Modern American beef cows spend the first six months of their lives with their mothers on pastureland getting their nutrition through nursing and grasses. They are then switched to an inexpensive, high grain and corn diet which encourages quick growth, specifically fat growth. Cows that were once ready for slaughter at four to five years old are now being taken at 14 months. A cow's digestive tract is not designed to digest corn, especially the corn mush byproduct that is often used as feed. To counterbalance this unnatural digestion that can lead to health complications and illness, cows are given antibiotics several times throughout their lifespan.

- There's more. We love our beef grilled and fried, leading to charred and blackened meat. These high-temperature cooking processes cause the formation of heterocyclic amines (HCAs) and polycyclic aromatic hydrocarbons (PAHs), which are chemicals found to cause DNA changes and may increase the risk of cancer. HCAs are only found in significant amounts in meats cooked at high temperatures; PAHs are found in smoked foods, cigarette smoke, and car exhaust fumes. Aside from potentially cancer-causing genetic mutations, charred meats have been shown to cause inflammation and weight gain.

- Modern breeding of cattle has also posed health issues. Australian researchers tested pre- and post-inflammatory markers in two groups: one after eating kangaroo (wild, lean game meat that has been consumed for over millennia) and the other after eating Wagyu beef (hybridized, fatty, modern livestock only available within the last few decades). Inflammatory markers were significantly higher after eating the Wagyu beef, as opposed to the lean beef eaters, who showed no increase in inflammation.

Are there better beef alternatives?

Yes. "Grass-fed" terminology means that cattle were allowed to forage and graze on pastures on their own to find food they are naturally intended to eat; grass-fed beef is often moved to a feedlot for grain-finishing before slaughter to increase fat mass. "Grass-finished" beef comes from cattle that spend their whole life foraging on pastures, including the time before slaughter.

PREFERRED

Go for grass-fed, grass-finished, organic, pasture-raised meat: Grass-fed, grass-finished cattle that are raised on open pastures, fed a natural diet of organic grass, hay, and forage, and are not administered antibiotics or growth hormones will provide the most health benefits and least environmental and ethical damage. Studies have shown grass-fed beef is lower in saturated fat, and higher in omega-3 fatty acids, vitamin E, beta-carotene, B vitamins, and conjugated linoleic acid (CLA), a nutrient associated with lower cancer risk. These animals are raised more humanely, given sufficient space and natural diets encouraging natural behaviors and healthy lives. Choose lean cuts of meat that are certified organic and/or local. First, cook meat at a high temperature but spend the most time using lower heat, being sure to continuously flip the meat to avoid charring.

Beef marinade recipe: Combine olive oil, garlic salt, lemon pepper seasoning, fresh lemon juice, and dried oregano. Add meat and cover. Marinade in the refrigerator for up to eight hours before cooking.

Look for the term Regenerative Agriculture. This is a rehabilitative approach to food and farming focusing on improving the health and vitality of farm soil. It focuses on increasing biodiversity, enhancing the ecosystem, topsoil regeneration, water conservation, supporting biosequestration, and increasing resilience to climate change.

What does "organic" mean?

Buying organic should guarantee that the food you are eating contains no toxic pesticides or chemicals, no synthetic growth hormones or antibiotics, no GMOs, no artificial additives or preservatives, and is grown/raised using organic farming methods. However, standards for this vary worldwide, *so consumer beware!*

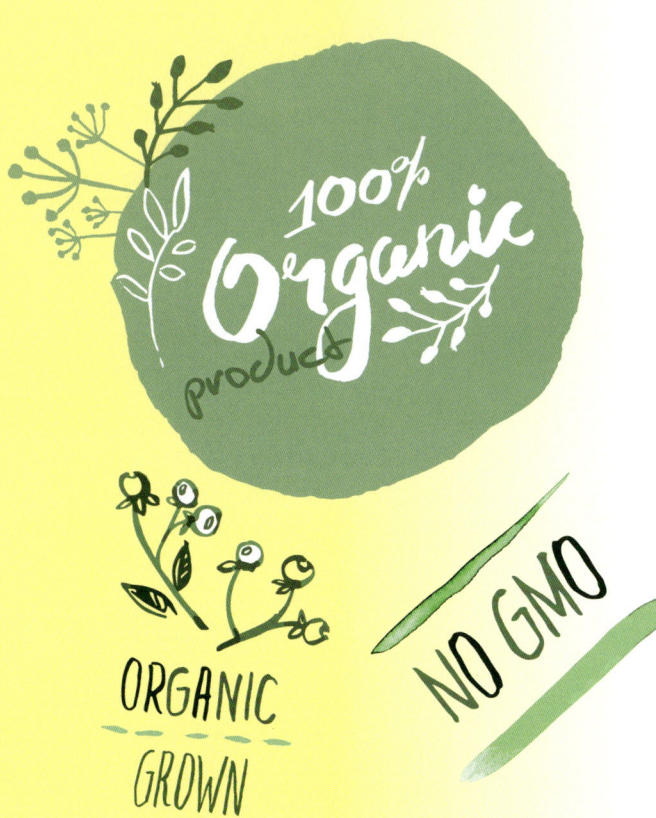

CHAPTER 11
Understanding Immunity and Allergy

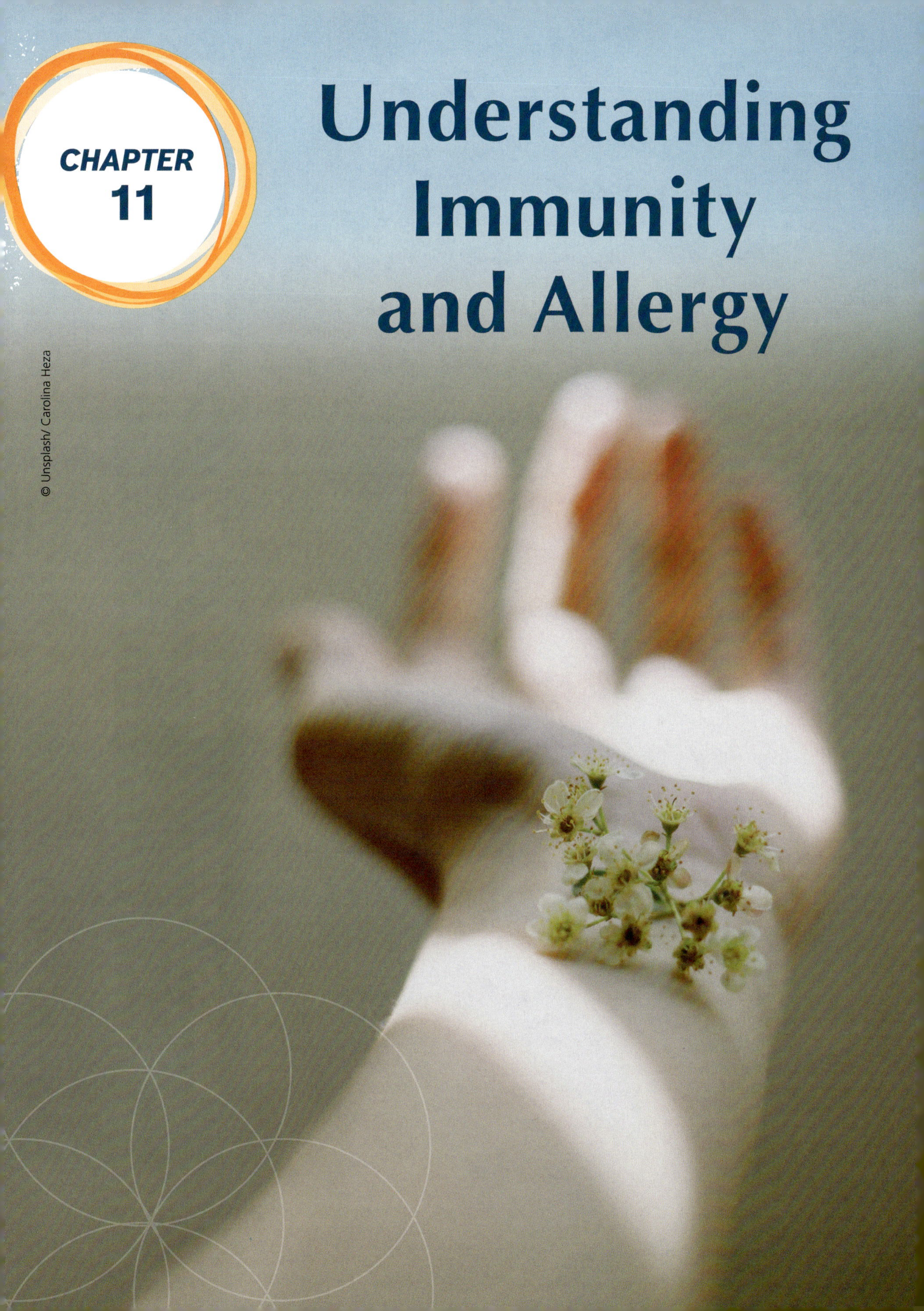

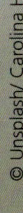
© Unsplash/ Carolina Heza

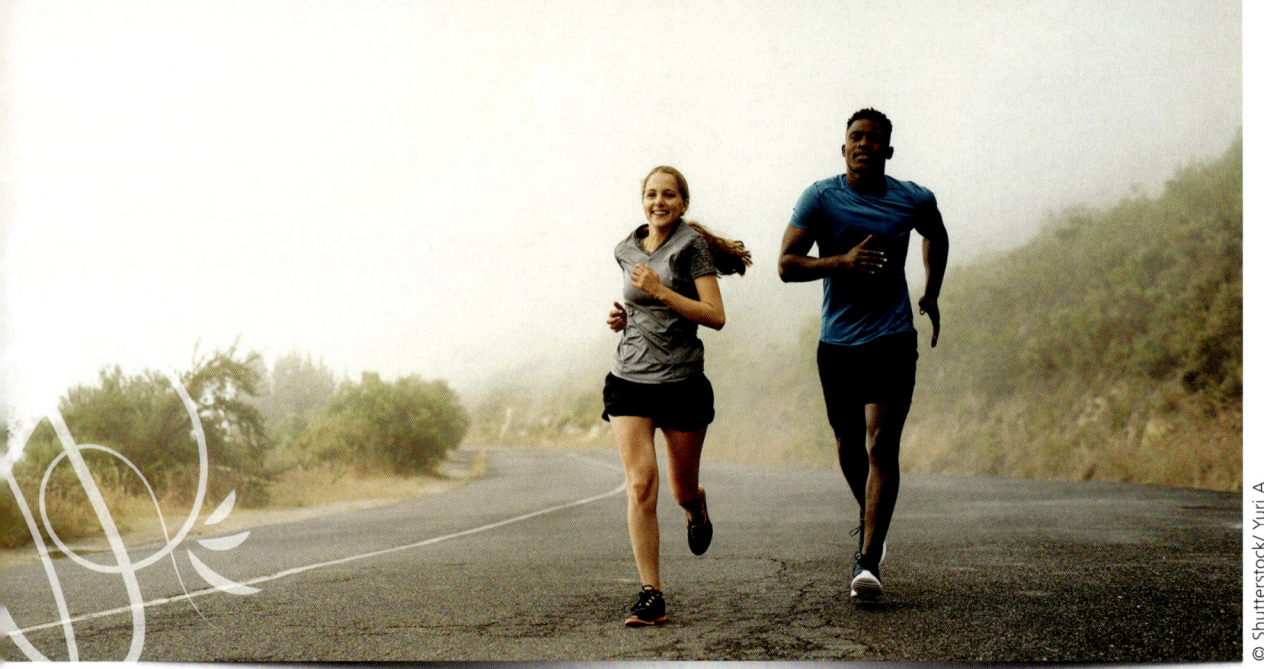

The human immune system is amazing. A complex network of barriers, specialized cells, tissues, and organs, it protects you against infection from pathogens and parasites and helps prevent and fight other diseases. It has four fundamental parts:

- *Your skin*, which is your body's largest organ, acts as a barrier to help keep germs from entering your body.

- *Mucous membranes*, another type of barrier, are the moist linings of some organs and body cavities, such as your nose, throat, airways, and intestines. They make mucus and other substances that trap and fight germs.

- *White blood cells* fight germs and create immunity against germs they have seen before.

- *Organs and tissues of the lymphatic system* include the thymus, spleen, tonsils, lymph nodes, lymph vessels, and bone marrow. They produce, store, and carry white blood cells.

All the parts of your immune system work together to create immunity against invaders. You have three types of immunity:

- *Innate immunity* **is the protection you're born with—your body's first line of defense against pathogens.** Innate immunity comes from barriers, such as your skin and mucous membranes, and from white blood cells that immediately attack invaders.

- *Acquired immunity,* **also called adaptive immunity, develops throughout your life as you're exposed to diseases or are vaccinated against them.** White blood cells called *T cells* and *B cells* attack pathogens that make it past the innate immune system. Active immunity is usually long-lasting. For many diseases, such as measles, it lasts your entire life.

- *Passive immunity* **happens when you receive antibodies to a disease from another source instead of making them through your own immune system.** This type of immunity protects you quickly but doesn't last long. Antibodies in breast milk, for example, give a baby temporary immunity to diseases the mother has been exposed to.

The immune system gets more complicated when we start looking at active immunity and the way things can go wrong with it, like allergies and autoimmune diseases. Stick with us as we explain.

White blood cells, also called *leukocytes*, are a key element in the immune system. White blood cells in the innate immune system are *phagocytes*, which literally chew up and spit out invading germs. They're part of the first-line immune response. White blood cells of the adaptive immune system are *lymphocytes*. These cells come in two types: *B cells* (because they're made in your bone marrow) and *T cells* (because they're made in your thymus gland). B cells are like guided missiles. Once they detect their targets (germs), they send defenses (antibodies) to lock onto them and tag them for destruction. Your body has two main types of T cells. *Killer T cells* are more like infantry. They march on the tagged invaders or on defective cells in your body and destroy them. *Helper T cells* signal other immune cells, such as phagocytes, telling them to fight harder. They also signal to B cells to join the battle.

The B cells work by detecting *antigens*, which are foreign proteins on the surface of pathogens. The guided missiles they send are antibodies, also known as *immunoglobulins*. B cells use antibodies to tag the germs for destruction, but they can't destroy them. That's the job of the T cells and phagocytes, who use the immunoglobulin tags to find their targets. After the B and T cells have done their job, they mostly die off, but a few stay around in your lymph glands just in case you need to fight the same germ again. These memory cells, as they're called, are what give you immunity to a disease like measles.

There are four main types of immunoglobulins:

- *Immunoglobulin A (IgA)* is found in the linings of your respiratory tract and digestive system, as well as in saliva, tears, and breast milk. It's there all the time and is part of your first-line defenses.

- *Immunoglobulin M (IgM)* is the first antibody you make when your body encounters a new infection.

- *Immunoglobulin G (IgG)* is the most common antibody in your blood. If you get sick or get a vaccine, you make large amounts of IgG, but the process takes a little time to get fully activated.

- *Immunoglobulin E (IgE)* is normally found only in small amounts in the blood, but if you have an allergy to something, you'll produce lots of IgE in a hurry when you're exposed to it.

When the Immune System Goes Awry

Over the past few decades, we have seen a huge rise in immune-related problems. There are many theories regarding this. (See the Hygiene Hypothesis sidebar below for one such theory.) Based on the work we have done in functional medicine, as well as work done by leaders in immunology such as Aristo Vojdani, PhD, we believe that multiple factors, including increased toxic burden and exposure, increased stress, a diet full of processed food, and an altered gut microbiome are causing the body to behave in an abnormal fashion. The result: the body's immune system begins to turn on itself. Dr. Vojdani has coined the term "environmentally induced autoimmunity" to aptly describe what is going on.

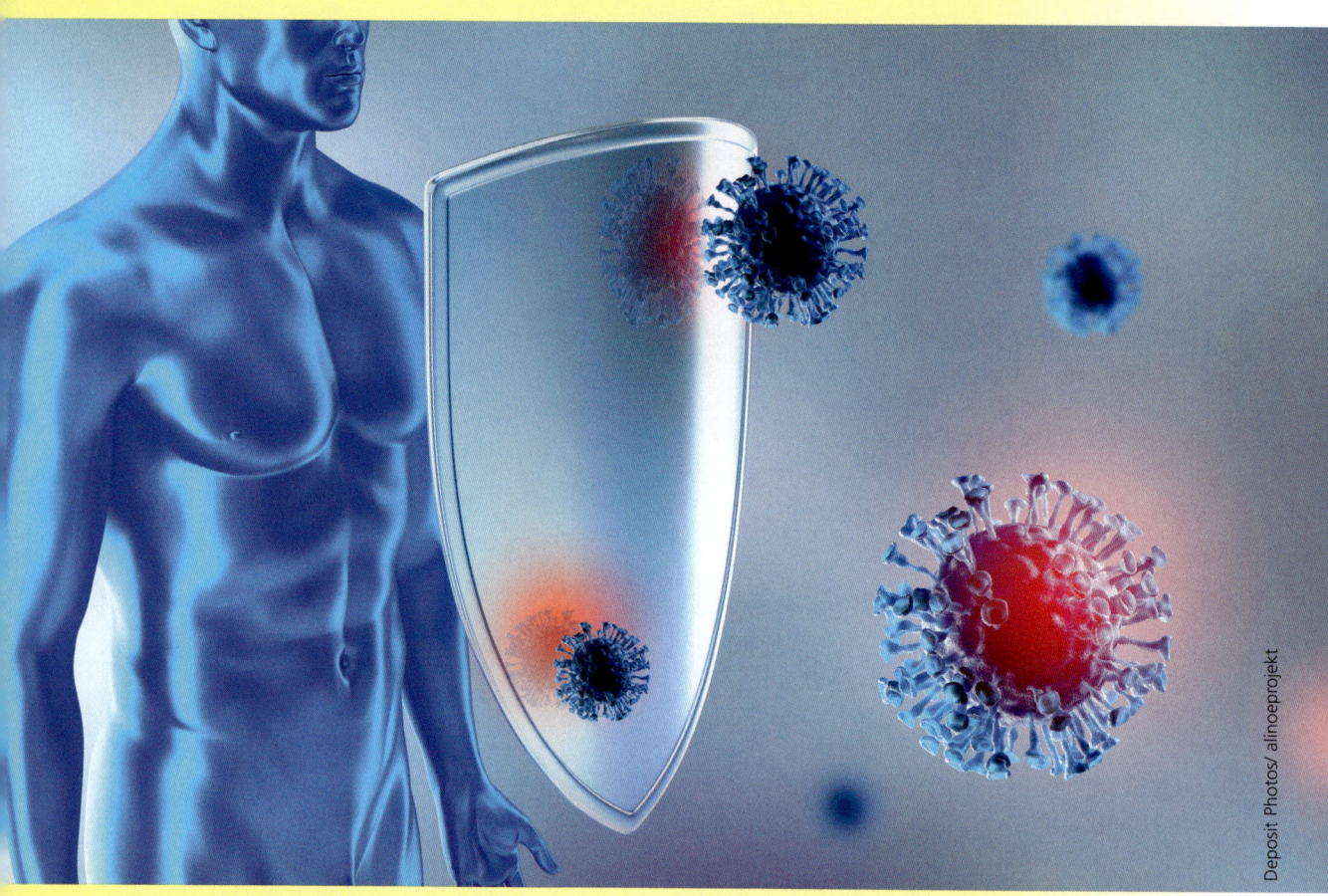

The immune system is an excellent area to showcase the different approaches of conventional medicine vs functional medicine:

In general, **conventional medicine tends to view the immune system in silos, focusing on specific pathways or mediators**. Allergists tend to focus on IgE responses. Hence, they focus on skin and blood testing for IgE-related allergies. They then treat the allergies with allergy shots, antihistamines, mast cell stabilizer drugs, steroids, and newer medications such as Xolair (omalizumab), a drug that binds to the IgE antibody.

Immunologists and rheumatologists look for autoimmune diseases and then treat the upregulated immune system. For many years the mainstays of treatment were immunosuppressant drugs such as prednisone or DMARDs (disease-modifying antirheumatic drugs) such as methotrexate, hydroxychloroquine, sulfasalazine, or cyclosporine. Today, much of their focus is on biologics, a class of drugs that bind to the cytokines that cause the inflammation seen in rheumatoid arthritis, lupus, and some other autoimmune diseases. These drugs include etanercept (Enbrel), infliximab (Remicade), and adalimumab (Humira). These drugs in general give excellent results. We often suggest them to patients after looking at the benefits, side effects, and cost. While biologics work well, they do nothing to stop the root cause of the illness. They are simply able to stop the inflammatory cascade.

Functional medicine has a different approach. It looks at these diseases from a systems biology standpoint. The first thing we usually see is that the immune system has reached a tipping point. It has arrived at the point of systemic overload! The tipping point may be an infection or some other stress with which the body can no longer cope.

Often environmental toxins have built up to the point where the body's detoxification systems can no longer cope. This leads to high oxidative stress. As discussed in previous chapters, these toxins can include plastics, pesticides, fertilizers, heavy metals, molds and much more. Sometimes emotional stress, trauma, or abuse may be a setup. Again, a genetic tendency to develop inflammation is an important contributing factor.

Gut function is often compromised. This usually starts off with an altered microbiome, so we see this more commonly in people who were not breastfed or have had multiple rounds of antibiotics or eat poorly, use alcohol, or take drugs that affect the microbiome.

The compromised microbiome and glycocalyx lead to a leaky gut. Inflammation starts happening at the level of the gut mucosa and undigested food particles and other intestinal contents that start entering the circulation. Secretory IgA levels start increasing—and the immune system is activated.

Typically, the immune system jumps to our defense when it detects danger. However, when the immune system sees undigested food particles as an enemy, it has an abnormal reaction.

The body starts developing IgA (surface antibodies), IgM (antibodies to a recent threat) and then IgG (chronically circulating antibodies). The whole immune system is activated and inflammation skyrockets! Later in this chapter we discuss CIRS (chronic inflammatory response syndrome). Then, as if this were not enough, the immune system develops cross-reactivity. At first, the antibodies may just be targeted to a set of proteins or antigens on the food itself. However, some foods share similar proteins, or antigens, to tissues in the body. As the body develops antibodies to foods, it also develops similar antibodies to certain tissues in the body, particularly the skin, joints, and organs. A classic example is celiac disease. As the immune system reacts to gluten, it also attacks joints (causing arthritis), the skin (causing dermatitis herpetiformis), and even the brain (causing "leaky brain") and mood changes. This is what Dr. Vojdani calls environmentally induced autoimmunity.

In functional medicine, we look at this entire process, try to figure out where it started and then how we can reverse it. This can be a big undertaking. Functional medicine doctors will often use drugs to treat the problem. At the same time, however, we continuously try to chip away at the underlying cause so that, if possible, the medications can one day be stopped.

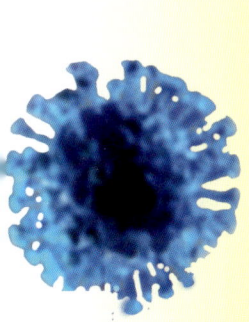

How Full Is Your Bucket?

Our bodies can only tolerate a certain amount of toxins before it starts to overload. Our natural detoxification mechanisms mean we can tolerate some exposure to environmental chemicals, stress, food additives, and other toxins. Unfortunately, we all have a tipping point where our system becomes overloaded, and our immune systems go awry. To avoid being overwhelmed, we need to minimize our toxin exposure, eat fewer processed foods, control our stress, and improve our defenses by getting sufficient sleep and exercise.

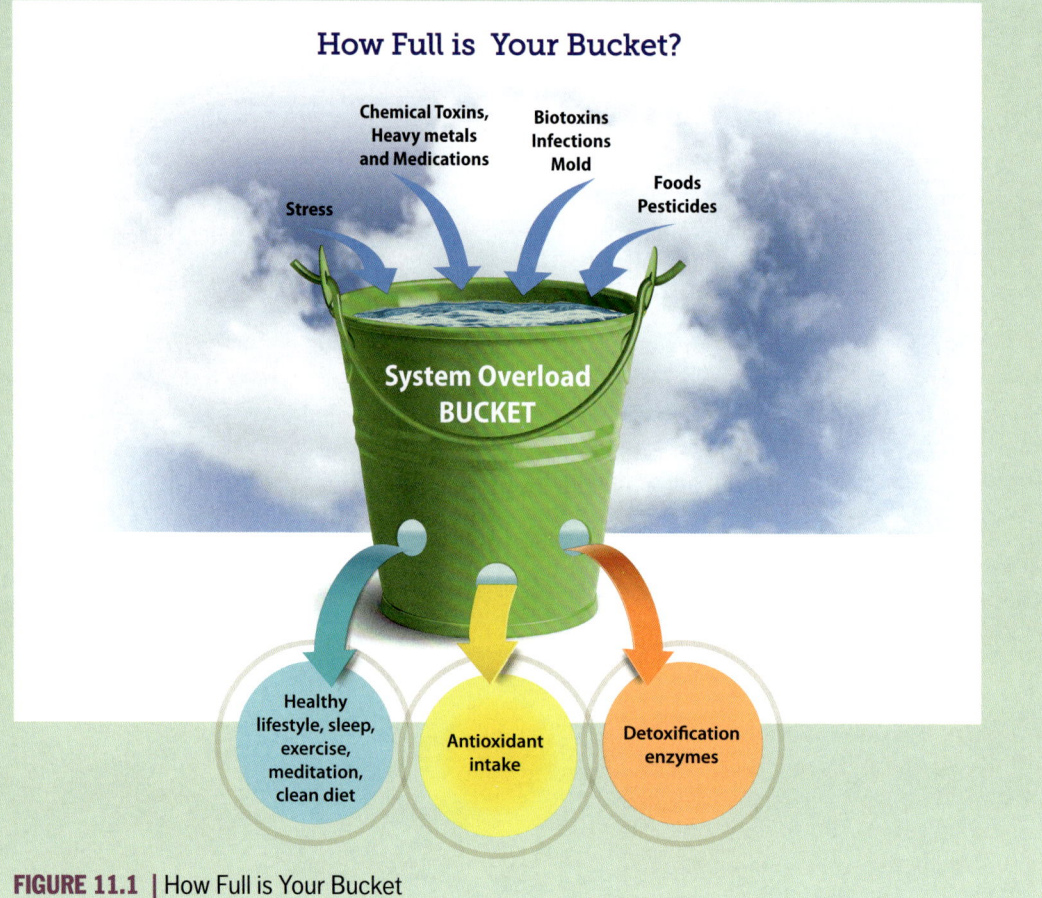

FIGURE 11.1 | How Full is Your Bucket

In autoimmune disease, your body mistakenly makes antibodies against itself, treating healthy cells and tissues as if they were foreign invaders. Simply put, your immune system confuses "friends" with "foes." This causes the inflammation and functional changes in your body that are the hallmarks of autoimmune diseases like rheumatoid arthritis and lupus.

In a similar case of confusing friend with foe, your body mistakes something harmless you have ingested or inhaled (pollen, for instance) as a dangerous invader and mounts an immune response to it. In other words, you have an allergic reaction.

The word "allergy" is derived from the Greek word *allos*, meaning "other." It was first used in 1908 to refer to an altered reaction by the body's immune system, where the body sees a harmless substance as a threat. While allergies involve the immune system and cause immediate reactions, you can be sensitive to almost anything and have a reaction that doesn't involve the immune system. In fact, most reactions involving food aren't allergies but sensitivities or intolerances.

In both cases, the body's immune system is unnecessarily upregulated and causes problems we don't need to have. If, on the other hand, your immune system becomes less effective at surveilling your body for aberrant cells and destroying them, your risk of cancer goes up, or you may be subject to frequent, recurrent, chronic, or unusual infections. The goal is a balanced immune system that reacts appropriately to protect you against infection.

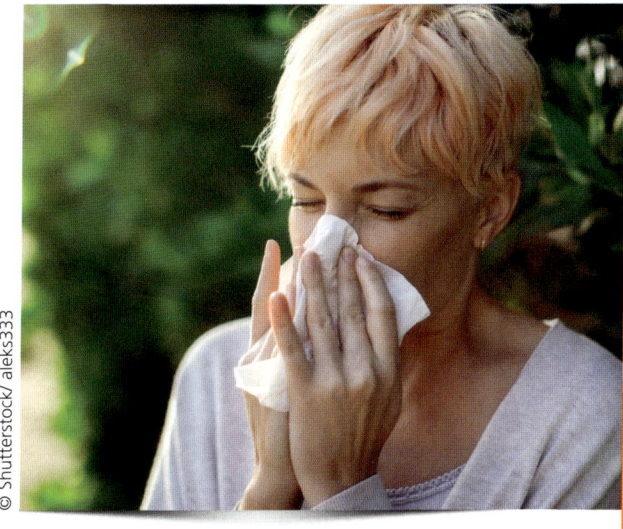

© Shutterstock/ aleks333

The Gut and the Immune System

Gut problems can make your immune system become over-responsive, causing systemic inflammation, allergy and food intolerance symptoms, decreased immunity, and a greater risk of autoimmune diseases.

Think of it like this: your immune system needs to constantly surveil the environment of your body, looking out for potential pathogens such as bacteria or viruses. It's not surprising, then, that immune system tissues surround your small intestine, your lungs, your sinuses, your tonsils, and your skin. These are all parts of your body that are exposed to the outside world. The immune system needs to be near them, poised to pounce on any dangerous pathogens that get in.

The gut lining strikes a tricky balance. It must be thin enough to allow in nutrients, but it must also provide enough defense to keep antigens and toxins from invading. In the small intestine, only a single layer of cells, about half the width of a human hair, separates your immune system from the food and potential pathogens that are within the small intestine. Lining the inside of this cell layer is a thin layer of mucus; lining the outside of the cell layer is the *gut-associated lymphoid tissue* or GALT. The GALT is there to trap any pathogens or toxins that escape through the intestinal wall. Its function is so important to your health that about 70 to 80 percent of all the immune cells in your body are found here.

Leaky Gut Syndrome and Food Sensitivities

The cells in the wall of the small intestine fit together, held firmly in place by what are known as *tight junctions*. Think of them as tiles forming a wall. The tight junctions between the cells open a bit to let digested food molecules out of the small intestine and into your circulation. Otherwise, they stay tightly closed to keep undigested food, bacteria, and toxins from entering your system. The tight junctions can open too widely, however, if your small intestine is stressed by illness, poor diet, alcohol, drugs, and a variety of other stressors, including stress itself. When the tight junctions open too widely, the cells drift apart, causing increased intestinal permeability. In other words, your gut becomes leaky. Large molecules of undigested food can now pass through the intestinal wall and enter the lymphoid tissue that lies just beyond. The immune cells waiting there to attack pathogens see these large molecules as foreign invaders. They're perfectly innocent food particles, but because they haven't been broken down enough, your immune system doesn't recognize them as the innocent bystanders they are. Of course, anything else that passes through, such as bacteria, also triggers your immune system.

The body's immune system is simply doing its job, but the consequences of a leaky gut have significant ramifications. The immune system goes on the attack, causing systemic inflammation and digestive problems such as abdominal pain, cramps, bloating, diarrhea, and food sensitivities. In the rest of the body, the inflammation can cause fatigue, muscle aches, joint pain, brain fog, and a range of other symptoms.

Leaky gut syndrome both causes food sensitivity and is triggered by reactions to food. It's a vicious cycle. Once you're sensitized to certain foods, you'll release antibodies every time you eat them. Removing the offending foods may help reduce symptoms, but you won't get better until you do something to heal the altered intestinal permeability.

Gluten and Wheat Sensitivity

Celiac disease is an autoimmune condition that causes the villi in the small intestine to be severely damaged when a sufferer eats the protein gluten. Ordinarily found in wheat, rye, and barley, gluten is also sometimes added to other products, including drugs, vitamins, supplements, cosmetics, and shampoos. Strict lifelong avoidance of gluten is the only treatment for celiac disease. Although celiac disease is uncommon, the symptoms are unmistakable, and most people are diagnosed in early childhood.

Gluten and wheat sensitivities aren't the same as celiac disease. People with gluten or wheat sensitivity react to foods that contain it, but their response doesn't damage the small intestine. Reactions can vary a lot from person to person but usually include some combination of bloating, diarrhea, stomach pain, fatigue, brain fog, headache, depression, and anxiety.

Sometimes the problem with wheat isn't gluten sensitivity but wheat allergy. Confusingly, the digestive symptoms tend to be the same, but wheat allergy symptoms also can include hives and nasal congestion. People who are sensitive to wheat can still eat other gluten-containing grains.

The Hygiene Hypothesis

In less-developed parts of the world, such as India and parts of Africa, poverty is high and the ability to sanitize things is limited. Infectious diseases are more common, but allergies and autoimmune diseases are significantly less common than in Westernized countries, where sanitization levels are high. Our superclean society means that young children aren't exposed to a wide range of germs in infancy and childhood, when their immune systems are developing. Not only is our environment highly sanitized, but our guts are subjected to more antibiotics. Our kids don't play outdoors as much and are exposed to fewer germs from the environment. The hygiene hypothesis says an environment that is overly clean cannot promote a truly healthy immune system. Lack of exposure to a wide range of germs causes a child's immune cells to be easily confused when they encounter some perfectly safe antigen. They respond inappropriately by attacking it—in other words, by causing an allergy or autoimmunity. The hygiene hypothesis tells us that letting your kids play outdoors in the dirt is a good thing that should be encouraged!

Treating Food Sensitivities and Intolerances

Because food sensitivities and intolerances are often an underlying cause of leaky gut syndrome, it's important to discover the source and try to eliminate it. That could mean avoiding the food altogether. For example, people who are allergic to eggs, tree nuts, or peanuts must strictly avoid all foods that contain them. Food intolerances are a bit easier to handle. Life-long complete avoidance isn't usually necessary. People with mild to moderate lactose intolerance, for instance, can often consume small amounts of lactose-containing foods as part of a larger meal. Over-the-counter lactase supplements can also help. Newer enzymes are now available that help people digest small amounts of gluten. For FODMAPs, gluten, and wheat sensitivity, avoidance is the best approach. (We'll discuss ways to reduce and treat food sensitivities in greater detail in Chapter 12.)

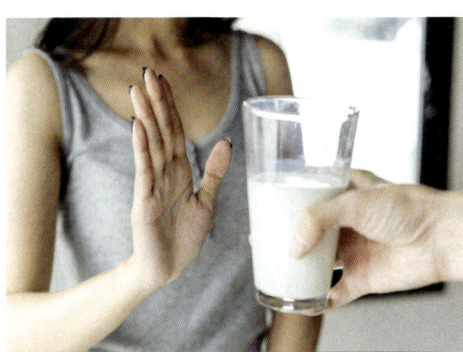
© Shutterstock/ Pormezz

High levels of stress alone can make your immune system go awry. Add in leaky gut syndrome, dysbiosis, or small intestinal bacterial overgrowth (SIBO), and you could develop serious health problems. Decreased immunity leads to infections and illness. Decreased immune surveillance for cells that are behaving incorrectly can lead to cancer. At the same time, digestive issues can cause the immune system to be wrongly activated, causing inflammation and all its consequences, increased allergic responses, and autoimmune diseases.

The Case of the Myßrious Rash

In her 50s, Kamiko developed a strange rash that would come and go. The rash started after a sinus infection and a period of prolonged stress and was originally attributed to the antibiotics she was taking. She saw multiple dermatologists and allergists to no avail. Skin tests for allergies weren't helpful. Neither were antihistamine medications. Her bowel movements had also changed. She suffered from alternating constipation and diarrhea, severe flatulence, and abdominal cramping. She also complained of a brain fog that would come over her at times. A gastroenterologist had done a colonoscopy, which was normal. Tests for celiac disease were negative. He diagnosed Kamiko with irritable bowel syndrome (IBS). Unfortunately, the usual medications for IBS didn't help. That was when she came to us, frustrated and angry.

IgG food sensitivity tests revealed high antibody levels to almonds and cashews. In her attempts to stay healthy, she had been eating almond or cashew butter daily. Removal of these foods from her diet resulted in a complete cure of her rash.

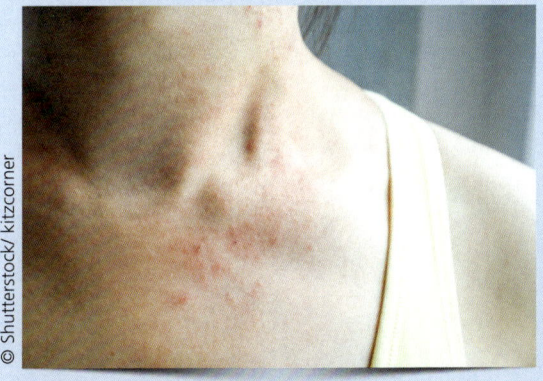
© Shutterstock/ kitzcorner

Chronic Inflammatory Response Syndrome

Chronic inflammatory response syndrome (CIRS) is a term coined by Ritchie Shoemaker, MD and is associated with an array of diffuse, non-specific symptoms. CIRS generally is due to an allergy to a type of mold common in many water-damaged homes, although there can be multiple causes, including tick-borne diseases. When you inhale tiny airborne mold spores, your body sees them as foreign invaders and has an allergic response. But in contrast to other histamine-based conditions, the allergic response is more severe and prolonged than expected in CIRS. The inflammation from the immune response stays with you and affects your whole body. Symptoms can include the usual itchy eyes, runny nose, wheezing, and sneezing, but some people also get brain fog, fatigue, achy joints and muscles, and other symptoms that can resemble other illnesses. The solution to CIRS is to treat biotoxins and remove mold from the home and to avoid it as much as possible elsewhere. Mold grows best in damp areas, so look for it in basements, bathrooms, and areas that have high humidity or water damage. Using dehumidifiers and HEPA air filters can help reduce your exposure to mold spores. Further treatments may include antifungal medications, far-infrared saunas, and antioxidants such as glutathione.

Common symptoms of CIRS include:

- Cognitive difficulties such as brain fog and trouble concentrating
- Fatigue and weakness or chronic fatigue syndrome
- Unexplained weight gain
- Frequent urination, excessive thirst, dehydration
- Fibromyalgia
- Visual insensitivity
- Postnasal drip and sore throat
- Numbness and tingling
- Digestive issues
- Mood swings
- Tinnitus
- Static shocks
- Vertigo
- Metallic taste in mouth

Autoimmune Disease and Environmentally Induced Autoimmunity

Environmentally induced autoimmunity is caused when genetically susceptible people are exposed to infections, toxins, poor diet, and other factors that trigger an autoimmune disease. We know, for example, that a viral infection often precedes type 1 diabetes, multiple sclerosis, lupus, and rheumatoid arthritis. Environmental toxins such as pesticides and other agricultural chemicals, methylmercury, and cigarette smoke are linked to some autoimmune diseases.

We don't know why environmental factors trigger autoimmunity in some people but not others. Endogenous factors, including immunity, genetics, diet, and by extension, the gut microbiome may all contribute to autoimmunity. Today, more and more evidence points toward dysbiosis as a potential cause or contributing factor. Low levels of vitamin D may also be a contributing factor. Many symptoms in autoimmune patients improve or sometimes disappear when we address dysbiosis and leaky gut issues and raise their vitamin D levels with supplements. In 2022, a study in the respected journal *The BMJ* showed that older adults who took vitamin D and fish oil had a significantly lower rate of autoimmune disease over five years compared with those who took a placebo. The vitamin D group saw their risk drop by 22 percent, while fish oil lowered risk by 15 percent. This study is particularly significant because autoimmune diseases are most likely to develop in people over age 50—and we now have a safe, easy, and inexpensive way to help avoid them.

Histamine, Allergies, and Illness

When you're sniffling and sneezing from seasonal pollen allergies or having an allergic reaction to some other allergen, it's because your body has released IgE, which in turn activates a type of innate immune cell called a *mast cell*. These cells are like tiny mines that float around in your body fluids and gather under your skin and your mucous membranes, just waiting for a pathogen or parasite to come along and try to get in. When a mast cell is activated, it degranulates—it literally blows up and dumps its contents on the invader. Mast cells contain histamine and inflammatory chemicals called leukotrienes. Histamine binds to receptors on cells found throughout your body and triggers allergy symptoms like a runny nose or itchy rash. Leukotrienes make you produce more mucus and fluid and cause airway muscles to tighten. To counter the allergic reaction, you may reach for an over-the-counter or prescription allergy medicine such as loratadine (Claritin), cetirizine (Zyrtec), or fexofenadine (Allegra). These products are antihistamines or drugs that block the histamine receptors in your cells and slow or stop the reaction.

Histamine isn't only triggered by allergies. Stress, infections, and toxins can all cause histamine release. In some cases, the mast cells may be unstable because of a disease called *systemic mastocytosis*. Histamine is involved in some unusual reactions in a wide variety of illnesses:

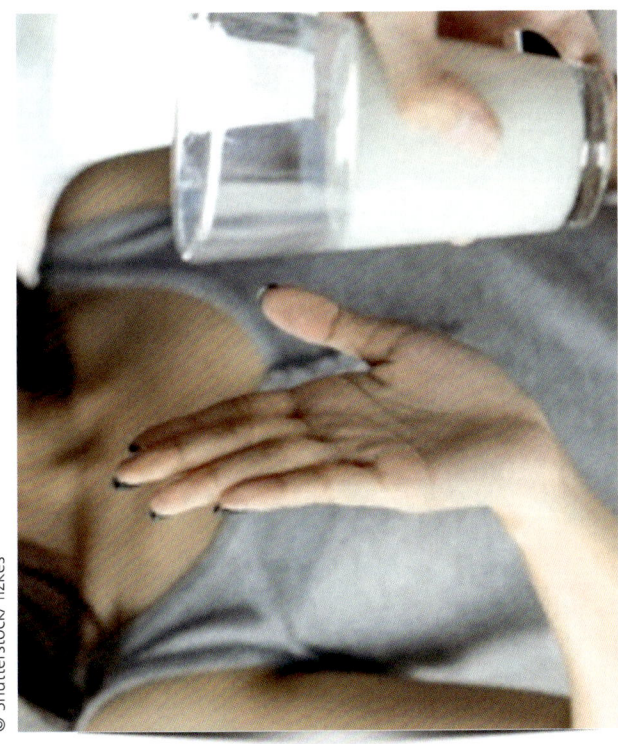

- **Musculoskeletal:** Ehlers-Danlos syndrome, fibromyalgia, and chronic regional pain syndrome

- **Respiratory:** Asthma, allergic rhinitis (hay fever)

- **Genito-urinary:** Uterine cramps, interstitial cystitis (bladder pain syndrome), and chronic prostate pain (prostadynia)

- **Gastrointestinal tract:** Leaky gut, SIBO, diarrhea

- **Central nervous system:** Restless legs syndrome, headaches, anxiety, insomnia, cyclic vomiting, depression, vertigo

- **Cardiovascular system:** postural orthostatic tachycardia syndrome (POTS), neurally mediated hypotension (NMH), anaphylaxis

- **Skin:** hives, itching, and rosacea

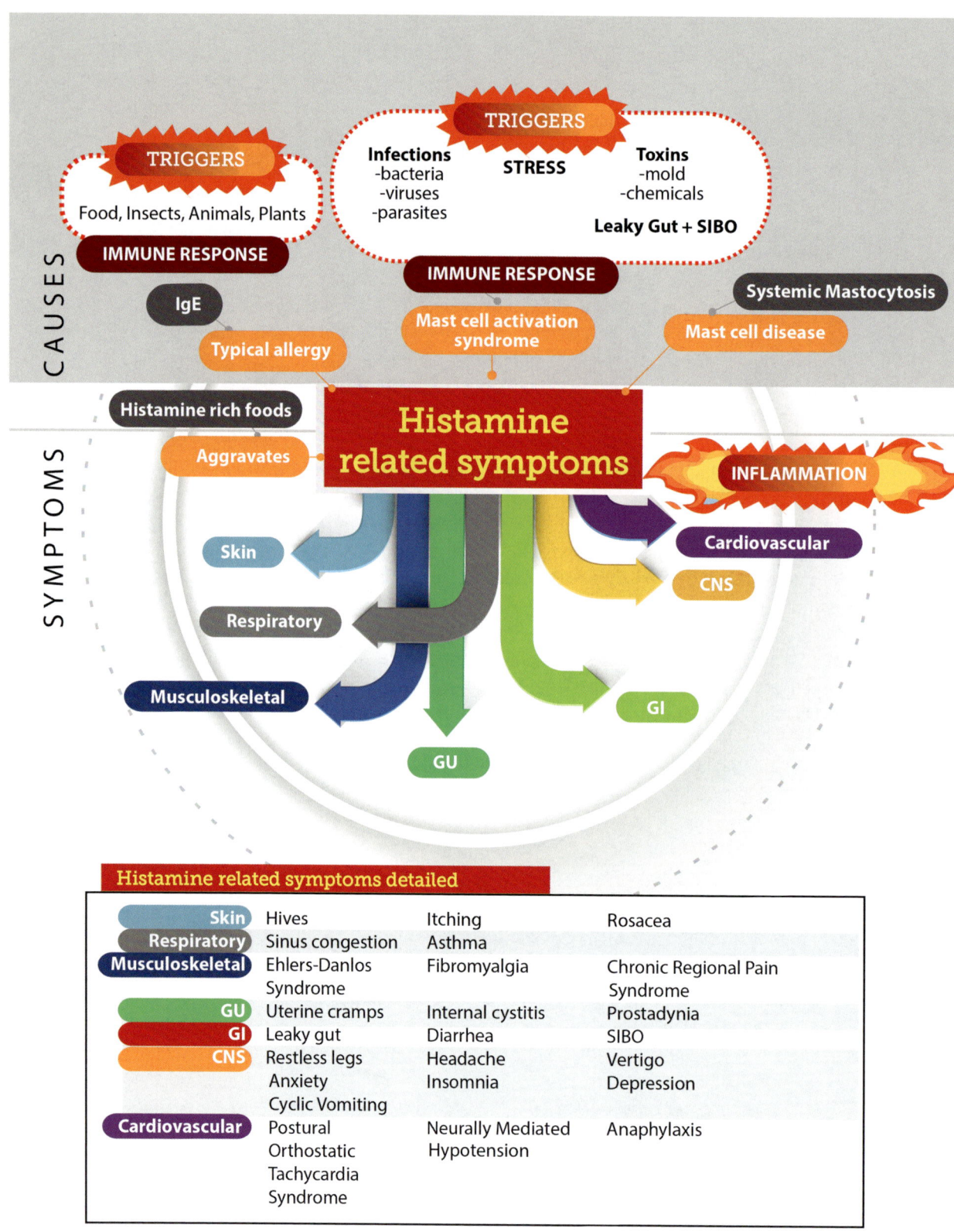

FIGURE 11.2 | Histamine related symptoms

Mast Cell Activation Syndrome

People in modern society, struggling with high levels of stress and eating poor diets, are increasingly prone to diseases caused in part by an imbalanced immune system. In addition to all the other immune problems that arise, we are seeing an increase in mast cell activation syndrome (MCAS).

For some people, mast cells aren't defenders—they're saboteurs. In their case, mast cells are triggered disproportionately or inappropriately by stress, mold, viruses, certain foods, chemicals or allergens—even exercise. The response creates allergy symptoms from histamine and inflammation from leukotrienes. In extreme cases, the mast cell activation response is so severe that the person goes into life-threatening anaphylactic shock.

In MCAS, we see a constellation of diseases and syndromes that all go together. Mast cells that line the sinuses and lungs cause sinus congestion or asthma when activated. In the gut, they may cause irritable bowel syndrome. In the nerves, activated mast cells may be behind pain syndromes such as fibromyalgia and reflex sympathetic dystrophy syndrome (RSDS, also known as complex regional pain syndrome). And in the urinary tract, mast cells may be behind interstitial cystitis and noninfective prostatitis. We've found that MCAS is sometimes the underlying cause of some cases of rosacea, POTS, restless legs syndrome, cyclic vomiting syndrome, multiple chemical sensitivities, and other illnesses that seem to have mysterious causes.

Histamine Intolerance

Histamine is found in all cells of the body. It's also naturally found in many foods, including yogurt, tomatoes, spinach, and alcohol. Complicating the diagnosis of MCAS is another possible problem called histamine intolerance (HIT). Two enzymes, diamine oxidase (DAO) and histamine N-methyltransferase (HNMT), are responsible for breaking down histamine. People who deal with HIT cannot produce either or both enzymes effectively.

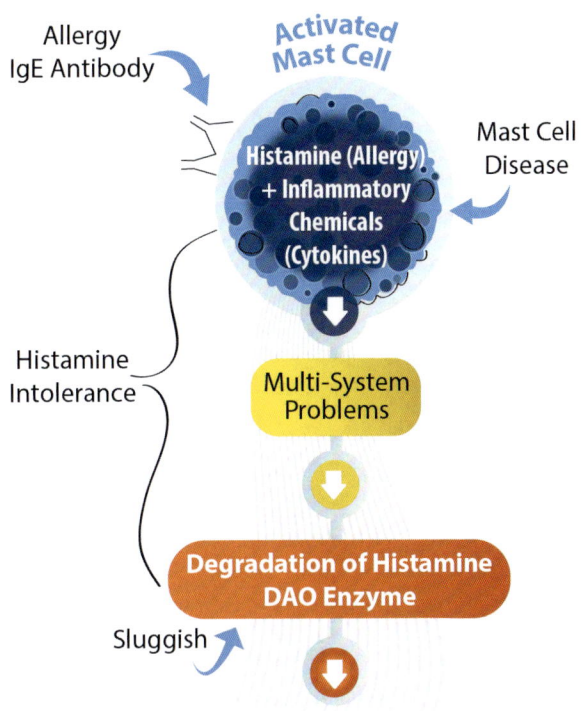

FIGURE 11.3 | Activated Mast Cell

Histamine intolerance can cause symptoms like those seen in MCAS—and if you have both conditions, the symptoms are worse. The most common symptoms resemble allergic symptoms, including rashes, hives, eczema, itchy eyes, runny nose, and congestion. Other symptoms include headaches, low blood pressure, and diarrhea. Specifically, gastrointestinal symptoms are related to faulty production of DAO, which takes place in the small intestine.

To diagnose HIT, we first try to eliminate other suspects, such as food allergies, mast cell activation syndrome, SIBO, gluten intolerance, and some other gastrointestinal disorders. Then we put you on an elimination diet that takes out high-histamine foods, like yogurt, tomatoes, spinach, and alcohol. If you get better, and we've eliminated the other possibilities, then HIT is probably the issue for you. We'll explain the details of a low-histamine diet in the next chapter.

Putting It All Together

As you can see in the diagram below, your immune system links to every other system in your body. When one aspect of your immunity is off, it affects everything else—it's like a trigger that sets off a myriad of problems. And if you have multiple triggers, the effect is magnified. The complex web of interacting triggers and stresses is a good example of systems biology at play.

When you have dysbiosis and a leaky gut, your body is inflamed because your immune system is activated. That constant activation weakens your immunity because your immune system is so busy handling the inflammation in your body that it can't deal with invaders effectively. As a result, you get frequent infections, colds, and digestive ailments. Skin injuries heal

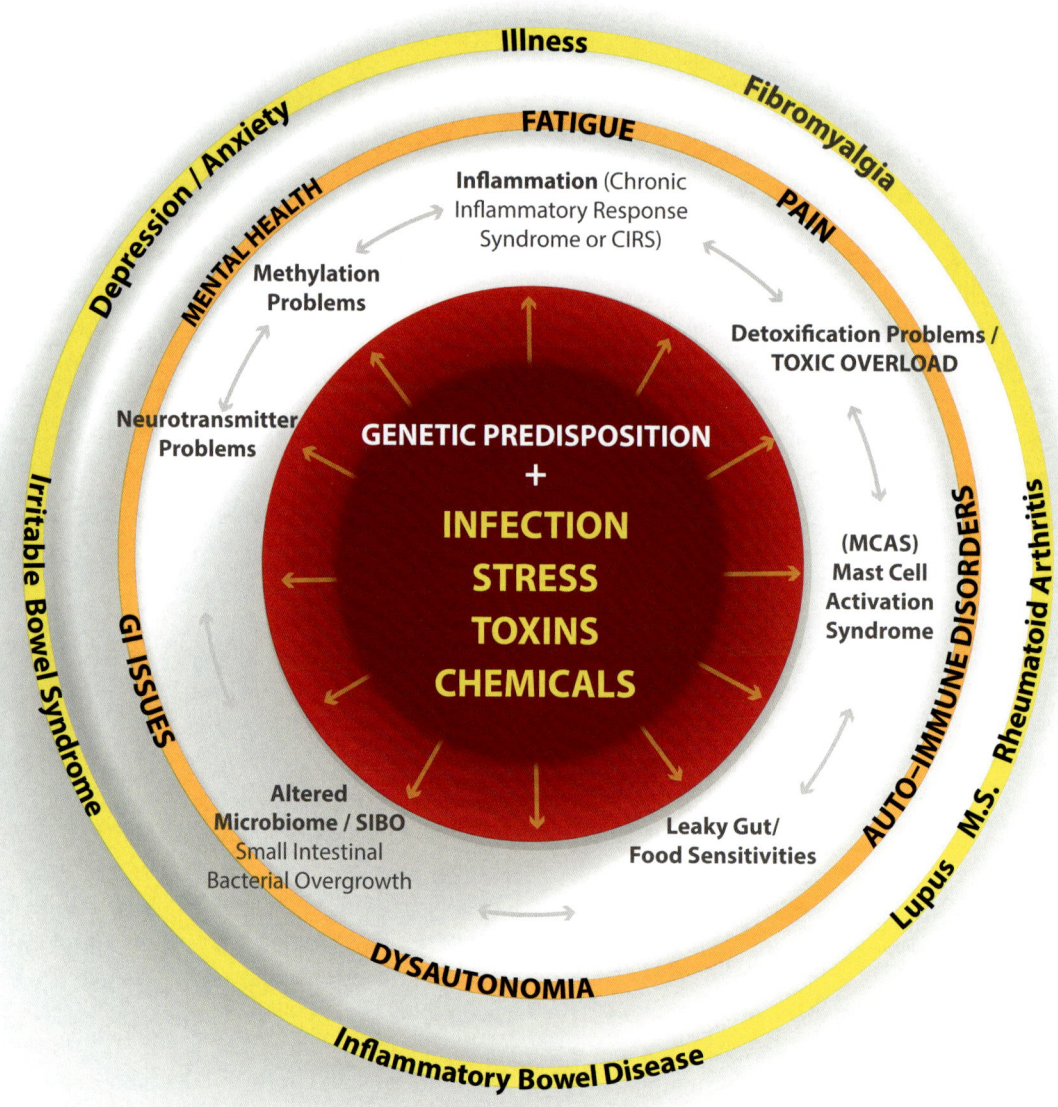

FIGURE 11.4 | The Complex Web of Interaction in Chronic Illness

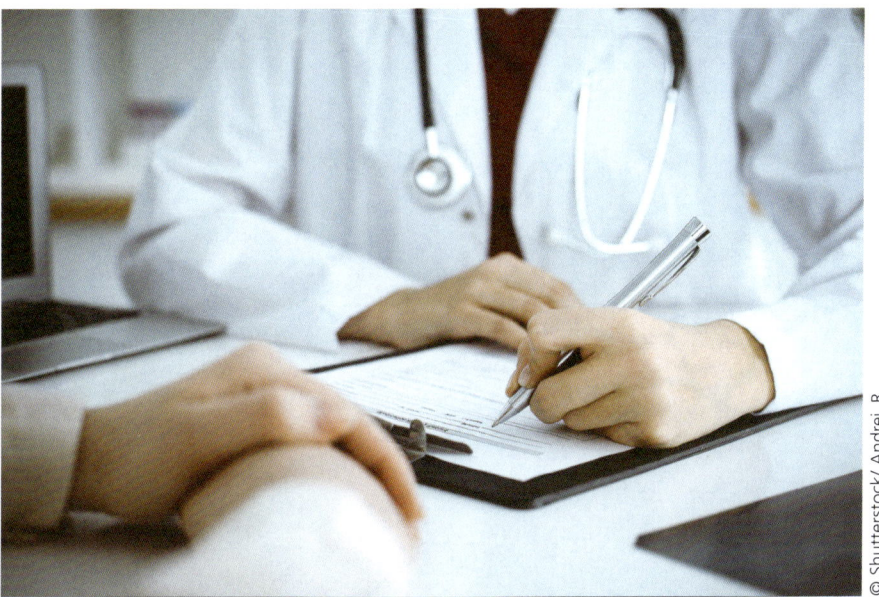

slowly. And not surprisingly, you feel exhausted all the time. Your risk of getting sick with something serious, like viral pneumonia, is greater. Functional medicine helps you get to the root cause and walk it back.

To restore your immunity and your energy, we need to look to your gut. Discovering and dealing with any food allergies and sensitivities is an important step. Food sensitivities are very individual, so they can be hard to track down. As we'll explain in the next chapter, testing can help us figure out your sensitivities, and fixing leaky gut problems can often help reduce them, to the point where some foods can be part of your diet again. After that, we can work on restoring a healthy balance in your gut microbiome and healing gut permeability. The process can take a while, but it pays off in the end.

Get well. Relax well. Move well. Live well.
Breathe well. Stay well. Sleep well.

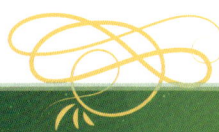

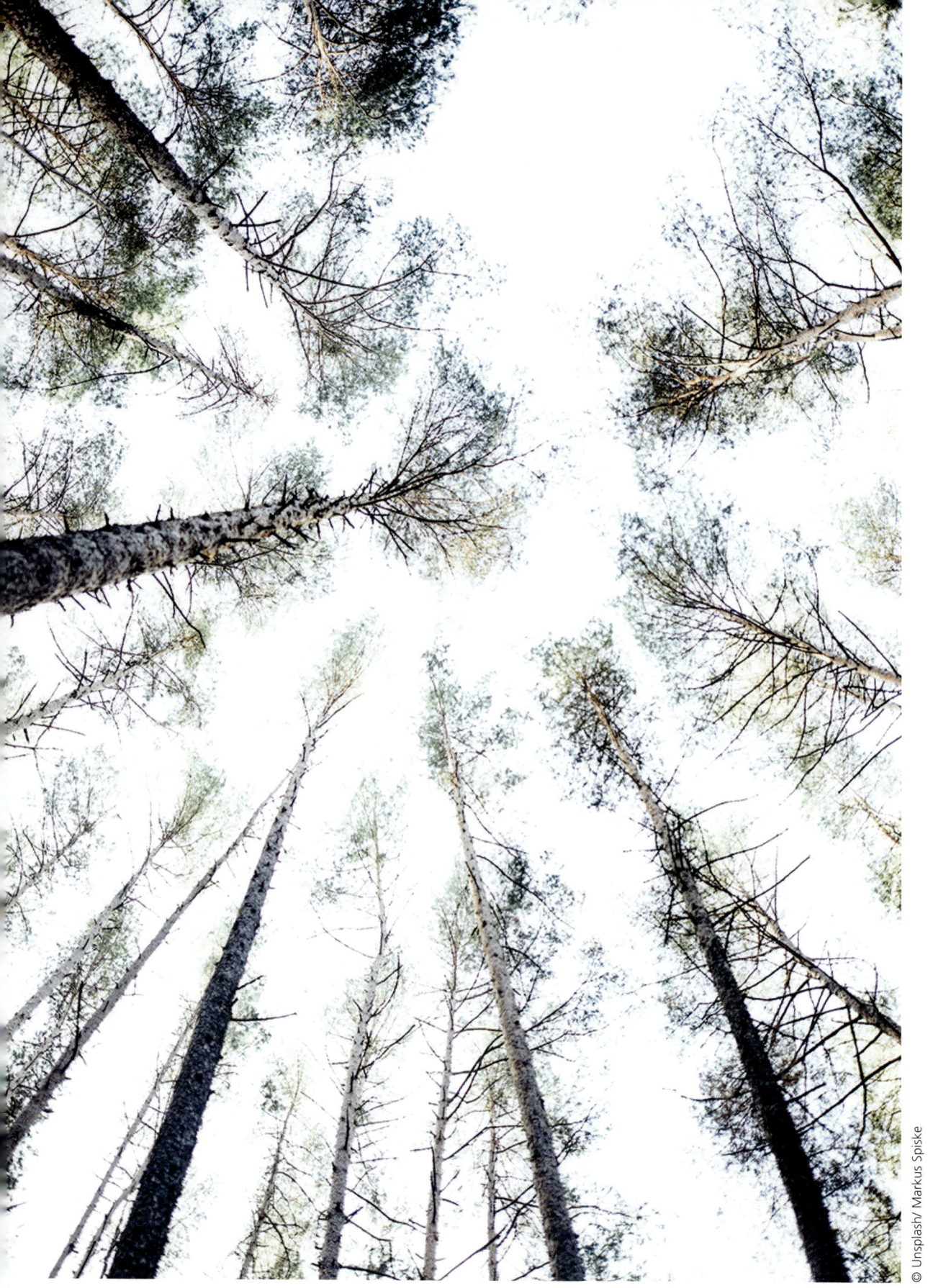

CHAPTER 12

Decoding Immunity and Treating Allergies and Sensitivities

Learning How to Normalize Immune Function

© Unsplash/ Ian Dooley

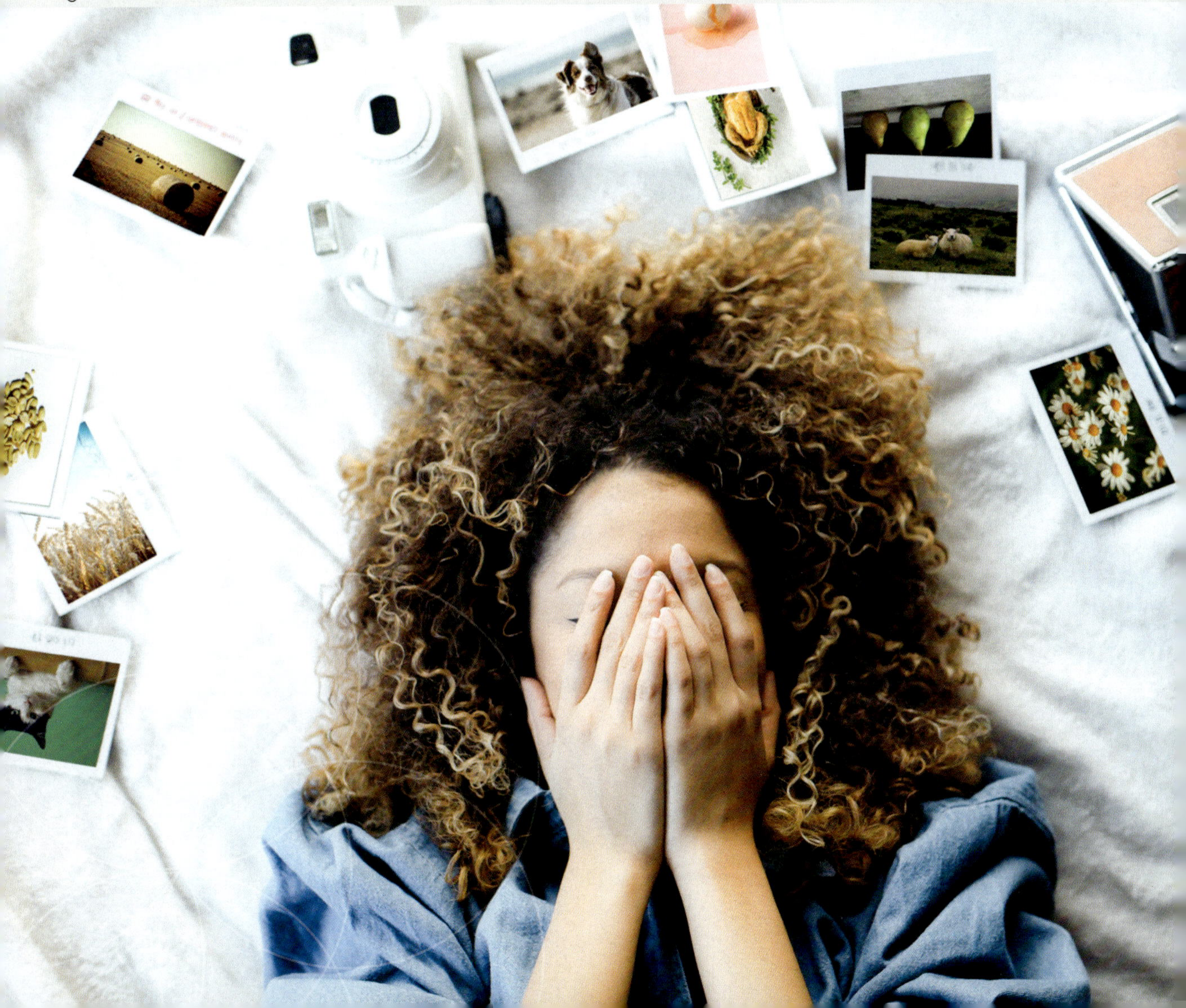

A good first step toward improving your immunity is to calm inflammation from food allergies and sensitivities. By minimizing inflammation, you can prime your body to mount a strong attack and improve your odds of having a good outcome in the event of an illness.

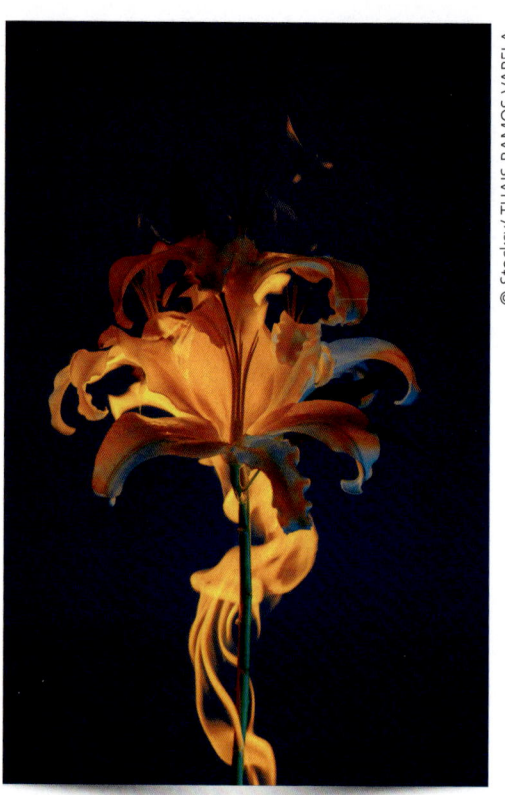

Testing for **Food Allergies** and **Food Sensitivities**

To treat food allergies and sensitivities, we first must identify them. Typically, doctors will check for food allergies using skin prick testing, although newer blood tests for IgE antigens are approaching the same sensitivity as skin tests. In our office, we use IgE blood testing to determine food allergies. We also sometimes use advanced functional lab tests to help determine food sensitivities. These tests can be expensive and aren't always covered by insurance. If finances are a concern, we can often track down the problem with an elimination diet (see below). While the only solution to food allergies is avoiding the food entirely, many food sensitivities can be reduced or even eradicated by improving digestive issues, especially leaky gut syndrome.

We can see how your immune system is responding to some foods by looking for the presence of specific immunoglobulins in your blood or saliva. We use antigenic intestinal permeability tests to detect leaky gut syndrome. These tests look for antibodies to substances that are released into the bloodstream when the intestinal barrier is damaged. Specifically, we test for antibodies for the proteins *zonulin* and *occludin*, which form the tight junctions that hold together the cells of the gut wall, and for antibodies to *actomyosin*, another protein released when the intestinal wall is damaged. Another test is for antibodies to lipopolysaccharide, the toxin released when harmful gut bacteria break down and cause inflammation and leakiness in the gut.

To help diagnose gluten sensitivity, we can use blood tests that look at your immunoglobulin response to gluten and related proteins such as gliadin and transglutaminases. The blood tests can give us a much better idea of how strictly you need to avoid gluten-containing foods and products. Standard celiac testing has low sensitivity; it doesn't always detect people with celiac disease. It also doesn't pick up all gluten sensitivity. We use a specialist lab that tests for thirty-two different proteins related to wheat and gluten; it also looks for cross-reactivity to foods contaminated with gluten.

Calming an overactive immune system usually means controlling leaky gut syndrome. We can do this with dietary changes and supplements. We give our treatment guidelines below, but every person is different—what helps one person may not be as effective for someone else. We suggest you work with a physician or dietitian with experience treating allergies and leaky gut syndrome.

Different Diets and How They Help

1. Elimination Diet for Food Sensitivities

We use an elimination diet to look for food sensitivities both to gluten/wheat and other foods. At its most basic, every elimination diet follows the same protocol. For example, an elimination diet for gluten and wheat issues is simple: avoid all foods containing wheat, barley, rye, malt and brewer's yeast for two to four weeks. During that time, keep notes on your symptoms. If gluten and wheat are a problem for you, your symptoms should improve. However, many other foods cross-react with antigluten antibodies. While eliminating gluten alone will help, you may also have to cut back on or eliminate some other foods. These include instant coffee, dairy, milk, chocolate, yeast, oats, millet, sorghum, corn, buckwheat, hemp, sesame, amaranth, quinoa, tapioca, teff, potato, eggs, and soy.

Other food sensitivities are trickier to track down. If you know or strongly suspect that a particular food is causing your symptoms, eliminate it from your diet completely for two to three weeks. If that food is the culprit, you should be feeling better after two to three weeks of not eating it. To be sure, you can try reintroducing it and noting if it triggers symptoms.

If you're not sure what foods are causing issues, your elimination diet should be broader.

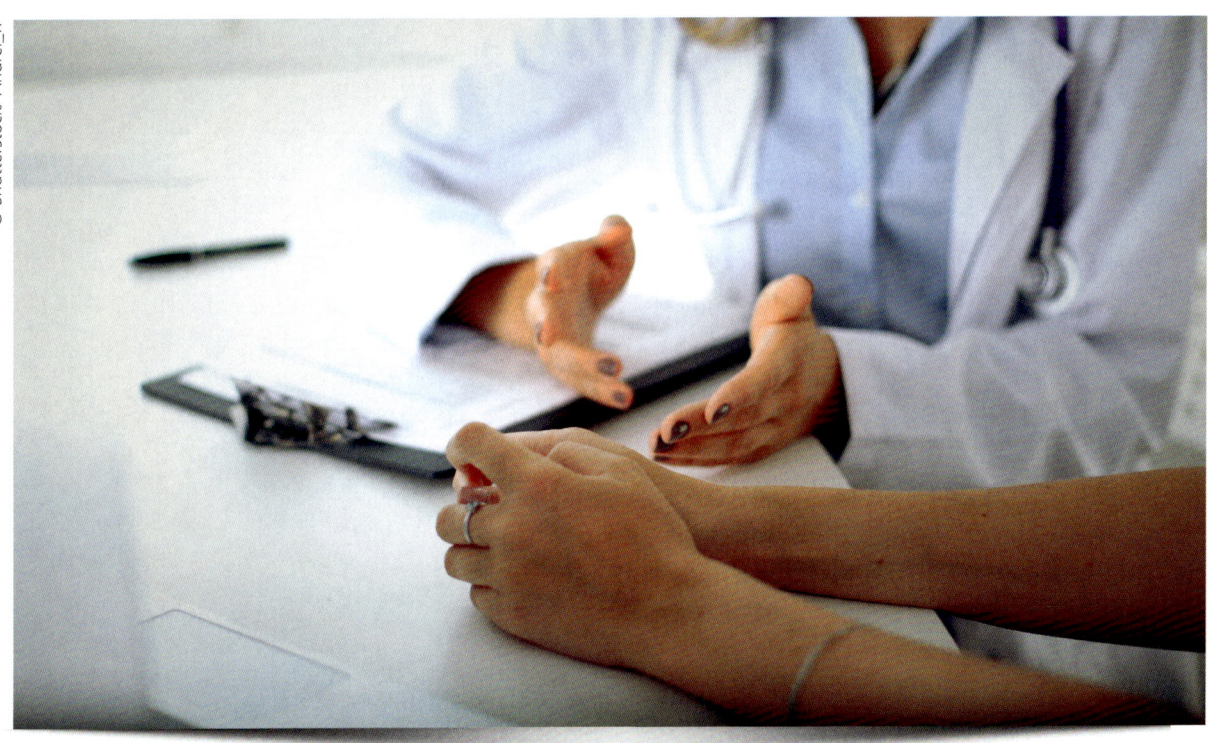

That means your diet will be restricted for about a month. The elimination phase starts with eliminating the foods you think you might be sensitive to, along with foods that are commonly problematic, including wheat and gluten, peanuts, corn, soy, dairy, citrus fruits, nightshade vegetables, eggs, and shellfish. This phase includes avoiding colorings, flavorings and preservatives, and processed food, especially processed meats like bacon and cold cuts. Aside from being bad for you in general, these foods contain additives and preservatives that can cause sensitivity.

By the end of one month without these foods, you should be feeling better, with less fatigue and brain fog and fewer digestive upsets, headaches, and sinus problems. We sometimes suggest continuing this elimination diet for up to three months if you're doing well on the diet. But at any point from one month forward, you may start slowly bringing eliminated foods back into your diet.

To reintroduce foods, start with any food group, such as citrus fruits, and eat a small amount every day for three days. Watch for symptoms such as a rash, fatigue, headache, diarrhea, stomach pain, and bloating. If they occur, it's likely that you're sensitive to the food. For optimal health, it's best to avoid it completely or eat it only in small amounts now and then. If nothing changes, then the food isn't a trigger and it's okay to add it back to your diet. Repeat with the other foods. The process can take several weeks to complete, but it's worth it in the end. (See Elimination Diet in the addendum.)

2. The Autoimmune Protocol (AIP Diet)

The Autoimmune Protocol (AIP) diet is sometimes used for patients with autoimmune disorders to heal their leaky gut and remove potentially problematic ingredients from their diet. The goal is to reduce inflammation, pain, and other symptoms. This diet resembles the Paleo diet but is a little stricter. Much like the elimination diet, you want to remove foods that may be causing a leaky gut and promoting inflammation.

On the AIP diet, you eliminate all grains, beans, legumes, nuts, seeds, nightshade vegetables, eggs, and dairy. You also eliminate all processed foods, refined or added sugar in all forms, artificial sweeteners, coffee, alcohol, and food additives. Acceptable foods are minimally processed meats, some vegetables and fruits, sweet potatoes, fermented foods such as sauerkraut, and green and black tea. Reintroducing foods on the AIP diet happens more slowly.

The AIP diet is a bit difficult to follow for long, but it can be very effective for people with autoimmune diseases. To make sure this diet is right for you and that you get good nutrition while following it, we recommend working with an experienced physician or dietitian.

3. The Gluten-Free Diet

If you've been diagnosed with celiac disease, you know you must follow a diet that's strictly gluten-free or else you'll quickly get sick with severe digestive symptoms. If you're sensitive to gluten or wheat, you also want to stay away from these foods, though you may not need to be as strict about complete avoidance.

Foods that contain gluten include anything made with wheat, barley, or rye. Other forms of wheat, such as semolina, bulgur, wheat berries, farro, triticale, and farina also need to be eliminated. That means avoiding wheat-based bread, pasta, baked goods, and snack foods, along with anything that contains barley or rye—including beer. Read the ingredients list for all processed foods carefully to avoid hidden wheat and added gluten. Many condiments and sauces, such as barbecue sauce, contain added gluten, so check the label. Many food manufacturers now put a gluten-free label on the package to help you choose.

Gluten Sensitivity

Wheat has been a cornerstone of the human diet for thousands of years. But many people are now saying they're sensitive to gluten and other wheat proteins, dealing with what is called non-celiac wheat sensitivity. Why is this so? The answer is that plant breeding has changed wheat significantly in the past fifty years. Wheat today contains more gluten and more of a protein called gliadin—the two proteins most likely to cause sensitivity. In addition, gluten is added to a surprising range of food products as a filler. It's even in cosmetics. We encounter it far more often than our bodies expect.

Gluten is a large, complex molecule that's hard to digest. People who naturally don't produce a lot of the enzymes needed to digest it might ordinarily still be fine—if they were to eat gluten-containing foods from years past. But eating such "gluten-enhanced" foods today, they have difficulty digesting it fully. Undigested bits escape through the gut barrier into the circulation and cause an immune response. Worse, once the body sees gluten and other wheat proteins as a problem, it often starts cross-reacting with foods that have a similar antigenic profile, such as corn, tapioca, and barley.

What can you eat on a gluten-free diet? Lots of healthy foods!

- Grains such as quinoa, rice, buckwheat, tapioca, sorghum, corn, millet, amaranth, arrowroot, teff and oats (if labeled gluten-free)
- Wheat-free pasta, such as chickpea or red lentil
- All unprocessed meats and fish (not battered or coated)
- Eggs
- All dairy products (although processed products may have added gluten)
- All fruits and vegetables, including potatoes and beans
- All nuts and seeds
- All vegetable oils and butter
- All herbs and spices

Today, many food manufacturers offer gluten-free products that are good substitutes, like chickpea pasta and gluten-free pretzels. Be aware, however, that gluten-free junk food is still junk food and may even be higher in calories than its gluten-containing counterpart.

When celiac disease or gluten sensitivity symptoms are not settling down on a gluten-free diet, it's possible you're cross-reacting to gluten-associated foods as discussed above. Work with your physician or dietitian to cut gluten-associated foods out of your diet and then reintroduce them to figure out which might be causing your continuing symptoms.

4. The Low Histamine Diet

If you have histamine intolerance, avoiding high-histamine foods can help reduce symptoms. The histamine content of a food is hard to quantify, and it's not listed on the food facts label. As a rule, fermented foods (sauerkraut, for example) and aged foods (like cheese) tend to be higher in histamine. So are cured foods (salami, for example), and foods that have preservatives and additives.

To address histamine intolerance, avoid these high-histamine foods:

- Fermented/aged dairy products, including yogurt, kefir, sour cream, buttermilk, and aged cheese. Some people find that eliminating all dairy is helpful.
- Fermented vegetables, including sauerkraut, lacto-fermented pickles, kimchi, and pickled vegetables
- Fermented soy products, including soy sauce, miso, tempeh, and natto
- Cured meats such as sausages, salami, ham, and liverwurst
- Canned fish
- Wine and beer
- Sourdough bread
- Vinegar
- Nuts
- Avocados, beans, eggplant, mushrooms, spinach, and tomatoes
- Bananas, citrus fruits, kiwi, pineapple, raspberries, and strawberries

What should you eat? Anything that isn't on the list, as long as it's fresh, unprocessed, or minimally processed, and doesn't contain additives, preservatives, or food dyes. If you have histamine intolerance, you should feel better within four weeks of being on this diet.

5. Dietary Changes for Seasonal Allergies

Dietary changes and supplements can help alleviate seasonal allergies. Avoid mucus-producing foods such as dairy products, sugary foods, and refined grains, which make secretions thicker. Drink plenty of plain water and herbal teas to stay hydrated and keep mucus thin. If you haven't identified food allergies that are contributing to your nasal congestion, we recommend doing so.

Foods high in bioflavonoids, such as citrus fruits and berries, help reduce the allergic response by strengthening mast cell walls so they don't break open and release histamine as easily. Bioflavonoids also help strengthen capillaries and keep histamine and other pro-inflammatory compounds in the bloodstream instead of leaking out into the tissues and causing allergy symptoms. Vitamin C from food and supplements also strengthens the cell walls of both capillaries and mast cells.

During allergy season, eating oranges and other citrus fruits can help with symptoms. Other foods high in both vitamin C and bioflavonoids include berries, red grapes, peaches, nectarines, peppers of all colors, broccoli, onions, and green tea.

We often recommend taking buffered vitamin C supplements (2,000 mg a day) and using a saline nasal rinse when necessary.

6. The Low FODMAP Diet

FODMAP stands for "fermentable oligosaccharides, disaccharides, monosaccharides, and polyols." These are all complex sugars found in dairy products such as milk, yogurt, and ice cream; wheat-based foods such as bread and breakfast cereal; beans; some vegetables such as onions, garlic, and asparagus; and some fruits, especially apples, peaches, cherries, and pears. High-fructose corn syrup and artificial sweeteners are also FODMAP foods. Many people have trouble digesting these foods because they can't break them down well in the small intestine. This is particularly a problem for people with irritable bowel syndrome (IBS), but many people are also just sensitive to fructose, lactose, and other natural sugars—they don't make enough or even any of the enzymes needed to break these complex sugars down. When FODMAP foods reach the colon, the undigested bits tend to absorb a lot of water. They also provide a real feast of partially digested food to your bacteria. The result is bloating, cramping, gas, diarrhea, constipation, and possibly dysbiosis.

A low FODMAP diet can help if you eat a diet high in nutrition from other foods. On the low FODMAP diet, you avoid eating:

- **Fruits** such as apples, applesauce, apricots, blackberries, cherries, canned fruit, dates, figs, pears, peaches, and watermelon
- **Sweeteners** including fructose, honey, high-fructose corn syrup, and sugar alcohols (e.g., xylitol, mannitol, maltitol, and sorbitol)

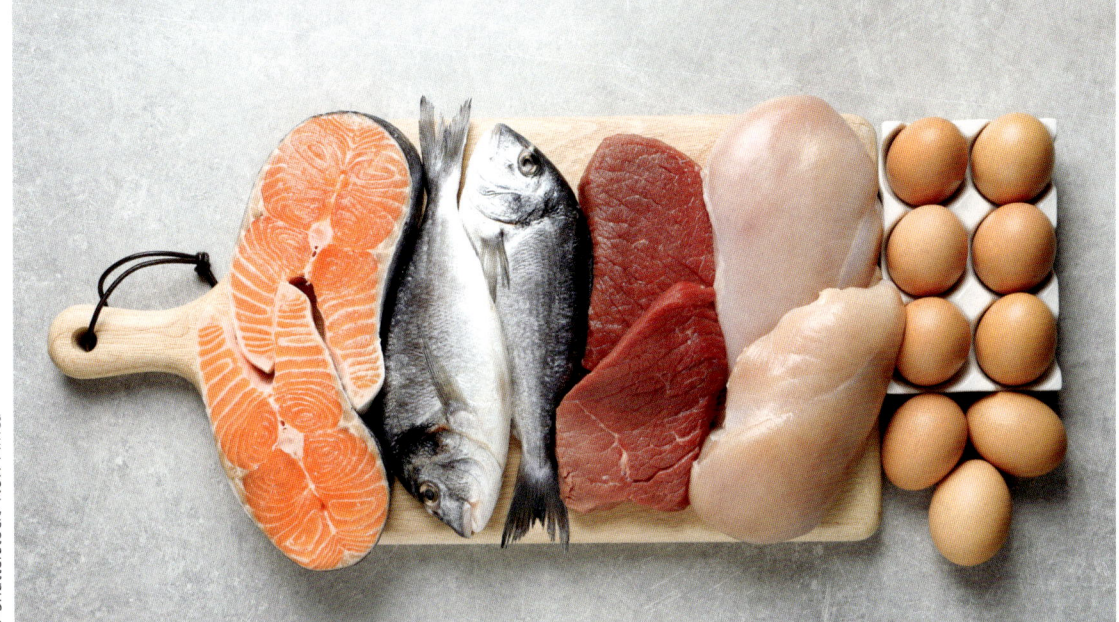

- **Dairy products** like milk, ice cream, yogurts, sour cream, soft and fresh cheeses (such as cottage cheese, ricotta, and farmers cheese)
- **Vegetables** such as artichokes, asparagus, broccoli, beets, brussels sprouts, cabbage, cauliflower, garlic, fennel, leeks, mushrooms, okra, onions, peas, and shallots
- **Legumes** including beans, chickpeas, lentils, red kidney beans, baked beans, and soybeans
- **Wheat product**s like bread, pasta, most breakfast cereals, tortillas, waffles, pancakes, crackers, and biscuits
- **Barley** and **rye**
- **Pistachios** and **cashews**
- **Beverages** such as beer, soft drinks with high-fructose corn syrup, soy milk, and fruit juices

Foods you can eat include:
- **Meats, fish,** and **eggs**
- **All fats** and **oils**
- **Most herbs** and **spices**
- **Nuts** and **seeds**: Almonds, peanuts, macadamia nuts, pine nuts, and sesame seeds
- **Fruits:** blueberries, cantaloupe, grapefruit, grapes, kiwi, lemons, limes, mandarin oranges, melons (except watermelon), oranges, passionfruit, raspberries, and strawberries
- **Sweeteners:** maple syrup, molasses, and stevia
- **Dairy products**: lactose-free dairy products, hard cheeses, and aged softer cheeses like brie and camembert
- **Vegetables:** bell peppers, bok choy, carrots, celery, cucumbers, eggplant, ginger, green beans, kale, lettuce, chives, olives, parsnips, potatoes, radishes, spinach, scallions, squash, sweet potatoes, tomatoes, turnips, and zucchini
- **Grains:** Corn, oats, rice, quinoa, sorghum, and tapioca
- **Beverages:** Water, coffee, tea, and herbal tea

The low FODMAP diet is a little restrictive, but it's a good way to figure out what foods give you the most trouble. As with the elimination diet, try slowly adding back foods to discover which you can tolerate and in what quantities. Remember, eating a low FODMAP diet is *not* the same as eliminating FODMAP foods! You only need to cut them down to a point where they don't cause symptoms! Many people find they can tolerate small amounts of FODMAP foods when eaten as part of a larger low-FODMAP meal. If you're having a flare-up of IBS symptoms, stick to the diet strictly for several weeks or until the symptoms go down, then add back small amounts of foods you can tolerate without triggering symptoms.

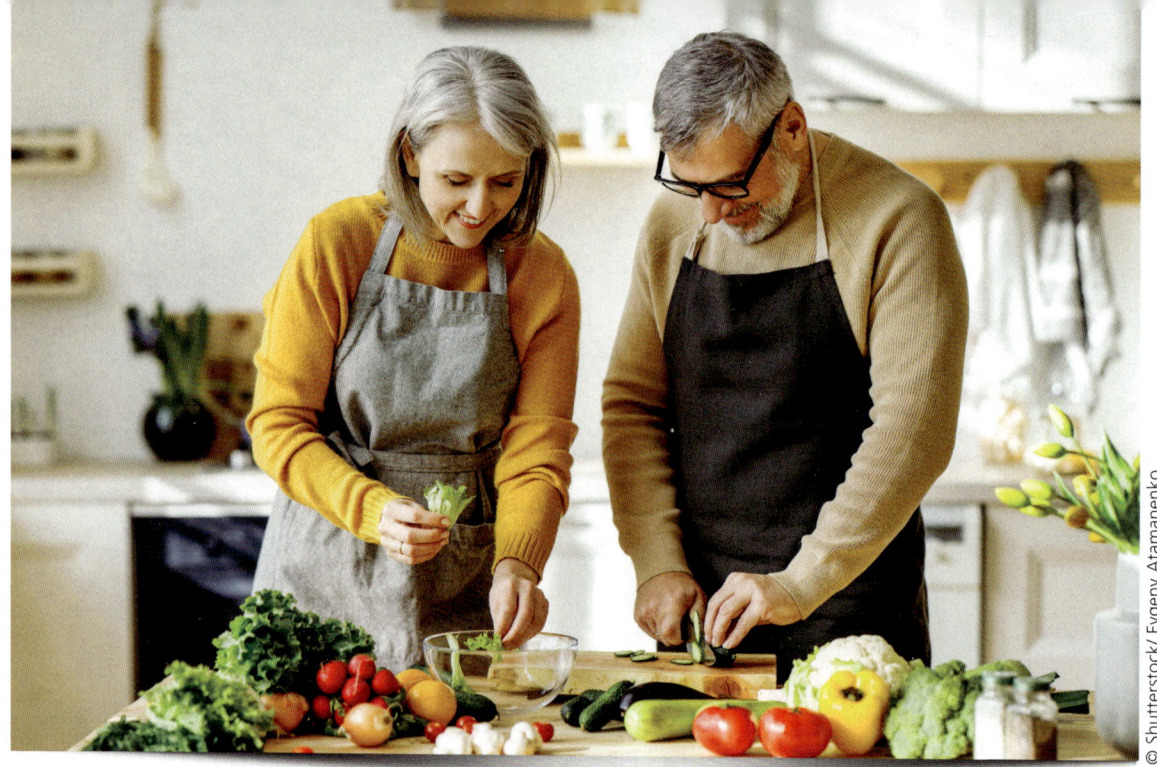

Diet, Lifestyle, and Supplements for Better Immunity

The dietary changes we talked about in earlier chapters usually help improve overall immunity by reducing systemic inflammation. If your immunity is weakened, it's particularly important to avoid simple sugars as much as possible. Simple sugars can suppress your immune system for up to four hours after you eat them—and if you follow the typical pattern of eating these foods at least once every few hours, your immune system is constantly being suppressed. Simple sugars include desserts, pastries, cake, soft drinks, candy, and other sweet treats. Processed foods made with refined grain products, like pasta and white bread, are quickly converted to glucose (blood sugar) and have as much of an impact on your immune system as sweet foods do.

Supplements that support your immune system include vitamin C, vitamin D, and zinc. Good levels of vitamin D are extremely important for your barrier defenses. Your body converts sunlight on your skin into vitamin D, but you need to be outside in the sun with exposed skin for about 20 minutes for that to happen. Most of us spend 90 percent of our time indoors, even in the summer—it's almost impossible to make enough vitamin D from sun exposure alone. Vitamin D is found naturally in fatty fish, eggs, and mushrooms, and it's added to milk, but the best way to be sure you're getting enough is with daily supplements. We recommend having your blood level checked and taking supplements to reach and maintain an ideal blood level of 50 to 75 ng/ml.

Take supplements of vitamins and minerals as needed or suggested by your doctor, but also increase your intake of fresh fruits and vegetables (the more colorful the better), leafy greens, beans, seeds, and nuts. Potassium-rich foods are also helpful for improving immunity—eat plenty of avocados, sweet potatoes, and bananas.

Lifestyle changes are also important. Getting more high-quality sleep, for example, helps give your body time to repair itself and rebuild its defenses. Another important step is get-

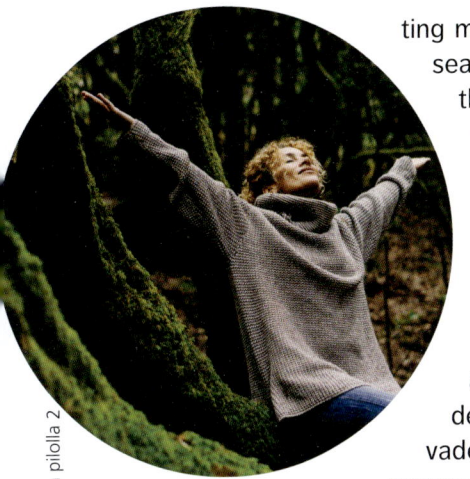

ting more exercise. Research clearly shows that people who stay active are much less likely to get sick. Moderate exercise increases the production of immune cells and improves your defense against invaders. This is a great reason to start a new fitness habit, but don't go too far—overly strenuous exercise can be detrimental. Keeping alcohol consumption to a minimum is also highly recommended. Yes, alcohol kills germs but only externally. And, of course, staying hydrated is crucial for optimal immune function. Drink plenty of plain water and herbal tea.

Some natural flavonoids and other compounds are great for helping to prevent and fight infection:

- **Quercetin:** This flavonoid powerfully modulates immune function and has direct antiviral actions. It's found in apples, berries, onions, and green tea.
- **Astragalus (*Astragalus membranaceus*):** This woody, neutral-tasting Chinese herb can also be added to soups and stews. It has long been touted for its ability to strengthen the immune system and prevent viral infection.
- **Medicinal mushrooms:** Mushrooms such as shitake, maitake, reishi and turkey tail can help prime the innate immune system, your first line of defense against pathogens.
- **Melatonin:** Besides helping you sleep, this is a powerful antioxidant and anti-inflammatory that helps minimize tissue damage caused by viruses.
- **Fish oil:** Increasing your intake of healthy fats can help boost your immune system. Supplement with 1,000 to 2,000 mg daily.
- **Green powder:** Enhance the antioxidant and bioflavonoid benefits of fruits and vegetables in your diet with a scoop or two of green powder added to smoothies or sprinkled over salad or pasta.

If you feel like you're getting sick, take immediate steps that will help you fight off the infection:

- **Quarantine.** Stay home from work and social events and stay away from vulnerable family members for a few days or until you're feeling better. This lets you rest and heal and keeps you from spreading the illness to others. If you feel you need a doctor's advice, ask if a telemedicine conference is possible.
- **Rest.** Give your body the time and energy it needs to heal.
- **Exercise?** If your symptoms are above the neck (e.g., sniffles, sore throat), exercise gently and only if you feel up to it. If your symptoms are below your neck and/or involve your whole body (e.g., fever, fatigue, muscle aches, cough, shortness of breath, abdominal distress), stay in bed.
- **Fast.** If you don't feel like eating, don't. Only eat light, easily digested food if you are hungry. This is a good time to avoid dairy, eggs, and raw vegetables.
- **Hydrate.** Drink plenty of water and clear fluids to keep your immune cells active. Liquids also keep mucus thin and easy to clear from the body. Fruit and vegetable juices (with no added sugar), clear soups, miso soup, and bone broth supply essential vitamins, minerals, and flavonoids that support immune function. Black tea, green tea, herbal teas, and electrolyte drinks are also good options.
- **Take honey.** This is a natural antimicrobial that soothes sore throats and has been shown in studies to be as effective as nonprescription remedies at decreasing cough. Pair it with lemon juice to add a dose of vitamin C to stimulate immune cells.

The AAT Approach for Allergies and Sensitivities

One of our secret weapons we use in treating allergy and sensitivity symptoms is Advanced Allergy Therapeutics (AAT). We once gave a talk on the Future of Medicine to a large group of scientists. As we typically do, we went round the audience asking how many people were familiar with, or utilizing alternative or integrative therapies. A multitude of hands went up. "What are you using?" we asked? They all replied almost in unison: "AAT!" They all said, "We don't quite understand it, but it works!" We concurred. So often when we felt sick, we were treated with AAT and twenty minutes later left feeling great.

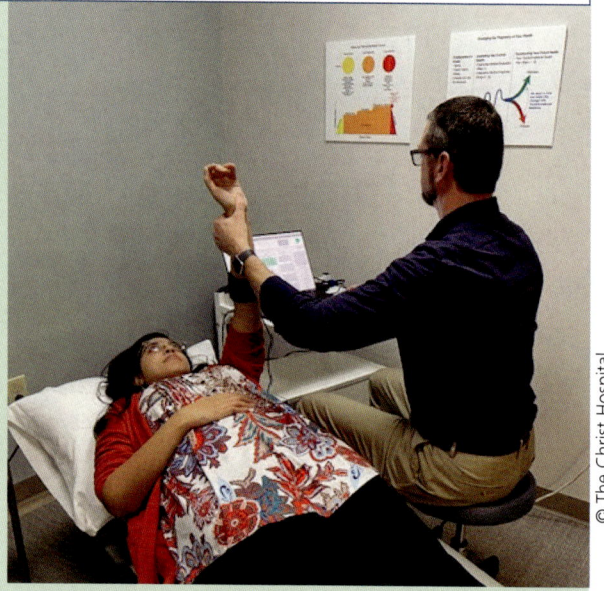

AAT is a unique and highly effective approach to treating the many symptoms associated with allergies and sensitivities. The nice thing about it is that it is safe, medication-free, not painful, and free of side effects. The technique combines the chiropractic approach of muscle testing, a special computer program that can check for multiple substances causing allergies and sensitivities, and stimulation of acupuncture points on the back with a mechanical vibrator. AAT also utilizes an acupuncture mindset in that it works directly with the relationship between the major organ systems and inappropriate reactions to harmless substances. A routine allergist visit usually involves testing for allergies using skin prick or blood testing and then treating with shots or drops. An old allergist friend of ours told us that he tells his patients that with allergy shots, "A third get better for good, a third get better for a while, and a third don't respond." In our office, we usually see about 70 percent responding well to AAT.

During the initial visit, the AAT practitioner tests for all the possible substances that could be responsible for the patient's symptoms, then treats a few at each visit until the patient feels better. With both sensitivities and allergies, symptoms typically stem from the organ system affected. For example, one person may react to soybeans by getting rashes, while another person may react with sinus congestion, heartburn, or IBS. The symptoms in each of these cases represent a different organ system. By treating the organ system(s) involved in a reaction, the body can respond more appropriately.

AAT can be very effective, but it doesn't test for or diagnose allergies, sensitivities, or intolerances. AAT doesn't cure allergies, nor does the therapy treat the immune system. The AAT system simply assesses what may be causing stress to the body. Then after the treatment, the body no longer treats a "friend" as a "foe." Not everyone responds to AAT treatment, but most patients respond quickly and achieve long-term results with the first few treatments. Typically, patients need five to twelve treatments.

Some supplements that help fight infection include:

- **Andrographis *(Andrographis paniculata)*:** An herb used in traditional Chinese medicine and Ayurvedic medicine, this plant has antimicrobial and anti-inflammatory actions. When used at the beginning of an illness, it can shorten the duration of symptoms.
- **Turmeric *(Curcuma longa)*:** The anti-inflammatory compounds in turmeric, especially curcumin, can help reduce symptoms such as aching joints. Turmeric has also been shown to help decrease the damage from a cytokine storm, caused when the immune system overreacts to a germ.
- **Pro-resolving mediators:** These are supplements made from a highly refined fish oil fraction. They help put the brakes on inflammation.
- **N-acetylcysteine (NAC):** This amino acid is one of the building blocks of glutathione, the body's most abundant antioxidant. It helps speed the repair of cells and tissues damaged by illness.
- **Chinese herbs** can help minimize symptom severity and help you feel better faster. A commonly used blend of Chinese herbs is called Yin Qiao.

Low-Dose Naltrexone for Immune Function

In low doses, the prescription drug naltrexone can help regulate a dysfunctional immune system, reduce pain, and fight inflammation. Low-dose naltrexone (LDN) is well-tolerated, cheap, safe, and non-addictive—and it isn't a narcotic or a controlled substance. Like the similar-sounding drug naloxone, naltrexone is used, in much larger doses, to treat alcohol and opioid addiction. LDN doses are a fraction of those used to treat addiction—they are typically only 1.5 to 4.5 mg taken at night instead of the 50 to 200 mg doses used to treat addiction.

In 1985, Bernard Biari, MD, a physician in New York City, was treating patients with naltrexone who both had HIV and were heroin addicts. He noticed that the naltrexone augmented the immune response in his patients. Based on this observation, Dr. Biari pioneered the use of low doses of naltrexone to improve immunity.

Benefits of LDN

Low-dose naltrexone can be valuable in many autoimmune diseases, especially when it is started soon after diagnosis. Autoimmune diseases it can help include:

- Alopecia areata
- Autoimmune thyroiditis (Hashimoto's disease)
- Diabetic peripheral neuropathy
- Inflammatory bowel disease (IBD), including Crohn's disease
- Irritable bowel syndrome (IBS)
- Lupus
- Multiple sclerosis
- Myalgic encephalomyelitis/chronic fatigue syndrome (ME/CFS)
- Rheumatoid arthritis

LDN may also be beneficial in cancer treatment, especially in conjunction with CBD (cannabidiol) and the natural anti-inflammatory supplement palmitoylethanolamide (PEA). It may also be helpful for weight loss, because it reduces appetite, improves insulin sensitivity, and may help modulate the body's set point. LDN is also very helpful for treating chronic pain (see chapter 16 for more on this).

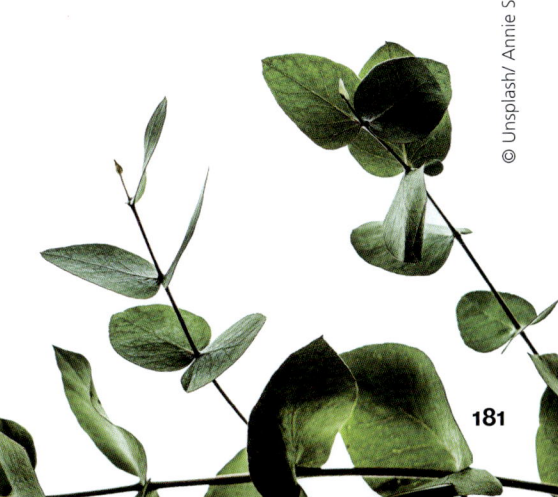

© Unsplash/ Annie Spratt

How does LDN work?

LDN works by blocking opiate (mu-opioid) receptors in the brain for just a few hours. The body responds by making more of these pain receptors, which makes you more sensitive to your body's own endorphins (natural pain-killing chemicals). This reduces pain.

LDN also has an antagonistic effect on non-opioid receptors (Toll-like receptor 4 or TLR4) that are found on macrophages and microglia. This mechanism reduces inflammation.

LDN also:

- Decreases oxidative stress via the NADPH oxidase pathway.
- May be neuroprotective and appears to modulate glial cells in the brain.
- Aids bowel peristalsis and helps repair a leaky gut.

LDN Cautions

LDN is an opiate antagonist. This means it blocks the effect of narcotic drugs such as codeine or hydrocodone. We suggest not taking opiate drugs if taking LDN.

We generally recommend taking LDN at night. However, some patients report sleep problems or vivid dreams when they take it before bedtime. In these cases we switch to a morning dose.

Remember, your immune system and your nervous system are intricately linked. We all know intrinsically that when we are stressed, we are more likely to get sick. This is another reason why handling stress correctly is so very important.

The Cell Danger Response

Conventional physicians have struggled to understand how genetics, toxic load, infectious burden, radiation and other factors we are exposed to, collectively called the Exposome, affect our health and lead to chronic illness. Robert K. Naviaux, MD, PhD, professor of medicine, pediatrics and pathology at University of California San Diego School of Medicine, has theorized that chronic disease is the consequence of the natural healing cycle becoming blocked, specifically by disruptions at the metabolic and cellular levels. He calls this the Cell Danger Response and has shown that environmental chemicals can now be correlated with annual and regional patterns of childhood illness and a broad array of chronic, developmental, autoimmune, and degenerative disorders. These disorders include autism spectrum disorders (ASD), attention deficit hyperactivity disorder (ADHD), asthma, atopy, gluten and many other food and chemical sensitivity syndromes, emphysema, Tourette's syndrome, bipolar disorder, schizophrenia, post-traumatic stress disorder (PTSD), chronic traumatic encephalopathy (CTE), traumatic brain injury (TBI), epilepsy, suicidal ideation, organ transplant biology, diabetes, kidney, liver, and heart disease, cancer, Alzheimer and Parkinson disease, and autoimmune disorders like lupus, rheumatoid arthritis, multiple sclerosis, and primary sclerosing cholangitis.

CHAPTER 13

Understanding Your Hormones

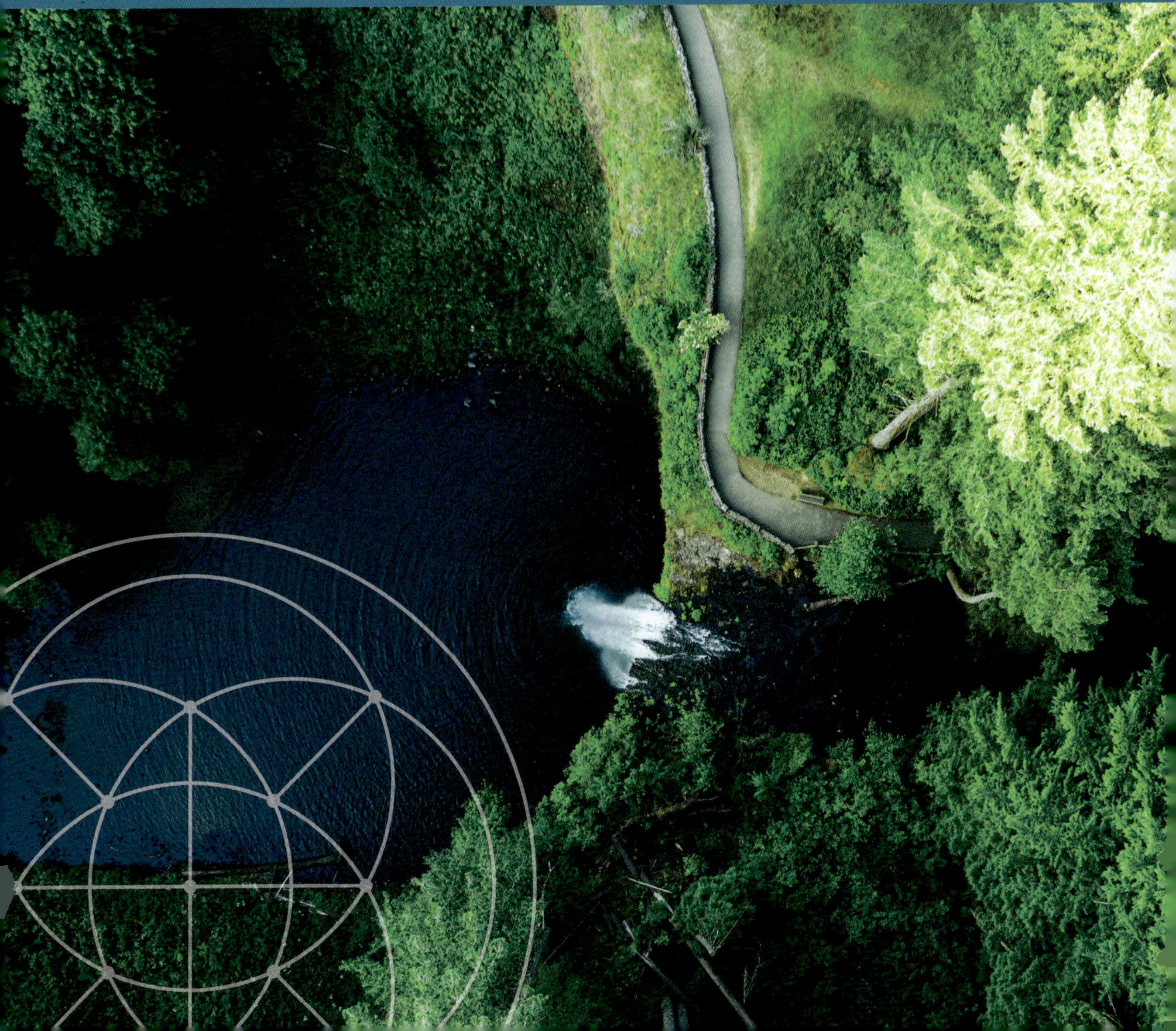

> Hormones get no respect. We think of them as the elusive chemicals that make us a bit moody, but these magical little molecules do so much more.
>
> —**Susannah Cahalan**

Hormones are chemical messengers—tiny molecules that serve as a means of communication between our cells, regulating body functions. Hormones are manufactured inside glands, such as the thyroid or pancreas, and are secreted into the body, usually directly into the bloodstream. The entire system of glands and the hormones they secrete is called the endocrine system.

In Greek, *hormon* means "to set in motion," and that is exactly what hormones do. They set in motion activity that ultimately affects every cell in our bodies. Our body chemistry is an invisible web of relationships—vast complex networks that ultimately make us who we are. Our hormones are always behind the scenes, calling the shots and defining everything that happens. They are everywhere at once, interacting with the microscopic receptors on every single cell in the body.

In this chapter, we explain hormone basics and discuss stress hormones, sex hormones, and thyroid hormones. In the next chapter, we'll go into the details of how to balance your hormones for better health and wellbeing. And in Chapter 15, we will discuss the hormone insulin, which controls our blood sugar.

Master Hormones

Many of our hormones, no matter where they are made or what they do, are controlled by a complex feedback mechanism that begins in the brain: the *hypothalamic-pituitary-adrenal (HPA) axis*. This mechanism begins in the hypothalamus, the part of the brain that links the nervous system to the endocrine hormone system through the pituitary gland. Among other crucial functions, the hypothalamus controls your body tem-

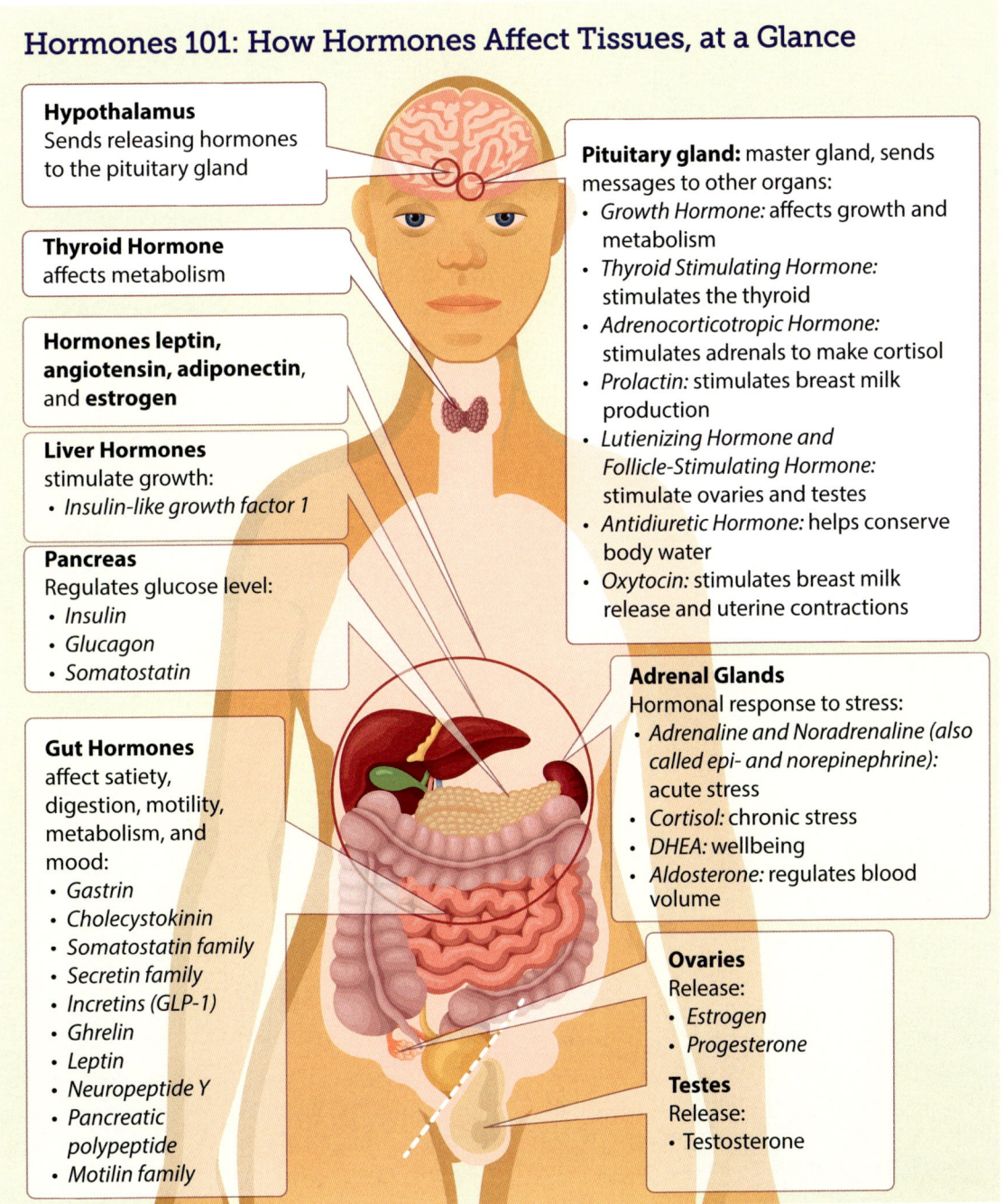

FIGURE 13.1 | Hormones 101

perature, your sense of hunger and thirst, and your sleep and circadian cycles. It also makes and secretes the hypothalamic-releasing hormones, also known as neurohormones. These hormones travel to the pituitary gland, where they may stimulate or inhibit the release of other hormones.

The pituitary gland is a pea-sized organ located in your brain, close to the hypothalamus. In response to hormones released by the hypothalamus, the pituitary gland produces pituitary hormones. Sometimes called the master gland, the pituitary orchestrates the entire symphony of hormonal chemistry. As the conductor, it sends messages to the adrenal gland, thyroid, testes, ovaries, breasts, uterus, kidneys, and other organs and tissues throughout the body.

Pituitary hormones send chemical messages to the adrenal glands, small organs that sit on top of each kidney. The adrenal glands respond by producing hormones that help us deal with stress (adrenaline, noradrenaline, and cortisol), produce sex hormones (estrogen and testosterone), and regulate our water and salt balance and control our blood pressure (aldosterone). The pituitary also sends signals to the thyroid gland to regulate the heartbeat, body temperature, and metabolism.

Stress Hormones

We tend to view stress hormones as harmful and stress as a negative. In reality, stress is simply how we adapt to our lives—it's part of being alive. The issue of stress is more a question of balance. How do we react to stress? Can we maintain a balanced response when stress intensifies?

Ultimately, we want to redefine stress as adaptation. Our stress hormones allow us to stay up all night to push through on a project that's due or study for an exam. This same response enables us to pull our child out of the path of danger in the blink of an eye. It is quite a marvelous survival mechanism.

Under acute stress, the adrenal glands secrete the hormones adrenaline (also called

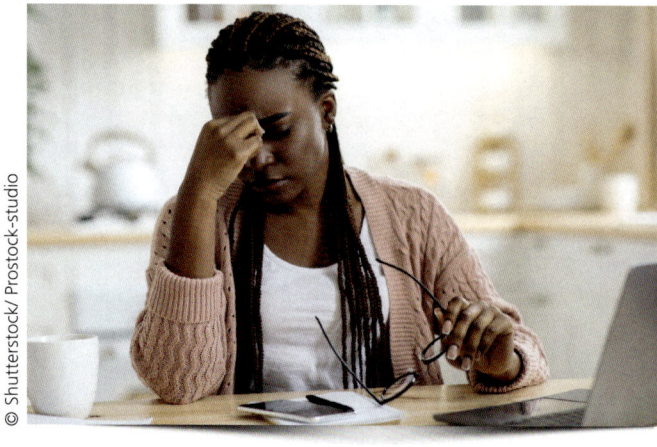

epinephrine) and noradrenaline (also called norepinephrine). Under chronic stress, the adrenals secrete the hormone cortisol. Stress hormones are essential to our adaptation and to our survival. Stress is fine—until it becomes relentless and depletes us. Then it can be dangerous to our health. (In chapter 2, we reviewed the changes that happen to cortisol under chronic stress.) In the end, it is always a question of balance.

Sex Hormones

Procreation is one of the primary drives for human beings. The sex hormones testosterone (produced primarily in the testes in men) and estrogen and progesterone (produced primarily in the ovaries in women) help us carry out this function. Sex hormones are also produced in smaller amounts by the adrenal glands. Although testosterone is the main male sex hormone, women also produce it in small amounts; similarly, men produce small amounts of the female sex hormone estrogen.

All sex hormones use cholesterol, a chemical steroid, as their main building block. Consequently, they are sometimes called the steroidogenic hormones.

Sex hormones fall into three major classes:

Androgens include testosterone and anabolic steroids, the primary hormones of the male body. Testosterone is needed to develop the male reproductive organs; it also gives men their male characteristics, including larger muscle mass, heavier bones, and body hair. Anabolic steroids build up the body's muscles and provide a sense of wellbeing. That's why so many athletes are tempted to take synthetic anabolic steroids to improve performance.

Estrogens are the primary sex hormones for women. The word estrogen comes from *estrus* (a period of fertility for female mammals) and *gen* (to generate). In other words, estrogen helps generate female fertility. It also produces female secondary sex characteristics, including wide hips and prominent breasts. Women produce three different forms of estrogen. The predominant estrogen type depends on the stage of a woman's life. For women who are still menstruating but are not pregnant, estradiol is the primary form. During pregnancy, estriol is the primary estrogen, and after menopause, the primary estrogen is estrone.

Progestogens include progesterone, which supports the health of the uterine lining. Low levels of progesterone can result in premenstrual syndrome (PMS) in younger women and can contribute to menopausal symptoms later in life. Progesterone appears to counterbalance some of the effects of estrogen.

Cholesterol is also the precursor for two other types of hormones: glucocorticoids (primarily the stress hormone cortisol), and mineralocorticoids (primarily the hormone aldosterone, which regulates the body's salt/water balance).

As we get older, the testes, ovaries, and adrenals begin to produce sex hormones at reduced levels. In women, menopause brings a significant reduction to estrogen production. Likewise, in men, testosterone production naturally dips.

Thyroid Hormones

The thyroid, a butterfly-shaped gland at the front of the neck, just below the voice box, produces the hormones that control the metabolic flame—turning the heat up or down. You could think of the thyroid as the thermostat of metabolism because it affects energy level, mental focus and function, sleep cycles, heart rate, digestion, muscle tone, and even strength. The thyroid has an impact on every system in the body.

Hormones Out of Balance

The elegant chemistry of hormones is like a beautiful symphony, with messages constantly feeding back to controller glands to balance and regulate the system, affecting the entire body and every aspect of its function. When a part of the endocrine system becomes out of tune, however, the result can be cacophony.

Physicians, especially the hormone specialists known as endocrinologists, are well trained to look for abnormal hormonal pathways. These vary from mild thyroid imbalances and type 2 diabetes to more complex hormonal problems, such as adrenal hyperplasia (resulting in excessive or deficient production of steroid hormones), pituitary tumors, and Cushing's disease.

We often see patients who are convinced that they have hormonal problems, yet their physicians have told them that all their conventional diagnostic tests are

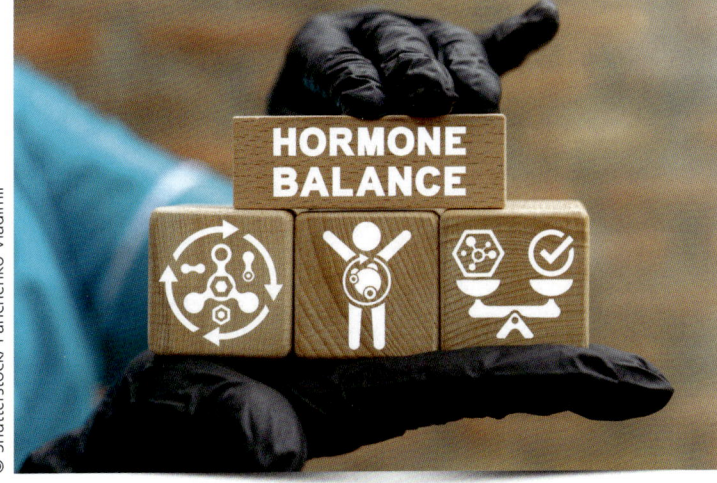

© Shutterstock/ Panchenko Vladimir

normal. This is due to one of two reasons. The patient may be attributing symptoms to a disease that simply isn't there. We often see patients, for example, who attribute their weight gain to thyroid problems, but they don't have thyroid disease. In these cases, the patient needs to look elsewhere, especially at lifestyle, for the cause of the problem. Alternatively, the patient may truly have a hormone imbalance, but conventional lab tests aren't detecting the problem. Hormones fluctuate from day to day and over the course of a month, so doing a single test may not reveal a problem. Often, the only way to diagnose a hormone problem is with more than one hormone test.

Our **Natural Steroids**

The hormones our bodies make from cholesterol are referred to as steroidogenic or steroid hormones. They are the natural steroids in our bodies—the same steroids that bodybuilders and athletes use to bulk up and enhance their performance. Our bodies make the very same hormones but in much lower doses—and they are essential to our wellbeing.

Steroid Pathways

Steroid hormones flow down two main pathways: the stress hormone pathway to form cortisol and the wellbeing hormone pathway to form dehydroepiandrosterone (DHEA), which makes testosterone and estrogens. DHEA is the most abundant steroid hormone in the body, produced mostly in the adrenal glands. DHEA is the basic hormone used by the body to manufacture testosterone and estrogens.

When we are living a balanced life, our hormones reflect this. We produce just enough cortisol (our primary stress hormone) to keep inflammation in check, and we make just enough of our wellbeing hormone, DHEA. People with high DHEA levels experience a sense of wellbeing and comfort in their bodies and have been found to have the lowest incidence of cancer, arthritis, and chronic disease.

But when we're dealing with intense stress—or relentless low-level chronic stress—the body will "steal" sex hormones so it can continue to produce higher levels of stress hormones. As a result, our levels of the wellbeing hormone DHEA drop. Testosterone levels go down, causing a decrease in libido and a loss of muscle mass and strength. Estrogen drops too, which is why menopausal women notice more hot flashes when they're stressed. You can see how the pathways flow and how stress affects them in the diagram on page 189.

How Our Bodies Wear Down— and **How They Get Restored**

Ideally, we have a balance between the two hormone systems—between the production of stress hormones and wellbeing hormones. Stress hormones tend to break our bodies down and are referred to as catabolic. In a famine or time of stress, the body needs to repair damage and find extra protein to make hormones and enzymes, so it breaks down muscle. It also needs to store fuel, so it builds fat. Is it any surprise that stress makes us weak and flabby?

Hormones that restore and heal us, such as DHEA, testosterone, estrogen, and human growth hormone, are anabolic. They build us up, make our muscles grow, and give us a sense of wellbeing.

The Effect of Stress On Cholesterol-Derived Hormones

```
                    Cholesterol
                         ↓
                  Precursor Hormones
                    /            \
                   /              \
     Wellbeing Hormones        Stress Hormones
          DHEA                     Cortisol
           ↓
     Testosterone → Estrogen
                    (Estradiol or "E2")
```

Chronic stress and inflammation result in increased demand for stress hormones.

A Balancing Act

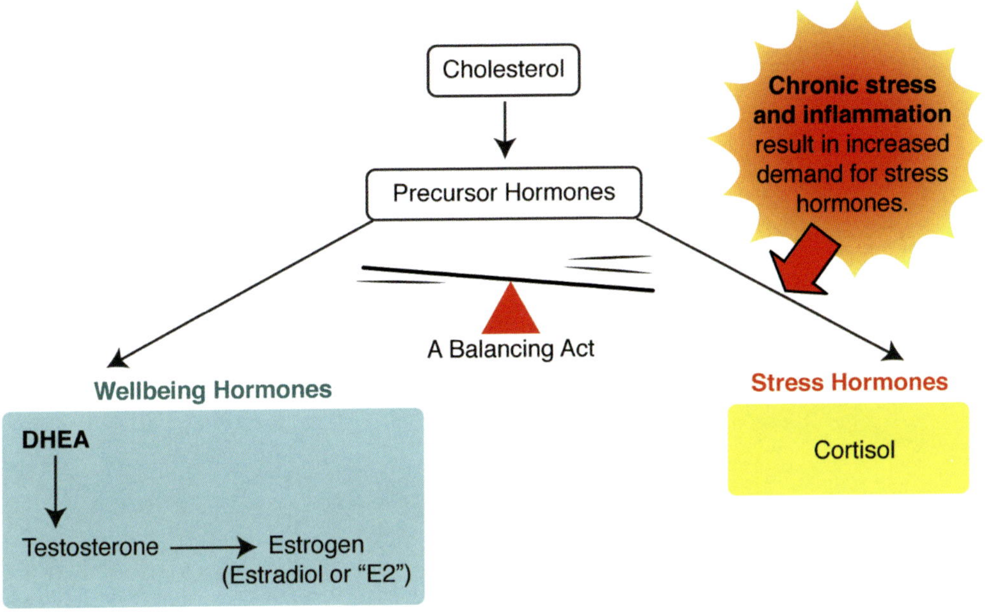

FIGURE 13.2 | The Effect of Stress on Cholesterol-Derived Hormones

Chronic stress is very different from acute stress. Acute stress triggers the production of adrenaline and noradrenaline, which give us a "fight or flight" response. These brief bursts of hormones are a survival mechanism that our bodies are designed to handle. However, when stress becomes chronic and long-term, our bodies eventually wear down. Cortisol initially climbs, but then bottoms out as our adrenal glands become overworked and depleted. The exhausted adrenals also result in low DHEA levels. Chronic stress is associated with higher inflammation and altered immunity. As the body shifts to produce more stress hormones, it also decreases the amount of wellbeing hormones it produces (DHEA, testosterone, and estrogen).

Sex Hormones in Midlife

For our ancestors, the cycle of life was quite different than it is for us today. In 1850, the average life span for women in the United States was just 40 years; in 1900, it was 48 years. Consequently, only a minority of women lived to experience menopause. Today, things are different. Most women reach menopause and may live several decades beyond it. Once women reach menopause, it's time to decide how to live the second part of their lives.

Similarly, in the past, men didn't have options as to how they would age. Until recently, we didn't hear much about erectile dysfunction and lower libido, because nothing could really be done about those conditions. In 1998, the erectile dysfunction drug sildenafil (Viagra) was approved and powerfully improved the sex lives of many men. But ED drugs work for only about 70 percent of men and can have some unpleasant side effects—and are very expensive even when covered by health insurance. Today, even with sildenafil (and similar drugs), men want better and different approaches to improve their virility.

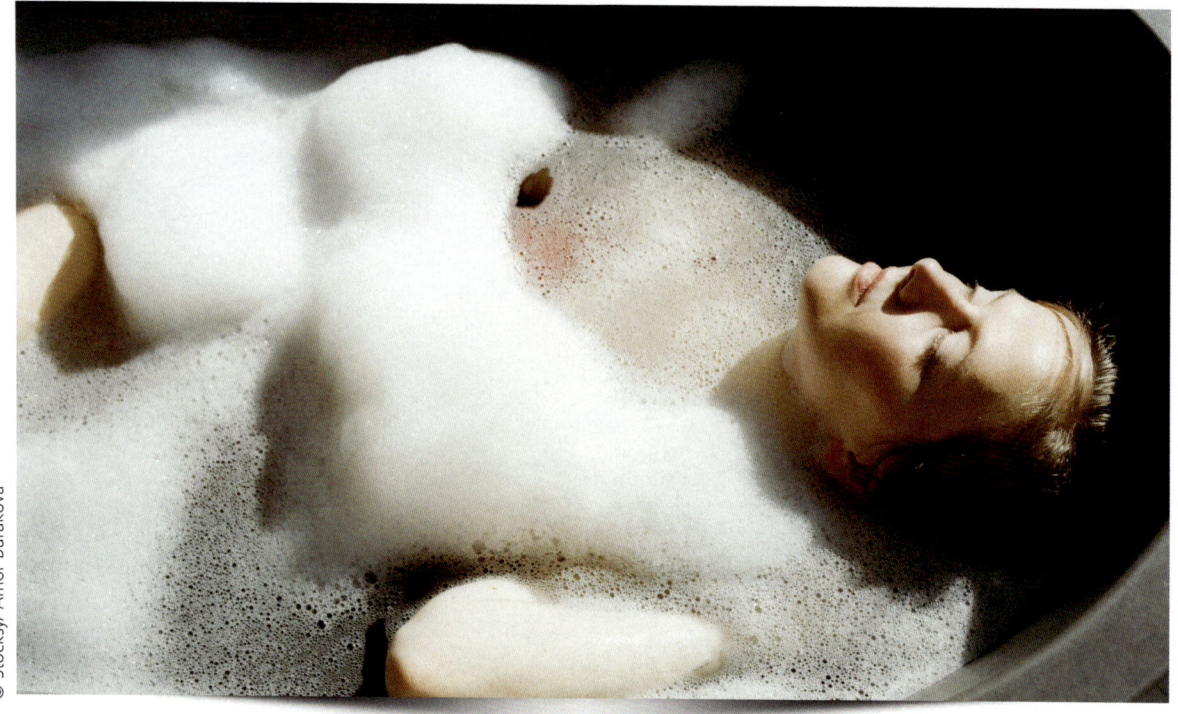

Menopause and Andropause

As the body ages, production of wellbeing hormones naturally begins dropping—we make less DHEA, testosterone, and estrogen. In both sexes, this results in a decreased sense of vitality and lowered libido. Men may notice more difficulty getting an erection or loss of muscle mass and strength.

In women, the typical symptoms of perimenopause (the time when menstruation begins to slow) and menopause—the complete stop of menstrual periods—include night sweats, hot flashes, mental fog, insomnia, vaginal dryness, and loss of libido. For most women, perimenopause begins in their late 40s; the average age for menopause is 51.

During perimenopause, a woman's ovaries become depleted and make less estrogen. Meanwhile, in response, the pituitary gland begins producing higher amounts of follicle stimulating hormone (FSH) as it tries in vain to get the ovaries to make more estrogen. In fact, a high FSH level is one of the normal signs of perimenopause. Once the ovaries start shutting down production, estrogen is still produced by the adrenal glands, but the adrenals must also still produce cortisol in response to stress. Since the adrenals don't produce much estrogen to begin with and have only so much capacity, when a postmenopausal woman is under stress, her adrenals will produce more cortisol and stop making estrogen. As a result, she will become catabolic, lose muscle, and gain weight. Her testosterone will also drop, so her libido will decrease.

The word andropause has become a popular term for the overall impact of lower testosterone in middle age. For men, hormone chemistry during andropause—the slow decrease in testosterone levels as men age—can vary widely. Andropause symptoms develop more gradually and less predictably than female menopause symptoms. A man may be less likely to notice the symptoms or to connect them with andropause. And though andropause is sometimes called "male menopause," it isn't really a good description; men don't experience the more dramatic changes that affect a woman in menopause.

In andropause, as testosterone levels drop, libido goes down and erectile dysfunction develops. In addition, men in andropause develop more body fat and have a higher propensity to develop insulin resistance. Decreasing testosterone levels also affect mood, mental functioning, endurance, bone health, and muscle strength. Of course, some men maintain high testosterone well into their later years. Others find their testosterone levels dropping in their forties, earlier than average.

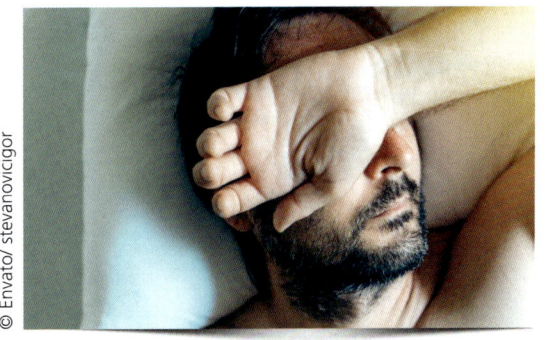

The Domino Effect of Stress in Men

Stress = need to cope = need for more cortisol
Testosterone "stolen" to make cortisol
Less testosterone = less protection against inflammation
More inflammation = more work-related injuries, sports injuries, and joint pain
Less testosterone = lower libido and erectile dysfunction

The Domino Effect of Stress in Women

Stress = need to cope = need for more cortisol
Body makes cortisol at the expense of DHEA, testosterone, and estrogen
More cortisol = more body fat
Less testosterone = lower libido
Less estrogen = lower serotonin = more depression and more irritability
In older women: less estrogen = more hot flashes and night sweats
In younger women: less estrogen = lower fertility

Measuring Your Sex Hormones

Sex hormones can be measured using blood, urine, and saliva tests. Each type of testing has its pros and cons. Because hormone levels naturally fluctuate with normal diurnal rhythms, the results can be different depending on what time of day the test is performed. In addition, estrogen and progesterone levels fluctuate with the menstrual cycle and the effects of approaching menopause. A single hormone test doesn't usually tell us enough—it should be repeated at least once.

Blood tests. Measuring FSH and the main form of estrogen (estradiol or E2) in the blood can be helpful in diagnosing menopause. Measuring testosterone levels can be helpful in determining if that is the reason men are suffering from erectile dysfunction.

Urine tests. We have found that urine tests correlate very well with patient symptoms, more so than blood tests. Urine tests help us determine how testosterone and estrogen are being broken down or metabolized in the body. We use this test to see whether unsafe estrogen metabolites, or by-products, are building up in the body or being safely cleared out.

Saliva testing. Saliva testing is an easy way to check hormone levels at different points throughout the day. All you have to do is collect saliva at regular intervals. Salivary testing is helpful in testing cortisol levels, but it might not be reliable for evaluating sex hormones.

We did an informal study in our own medical office. Some of our female physicians collected their saliva samples on the same day and then sent them off for estrogen and progesterone testing at three different laboratories. The results from the three laboratories were completely different for each physician, even though the samples were all taken at the same time. One of the physicians also had blood hormone levels drawn at the same time and sent off samples to two different labs. The results on the blood samples were almost identical.

Estrogen Byproducts and Cancer

As estrogens are naturally broken down by enzymes in both the female and male body, they are converted into metabolites that can sometimes be harmful. The chances that the byproducts will be harmful are increased if the body's detoxification pathways are not working well.

Breast Cancer

The lifetime incidence of breast cancer has tripled. In 1960, one in 20 women could expect a diagnosis of breast cancer; today, that figure is one in eight. In 2021, about 281,550 new cases of invasive breast cancer were diagnosed; about 49,290 new cases of ductal carcinoma in situ (DCIS) will be diagnosed; and about 43,600 women will die from breast cancer.

Breast cancer is currently the eighth leading cause of death in women in the United States and the second leading cause of cancer death; only lung cancer kills more women. In 2021, the chance that a woman would die from breast cancer was about 1 in 39, or about 2.6 percent. Although since 2007, death rates have been steady in women under 50, they have been decreasing steadily for women over 50. The death rate from breast cancer for women of all ages decreased by one percent per year from 2013 to 2018, and it continues to drop. Treatment advances and screening resulting in earlier detection appear to be the fortunate causes of the decreased death rates.

For decades, women had been urged to take estrogen hormones during menopause to relieve hot flashes and prevent osteoporosis. Some doctors even touted these hormones as a way to remain youthful. Everything changed when the Women's Health Initiative results were published in 2002. The Women's Health Initiative (whi.org), a study that looked at over 16,000 women over 10+ years, showed that taking a combination of synthetic (not bioidentical) estrogen, Premarin, and a synthetic progestin, Provera caused an increased risk of blood clots, heart attack, strokes, and breast cancer in women who started taking the hormones after menopause. Millions of women panicked and stopped taking their hormone supplements. Suddenly, the elixir of youth had become a toxin to be avoided. Women began to realize that the decision to use hormone replacement therapy should not be taken lightly.

Thankfully, we have come a long way since that time. Subsequent reanalysis of data from the WHI dividing patients by their time from menopause, plus newer studies, now consistently show reductions in cardiovascular disease and mortality when hormone replacement therapy is initiated soon after menopause. In younger, healthier women (age 50-60), the risk-benefit balance is positive for using HRT, with risks considered rare. It is also reassuring that a 2022 National Institutes for Health (NIH) study showed that women 65 and older on estrogen-only therapy have statistically fewer of all five cancers studied (breast, ovarian, uterine, lung, and colon). They live almost 20 percent longer/healthier lives and have less heart disease (unless on oral estrogens) and less dementia (Seo et al. 2022). Adding synthetic progesterone slightly increases the risk of breast cancer, but it is unknown if natural progesterone has the same increased risk. Progesterone is given with estrogen to prevent uterine cancer in women who have their uterus.

While not all women are a candidate for estrogen therapy, and elevated levels of estrogen and its metabolites can potentially increase breast cancer risk, it should not cause the intense fear it once had and is often used to improve quality of life, reduce symptoms of perimenopause and menopause, and potentially to increase healthspan.

Other risk factors for breast cancer include a family history of breast cancer in a first-degree relative (mother or sister), increasing age, dense breasts, prior radiation therapy for an earlier cancer, a sedentary lifestyle, being overweight or obese after menopause, and excessive alcohol consumption. In addition, endocrine disruptors appear to have an influence.

Some risk factors are typically modifiable, such as body weight, alcohol consumption, and activity levels. Other risk factors like aging, a previous history of radiation, and dense breasts can't be changed. But what about the genetic risk factors? We know that gene mutations such as BRCA1 and BRCA2 predispose women to breast cancer and other cancers. Women with these genes who were born before 1940 had a 24 percent lifetime risk of breast cancer, while those born after 1940 have a 67 percent risk. And even though the incidence of breast cancer in women with these gene variants has gone up over the years, not everyone who inherits a BRCA1 or BRCA2 mutation will get breast cancer. This suggests that something in the environment is affecting the way breast cancer genes turn on. While medicine has focused on what causes women to develop breast cancer, no one seems to have looked at the flip side. We know that BRCA1 and BRCA2 variants confer a greater risk on women for breast cancer. Women with BRCA1 have a 50 to 80 percent risk of developing breast cancer, while those with BRCA2 have a 40 to 70 percent risk. So the question we should ask is: Why are some of these women *not* getting breast cancer? What are they doing differently, and what can we learn from them? Are they less exposed to estrogen-disrupting chemicals in the environment? Do they eat a diet higher in detoxifying fruits and vegetables? Do they get more sun exposure, resulting in higher vitamin D levels? Do they detoxify estrogen metabolites better? Do they get more exercise and maintain a healthy weight? We don't know for sure. But there's clearly more to breast cancer than just genetic susceptibility.

Prostate Cancer

About one in six men will develop prostate cancer during his lifetime—aside from skin cancer, it is the most common cancer in American men. Prostate cancer is the second leading cause of cancer deaths in American men over the age of 45 (behind lung cancer), but only one man in 41 will die of it. By the age of 85, 85 percent of all men will have prostate cancer, but at that age, very few will die of it or even have troublesome symptoms.

The largest long-term outcome study of intermediate-grade prostate cancer confirmed that early treatment improves survival rates significantly. Early treatment means early detection, but the guidelines for prostate cancer screening using a blood test for prostate-specific antigen (PSA) levels are a little confusing. PSA is a protein that can be produced by prostate cancer cells. Unfortunately, normal prostate cells stimulated by inflammation or infection can also produce an elevated PSA, as can benign prostatic hyperplasia (BPH), a relatively common but noncancerous change in the prostate that occurs with age. In other words, elevated PSA doesn't always mean cancer. Screening offers the small potential benefit of reducing the risk of death from prostate cancer in some men, but it also has potential harms, including false positives that lead to unnecessary treatment. The US Preventive Services Task Force (USPSTF) recommends that, in the absence of symptoms, we screen men aged 55 to 69 with a PSA test if they request it but only after talking over their family history, other factors such as race, and the risks and benefits of doing screening. For men over 70, the USPSTF does not recommend screening. The reasoning here is that even if they turn out to have prostate cancer, they will probably die of something else, and the cancer is so slow-moving that it doesn't need treatment. In practice, this does not usually happen as most men want a PSA test.

Early Detection Isn't the Same as Prevention

PSA levels and mammograms can be helpful for early detection of prostate and breast cancer. But while these tests have saved thousands of lives, they are not perfect. They only pick up cancer that has already developed. They also have false positives, which can lead to unnecessary procedures and overtreatment. About 12 percent of abnormal mammograms are false positives.

What about going one step further than early detection? Can we prevent these illnesses?

Detoxification and Cancer Prevention

The human body is more complex than any factory system ever developed. Every substance that passes through the body must be broken down and disposed of safely. That applies to toxins we breathe in, foods we eat (healthful and unhealthful), and medications we take—as well as our own hormones.

The body's ability to fully detoxify hormones depends on several factors:

- **Genetic predisposition**
- **The level of toxins produced within the body**
- **The toxic burden from the environment**
- **The body's ability to detoxify the hormones**
- **A diet rich in nutrients that support detoxification**

When the harmful byproducts of hormone metabolism are not broken down completely and quickly, they may contribute to conditions such as breast cancer and prostate cancer.

The Good, the Bad, and the Ugly Estrogens

Both men and women produce estrogen, although women produce far more of it. In both sexes, the primary active form of estrogen is estradiol, or E2. When estradiol is metabolized, it is broken down into three different metabolites, which we term "the good" (2-hydroxyestrone or 2-OH E1), "the bad" (16-hydroxyestrone, or 16-OH E1), and "the ugly" (4-hydroxyestrone, or 4-OH E1).

Good estrogen (2-hydroxyestrone) has a naturally protective effect on the breast and prostate. Bad estrogen (16-hydroxyestrone) has a damaging effect on breast and prostate tissue. Ugly estrogen (4-hydroxyestrone) can be converted to a quinone, a toxic byproduct found in high amounts in cancerous breast and prostate tissue. Some people are genetically prone to producing more quinones.

Estrogen is detoxified in the liver by phase I and phase II pathways. (Chapter 7 has more information on detoxification pathways.) Genetic variants can produce glitches in the detoxification pathways that result in more bad and ugly estrogens, as well as unsafe metabolites. Fortunately, the good, the bad, and the ugly estrogens can all be safely converted to what we call "safe exhaust fumes," or byproducts that can be excreted from the body before they do any damage. For example, bad estrogen is successfully detoxified into estriol (E3), which appears to protect against benign breast disease, breast cancer, and endometrial cancer.

In the next chapter, we'll talk about ways to influence your detoxification pathways so they are more likely to convert estrogen to harmless metabolites.

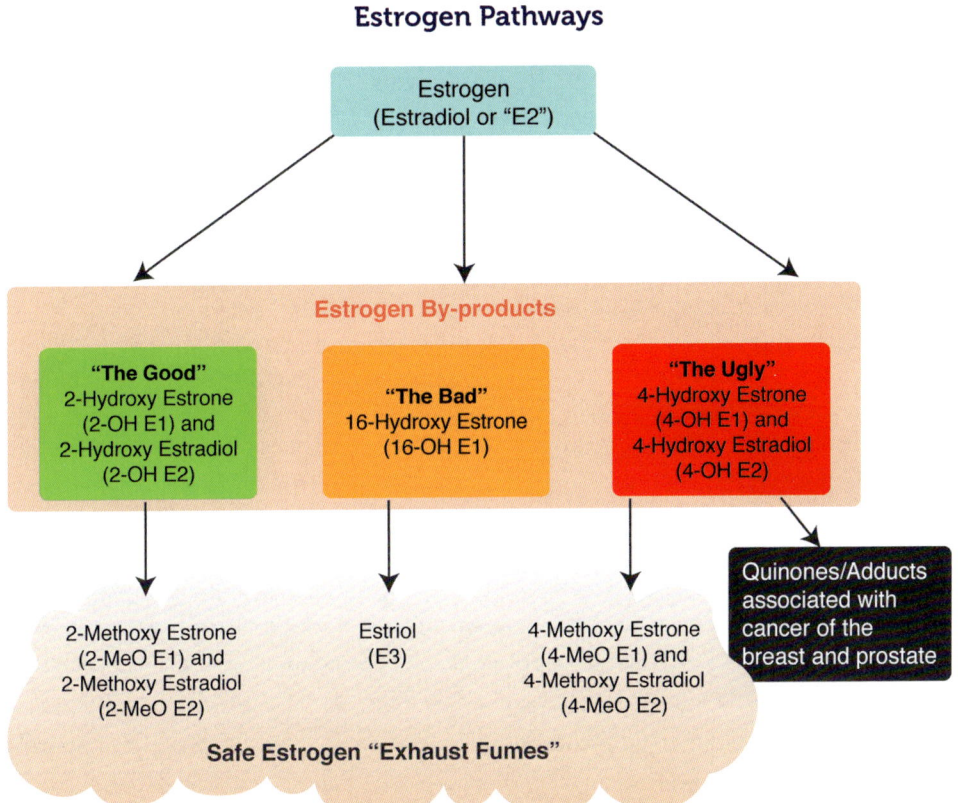

FIGURE 13.3 | Estrogen Byproducts and Breast and Prostate Cancer Risk

Genetic Variants in Phase I Detoxification:

- CYP1B1 results in more of the ugly estrogens (4-hydroxyestrone).
- CYP3A4 results in more of the bad estrogens (16-hydroxyestrone).

Genetic Variants in Phase II Detoxification:

- Catechol-O-methyltransferase (COMT) decreases the ability to convert or methylate the good estrogen (2-hydroxyestrone) to its safe byproduct (2-methoxyestrone) as well as the ugly estrogen to convert to its safe byproduct (4-methoxyestrone).
- Glutathione-S-transferase (GST) metabolizes ugly estrogens into the toxic quinones that are found in high amounts in cancerous breast and prostate tissue.
- NAD(P)H quinone oxidoreductase 1 (NQO1) decreases the ability of the liver to convert the unsafe quinones to safe byproducts for excretion.

More on Estrogen Disruptors: Toxins in the Environment

Estrogen disrupters are chemicals that we are exposed to in our environment, including chemicals from plastic bottles, automobile exhaust, pesticides, and herbicides. They all affect the body by mimicking estrogen, but unlike estrogen they can hang around in the body for years. In young girls, estrogen disrupters can cause early puberty, causing the development of breasts and menstruation at an early age. This prolonged estrogen stimulation should be taken seriously. Estrogen disruptors are associated with an increased risk of breast cancer in women and an increased risk of prostate cancer in men.

Estrogen Replacement or Hormone Therapy

Estrogen replacement therapy, now more commonly known as hormone therapy (HT), is sometimes recommended for women as a treatment for severe menopause symptoms such as disruptive hot flashes, night sweats, and vaginal dryness. It is being studied to improve mood and reduce pain that feels similar to fibromyalgia. Estrogen therapy is also being studied for both bone health and brain health. Researcher and author, Dr. Lisa Mosconi, who studies the female brain, reports that estrogen therapy may be included as part of a plan to reduce dementia risk and preserve brain volume. There are some side effects to using estrogen. Oral estrogen pills do come with a slight increased risk for blood clots and stroke, which is why transdermal estrogens are usually recommended as they do not pose the same risk. If a woman still has her uterus, progesterone is prescribed at the same time as estrogen to reduce or eliminate the risk of uterine cancer. (We will look at the pros and cons of HT in the next chapter.)

The Thyroid: Revving Your Body's Engine

The thyroid, a butterfly-shaped gland at the front of the neck, just below the voice box, produces the hormones that control the metabolic flame. It works with the hypothalamus and the pituitary gland to regulate energy level, mental focus and function, sleep cycles, heart rate, digestion, muscle tone, and even strength. This complex process begins with the hypothalamus telling the pituitary gland to secrete *thyroid-stimulating hormone* (TSH). As the name suggests, TSH stimulates the thyroid to make the hormone *thyroxine*, or T4, which is key to controlling how much energy your body uses—your metabolic rate. The thyroid also produces a hormone called *triiodothyronine*, known as T3. These hormones work together to regulate your body's temperature, metabolism, and heart rate.

TSH and T4 work in a feedback loop. Normally, when T4 blood levels are low, this will activate the pituitary gland's "on switch," and TSH will rise, stimulating the thyroid to produce more T4. When T4 levels are high enough, this will kick the "off switch," and the pituitary gland will stop secreting TSH. This loop is how the body keeps thyroid levels within a normal range.

Common Thyroid Conditions

The most common thyroid condition is *hypothyroidism*, or low thyroid function. When the thyroid isn't producing enough T3 and T4, the body's metabolism slows, making you feel tired and weak. Hypothyroidism can also cause depression, weight gain, memory problems, dry skin and brittle nails, cold intolerance, constipation, and menstrual irregularities.

Killing Itself Slowly: Hashimoto's Thyroiditis

Hashimoto's thyroiditis is an autoimmune disease in which the body attacks its own thyroid gland. Autoimmune diseases of the thyroid gland are the most common of all autoimmune conditions, and Hashimoto's thyroiditis is the most common cause of hypothyroidism, which affects about one in 20 Americans. Probably for hormonal reasons, Hashimoto's thyroiditis is somewhere between four and ten times more common in women than men and most often develops in women aged 30 to 50. This disease usually comes on very slowly, taking years to damage the thyroid enough to reduce hormone production. Patients might think that their forgetfulness and tiredness, for instance, are just from getting older, but it could be that Hashimoto's thyroiditis is finally causing noticeable symptoms.

Catching on Fire, Then Fizzling Out: Graves' Disease

Graves' disease is another autoimmune condition of the thyroid. In contrast to the low thyroid production characteristic of Hashimoto's thyroiditis, Graves' disease initially causes excessive thyroid production, or hyperthyroidism. It's the most common cause of hyperthyroidism in the United States, affecting about one in 200 people. Graves' disease usually affects people aged 30 to 50. It's seven to eight times more common in women than men.

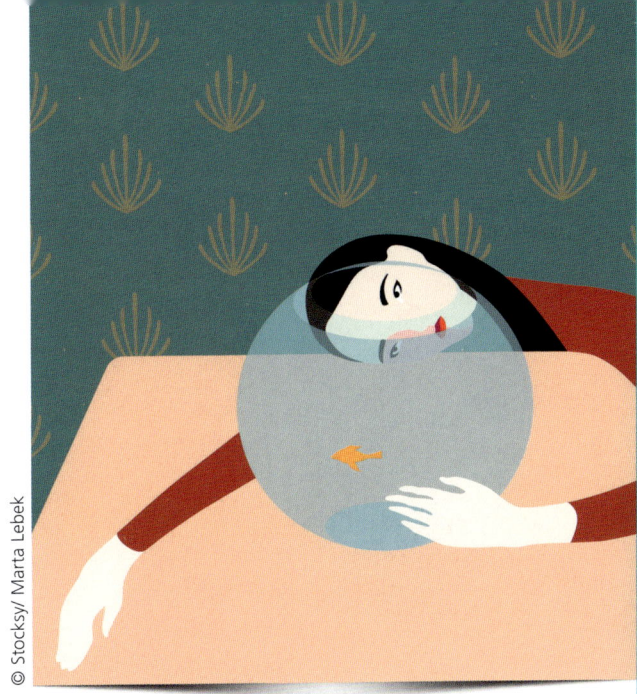
© Stocksy/ Marta Lebek

In early stages, patients usually have heart palpitations, insomnia, diarrhea, and unexplained weight loss. Their symptoms are triggered by high thyroid levels amping up their metabolism. The patient may develop an enlarged thyroid gland (goiter) and may also develop a protrusion of one or both eyes. Like Hashimoto's disease, Graves' disease has a genetic component.

Fortunately, as we'll discuss in chapter 14, problems with thyroid hormones can be detected with accurate blood tests and can almost always be successfully treated.

A Final Note on Hormones

Our body's endocrine system functions in tandem with the neurological and immune systems. Stress and depression can have a major effect on our hormones, as can detoxification, oxidation, and inflammation. Together, all these processes affect our metabolism.

The important thing to understand is that altering hormonal balance isn't just accomplished by using medications. By changing lifestyle, diet, and environment, using appropriate nutritional supplements, and dealing with stress, you can make a dramatic difference in how you look, feel, and age.

When the hormones are in balance, they maintain the normal function of the body. If they are imbalanced, we want to know why. When we look for hormonal imbalances, we do so while looking at the patient's body and their life as a whole—and then we help them regain balance.

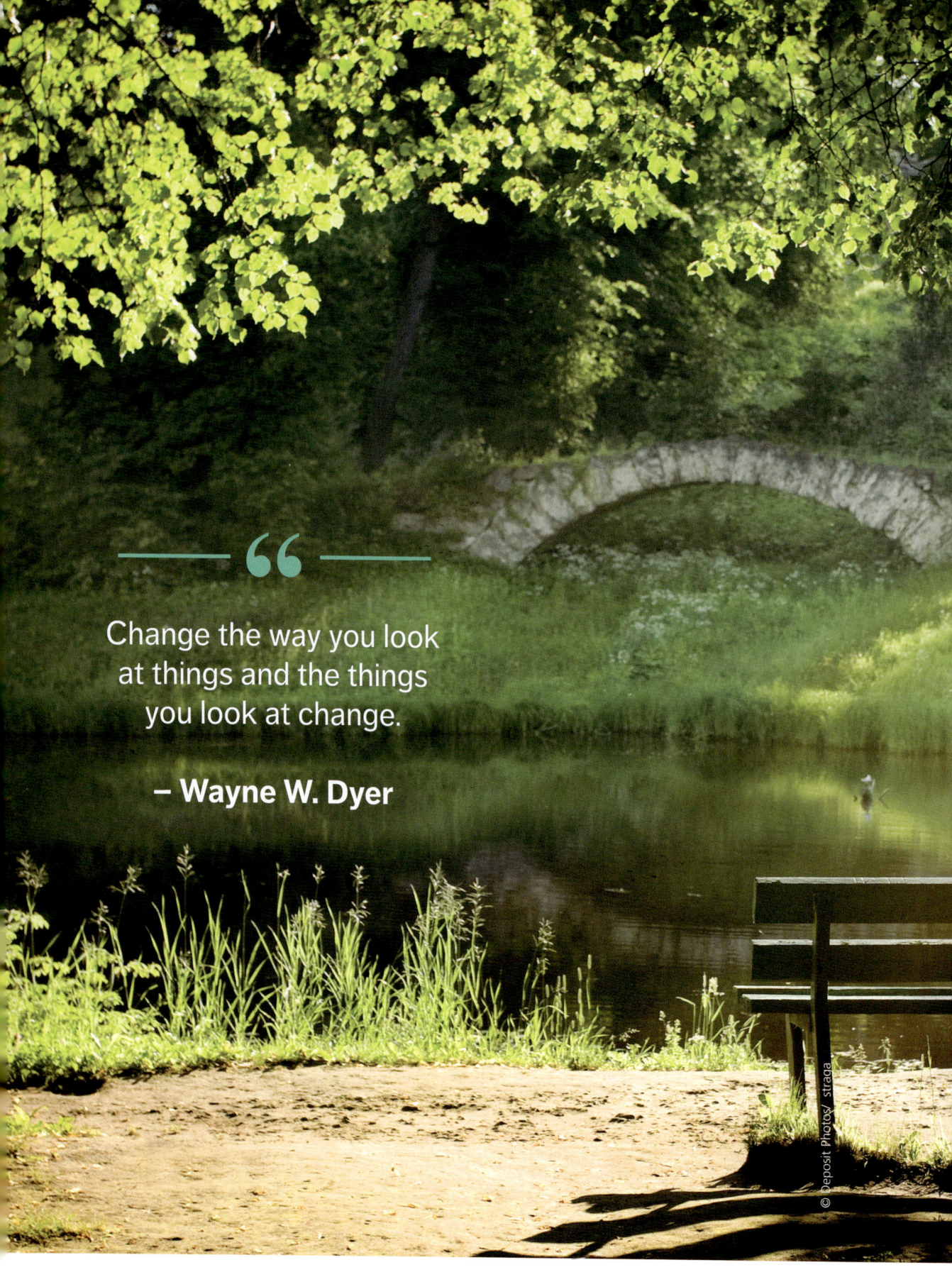

CHAPTER 14
Optimizing Your Hormonal Balance

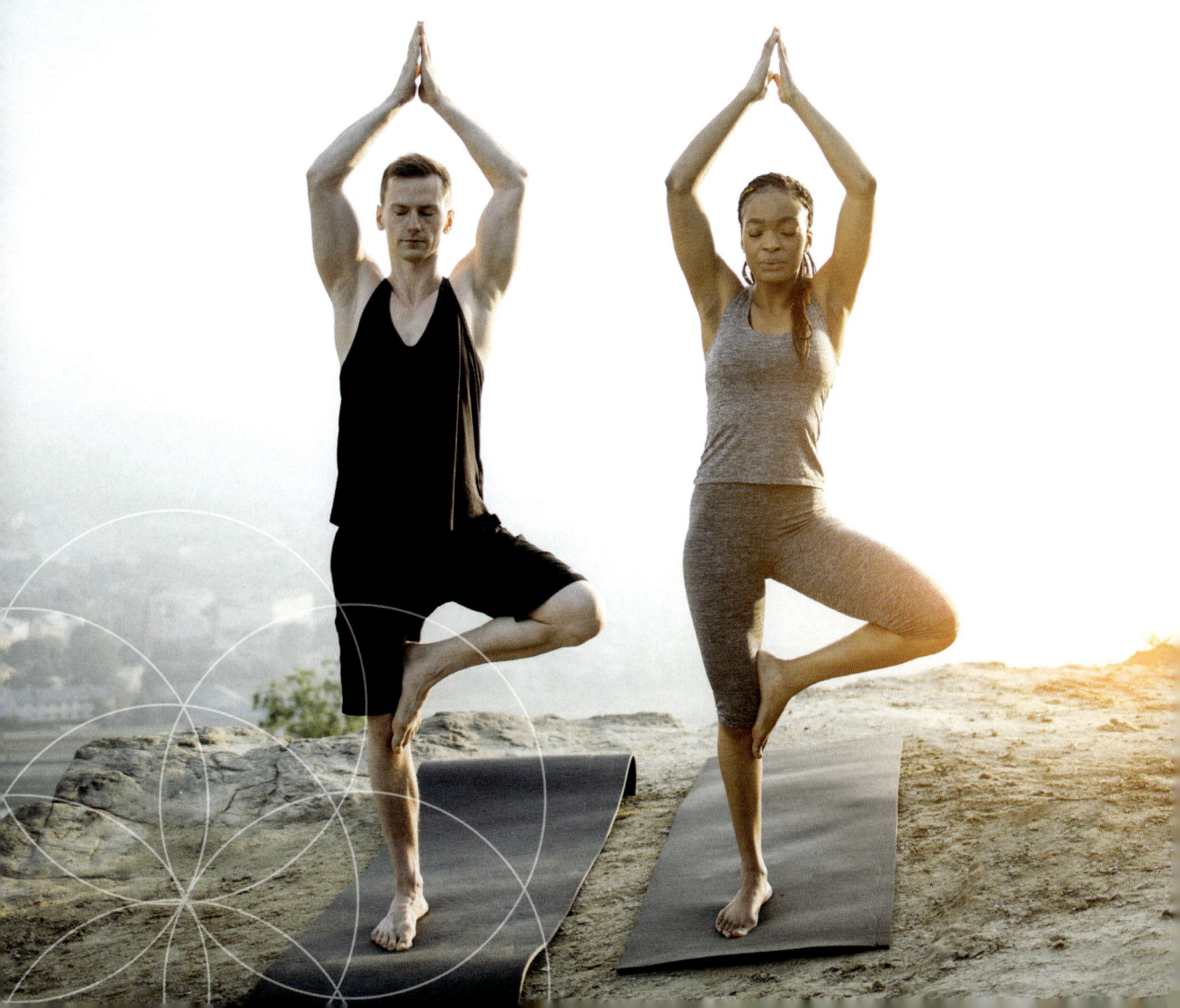

We have been primed to think that the only way we can help our endocrine system is to take supplemental hormones. This isn't necessarily true! If certain hormones are deficient, as they might be with low thyroid, taking replacement hormones is necessary. If you have type 1 diabetes, you need to replace the insulin your body can no longer produce with injections. But for many conditions, we can work with you to improve your quality of life using other approaches, especially if you're in the early stages of midlife changes.

Some diseases do need medical treatment to replace deficient or missing hormones. Congenital adrenal hyperplasia, Addison's disease, Cushing's disease, Conn's syndrome, Hashimoto's thyroiditis, and Graves' disease are not uncommon, and several other rare diseases should also be ruled out. We suggest you start addressing potential hormonal issues with a thorough evaluation by a medical practitioner who understands how to diagnose and treat endocrine issues. The practitioner can then tell if you have an outright endocrine disease or just a mild dysfunction implying your hormones are simply out of balance.

Five Steps to Balancing Your Hormones

Once we've ruled out a disease as the cause of our patients' symptoms, we help them with a five-step approach to balancing their hormones.

Step 1. Reduce stress to help balance your stress hormones.

Step 2. Conquer insulin resistance.

Step 3. Balance your wellbeing and sex hormones.

Step 4. Protect against breast cancer or prostate cancer by optimizing estrogen metabolites.

Step 5. Balance your thyroid hormones.

call the "wellbeing" or sex hormones: dehydroepiandrosterone (DHEA), testosterone, and estrogen. Our bodies are designed to handle chronic stress by shunting hormone production toward cortisol and away from wellbeing hormones. (Refer to the diagram on page 185 in Chapter 12 to see how this works.) Think of it this way: In times of famine, our ancestors would have needed to survive, not make babies. Their bodies made more cortisol to store fat and survive. Although times have changed, our bodies have not. We still handle stress in the same way—by reducing our sex and wellbeing hormones and increasing our cortisol production. But now we complain that stress is making us fat and giving us hot flashes! We can't change our hormonal responses, but we can learn how to modify them. Let's look at what else we can do to balance hormones.

Step 1. Balancing Stress Hormones

We consider good stress management the essential first step in balancing your hormones. You want to manage stress effectively, because your body uses the same cholesterol as the building block for both stress hormones, such as cortisol, and what we

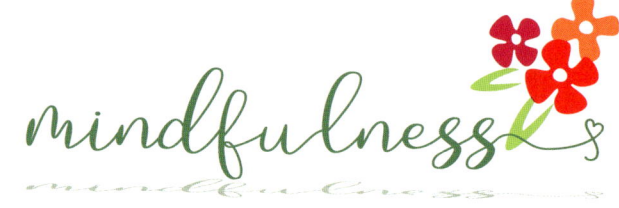

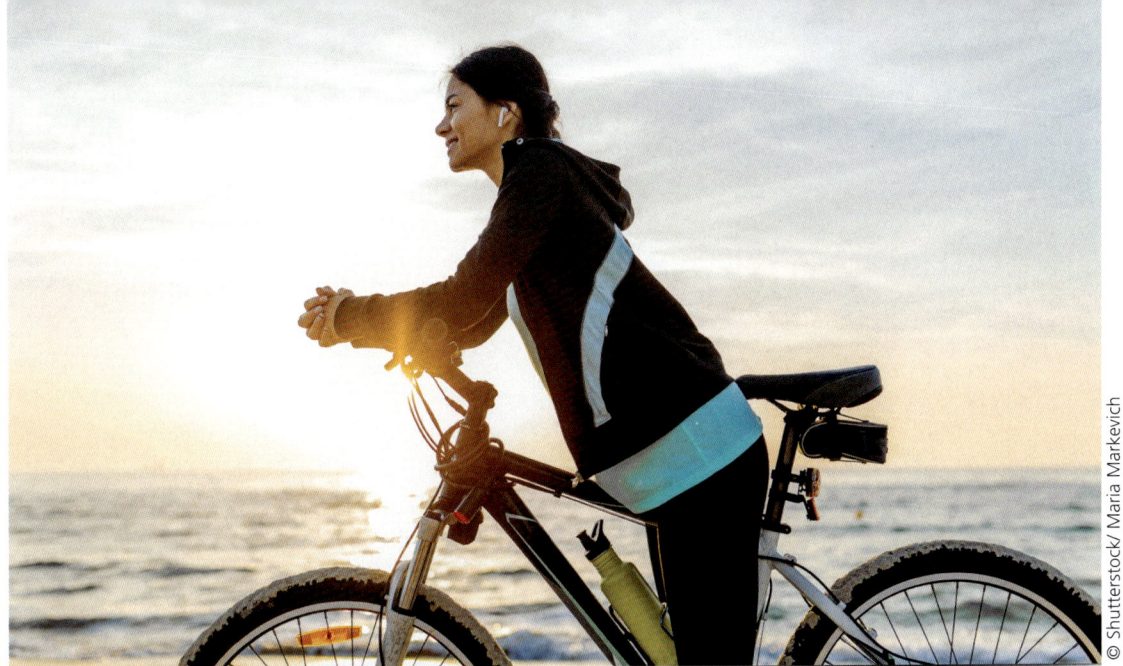

Step 2. Conquering Insulin Resistance

If blood glucose problems are a concern for you, refer to Chapter 15 for a discussion of ways to change the insulin resistance dynamic.

Insulin is a hormone produced by your pancreas. Insulin carries glucose (blood sugar) into your cells, where it can be burned for energy. In insulin resistance, the insulin receptor is faulty. If we think of insulin as a key, and the insulin receptor as a lock it fits into, then in insulin resistance, the lock isn't working properly, so insulin can't do its job properly. If you become resistant to the effects of insulin, you can't use glucose efficiently. At first, when you simply have mild insulin resistance, you might not have any symptoms, but unless you take steps to stop it, insulin resistance slowly gets worse over time and eventually causes type 2 diabetes. Excessive glucose increases your blood sugar, causes weight gain, and causes vascular changes and damage in the tiny blood vessels of your heart, kidneys, eyes, and elsewhere.

A better diet (preferably a plant-forward, high-fiber, low-carb eating pattern) and weight loss are crucial for preventing and treating insulin resistance. Just watching calories isn't usually enough, however. Regular physical activity and stress reduction are the other parts of the equation.

Step 3. Balancing Your WellBeing Hormones

Sometimes just treating stress will normalize the production of wellbeing hormones. Hot flashes go away, erectile dysfunction resolves, and libido returns. However, in menopause or andropause, estrogen and testosterone levels naturally begin dropping, regardless of stress levels. For any person hitting midlife and beyond facing lowered hormone production that is affecting their quality of life, using supplemental hormones may be an option. After the WHI study that came out in 2002, practitioners were told to use the lowest dose for the shortest amount of time. Often though, men and women prefer to stay on hormone therapy. The North American Menopause Society (NAMS) has updated their recommendations to state that women can stay on hormones over 65 if they still have symptoms as long as they are regularly evaluated by their doctor. We always check their estrogen metabolites, optimize their nutritional balance, and ensure they understand the risks as well as the benefits.

When Are Hormones Needed?

We consider several issues before recommending hormones. The first step is to do a thorough lab evaluation. We want to know the cause of your hormone imbalance and make sure you don't have a serious underlying problem.

In particular, we want to rule out hypogonadism as the cause. For both men and women, when your sex organs (also known as gonads) don't produce enough hormones, it can either be due to a central (hypothalamic or pituitary) or a gonadal problem. The gonadal problem could be due to a genetic disorder (Klinefelter syndrome, for example), an infection, trauma, an autoimmune disease, some types of liver or kidney disease, radiation, or chemotherapy. Your brain is still sending your organs the message to produce hormones, but they can't make them. If this is the reason for low hormones, then you have primary hypogonadism. In contrast, when the sex organs are working normally but your hypothalamus and pituitary glands aren't sending the message to make hormones, you have secondary hypogonadism. Many conditions and situations can cause secondary hypogonadism, including pituitary tumors, tuberculosis, HIV/AIDS, steroid use, and obesity.

To see if you have primary or secondary hypogonadism, we use blood tests to check your levels of luteinizing hormone (LH) and follicle-stimulating hormone (FSH). In both men and women, high LH and FSH suggests primary hypogonadism. If LH and FSH are normal or low, that suggests secondary hypogonadism. We also screen estrogen, testosterone, DHEA, prolactin, and thyroid levels to see the whole hormonal picture.

In some cases, lab tests for LH and FSH are normal for your age and sex, but other hormone levels are too low. If we find that self-help measures and nondrug alternatives aren't sufficient, we will then review the pros and cons of hormone therapy (HT). When we use HT, our goal is to use the lowest possible dose that controls symptoms. Both women and men taking supplemental sex hormones should be seen regularly by their primary care doctor or gynecologist.

Hormone Delivery

Hormones can be delivered to the body using pills, creams, gels, patches, pellets, and injections (testosterone). We usually recommend using estrogen or testosterone patches, gels, or creams.. This way, a measured amount of hormone is absorbed directly into the bloodstream through the skin. Transdermal absorption ensures that the hormones go directly into the bloodstream at a steady rate and aren't first metabolized by the liver, as they would be in pill form. This decreases the risk of side effects such as blood clots. They still must eventually go through estrogen metabolism in the liver, which is why we believe testing for those estrogen metabolites, as mentioned, is so important.

We generally recommend against hormone implants that are placed under the skin and left there for several months. Because these products release the hormone continuously, you can accumulate them at excessively high levels. Too often we see women come in with hair loss and clitoral enlargement from using too high a testosterone dose. Using a patch instead of an implant also allows you to adjust the dose as we figure out what the most effective amount is for you.

It is imperative that you discuss benefits and risks of hormone therapy with your physician.

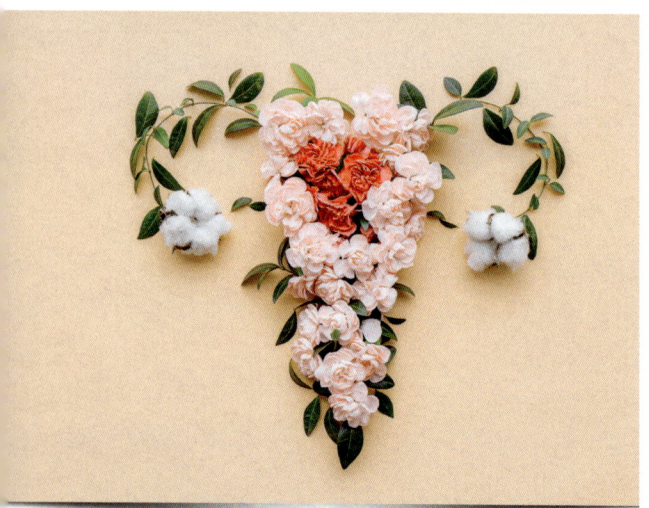

Is Hormone Therapy Safe?

In Chapter 13 we discussed the results from the Women's Health Initiative (WHI) study of HT, published in 2002. This was the largest study (at the time) ever undertaken to evaluate HT, and the results were unsettling and unfortunately, incompletely analyzed when reported. According to the authors, hormonal treatment with Premarin (conjugated equine estrogen) and Provera (synthetic progestin) resulted in an increased risk of blood clots, heart attack, strokes, and breast cancer. When women stopped their hormones abruptly to avoid these risks, they were often devastated by a resumption of hot flashes and other menopausal symptoms. It also plunged them back into the risks of bone loss, brain volume loss, and more. As mentioned, there were many issues with this study. These women were not taking bioidentical hormones, and many of the women in the study started taking the hormones on a long-term basis 10 or more years after menopause. Lastly, the authors reported that the risk of breast cancer for the combination estrogen and progestin group was essentially a significant increase. In reality, it was 8 extra cases of breast cancer per 10,000 women.

As stated in Chapter 13, we've come a long way since the WHI study but it's taking time to re-educate both women, prescribing practitioners, pharmacists, etc. If you and your doctor decide hormones are right for you, consider using bioidentical estrogen transdermally. Ideally, oral micronized progesterone (OMP) which is also bioidentical should be added for women with a uterus to prevent thickening and precancerous changes of the uterine lining. Please note, some women prefer to start with progesterone especially in perimenopause to support mood, sleep, and heavier periods, then add estrogen at a later date. ==When used appropriately, the combination of topical estradiol and micronized progesterone is safe and has minimal risk of breast cancer in women near the age of menopause.==

Testosterone therapy for men is usually safe to continue indefinitely, but regular testing is needed to make sure side effects, such as increased red blood cells and increased risk of clotting, are under control. Testosterone therapy has been associated with an increased risk of heart attacks, so this should be carefully considered before starting treatment. And while testosterone may aggravate the symptoms of benign prostatic hyperplasia (BPH), it has not been associated with an increased risk of prostate cancer. Testosterone also appears to help improve insulin resistance. If you need to stop the hormone, we recommend you taper it off gradually under the guidance of a physician.

Bioidentical Hormones

We prefer to use hormones that are structurally the same as the ones your body produces. These are called bioidentical hormones. We feel they are metabolized better by the body and don't create toxic byproducts when they are broken down for removal.

There is a misconception that only compounding pharmacies can produce bioidentical hormones. These hormones are also made by many pharmaceutical companies. While they can be made to order by compounding pharmacies in preparations of various strengths and combinations, this practice is controversial because the compounding pharmacy may not offer the same reliable dosing and quality controls (such as batch testing) as a pharmaceutical company does. Compounded pharmaceuticals also aren't necessarily less expensive, better, or natural. On the other hand, compounded hormones can be highly personalized to each patient. The most important thing is getting the bioidentical hormone delivered to where it needs to go. Again, this should be discussed with your physician.

==While it seems that bioidentical hormones have less risks than synthetic versions, we must still consider how our genes interact with medications, environmental toxins, life stress, and diet. Here are some details to consider, especially with estrogen and testosterone replacement.==

Genes governing the way you detoxify hormones: If you have genetic variations of the cytochrome P450 enzymes CYP1B1, CYP1A1, CYP3A4, COMT, NQO1, and GST, you're more likely to make carcinogenic compounds when you detoxify estrogen in your liver.

Genes governing clotting: Some genetic variants increase the risk of blood clots. These include the genes for clotting factor II (prothrombin), clotting factor V, and GP3A Pl(A), which affects platelets. A woman with one or more of these variants who takes estrogen is more likely to suffer from clotting problems such as deep vein thrombosis (DVT), pulmonary embolism, heart attack, and stroke. On the other hand, a genetic variant called PAI-1, which increases the risk of clotting, is actually inhibited by hormones such as estrogen or DHEA, decreasing the risk for clotting. So, depending on your genetics, estrogen may be bad or good. And if you have a mixed picture, the answer is even murkier.

Excessive exposure to estrogen or estrogen-disrupting chemicals: Between 1940 and 1970, pregnant women were often given a synthetic estrogen called diethylstilbestrol (DES) in the mistaken belief that it would reduce miscarriages. Worse, women who were exposed to DES had a higher risk of breast cancer. Their daughters were at higher risk for uterine anomalies that could cause preterm births and breast, vaginal, and cervical cancers. Their sons were at higher risk of urogenital abnormalities as well. DES was banned in 1971, but rodent studies and some small human studies suggest that epigenetic changes from this chemical can persist into the third generation. And although DES is no longer used, synthetic estrogens and estrogen-disrupting chemicals such as pesticides and industrial solvents have been associated with illnesses such as reproductive disorders, endometriosis, breast abnormalities and cancer, polycystic ovary syndrome (PCOS), and even breastfeeding problems.

Nutritional factors, lifestyle, and behavioral factors: Diets high in broccoli and other cruciferous vegetables contain antioxidants and other natural chemicals that help improve hormone detoxification through the liver and help prevent cancer. Smoking, stress, an inflammatory diet, and dehydration can aggravate the risk for clotting, while a diet high in fish oils will help prevent clotting.

How Do You Know What to Do?

There is no way that the gold standard of studies—the double-blind, placebo-controlled crossover study—can answer whether HT is "good or bad" for you. There are too many individual variables, and you must still remember to use hormones as part of a full plan to optimize your overall health. If you are considering HT, discuss the risks and benefits with your doctor and get a proper laboratory workup. Starting HT before or close to the menopausal transition for women appears much more beneficial with fewer risks than waiting until the later decades. If men or women want to stay on HT long term, guidelines suggest this can be quite beneficial in the long term as long as they understand possible risks and know how to monitor for them.

Testing for the genetic variants involved in the breakdown of estrogen, as well as the estrogen metabolites themselves, can help you better understand your risks. A physician who understands these mechanisms can then advise how to individually mitigate your risk factors by using appropriate HT alongside diet, nutritional supplements, stress reduction, and lifestyle techniques.

DHEA: The Wellbeing Hormone

Dehydroepiandrosterone, or DHEA, is a hormone made in the body by the adrenal glands—it's the most abundant hormone they make. DHEA is the precursor hormone for both estrogen and testosterone. Your DHEA production naturally drops by about 10 percent for each decade after about age 20. By the time you're in your 70s, your DHEA production is only about 20 percent of what it was when you were 20. Overall, higher natural levels of DHEA are associated with lower levels of cancer, heart disease, metabolic syndrome, arthritis, and chronic disease. Low DHEA causes fatigue, trouble concentrating, and a diminished sense of wellbeing. We can use a blood test to check if your DHEA is too low for your age. Using supplements to raise DHEA if it's low can help sexual function (particularly erectile dysfunction), depression, immune function, and inflammation.

Even though DHEA is readily available as a nonprescription supplement, it still must be used with caution. Because it is metabolized into both testosterone and estrogen, supplemental DHEA may increase the risk of hormone-sensitive cancers affecting the prostate, breasts, uterus, or ovaries. On the other hand, higher levels of DHEA inhibit the action of enzymes that break sex hormones down into toxic byproducts. In other words, higher levels of DHEA might help prevent breast and prostate cancer. Unfortunately, there are no definitive studies on which situation is the case.

Typically, DHEA dosage usually ranges from 25 to 200 mg a day. We prefer to use low doses, ranging from 25 to 50 mg. Because DHEA is converted into testosterone, high doses of DHEA can be associated with typical symptoms of high testosterone such as alopecia (balding), as well as increased facial hair, acne, prostate enlargement, and irritability. In addition, DHEA should not be used by patients already using HT or by women who are taking tamoxifen to treat breast cancer or prevent a recurrence.

Testosterone

Low testosterone ("low T") has become a more common diagnosis in men because drug company advertising campaigns have increased awareness of it. But is it as common as the ads suggest? Probably not. Erectile dysfunction, for example, is a symptom of low testosterone, but it can have other causes. However, when accompanied by low sex drive, fatigue, decreased muscle mass, and growth of male breast tissue, we suspect low T.

To treat the symptoms of low testosterone, we need to figure out where the problem lies. That starts with testing your testosterone level. To get an accurate reading, we test both your blood and your urine. The blood test is done early in the morning when your testosterone levels are naturally at their highest and should be repeated 2 to 3 times, as it is not uncommon to see a low level of testosterone episodically in

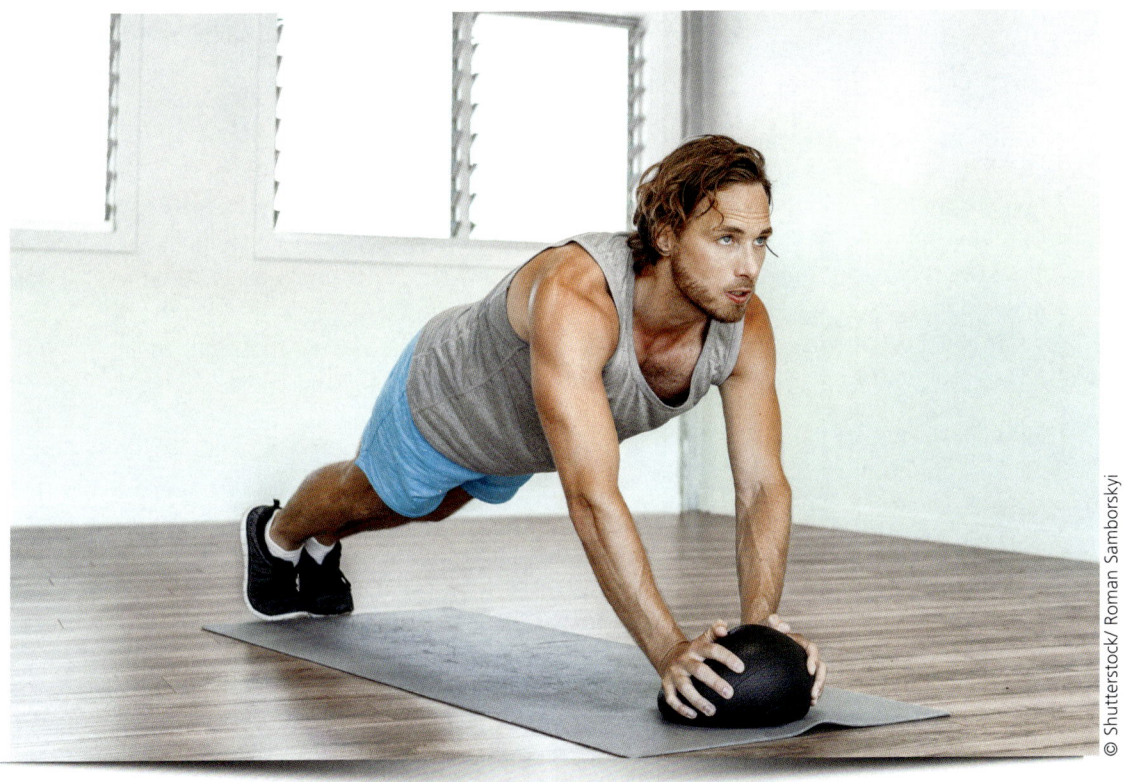

© Shutterstock/ Roman Samborskyi

normal patients. The problem with the blood test is that it's only a snapshot of your level at that moment, while your testosterone levels vary over the course of the day and even over the course of several days. To get a fuller picture of your levels, we also use a urine test that measures the average level over a 24-hour period.

If your testosterone is low, you have several good treatment options. Because your overall health affects your testosterone level, we start with lifestyle changes.

- **Reduce stress** to let your body shift from making excessive stress hormones to making more testosterone.
- **Get more sleep** to help shift the balance away from stress hormones and toward testosterone.
- **Lose weight,** especially belly fat. Adipose tissue increases your estrogen production. Weight loss also improves insulin sensitivity.
- **Increase your lean muscle mass** through exercise and resistance training. This increases the improvement from weight loss.
- **Remove the burden of environmental toxins** on your body.
- **Increase your protein intake.**
- **Quit smoking.**
- **Minimize alcohol** consumption.

About 40 percent of the testosterone in men is produced by the adrenal glands. Excess stress for a prolonged period can cause adrenal fatigue and low testosterone levels. We'll discuss ways to treat this important aspect of hormonal health later in this chapter.

Testosterone Therapy in Men (and Occasionally Women)

If basic self-help and lifestyle steps aren't helping enough, we can add supplemental DHEA or even other supplements that can increase testosterone. Only when we've tried all the non-drug approaches do we recommend testosterone supplementation. We prefer using a transdermal cream or gel instead of patches, pills, implanted

> "You'll never change your life until you change something you do daily. The secret to your success is found in your daily routine
>
> —John C. Maxwell

pellets, or injections. The dose is easier to control with the cream and the hormone enters your bloodstream directly. In appropriately low doses, testosterone can sometimes be helpful for postmenopausal women, but this is an off-label use not approved by the FDA. For men and women, we find testosterone is often helpful in correcting low libido, fatigue, and poor muscle tone.

Another way to raise testosterone is to stop it from being converted to estrogen. Testosterone is the precursor of estrogen in the form of estradiol. It's converted into estradiol by an enzyme called aromatase. If you inhibit the production of the aromatase enzyme, less testosterone gets converted to estrogen and more is retained in the body for other functions. In fact, this strategy is used in drugs that help prevent the recurrence of hormone-sensitive breast cancer in women. We can use aromatase-inhibiting drugs such as anastrozole (Arimidex), letrozole (Femara), and exemestane (Aromasin) to block the conversion of testosterone to estrogen in men as well. This approach is used very cautiously in men, but may be needed if testosterone therapy side effects such as gynecomastia (male breast development and enlargement) or edema (fluid retention in the extremities) develop. Aromatase inhibitors should be used in women only as a treatment to prevent breast cancer recurrence.

Many natural products can also slow conversion of testosterone. These include chrysin, stinging nettles (*Urtica dioica*), soy isoflavones, procyanidins, ECGC (a green tea extract), and vitamin C. If a zinc deficiency is affecting testosterone levels, zinc supplementation will also help.

Testosterone Warnings

Supplemental testosterone can have some potentially serious side effects. When a man starts testosterone therapy, his testes gradually produce less of their own. This makes coming off the hormone difficult because the testes need some time to start producing it again. Once a man starts testosterone therapy, he will probably need to continue it indefinitely. Side effects of the hormone can also include acne, breast swelling, high red blood cell counts, and increased risks for heart attacks, strokes, and clotting.

In some men, testosterone is converted too rapidly to the form dihydrotestosterone (DHT). High DHT levels are associated with baldness. Drugs now used to treat both baldness and prostate enlargement (benign prostatic hyperplasia, or BPH) work by inhibiting production of the enzyme 5-alpha reductase, which converts testosterone to dihydrotestosterone (DHT). Drugs that inhibit 5-alpha reductase conversion keep the testosterone from being converted, leaving more to circulate in the body. These medications include finasteride (Proscar and Propecia) and dutasteride (Avodart). Natural supplements such as saw palmetto (*Serenoa repens*), pygeum (*Prunus africana*), and stinging nettles also appear to reduce DHT activity.

Side effects are more likely to occur in men who are obese, stressed, inflamed, or have insulin resistance. These conditions lead to increased production of the enzymes aromatase and 5-alpha reductase, raising levels of estrogen and DHT.

We can manage the side effects by starting with a low dose of testosterone and gradually increasing it until symptoms improve. If side effects develop, cutting the dose back until they go away usually works well.

Adrenal Fatigue

When you're under prolonged stress, your adrenal glands work overtime to produce the stress hormone cortisol. If the stress goes on long enough, the adrenals can get so overworked that they stop functioning well. When this happens, they can't produce hormones like cortisol, testosterone, and estrogen in adequate amounts. This results in fatigue, aches and pains, low blood pressure, sleep disruption, brain fog, and an overall feeling of being unwell. It's important to catch and treat adrenal fatigue before it does more damage to your body. We check for it using saliva and blood tests.

Treating low-functioning adrenal glands focuses on stress reduction, as we've discussed in Chapter 6. Sometimes, neurofeedback and eye movement desensitization and reprocessing therapy are useful as nonpharmaceutical approaches to help with anxiety and depression. Improving the diet and cutting back on alcohol, as explained in Chapter 9, are also extremely important. Your body needs good nutrition and plenty of micronutrients to build hormones. Getting more sleep is also key to reducing stress

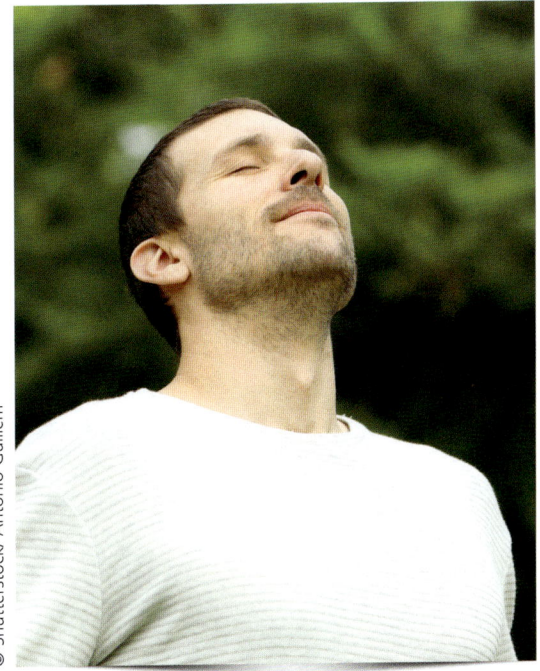

© Shutterstock/ Antonio Guillem

and restoring balanced hormone levels.

To give your body the raw materials it needs to build adrenal hormones, we suggest supplementing with B vitamins, vitamin C, zinc, and magnesium. Adaptogenic herbs such as licorice (*Glycyrrhiza glabra*), ashwagandha (*Withania somnifera*), tulsi or holy basil (*Ocimum tenuiflorum*), Korean ginseng *(Panax ginseng)*, and rhodiola (*Rhodiola rosea*) can be very helpful. Finally, supplementing with DHEA to support your natural production of this important precursor hormone can also help.

Managing Menopausal Symptoms

Women who reach menopause often come to us for help. "I feel desperate," a woman will tell us. "My hot flashes wake me up at night. The bed is sopping wet. I feel moody and depressed. My libido has disappeared, and when I do have sex, it's painful." Fortunately, there's a lot we can do—safely and easily—to help women manage their symptoms as they move through and beyond menopause. Before we start any treatment for menopausal symptoms, however, we check FSH, estradiol,

Are You Catabolic or Anabolic?

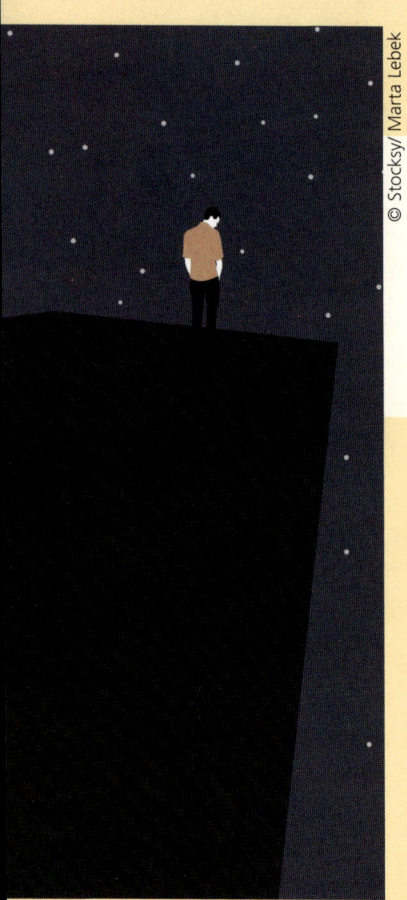

Anabolic steroids are the illegal substances that athletes and bodybuilders use to enhance their performance and make their bodies grow exceptionally big and strong. The word anabolic refers to building up muscles as part of the normal growth and healing response. We need—and indeed, produce—natural anabolic hormones in low quantities to help us repair and rebuild, but too much is not good. Although bodybuilders may think they look great, they are putting themselves at risk for problems. When some men take illegal anabolic steroids, they grow small breasts, and their testicles shrink. Likewise, women on steroids can develop clitoral enlargement and a variety of hormonal abnormalities. We need our bodies to make our own anabolic steroid hormones. If they don't, injuries won't heal, and we feel tired and depressed.

The opposite of anabolic is catabolic, meaning "breaking down." When you suffer excessive wear and tear or are seriously ill, you are in a catabolic state—you are breaking down your body faster than it can repair itself. In general, we become somewhat catabolic as we get older and when we are under prolonged or excessive stress. Our muscles become weaker and smaller, and we develop more fat around our bellies.

By measuring the ratio between your stress hormones and your wellbeing hormones, we can learn where you fall on the anabolic-catabolic continuum. Then we can balance these hormones through lifestyle changes and by using supplements and/or hormone treatments. These measures can help you thrive through your older years.

progesterone, DHEA, and testosterone levels. Let's look at why.

FSH is a hormone released into the bloodstream by the pituitary gland. In men, FSH acts on the testes to stimulate sperm production. In women, FSH stimulates the release of estrogen in the form of estradiol and the growth of ovarian follicles in the ovary. The buildup of hormones leads to ovulation when an egg from one of the follicles is released. After ovulation, the ovarian follicle re-forms as the corpus luteum, which releases both estrogen and progesterone. These hormones in turn signal the pituitary gland to stop FSH production.

Levels of FSH, estradiol, and progesterone naturally rise and fall as a woman goes through her menstrual cycle. As menopause develops, ovulation slows as the total number of eggs in the ovary decreases. FSH levels still rise, but estrogen and progesterone production drop so much that the signal to turn off FSH production can't be sent, and the pituitary gland keeps releasing it. During the years of the menopause transition, FSH levels start to go up and down unpredictably, causing estrogen levels to fluctuate as well. To get an accurate idea of your levels, we need to test more than once.

A woman's progesterone level may also be low. If this is the case, and a patient is having annoying symptoms in early perimenopause, trying a low dose of progesterone alone (without estrogen) often helps.

Estradiol is the main form of estrogen found in premenopausal women. Estradiol levels naturally drop as women reach their 40s. Women who exercise strenuously, such as marathon runners, dancers, and high-level athletes, can suppress their estrogen levels and have irregular periods or even stop menstruating. They may also have low estrogen if their body mass index is too low. As menopause progresses, estrogen levels drop even further. When women reach full menopause—when they have experienced no menstrual period for a year—their estrogen levels fall to an extremely low level.

The next step is to check DHEA levels. If a patient isn't making much DHEA, it can't be converted to estrogen, so estrogen levels drop. Remember that high stress can lead to low DHEA levels.

Non-Medication Options for Menopausal Symptoms

Women in perimenopause and menopause have several good options for treating symptoms such as hot flashes, vaginal dryness, and low libido without estrogen replacement or HT.

We recommend starting by checking your stress level. When you're stressed, your body prioritizes making stress hormones and cuts back on making estrogen. The stress reduction techniques brought up in Chapter 6, as well as acupuncture, can be very helpful in reducing hot flashes.

DHEA supplementation can help provide more of the foundation for making estrogen. But while supplementing DHEA, women need to watch for increased facial hair, as well as hair loss. If that happens, the dose needs to be reduced or stopped.

If progesterone is too low, herbal supplementation with chaste tree berry extract (*Vitex agnus-castus*) can help. Progesterone creams and patches can be helpful, although the ability to absorb progesterone through the skin may vary considerably. We recommend either a bioidentical pharmaceutical progesterone pill called Prometrium or micronized progesterone. It is also possible to compound a progesterone cream or vaginal troche (a lozenge that dissolves in the vagina), but the dosing is less predictable, and the cost can be significantly higher. If your hot flashes are so severe that they're substantially disrupting your life and we need to prescribe estrogen for you, we also prescribe Prometrium to lower your risk of endometrial cancer (if you still have a uterus).

For older women with normal estrogen loss, we often suggest an herbal or nutritional supplement. Herbs such as red clover (*Trifolium pratense)*, and sage (*Salvia officinalis*) have mild estrogenic effects. Black cohosh (*Actaea racemosa*) also is very helpful in menopause, and its benefits are mediated via its effect on the central nervous system, rather than on estrogen, so it is useful in treating patients with breast cancer. Soy isoflavones also appear to be helpful, especially when they come from organic soy foods such as tofu or miso. Heavily processed soy foods such as soy milk and soy-based meat substitutes may be less helpful and not as safe. Rhapontic rhubarb (*Rheum rhaponticum L.*) root extract, sold as the nonprescription pill Estrovera, made by Metagenics, is a plant estrogen that has been clinically demonstrated to help relieve hot flashes, sleep disturbances, and mood problems in menopausal women. This supplement is safe to use in breast cancer.

Hormone Therapy

We cannot overemphasize the importance of being under the care of a physician who is familiar with hormones and their metabolites—and with you and your health. This is not the time to experiment on your own with nonprescription products or work with a physician remotely. You need to have regular pelvic exams and gynecologic care whether you're on prescription hormones or over-the-counter supplements.

For estrogen supplementation, we usually recommend using a skin patch or gel containing bioidentical estradiol, whether from a pharmaceutical company or a compounding pharmacist. For progesterone supplementation, we usually recommend micronized progesterone pills (Prometrium), a compounded progesterone cream, or a vaginal troche. The hormones can be taken together throughout the month, or the progesterone can be cycled for 10 to 14 days each month. Women with insulin resistance tend to have better glucose control when they maintain monthly menstrual periods by cycling estrogen and progesterone levels, although many gynecologists feel that the endometrium is better protected by continuous progesterone.

Testosterone can sometimes be helpful for women. Replacement therapy was discussed earlier.

Healthy Menopause

Once a woman's hormone levels drop, she no longer has the protection provided by estrogen against heart disease and osteoporosis. If you are at that point, appropriate lifestyle modifications become even more important to protect your health. We suggest confronting risk factors such as smoking, high blood pressure, high blood cholesterol, diabetes, physical inactivity, and being overweight or obese. If necessary, consider medications to control high blood pressure, high blood cholesterol, and prediabetes or diabetes.

The risk of osteoporosis (brittle bones that break easily) increases with age, especially if you have a family history or are a current or former smoker. We recommend a bone density screening for all women at menopause to check for bone loss, especially if you're at high risk for osteoporosis. Some bone loss, or osteopenia, is normal, but if you're losing bone faster than normal, we want you to start taking steps to slow it down. To help prevent osteoporosis, one key step is to follow an eating plan that is rich in calcium and vitamin D and also includes plenty of fresh fruits and vegetables. The many different micronutrients in these foods, including vitamin C, vitamin K, carotenoids, folate, magnesium, strontium and potassium all contribute to bone health and reduce bone loss over time.

Regular weight-bearing exercises help strengthen bones. Don't smoke and limit alcohol consumption. While there is a positive link between moderate intake of red wine and beer and bone health, going beyond moderation increases

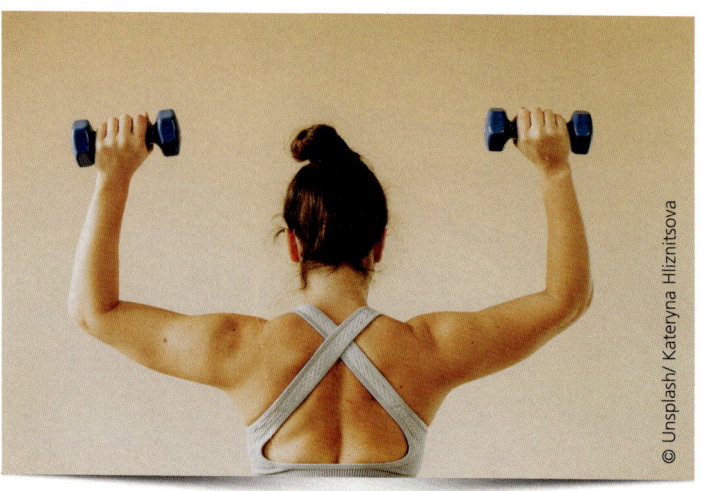

bone loss. Adequate protein intake is also important for maintaining healthy bones. However, red meat and processed meats are detrimental. Aim to get your protein from fish and seafood, poultry, tofu, and dairy products.

A good diet, vitamin D supplements, and natural remedies may help slow down bone loss early on. If you progress to more severe osteoporosis, however, medication may well be needed. Today we have many good options. Discuss the possibilities with your doctor to decide which is best for you.

Your bones act as a kind of "calcium bank" for the body. Bone is constantly being remodeled. If your bones are healthy, you have a dynamic balance between bone being formed and resorbed by the body. If not enough bone is being formed, osteoporosis can develop. That's why calcium, vitamin D, and other micronutrients are so important as a first line of prevention and treatment. What is just as important, however, is limiting inflammation, which contributes to bone resorption. Stress, poor diet, and inflammatory diseases can all contribute to inflammation and the acceleration of bone loss. Genetic variants that make you produce higher levels of inflammatory cytokines such as interleukin-6 and tumor necrosis factor alpha can increase your risk for inflammation. Counter these genetic tendencies with an anti-inflammatory diet.

Over and over, we see the benefit of a Transformational Medicine approach. The same approach that helps one problem can also help many others. Here again we see how reducing stress (Chapter 2), reducing inflammation, and improving your diet (Chapter 4) helps yet another problem: osteopenia, and osteoporosis.

Conquering PMS and Irregular Periods Naturally

Symptoms of too much estrogen, known as estrogen dominance, include irregular periods, premenstrual syndrome (PMS), breast tenderness, bloating, irritability or anxiety, migraines, and weight gain. Chronic estrogen dominance can result in heavy periods, infertility, fibroids, and even uterine cancer.

Estrogen dominance may be caused by excess estrogen produced by the body, excess foreign estrogens from endocrine-disrupting chemicals (endocrine disrupters), or inadequate estrogen detoxification in the liver. In some cases, estrogen dominance may be due to a relative deficiency of progesterone.

The conventional medical approach to these problems is to prescribe birth control pills, which increase the level of synthetic progestin in the body. If a woman wants to get pregnant, however, birth control pills are obviously not appropriate. Also, birth control pills can cause dangerous blood clots. Our approach is to first try to increase the level of progesterone by natural means.

We look for clues of estrogen or progesterone excess or deficiency, then check hormone levels with standard lab tests. We also discuss lifestyle, stress, exercise, and diet.

If estrogen levels are too high, we use supplements that reduce aromatase activity. We usually recommend green tea extract, flaxseed (*Linum usitatissimum*), vitamin C, and chrysin. We also use nutritional supplements that improve estrogen metabolism. These include isoflavones from natural soy products, rosemary leaf extract (*Salvia rosmarinus*), folic acid, vitamin B6 (pyridoxine), vitamin B12 (as methylcobalamin and cyanocobalamin), trimethylglycine (vitamin B15, also called pangamic acid), and resveratrol.

If progesterone is too low, we may suggest an herbal supplement such as chaste tree berry or an over-the-counter progesterone cream. Acupuncture can also be useful in normalizing menstrual cycles, and the stress reduction techniques outlined in Chapter 6 can be helpful in reducing mood swings.

Endometriosis

Endometriosis, where tissue similar to the lining of the uterus grows in other places in your body, causes dysmenorrhea (severe menstrual cramps and sometimes heavy bleeding during your period), pelvic pain, and possibly infertility. Doctors often suggest birth control pills to treat

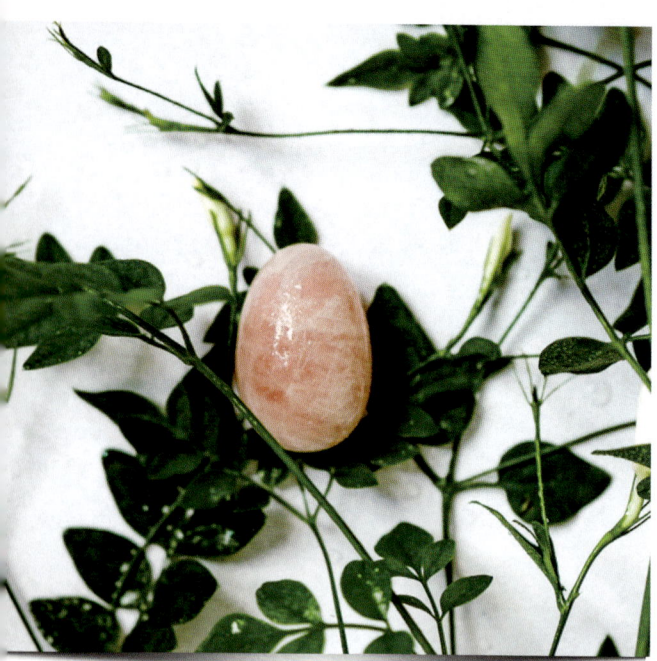

endometriosis and even recommend surgery in severe cases or if the disease is causing infertility. We suggest trying other approaches first.

Research suggests a link between dysbiosis (leaky gut syndrome) and endometriosis. The systemic inflammation caused by dysbiosis can aggravate endometriosis symptoms such as pain and bloating. It's unclear whether endometriosis triggers leaky gut or vice versa, but fixing leaky gut often results in a reduction of endometriosis symptoms.

The causes of endometriosis aren't fully understood, but estrogen dominance seems to play a role. Treating estrogen dominance and reducing high levels of aromatase to inhibit the conversion of androgens to estrogen may help.

Reducing your overall level of inflammation with an anti-inflammatory diet and moderate daily exercise helps reduce endometriosis symptoms. Turmeric (*Curcuma longa*), in capsules or as a tea, helps reduce inflammation in general and has also been shown to reduce excess estradiol, which helps endometriosis symptoms.

Sometimes estrogen dominance happens because it's not being metabolized properly in the gut or the liver. Upregulating phase 1 and phase 2 liver enzymes (see Chapter 7) and working to resolve gut dysbiosis often helps with estrogen detoxification and reduces estrogen dominance. And if estrogen dominance doesn't respond enough to the other approaches, progesterone cream can be very helpful.

We have just discussed multiple estrogen-dominant conditions and recommended treatments. If none of those options works well enough to eliminate your symptoms or reduce them to an acceptable level, consider using birth control pills. We usually recommend a low-dose progestin minipill.

Polycystic Ovary Syndrome (PCOS)

Polycystic ovary syndrome (PCOS) occurs when a woman's ovaries or adrenal glands produce more male hormones than normal. The imbalanced hormones cause a range of symptoms that include irregular menstrual periods, infertility, pelvic pain, excessive hair growth, acne, and as the name implies, cysts on the ovaries. The imbalance can cause metabolic problems including insulin resistance, weight gain, metabolic syndrome, and diabetes and can lead to heart disease later in life.

About one in ten American women have PCOS. It's the most common cause of female infertility—and fortunately, the most treatable. Most women find out they have PCOS in their 20s and 30s, when they have problems getting pregnant and consult with their doctor. Others find out sooner when they see their doctor for unwanted facial hair and acne or irregular periods.

To diagnose PCOS, we look for high androgen levels, irregular or absent menstruation, and evidence of polycystic ovaries. If a woman has two out of three, or all three, she likely has PCOS—as long as other causes have been ruled out. Insulin resistance is a key factor. Diagnostic tests may also include checking the following: your insulin levels; thyroid hormones; the fertility hormones prolactin, FSH, LH, and anti-Müllerian hormone; and the adrenal hormone 17-OH progesterone (in case of a condition called congenital adrenal hyperplasia). We also do a pelvic ultrasound to image the ovaries and see if they look cystic or have a classic "string of pearls" image along the edge of the ovary, which suggests PCOS. Other tests may include checking the leptin level and lipid profile.

The cause of PCOS is unknown. Genetics probably plays a big role in androgen excess, but other factors such as stress, diet, and obesity are often also involved. Many women with PCOS have a family history of type 2 diabetes, another inherited risk factor. But women with PCOS are also often overweight or obese, have a poor diet, and don't get much exercise. Fixing these issues helps prevent weight gain, insulin resistance, and diabetes in PCOS.

There's no cure for PCOS, but the condition, including any resultant infertility, can be successfully treated with a combination of lifestyle and dietary changes—and medication if needed. Weight loss and dietary changes to manage insulin resistance are essential first steps. Sometimes even modest weight loss, along with dietary improvements (especially eliminating sugar) and more exercise, are enough to reduce symptoms, normalize the menstrual cycle, and restore fertility.

Because stress can cause some of the hormonal imbalances associated with PCOS, stress reduction and improving adrenal gland function can be helpful. The same steps that improve insulin resistance also help block androgens, which helps improve skin problems and hirsutism. In some cases, we prescribe the drug metformin, which improves insulin resistance.

Women with PCOS have elevated testosterone and DHEA. In women, testosterone is produced in the ovaries and DHEA is produced in the adrenal glands. Sometimes the levels of both these androgens are elevated because of insulin resistance. When the pancreas releases a surge of extra insulin to try to force muscle cells to let it in, this signals the ovaries to produce extra testosterone. Normalizing insulin resistance through dietary changes, more exercise, supplements such as alpha lipoic acid, inositol and berberine, and drugs such as metformin can lead to a reduction in testosterone that's enough to restore normal menstrual periods.

About 10 percent of the testosterone in adult men and women gets converted in the liver into an androgen called dihydrotestosterone (DHT). In the body, DHT has many of the same functions as testosterone, but it's even stronger—it binds to androgen receptors on your cells longer and has a more powerful impact.

Women with PCOS have more androgens, so they produce more testosterone and more DHT. The extra DHT is what causes many PCOS symptoms, including acne, facial hair, thinning scalp hair, and irregular periods. Stress, inflammation and insulin resistance predispose the body to convert testosterone to DHT.

That's why reducing stress and lowering insulin resistance through a better, anti-inflammatory diet and more physical activity helps lower the production of active DHT and reduces PCOS symptoms.

Once we have done all this, we also look at estrogen metabolites. High levels of the bad estrogen 16-OH estradiol can cause breast tenderness. We can decrease this with a broccoli extract or the supplement diindolylmethane (DIM), a compound commonly found in cruciferous vegetables such as broccoli and cabbage.

Lowering Androgens

Birth control pills are often prescribed for treating PCOS. They're effective because they stop follicular development. But before using birth control pills, we suggest trying botanical supplements that inhibit DHT production, including the medicinal mushroom reishi (*Ganoderma lucidum*), spearmint (*Mentha spicata*), and saw palmetto. If HT is needed, progesterone cream is often helpful. It has the advantage of improving sleep and reducing anxiety and is helpful to optimize the metabolization of testosterone.

Improving Insulin Resistance

Insulin resistance is a very common aspect of PCOS. Reducing it lowers insulin levels in the blood, helps with weight loss, and reduces inflammation. Taking berberine, a component of the herbs goldenseal (*Hydrastis canadensis*), Oregon grape (*Mahonia aquifolium*), and barberry (*Berberis vulgaris*) is an effective natural way to increase insulin sensitivity. Other natural compounds that can help improve insulin sensitivity include inositol, d-pinitol, chromium picolinate, and fish oil.

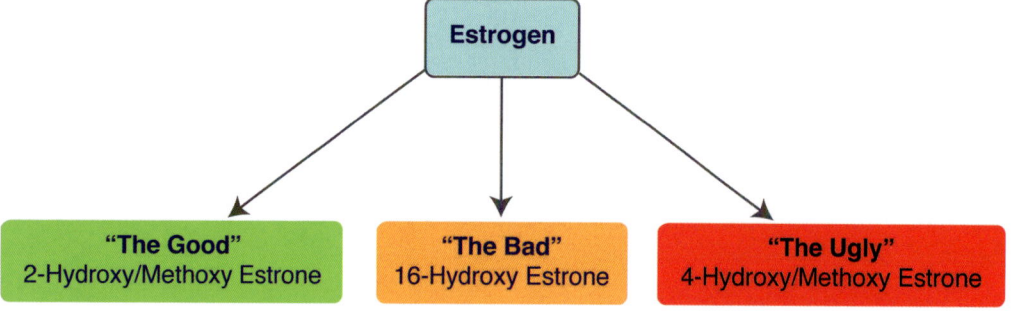

FIGURE 14.1 | Protect Yourself from Breast and Prostate Cancer

Step 4. Enhanced Protection Against Breast and Prostate Cancer

In addition to regular conventional screening and examination, we recommend some extra steps to protect yourself against the risk of breast or prostate cancer.

When estrogen (in men and women) isn't metabolized well by the body, its byproducts can be harmful. Specifically, these hormones can trigger breast cancer and prostate cancer.

The genes that increase the risk for breast cancer in women are similar to those that cause prostate cancer in men. What has become clear in recent years is that we each have a unique genetic signature that controls how we detoxify and remove estrogen from our bodies. Some pathways of metabolism result in metabolites that are safer and less likely to cause DNA damage and cancer in our cells, while other pathways result in metabolites that are less safe.

We can influence the pathways toward safer metabolism simply by providing plenty of the raw materials used by the body in estrogen metabolism. Specifically, this means eating more cruciferous foods such as broccoli or taking cruciferous extracts, including indole-3-carbinol or DIM, which help improve the ratio of good to bad estrogen metabolites. A diet high in antioxidants, especially those found in pomegranate juice and lycopene from tomatoes, appears to help by reducing production of the byproducts.

In Figure 14.1 on page 214, you can see some of the factors that promote estrogen byproducts, both good and bad.

Removing Endocrine Disrupters from Your Environment

In earlier chapters we discussed the effect of environmental chemicals on metabolic pathways and detoxification. Unfortunately, many of these chemicals are widespread in our environment. Examples include herbicides, pesticides, solvents, cleaning agents, plastics, cosmetics, cooking utensils, flame retardants, synthetic fabrics, and food packaging materials. Because these chemicals don't break down in the environment or in your body, they're also known as persistent organic pollutants (POPs). In particular, POPs accumulate in the food chain, so they can be found in our food. It's impossible to eliminate our exposure to these chemicals in the environment. For example, studies show that bisphenol A, an estrogen disrupter, is detectable in most humans. So, what should you do?

Here are some steps to reduce your exposure to endocrine disrupters in the environment:

- Use green cleaning products that are natural, nontoxic, biodegradable, and made without petrochemicals.
- Avoid heating food in plastic containers. Use glass or ceramic containers instead, especially when using a microwave oven. Heated plastics release more endocrine disrupters into your food.
- Air out dry-cleaned garments, mattresses, and fabrics that have been chemically cleaned or treated.
- Many cosmetics, shampoos, lotions, nail polish, sunscreens, perfumes, and chemical air fresheners contain parabens and phthalates, which are known estrogen disrupters. Try natural or organic products free of these compounds.
- Nonstick cookware coatings contain PFOA (perfluorooctanoic acid or C8), a heat- and grease-resistant chemical that can affect thyroid hormones and may increase obesity. In addition to cookware, this chemical is found in some microwave containers and pizza boxes. If you use nonstick cookware, discard it if it becomes scratched. Never scrape nonstick cookware with a metal spatula.
- Eat organic foods whenever possible. Choose beef, pork, poultry, fish, dairy products, and eggs from animals raised without antibiotics or hormones.
- Enhance your detoxification systems as discussed in Chapter 7.

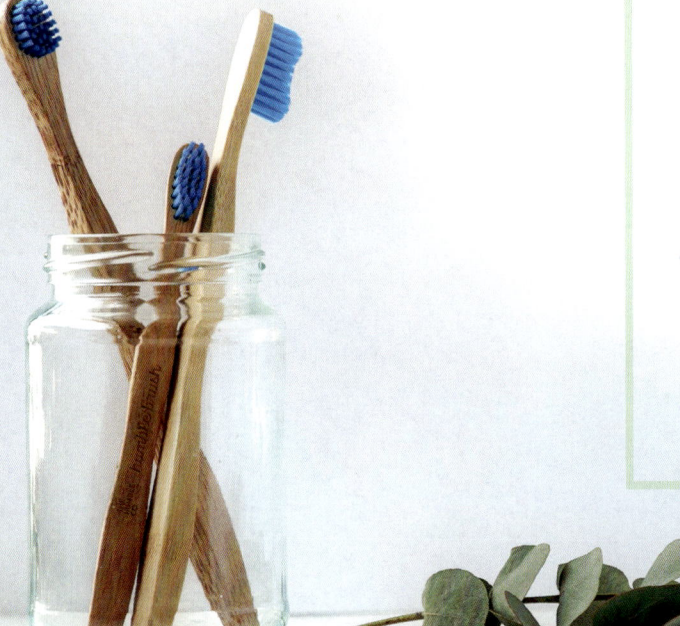
© Unsplash/ The Humble Co.

Step 5: Balance Your Thyroid Hormones

When we experience chronic stress, the thyroid gland can be sluggish. The thyroid gland can also stop producing enough hormones if you have Hashimoto's thyroiditis.

If your thyroid is sluggish, blood tests will show that you are producing slightly more thyroid stimulating hormone (TSH), but your levels of free T3 and free T4, the two hormones you need for good thyroid function, will be normal. Ideally, your TSH will be under 2.5 mU/L and your T3/T4 will be within normal limits. You also won't have any antithyroid antibodies.

Antithyroid antibodies in a blood test mean you probably have Hashimoto's thyroiditis and are no longer making enough T3/T4 hormones. In that case, we need to replace the missing hormones with medication.

Treating Hypothyroidism

Supplements can often help return the TSH level to normal. We usually suggest vitamin A (in the form of palmitate), vitamin E, vitamin D, iodine, iron, selenium, and zinc. Herbal remedies that are helpful include ashwagandha and rhodiola.

For Hashimoto's thyroiditis, we prescribe levothyroxine (Synthroid), which is bioidentical to T4. Your body converts some of your T4 to T3, so taking levothyroxine should raise the levels of both hormones. If necessary, we add Cytomel (liothyronine sodium), a bioidentical synthetic form of T3. Many integrative medicine practitioners like to use Armour thyroid (also called desiccated thyroid extract) because it's natural (derived from pig thyroid glands) and because it contains both T3 and T4. We believe that while this product may be natural, it is not bioidentical to human thyroid hormones. Your body takes it up more slowly and it is more likely to cause side effects.

To find the levothyroxine dose that's right for you, we start with a low dose and gradually increase it until you feel better and your blood test results improve. You will have to take thyroid medication for life, so it's important to get your hormone levels checked regularly.

Achieving a More Balanced Life

Balancing your hormones can help you achieve a more balanced life and vice versa. It is crucial, though, to start with an accurate medical diagnosis based on a physical examination and laboratory testing. If prescription drugs are needed, you need regular follow-up visits to monitor your response.

We are often asked, "How do you know if balancing the hormones is working?" The answer is simple. When you aren't feeling right, your symptoms let you know. Then you need lab tests to confirm what you feel. When you are better, you feel better, and the results on the lab tests will reflect this.

The body is a complex matrix of systems. Even when replacing hormones, it's still a good idea to look at the body as a whole. This is a perfect example of how the functional medicine systems approach provides a more com-

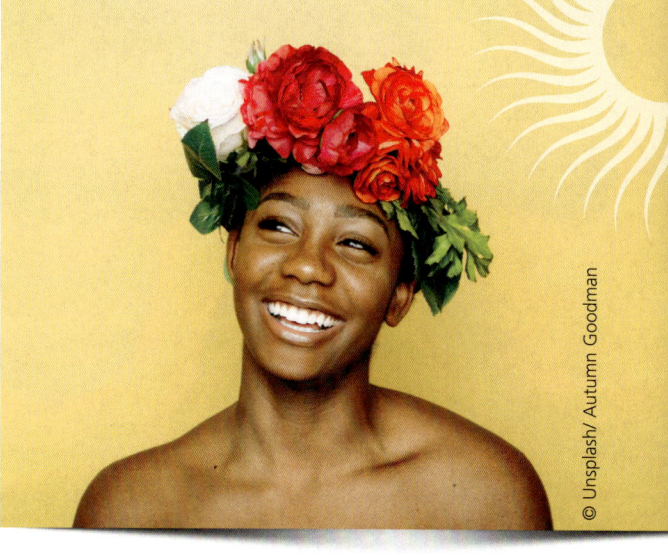

plete understanding of your health. By supporting lifestyle, diet, oxidative stress, and detoxification processes, we support healing and balance.

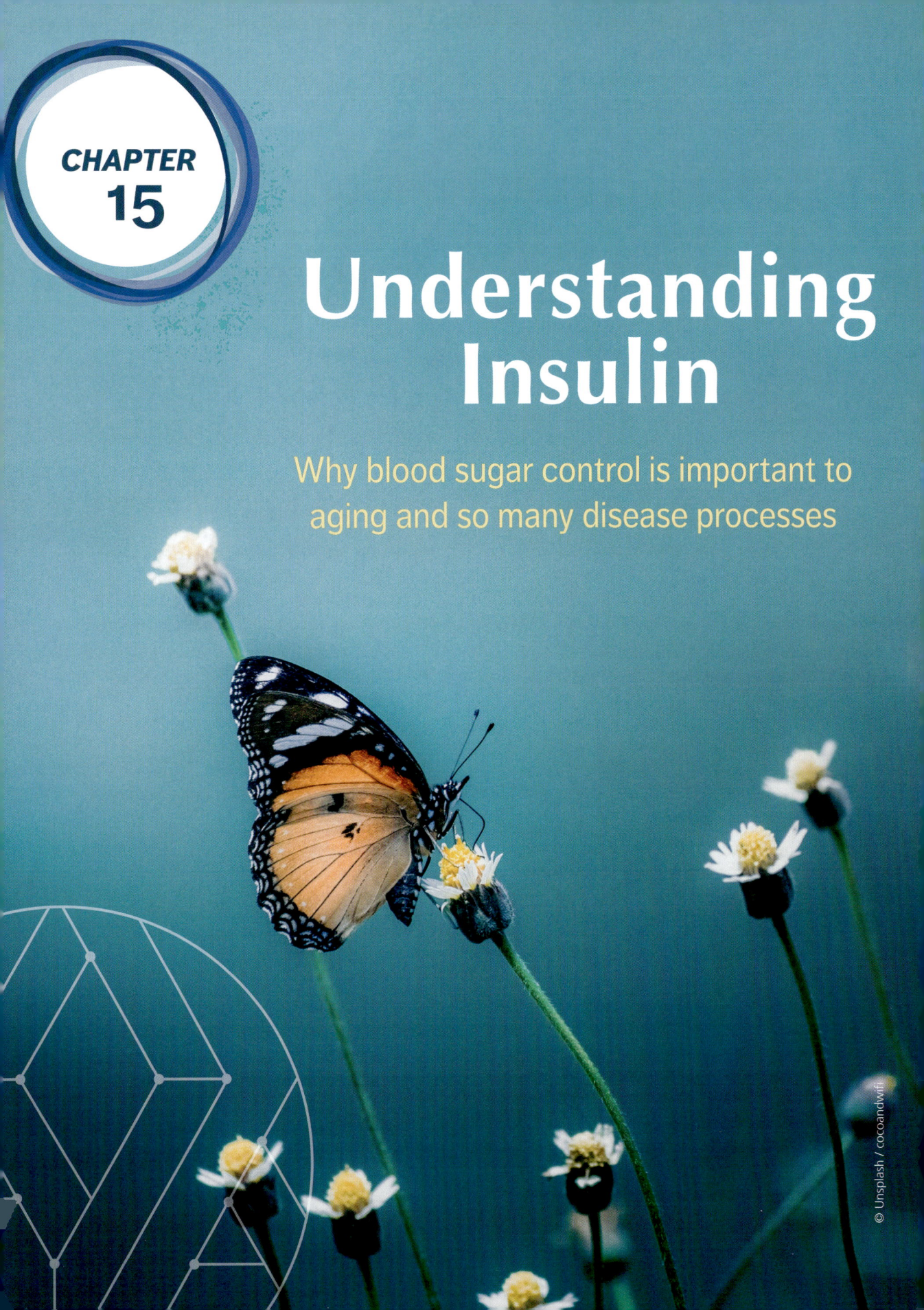

CHAPTER 15

Understanding Insulin

Why blood sugar control is important to aging and so many disease processes

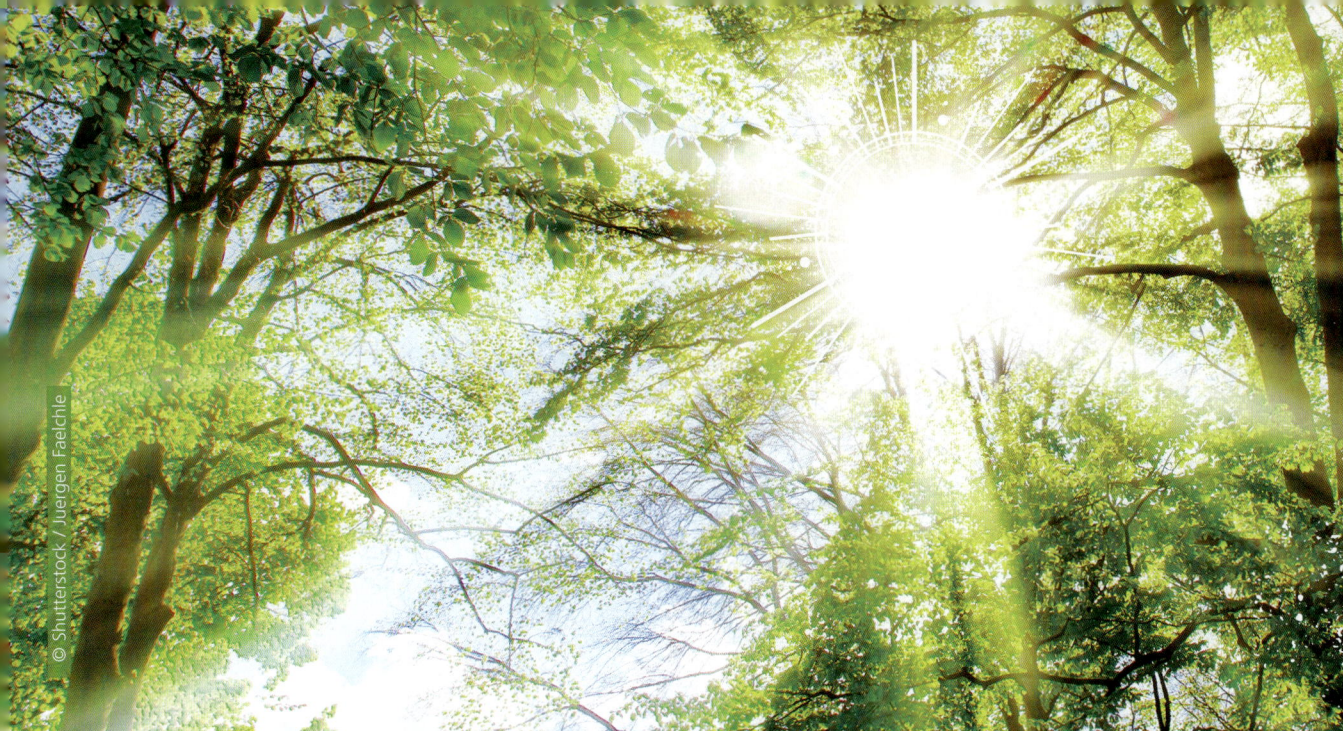

The hormone insulin controls how your body uses glucose, or blood sugar—its primary fuel. Understanding insulin is key to understanding and treating blood sugar problems such as insulin resistance, metabolic syndrome, prediabetes, and type 1 and type 2 diabetes. It's also key to understanding the link between blood sugar, insulin resistance, and weight gain.

Today, prediabetes and type 2 diabetes are prevalent—and largely preventable. These conditions have very serious long-term consequences for your health. In this chapter, we'll explain the basics and how we work with our patients to reverse insulin resistance.

How Insulin Works

> **Think of insulin as a key, which fits into a lock (the insulin receptor). When insulin turns the lock, glucose moves from the blood into the cell.**

When you eat sugary or starchy foods (i.e., carbohydrates), they enter the bloodstream as glucose. A rise in blood glucose stimulates the pancreas to produce insulin, which then carries the glucose into cells, where it can be used for energy. If the glucose/insulin feedback loop is working properly, enough glucose enters the cells to keep them fully fueled. Excess glucose gets carried off to be stored as glycogen in the liver (your body's fallback glucose supply) and as fat. When this happens, the blood glucose level drops down to a baseline until you eat carbohydrates again. Your blood sugar normally rises after you eat and returns to baseline within a couple of hours.

The glucose/insulin loop can be disrupted. Some people simply don't produce enough insulin to carry glucose into their cells. More commonly, some people develop resistance to the effect of insulin. In either case, these people have diabetes mellitus, a disease marked by high blood sugar levels.

In type 1 diabetes, an autoimmune disease, the insulin-producing beta cells of the pancreas are destroyed and can no longer produce insulin in adequate amounts or even at all.

The disease, once named Juvenile Diabetes, can strike at any age, not just during adolescence. " Emerging data indicates that up to 62% of T1D new diagnoses are in adults over 30. To survive, someone with type 1 diabetes must replace their missing insulin with daily injections of the hormone. About 1.6 million Americans have type 1 diabetes.

The hallmark of type 2 diabetes is insulin resistance. The causes of insulin resistance are complex and not fully understood, but obesity and a sedentary lifestyle play a significant role in most cases. People with this disease have insulin levels that are normal or even elevated but have trouble carrying glucose into cells. This is because receptors in the cells don't open correctly to allow the insulin to enter and carry glucose with it. Instead, glucose floats around in the bloodstream in abnormally high amounts. The excess glucose clogs the tiny blood vessels of the body, eventually damaging organs such as the kidneys, heart, and eyes.

About 35 million Americans, or more than 10 percent of the population, have type 2 diabetes. But only about 26.8 million have been diagnosed with the disease—the rest don't know they have it yet. That's because the symptoms of type 2 diabetes aren't obvious at first. A person can have it for years while it quietly damages the heart, kidneys, eyes, and blood vessels. Sadly, many people only discover they have diabetes as they are being treated for a heart attack in the emergency room.

An additional 88 million Americans have prediabetes; insulin resistance is making their blood glucose levels rise higher than normal but not yet high enough to be diagnosed as type 2 diabetes. Most people with prediabetes don't know they have it, but unless they make changes, they will almost certainly progress to type 2 diabetes within ten years.

The single biggest risk factor for type 2 diabetes is being overweight or obese. As a person puts on more weight in the form of adipose tissue, their muscle and tissue cells become more resistant to their own insulin. Even if their weight is normal, they are at higher risk for diabetes if their diet is high in low-fiber processed foods and they get little exercise.

Age is another risk factor for diabetes. Among Americans aged 65 and older, about 27 percent have diabetes, including many who are undiagnosed.

Insulin Resistance: When Sugar Becomes a Poison

Why is it so easy to gain weight and so hard to take it off—and keep it off? One reason weight gain can be so difficult to reverse is that it's often caused by insulin resistance or prediabetes. If you have high blood glucose from insulin resistance, you're also likely to have low levels of HDL (the "good" cholesterol), high triglycerides (tiny fat droplets) in the blood, high blood pressure, high inflammation markers, and a large waist circumference (often referred to as an apple-shaped body). This group of signs and symptoms occurs together so often that they are called metabolic syndrome. Having most or all of the syndrome characteristics is the first leg of the journey on the road to diabetes.

The Snowball Effect of Weight Gain

If we look at the data on obesity and diabetes incidence, we see that they parallel each other. In other words, the fatter we get as a nation—and over 70 percent of all Americans are now overweight or obese—the higher our incidence of type 2 diabetes. We used to call type 2 diabetes adult-onset diabetes. Unfortunately, these adult-onset conditions now affect children as well—and are affecting them at younger ages. Children as young as 8 are being diagnosed with type 2 diabetes, a disease that will almost certainly cut their lives short.

Insulin resistance describes an aspect of our body chemistry that probably evolved as a way for our bodies to adapt to alternating periods of food abundance and food scarcity. Thousands of years ago, people who had insulin resistance were more likely to survive periods of starvation. When carbohydrate-rich food such as ripe fruit was plentiful, insulin resistance meant they could gorge on the food while it was available and quickly add fat around their bellies. Later, when food was scarce, the stored fat helped them survive.

Fast forward to current times. In wealthier countries, starvation is rare or non-existent. We live in a land of plenty—more than plenty, in fact. We get about three-quarters of our daily calories from ultraprocessed foods that almost always include added sugar. Today, the average American consumes about 152 pounds of sugar in one year—more than the body weight of most people. This amount of sugar works out to 3 pounds (or 6 cups) every week. About a third of all that sugar comes from sodas—an average can of soda has 10 to 12 teaspoons of sugar, and half of all Americans drink at least one can a day. Another 10 percent of the sugar we consume comes from sweetened fruit juices. An additional 15 percent comes from baked goods like cookies and breakfast pastries.

Our bodies are genetically adapted to a lifestyle of scarcity, not abundance. The bodies of people who are genetically inclined toward insulin resistance react to all that sugar as if the growing season that year had been especially good. Their insulin resistance kicks in, and their bodies store the excess sugar as fat in anticipation of the scarce food supply that is sure to follow any period of abundance. But if the abundance never ends, insulin resistance stops being a survival mechanism and instead becomes a disease that leads to increasing complications, disability, and premature death. Not only that, but insulin may also be a tumor growth factor, making people with high insulin levels more likely to get cancer or making their cancer worse if they get it.

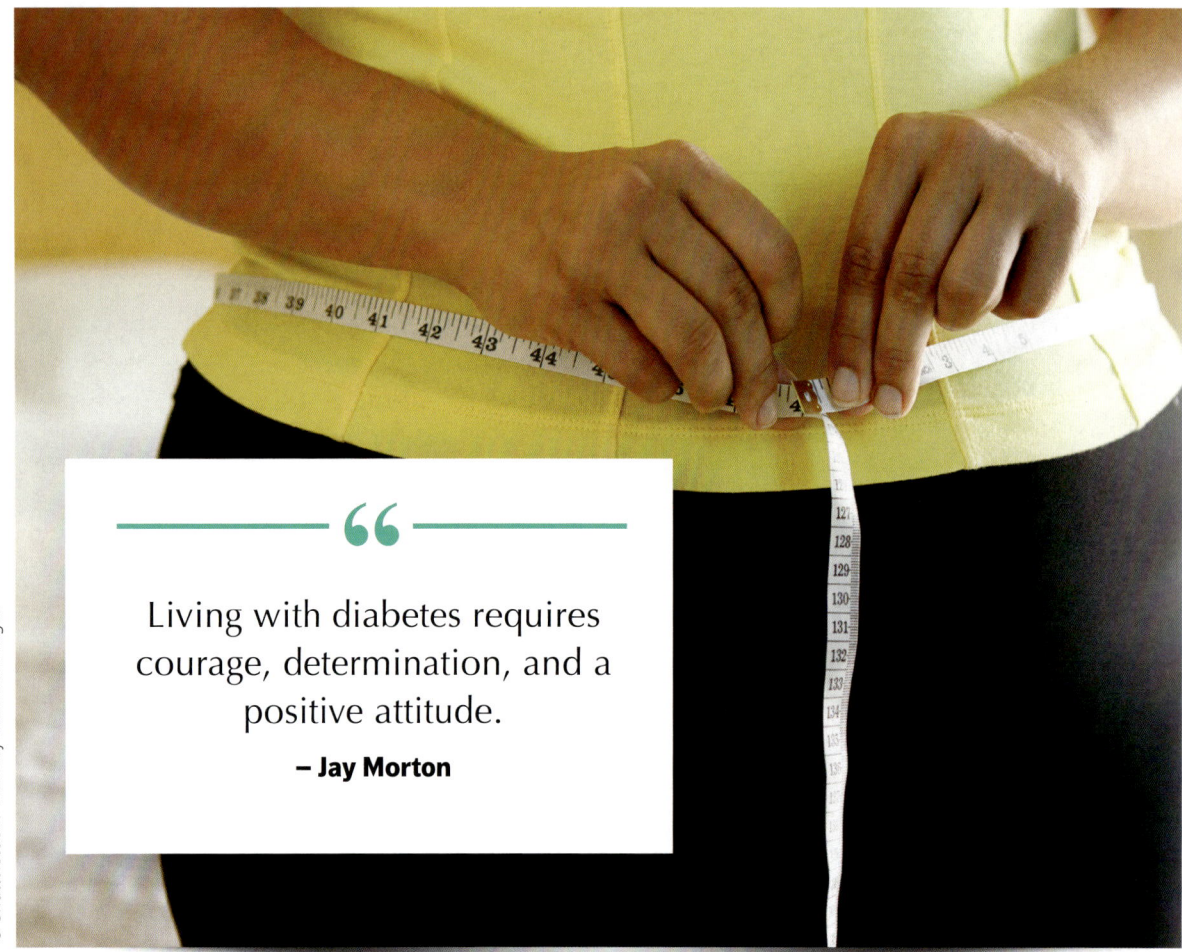

> "Living with diabetes requires courage, determination, and a positive attitude."
> – Jay Morton

220 CHAPTER 15 | Understanding Insulin

The Path to Diabetes

In general, the tendency to develop type diabetes 2 starts with insulin resistance. Think of insulin as a key fitting into an insulin receptor as a lock. Imagine the lock being rusty. So, insulin tries to turn it, but it just doesn't work properly. As a result, sugar levels rise in the bloodstream, which the body turns into fat, depositing it in organs (think fatty liver) or adipose tissue. This fat creates further insulin resistance, which in turn aggravates the problem. Although insulin resistance is associated with obesity, refined food, and poor exercise habits, the actual cause is not well understood. It definitely has a genetic underpinning (initially called "the thrifty gene"), but other causes are emerging. The primary issue appears to be chronic exposure to sugar in all its forms. Insulin resistance can also develop after exposure to toxins called obesogens. Microbiome imbalance, especially a deficiency of *Akkermansia*, and liver dysfunction all appear to cause or add to insulin resistance.

Medically, there is a progression from normal to metabolic syndrome to prediabetes and then diabetes.

Normal → Metabolic Syndrome → Prediabetes → Diabetes

We discuss each of these briefly below:

Metabolic Syndrome

According to the American Heart Association and the National Heart, Lung, and Blood Institute, metabolic syndrome exists if you have any three of the following five conditions:

- **Waist measurement** > 40 inches for men; >35 inches for women
- **Triglyceride levels** >150 milligrams per deciliter (mg/dL), or taking medication for elevated triglyceride levels
- **HDL, or "good," cholesterol level** < 40 mg/dL for men and < 50 mg/dL for women, or taking medication for low HDL levels
- **Blood pressure levels** >130/85 mmHg, or taking medication for elevated blood pressure
- **Fasting blood glucose levels** >100 mg/dL, or taking medication for elevated blood glucose levels

Similar definitions have been developed by the World Health Organization and the American Association of Clinical Endocrinology. Individuals with metabolic syndrome are at high risk for type 2 diabetes, heart disease, peripheral vascular disease, and stroke. Having metabolic syndrome doubles your risk of coronary artery disease and increases your risk of stroke, fatty liver disease, and cancer, especially breast cancer.

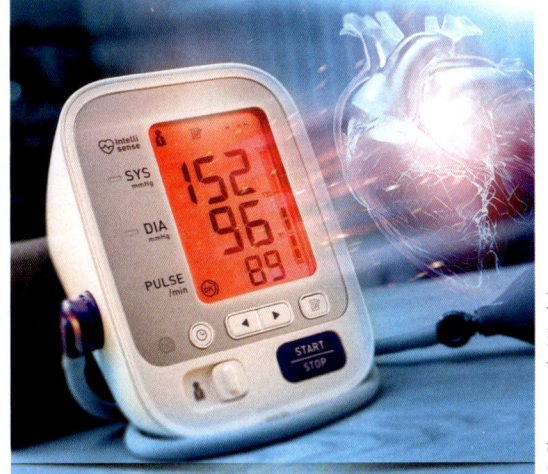

Prediabetes

When your blood sugar levels are higher than normal, but not yet high enough to diagnose you with type 2 diabetes, you have prediabetes (sometimes called borderline diabetes), impaired glucose tolerance, or impaired fasting glucose. About forty percent of American adults have prediabetes—and most of them don't know it. Prediabetes doesn't usually have any obvious signs or symptoms, but it puts you at an increased risk of developing type 2 diabetes. With that increased risk comes an increased risk of a heart attack or stroke.

Your risk of prediabetes is greater if you are:

- Overweight or obese
- Over age 45
- Have a parent or sibling with type 2 diabetes
- Are physically active less than three times a week
- Had gestational diabetes (diabetes during pregnancy) or gave birth to a baby weighing more than nine pounds
- Have polycystic ovary syndrome (PCOS)

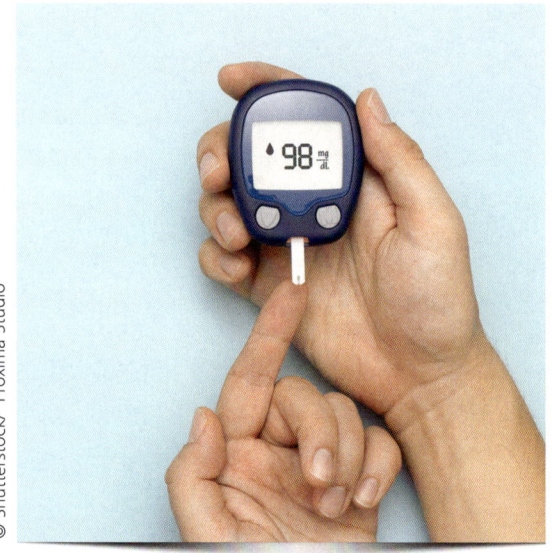

© Shutterstock/ Proxima Studio

Prediabetes is usually diagnosed by testing your blood glucose. We have several different ways to do this, but the easiest is a simple blood test that looks at your hemoglobin A1C level (sometimes referred to as just A1C). This test measures your average blood glucose for the past two to three months. You don't have to be fasting for it. Normal A1C is less than 5.75 percent; the prediabetes level is 5.7 to 6.4 percent. You have type 2 diabetes if your A1C is 6.5 percent or higher.

We can also use a simple finger prick that looks at your blood glucose after you've been fasting for eight hours. Fasting blood glucose of 100 to 125 mg/dl suggests prediabetes. We like to repeat this test a few days later to make sure the fasting number is consistently high.

If you have prediabetes, you won't automatically go on to develop type 2 diabetes—we like to say that the "pre" part of prediabetes stands for "prevention." You can head off diabetes if you take steps now to lose weight and exercise more. You don't even need to get down to your ideal body weight. You can cut the risk by more than half by losing only about 7 percent of your weight. So, if you weigh 200 pounds, losing 15 pounds will make a big difference. Even losing 10 pounds will help. We strongly recommend losing weight by following a low-carbohydrate, plant-based diet (see chapter 9 for details).

Exercising more is the other half of fixing prediabetes. You don't need to train for a marathon or even start hitting the gym. A brisk walk, a bike ride, or some other moderate activity (following a step aerobic video, for example) for 30 minutes most days is enough to help normalize your blood sugar. If you've been very sedentary, you should work up to this activity level gradually.

You may find that the steps you take to treat your prediabetes also improve other health issues you might have, such as high blood pressure and high cholesterol. You may still need medication for these conditions, however.

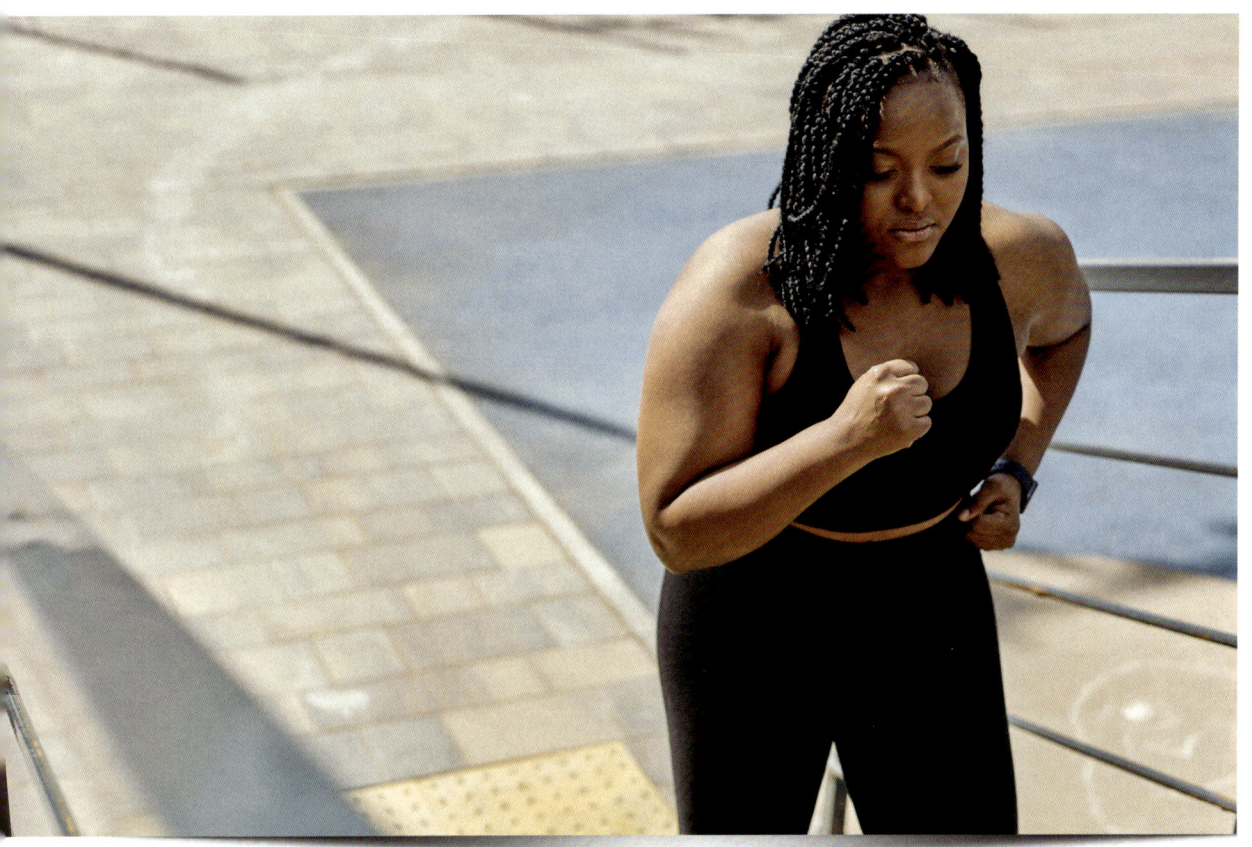

Type 2 Diabetes

You've officially tipped over into type 2 diabetes if your A1C blood test is 6.5 percent or higher, if your fasting blood glucose is 126 mg/dl, or if a random sample of your blood while you aren't fasting is 200 mg/dl or higher. You are more likely to develop diabetes if you are:

- Overweight or obese
- Age 45 or older
- Have a family history of diabetes (parent or sibling)
- Black, Native American, Asian American, or Hispanic/Latinx

Other risk factors include:

- High blood pressure
- Low level of HDL (good) cholesterol
- High triglycerides
- History of gestational diabetes
- Sedentary lifestyle
- History of heart disease or stroke
- History of depression
- History of PCOS

The treatment for type 2 diabetes is the same as for prediabetes, just more so. Now it's more important than ever to eat a healthy low-carbohydrate diet, lose some weight, and be more physically active. It's also more important than ever to control other health issues such as high blood pressure. Your doctor may want you to add an oral drug such as metformin to lower your blood glucose and may also want you to take medications to lower your blood pressure and your cholesterol. Our goal is to help you stabilize your blood sugar and keep it from getting worse. Then we work with you to take the steps that will help bring it down. We want to help you avoid needing to take several prescription drugs for the rest of your life.

Endocrine Disrupting Chemicals and Obesogens: Substances that Can Make Us Sick and Fat

Hormones are chemical messengers that turn processes on and off in our bodies. Just as a key fits into a lock, a particular hormone fits into receptor sites on the cells to set the process in motion or turn it off. Some chemicals in our environment can do the same thing because their molecular structure is very similar to the molecular structure of some natural hormones, such as estrogen. These chemicals are called endocrine disrupters, because they can mimic and disrupt the body's normal endocrine system. Unlike hormones, which break down when they're no longer needed, endocrine disrupters break down slowly and persist in the body for a long time. They turn the lock to the on position and leave it stuck there, possibly for years.

What are these chemicals and how are they gaining access to our bodies? Endocrine disrupters are in the artificial hormones and antibiotics used to process our meat, fish, and milk, the pesticides on our fruits and vegetables, the additives in our processed food, the plastics in our bottles and containers, and the solvents in the cleaning fluids we use. Examples of these chemicals include plastics such as bisphenol A (BPA), perfluorooctanoic acid (PFOA or C8), and PVC. BPA is a synthetic estrogen found in some polycarbonate plastic bottles (usually marked with the recycle numbers 3 or 7) and in the lining used in some tin cans. Fortunately, BPA is gradually being replaced as the tide of public opinion turns against it. However, we still have yet to know if the replacement plastics are that much safer! C8 is found in nonstick pans, spatulas, and serving spoons; microwave popcorn containers; and pizza boxes. PVC contains chemicals called phthalates that lower testosterone and affect metabolism. PVC is found in the plastic wrap on commercial meat products, shower curtains, and air fresheners. Atrazine, a common food additive, can affect thyroid hormones. Tributyltin, which has been linked to obesity, is a fungicide used on the bottom of boats; as it leaches into the water, it then enters the food chain as it is taken in by fish.

What happens when we place a bigger load of endocrine disrupters on the detoxification system than it can handle? Many solid studies now link endocrine disrupters to type 2 diabetes, heart disease, hypertension, breast and prostate cancer, PCOS, and infertility. BPA, for example, hijacks the body's chemical messengers and acts directly on pancreatic cells, triggering insulin resistance. Endocrine disrupters also have an adverse effect on detoxification. (Refer back to chapter 7 for more on detoxification.)

In 2015, the Endocrine Society, the leading expert organization for hormone study, released a statement acknowledging that endocrine disrupters pose a significant harm to human health and that exposure to them is linked to diabetes and obesity.

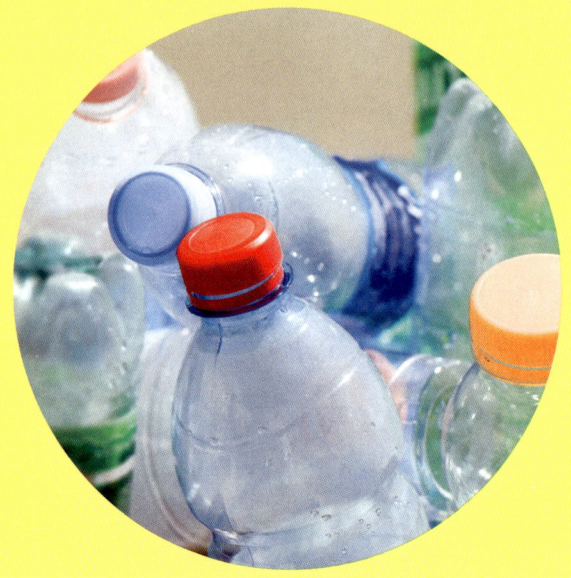

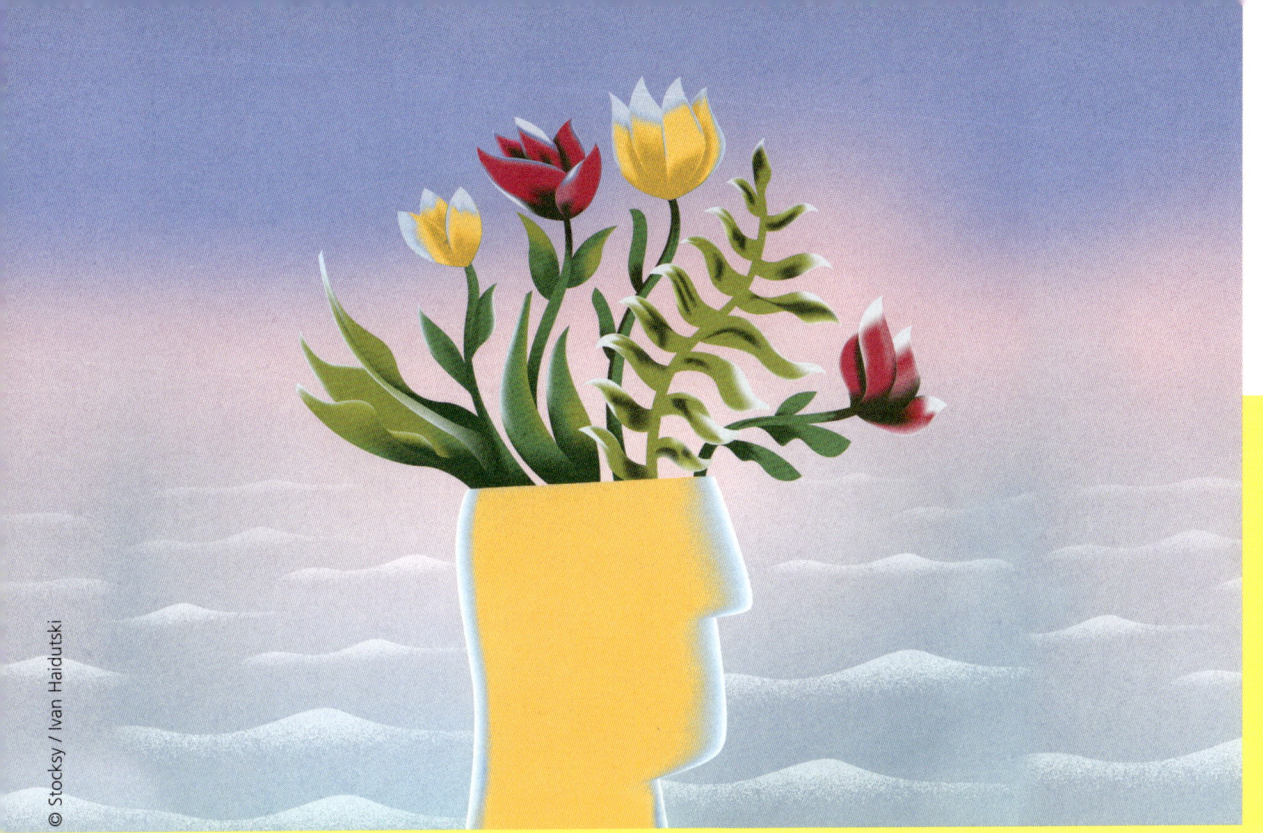

Why it's so difficult to lose weight when you're stressed

Have you ever tried to lose weight when you were also in a stressed state? Did you find it was difficult? If weight loss was as simple as lowering caloric intake, we wouldn't be facing this current epidemic of obesity. Despite calorie cutting, some people just seem to gain more weight. Clearly, evaluating insulin resistance and lowering calories are important aspects of weight loss, but more needs to be taken into consideration.

Trying to lose weight by dieting during a stressed (and catabolic) state simply amplifies the message that starvation is imminent, piling another stress on an already stressed body. The body reacts by increasing cortisol levels, making it more difficult to lose weight. Emotional stress can affect your cortisol balance, causing you to go into storage mode to retain fat. In addition, emotional overeating is likely to cause you to binge on comfort foods, which are usually high in calories and low in nutrients. Being stressed and inflamed will make things even worse. The increased inflammation aggravates the insulin resistance, resulting in another vicious cycle. So losing weight is more than just reducing calories!

To truly optimize your chances of losing weight successfully, you need to do more than just count calories and address insulin resistance. It is also vital that your stress hormones are balanced and that your thyroid hormones are normal. Inflammation, oxidative stress, and detoxification problems can play a role in weight gain and weight loss. Normal gut flora seems to be an important component of a weight loss program. And you need to remove chemicals known as obesogens from your life by limiting your chemical exposure wherever possible. (We discuss these later in the chapter.)

It's Not Just About the Insulin!

Much more than just insulin is involved in regulating appetite, weight gain, glucose and lipid metabolism, and metabolic syndrome. Enteroendocrine cells, specialized cells lining the stomach, intestines, and pancreas, secrete peptide hormones, which in turn help regulate our metabolism, mood, gut motility, and immune system. Your body's ability to regulate these hormones is key to maintaining a healthy metabolism.

When an obese, fasting diabetic patient is admitted to hospital overnight and given isotonic fluids, it is rare to see any changes in blood pressure, blood sugar, or insulin levels. But if a similar patient has bariatric (weight loss) surgery that places a band around their stomach to reduce their stomach capacity, on the same IV drip their blood pressure, blood sugar, and insulin level drop significantly—and almost immediately after the surgery is finished. Why? The mechanical squeezing of the stomach effects the production of a group of hormones called peptides. Your stomach produces a lot of these. Some hormones, like GLP-1 (glucagon-like peptide-1), GLP-2 (glucagon-like peptide-2), PYY (peptide YY), leptin, oxyntomodulin, glucagon, cholecystokinin (CCK), and pancreatic polypeptide are *anorectic,* or causing a decrease in appetite. These counteract the effect of peptides such ghrelin, which is *orexigenic,* or stimulating appetite.

When someone becomes obese, they lose the ability to regulate the balance between anorectic and orexigenic peptides. To us, this isn't a mystery. These peptides are produced as the microbiome interacts with the enteroendocrine cells. And as we eat a progressively more refined diet, packed with fast foods and processed foods full of colorings, preservatives, antibiotics, and other additives, and very low in fiber, our microbiome has changed! The normal interplay between the microbiome and the enteroendocrine cells is disrupted.

Pharmaceutical companies are obviously very interested in drugs that can manipulate the gut hormones. GLP-1, for example, appears to be very helpful in controlling glucose, appetite, and weight. In fact, a number of drugs that block the GLP-1 receptor (agonists) are used for both diabetes and weight loss. These include dulaglutide (Trulicity), exenatide (Byetta, Bydureon), semaglutide (Wegovy), liraglutide (Victoza, Saxenda), and lixisenatide (Lyxumia) Of these, semaglutide appears to be the most effective in helping patients lose weight. A study showed that Tirzepatide (Monjouro), a GLP-1 receptor agonist, together with GLP (glucagon-like peptide-1) receptor agonist resulted in a 22 percent weight loss.

More Natural Ways to Help Weight Loss

We know that dietary fiber from fruits, vegetables, and whole grains raise PYY levels. We also know that prebiotics, nondigestible carbohydrates found in dietary fiber, raise GLP-2 and PYY levels. The probiotic bacteria *Akkermansia muciniphila* also raises GLP-2 and PYY. In other words, eating more fiber and changing our microbiome is a natural way to control our appetite.

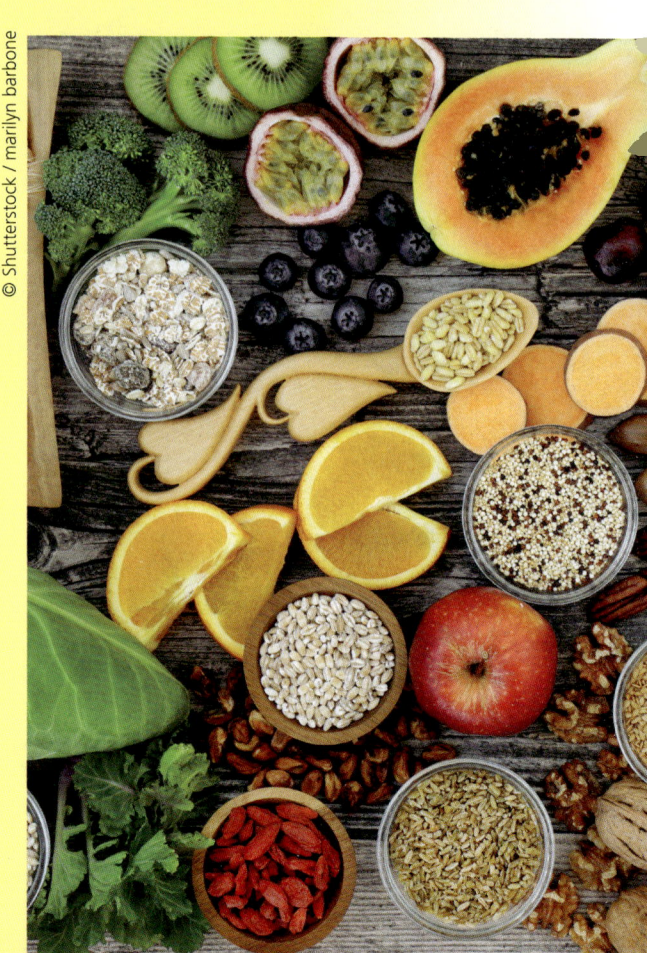
© Shutterstock / marilyn barbone

Treating Insulin Resistance

In its early stages, insulin resistance is easily treated with three key steps: dietary improvements, weight loss if needed, and more exercise. In its later stages, even for people with long-term type 2 diabetes, these steps are still the foundation of treatment, although drugs may now be needed to treat related problems, such as high blood pressure.

If you have insulin resistance, you may also be likely to have episodes of hypoglycemia, when your blood sugar drops too low. Symptoms of hypoglycemia include irritability, jitteriness, or unhappiness. Low blood sugar can make you feel lightheaded or confused and can trigger an uncomfortable cold sweat. When you're having a hypoglycemic episode, you instinctively want to eat something sugary or starchy to raise your blood sugar. If you do, it does raise your blood sugar quickly, but the sudden spike of blood sugar also stimulates your pancreas to release a lot of insulin to compensate. This then drives your blood sugar down again, which can trigger another hypoglycemic episode. Switching your diet to include more nutrients and fewer refined carbohydrates and processed foods will help you get off this endless roller coaster of blood sugar highs and crashes.

Just watching calories usually isn't enough to help insulin resistance. We need to do more to make food and lifestyle work for us, not against us. Remember, insulin resistance probably evolved as a way to store excess sugar (mostly fructose) in the diet as fat for energy later, when food might be scarce.

Today, in the land of plenty, we no longer need our bodies to store fat as insurance against food scarcity, but our genes are still programmed to do this. We can't reprogram our genes, so instead we need to be much more selective about the types and amounts of food we eat.

Dietary Changes

A better diet should be the first line of attack against insulin resistance and weight gain. Not only do you need to change what you eat, but how you eat as well. We strongly recommend working with a dietitian for this. Nutrition is a complex subject, and everyone has individual needs and personal food preferences. A nutritionist can help you work out a meal plan that puts you on a better path while still letting you enjoy your favorite foods.

Use Diet to Lower Insulin

In Chapter 9, we discussed the low-carbohydrate diet, which we suggest as a first-line treatment for insulin resistance. If your blood sugar levels still aren't responding, we recommend time-restricted eating as an effective way to get insulin resistance, prediabetes, and diabetes under control. We suggest you start by fasting for 14 hours after your last meal of the day and limiting your eating window to 10 hours. If possible, then move toward a 16/8 schedule (fast for 16 hours, eat during the eight-hour window). If you need a snack between meals or during the fasting period, aim for small portions of low-carbohydrate foods such as veggies, fruit, nuts, cheese, or protein.

For severe insulin resistance, consider following a ketogenic diet for a few months until your blood sugar improves. This helps improve metabolic flexibility—your body's ability to easily switch from burning glucose to burning ketones. Once insulin resistance is improved, the ketogenic diet restrictions can be relaxed a bit and you can add more carbohydrates.

For most people, we suggest the Prolon® five-day fasting mimicking diet (FMD), developed by Dr Valter Longo, Director of the Longevity Institue at the University of Southern California. This diet, followed for five days a month, has been shown to help patients reverse diabetes and help them get off medication. The Prolon® FMD has also been shown to reduce markers (risk factors) for aging, cancer and cardiovascular disease, promote multi-system regeneration, enhance cognitive performance and healthspan, improve skin hy-

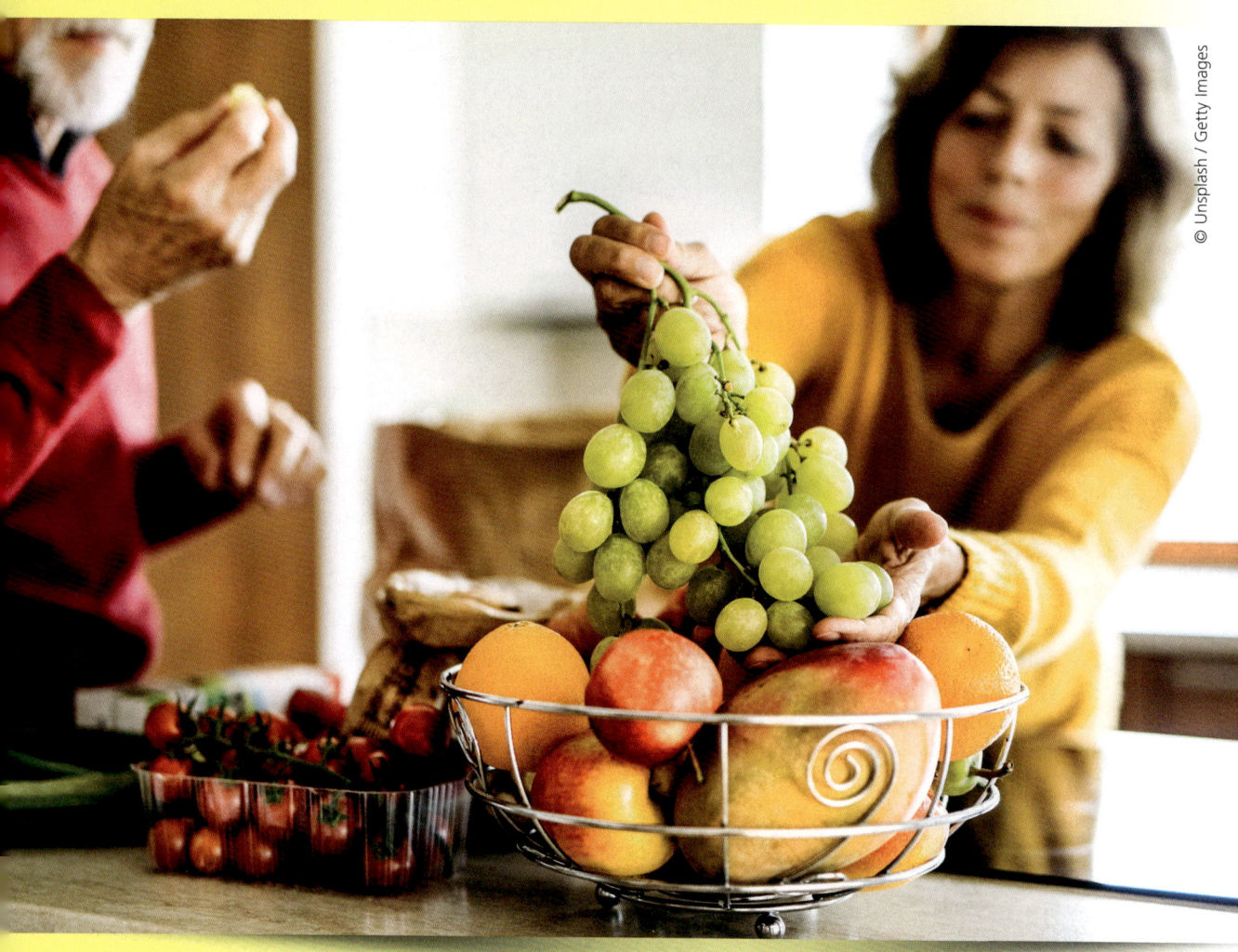

dration and texture, improve diabetic nephropathy, induce breast cancer regression, reverse auto-immune disease and immune aging, promote stem cell regeneration and even reverse aging. *What a proof of concept that something as simple as changing your diet can do so much!*

Avoid the Terrible Twins and Their Horrible Children!

Avoid foods that contain added glucose, sucrose (table sugar), fructose (fruit juice or fruit-sweetened foods), and high-fructose corn syrup. Some sort of sugar is added to almost all processed and ultraprocessed foods. If these culprits are listed on the food label in the first five ingredients, stay away. (Even better, stay away from processed and especially ultraprocessed foods altogether.) Added sugars are so prevalent in our food supply that you get much more than enough of them without trying. It takes effort and attention to keep your intake down. We suggest you keep your sugar intake below 25 grams (about six teaspoons) a day and no more than 10 grams per meal.

Eat in Order

Eat your foods in this order:
- Fiber (veggies) first,
- Then proteins and fats,
- Then carbs/starch last.

By eating fiber first, you create a viscous mesh that soaks up glucose and fructose, slowing how quickly they enter your bloodstream. Fiber also slows gastric emptying, giving you a greater sense of satiety, as well as slowing down the action of the enzyme alpha amylase, which breaks down starch. Adding a green salad or veggie starter to all your meals will help remind you to do this. Beans, leafy greens, and most vegetables will help you reduce glucose spikes without really trying.

Don't Let a Sugar Spike Ruin Your Day!

As a culture, we have learned from food companies to start the day off with a sugary cereal or a pop-tart of sorts. This is the worst thing you can do, as the sugar spike is then likely to lead to insulin surge, then a sugar drop (hypoglycemia) and you are off to the races toward your own Snickers bar moment. What you want is a low (but normal) glucose level while your metabolism revs up and thus can keep it in the normal range throughout the day.

One way you can do this is to use a high-fat, low-protein bar or shake. Research has shown that the Fasting Bars or Shakes by Prolon® for breakfast will help you stay in ketosis even though you are eating. This is a great idea if you're trying to lose weight or conquer insulin resistance.

Another way is to make your first meal of the day one high in protein, along with some healthy fats. A vegetable omelet with avocado on the side is infinitely better than a bowl of sugary breakfast cereal in milk. Other ideas for a high-protein breakfast include full-fat Greek yogurt with nuts, a tofu scramble, fish, chicken, meat (but not processed meat like bacon), protein powder, nuts, seeds, nut butters, and eggs in all forms. If you must have carbs, have steel-cut oats with some full fat yogurt and nuts, or a whole-grain dark bread with nut butter. If you want fruit, have some berries or an apple. They're high in fiber and low in fructose, so are less likely to cause a glucose spike.

Finally, you can just eat a breakfast of complex carbohydrates. A good example here is steel-cut oatmeal, which will not spike your glucose. Sprinkle some nuts, sunflower or pumpkin seeds and a few berries on the top for a delicious breakfast.

Eat Carbs with Protein or Fat

If you're eating a high-carbohydrate food, keep your blood sugar from spiking by also eating something with fat and/or protein. When carbs are eaten on their own, they can cause a glucose spike. By adding protein and fats, you blunt the glucose response.

What to Drink

We suggest drinking plain, filtered water as your primary beverage. Coffee, green tea, black tea, and herbal teas are all good choices. Avoid adding large quantities of sugar, sweetened flavorings, and dairy/plant-based milks or creamers to your beverages. These add sugar and a lot of calories.

Avoid Artificial Sweeteners

Artificial sweeteners such as aspartame (NutraSweet, Equal), saccharin (Sweet'N Low), and sucralose (Splenda) taste sweet but have no calories or nutritional value. The taste sets off a cascade of signals to let your body know something sweet is coming down, but the calories never arrive—so your body produces insulin that isn't needed. Artificial sweeteners may increase your risk of cancer and heart disease and disrupt your gut microbiome.

Drink Apple Cider Vinegar

Drinking some vinegar a few minutes before a meal can help prevent or reduce a glucose spike. We suggest using apple cider vinegar for this because it has a milder flavor. Add 1 to 2 tablespoons of vinegar to 8 ounces of water and sip through a straw to avoid damage to your tooth enamel. Aim to drink the vinegar up to 20 minutes before you eat. Why this works isn't fully understood, but it probably slows how quickly your stomach empties into your small intestine, which slows how quickly you break down and absorb carbohydrates and reduces the glucose spike. If you don't like the taste of vinegar, eating a handful of almonds before a meal has also been shown to reduce the sugar spike.

Detox Your Liver, Improve Your Microbiome

Dark green leafy vegetables, brightly colored vegetables, and root and cruciferous vegetables are all helpful for improving your liver detoxification processes and keeping your gut microbiome healthy. Broccoli, cauliflower, artichokes, onions, and garlic are particularly helpful. Insulin resistance improves when your liver and gut are healthy.

Akkermansia mucinophilia is a keystone species of probiotic bacteria inhabiting the intestinal mucus layer. Low levels are associated with inflammation, liver dysfunction and metabolic abnormalities such as insulin resistance. Raising *Akkermansia mucinophilia* levels improves satiety, decreases inflammation, improves insulin sensitivity and improves gut health, even lowering LPS levels. If you are going to supplement with this, a study has shown that using a pasteurized product at a dose of 30B works better than the live bacteria.

Try Supplements

Some supplements may help improve insulin sensitivity. These include *Akkermansia mucinophilia*, berberine, cinnamon, green tea, chromium picolinate, alpha lipoic acid, L-carnosine, and the herb gymnema (*Gymnema sylvestre*). The improvements are usually small, however, and results vary from person to person. Supplements will help much more if you use them in conjunction with the other approaches we discuss here.

Take a Walk

If possible, take a brisk walk for at least ten minutes right after eating. Glucose is quickly converted to adenosine triphosphate, or ATP, the fuel that runs your body. If you use your muscles after eating, you convert glucose to energy instead of sending it to your liver or your fat cells for storage. In addition, be sure to get at least 30 minutes of physical activity a day. Aside from its other benefits, aerobic exercise or resistance training (weight training) helps improve insulin sensitivity.

Avoid Self-Blame

Sticking to a diet and all the other steps that help insulin resistance is hard. Everyone slips now and then. How can you say no to birthday cake or holiday treats? Illness or an injury can keep you from exercising. When life gets in the way of your good intentions, don't waste emotional energy on guilt or self-blame. Just get back on your healthy path as quickly as you can and try to stick with it for the next day. That will help reset your metabolism and mind-set back to where it was and get you back on track. The longer you've been following a healthy lifestyle, the less likely you are to go off it in a significant way and the easier it is to get back when you do.

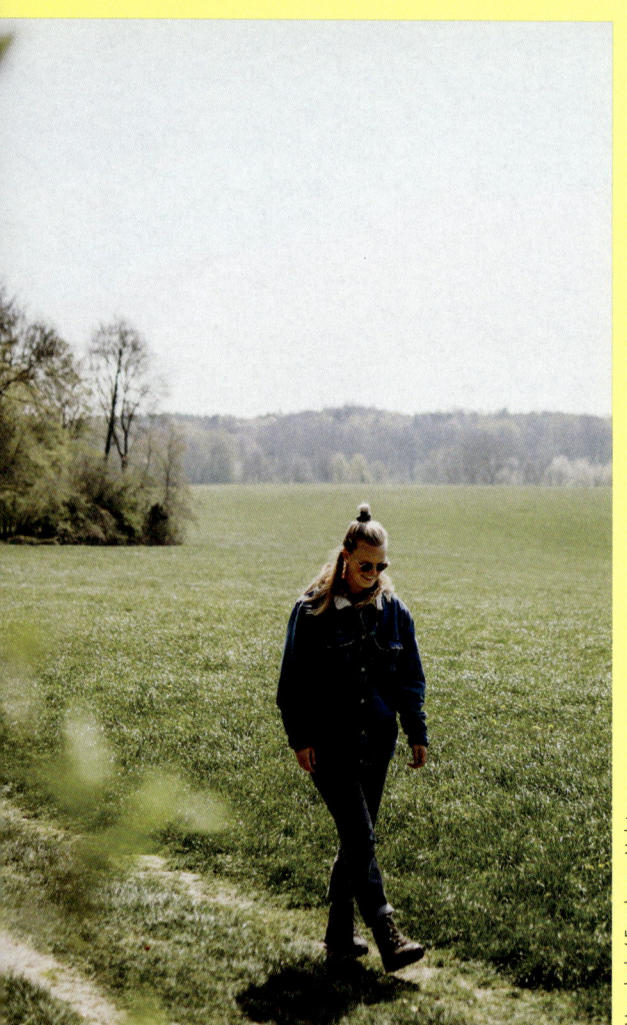

© Unsplash / Frank van Hulst

Use a Continuous Glucose Monitor

You wouldn't drive a car without a speedometer, right? A continuous glucose monitor is like a speedometer for your blood sugar. It lets you track how your food choices affect your blood sugar. It can tell you how blood sugar fluctuates over the course of the day, before and after meals, after specific foods, and at night while you sleep. If you're willing to pay for it yourself, you may be able to sign up directly for a CGM service without a doctor's prescription. If you have type 1 diabetes, type 2 diabetes, or serious trouble controlling your blood sugar, your doctor can prescribe a CGM so your health insurance pays for it. In her books *Glucose Revolution: The Life-Changing Power of Balancing Your Blood Sugar* and *The Glucose Goddess Method: The 4-Week Guide to Cutting Cravings, Getting Your Energy Back, and Feeling Amazing,* Jessie Inchauspé explains how using a CGM helped her and her clients have breakthroughs in controlling their sugar spikes.

Lose Weight, But Slowly

Losing weight too rapidly puts a lot of stress on your body. We suggest aiming to lose no more than 1 to 2 pounds a week. Losing weight any faster risks losing muscle mass in addition to fat. It may also raise your risk of gallstones.

Consider Medication

If all the above ideas don't help control your insulin resistance, or don't help enough, discuss adding an antidiabetic medication with your doctor. We usually begin by prescribing metformin, a safe, well-tolerated drug that helps your cells take up more glucose, decreases the amount of glucose made by your liver, and decreases the amount of glucose you absorb from your small intestine.

If you need an additional or different drug, we have a lot of possible options, with varying benefits and side effects. The GLP-1 drugs that became widely available starting in 2022 are

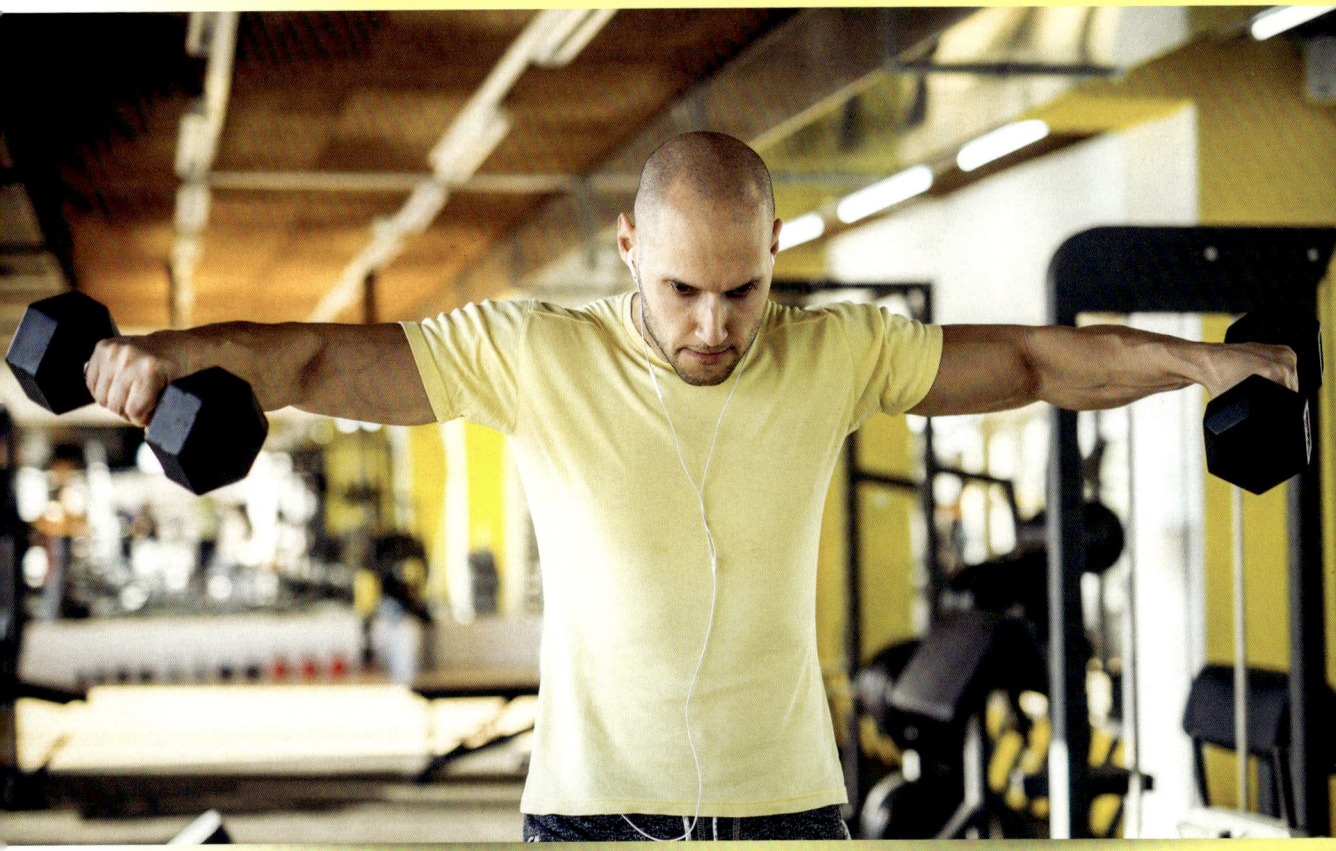

one possible choice. This class of drugs includes tirzepatide (Zepbound), dulaglutide (Trulicity), exenatide (Byetta), semaglutide (Ozempic and Wegovy), and liraglutide (Victoza). These drugs mimic the action of a hormone called glucagon-like peptide 1 (GLP-1). When your blood sugar starts to rise after eating, the drug stimulates your body to release more insulin, which in turn lowers your blood sugar. What makes these drugs so popular, however, is that they also lead to weight loss without hunger or cravings.

GLP-1 drugs seem to be generally safe with few serious side effects, but they have some drawbacks. They can cause significant impaired motility of the intestines as well as loss of muscle mass. Most must be injected once a week, they are very expensive and may not be covered by health insurance, and their benefits for blood sugar and weight loss stop when you stop taking them. Most people who stop these drugs regain the lost weight. Finally, they result in loss of muscle mass which can be difficult to regain. That is why exercising when on these drugs is so important.

These and subsequent weight loss drugs are financial blockbusters. Expect new and improved drugs to continually appear on the horizon.

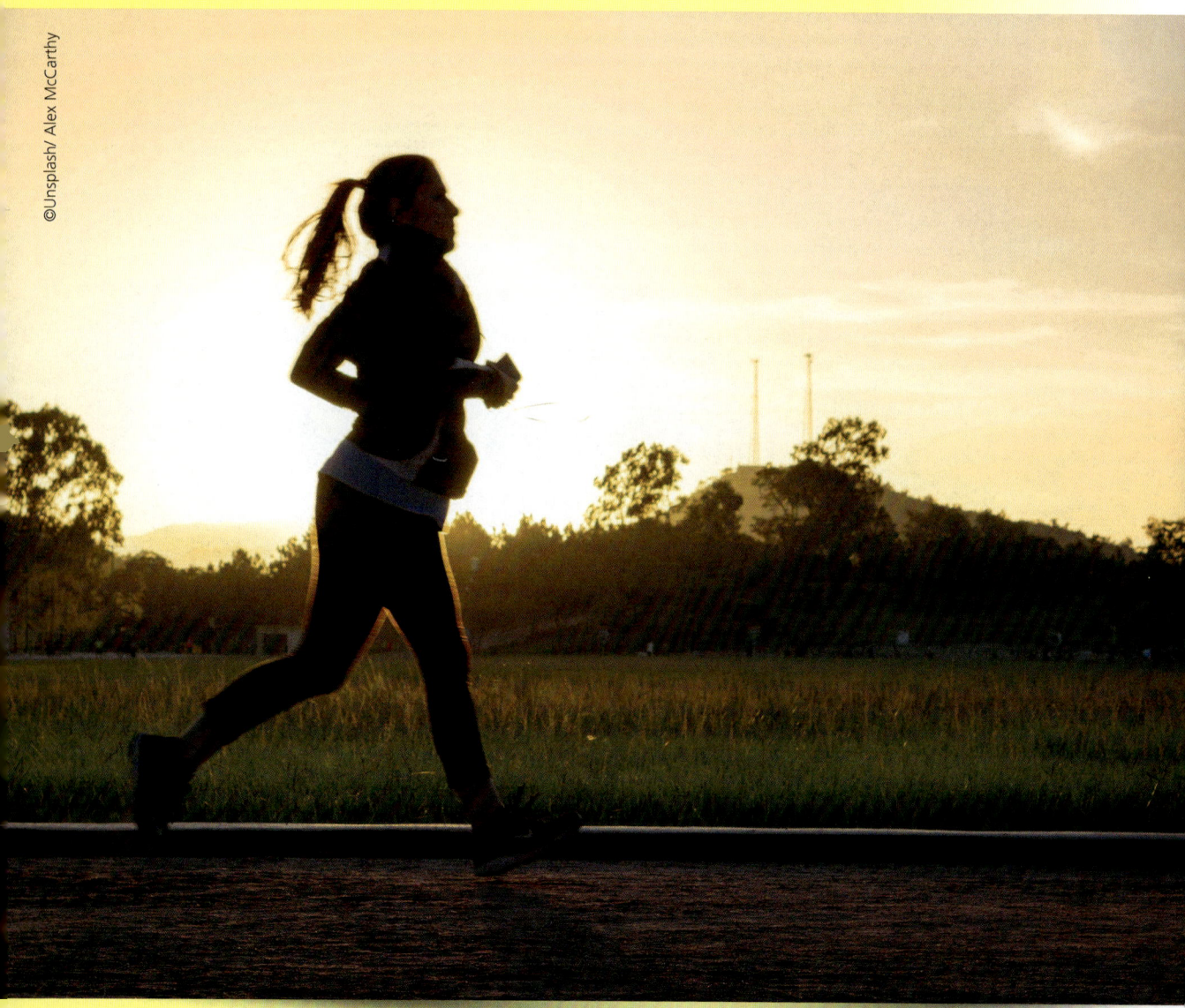

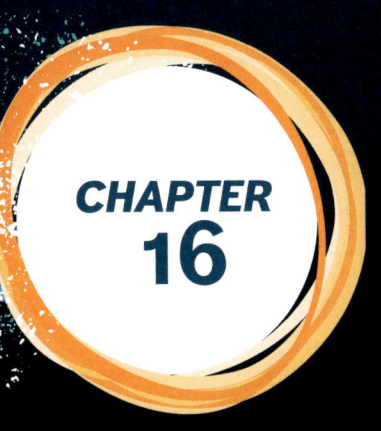

CHAPTER 16

The Legacy of Our Standard American Diet (SAD) and Lifestyle:
The SAD Diseases

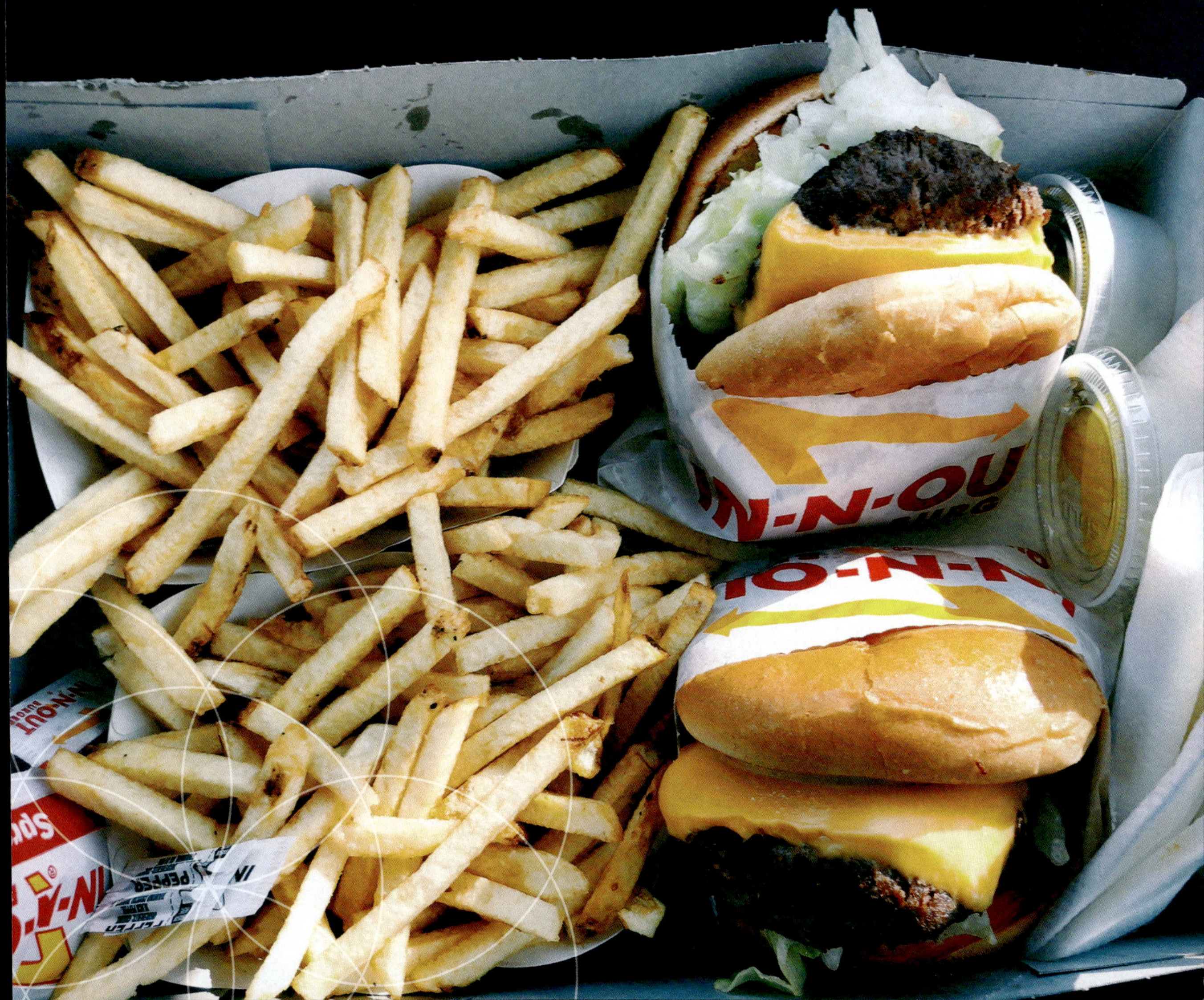

As we have tried to show you throughout this book, diseases don't happen randomly. Seemingly different diseases are connected by common metabolic pathways. At the core appears to stand a giant called the mechanistic Target of Rapamycin, or mTOR for short. This key pathway coordinates cell growth and metabolism with environmental inputs, including nutrients and growth factors. An enzyme complex, mTOR plays a central role in regulating many basic cell activities that are fundamental to survival, such as promoting the growth and development of tissues. The pathway is stimulated by glucose, carbohydrates, and protein. Ideally, it should turn on intermittently, only after eating foods that stimulate it. The problem is that today, with our superabundance of food, the pathway is constantly stimulated. And the single biggest culprit: the highly refined, ultra-processed, carbohydrate-laden, high-sugar, high-protein, high-saturated fat, Standard American Diet (SAD), which is now consumed by much of the developed world.

Deregulated mTOR signaling is implicated in a wide array of illnesses. You will recognize them easily. They fill our doctors' offices and overburden our medical system. And as much as powerful medications are helpful in mitigating each of these on their own, they have done little to eradicate them. Instead, we are burdened as a nation with their incredible costs. So, what are these diseases? Insulin resistance, metabolic syndrome, prediabetes and diabetes, obesity, hyperlipidemia, coronary artery disease, non-alcoholic fatty liver disease (NAFLD), chronic kidney disease (CKD), certain neurodegenerative diseases including Alzheimer's disease, osteoporosis, certain cancers, depression, and more, including the aging process! We call them SAD diseases because we can trace them back to the SAD and the way it constantly stimulates the mTOR pathway.

We are now, for the first time in a century, seeing a generation that isn't living as long or longer than previous generations. This is alarming!

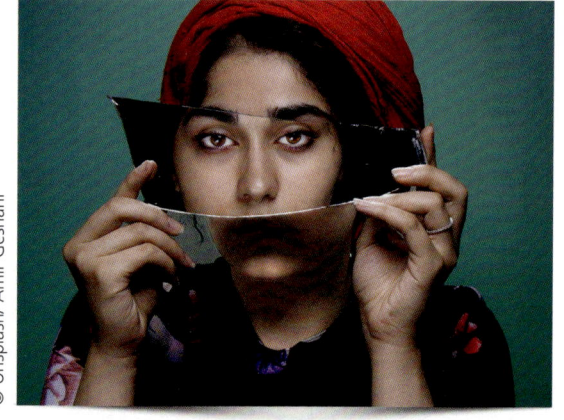

The mTOR Pathway

The kinase mTOR is a well-known target molecule in the race to stop and reverse aging. The mTOR kinase enzyme system is responsible for cell growth and protein synthesis. It senses growth factors and amino acids. mTOR activity is stimulated by insulin, protein kinases (PK) from both protein and carbohydrates, and growth hormone (IGF-1). Stimulants of growth hormone include animal proteins, milk, carbohydrates, and certain B vitamins. When any of these are present in abundance because of what you eat, mTOR is activated. Your cells go into anabolic, or building-up, mode and start to grow and divide. This is good if we are growing or healing.

mTOR Stimulation and the SAD Diseases

When the mTOR pathway is constantly activated from sensing an abundance of nutrients, the continuous growth mode can have harmful downstream effects that can decrease longevity and lead to the SAD diseases. If we can reduce mTOR production, we may be able to increase longevity and healthspan! Of course, shutting off mTOR completely would mean shutting down anabolism, the process that is essential for cell maintenance and growth. If we have too little mTOR we can't grow or maintain muscle. Instead, we want to manage mTOR production and decrease the constant on-state. So, in an ideal world, mTOR needs to be intermittently lowered. This mimics the normal balance of feast and famine our bodies have evolved to expect.

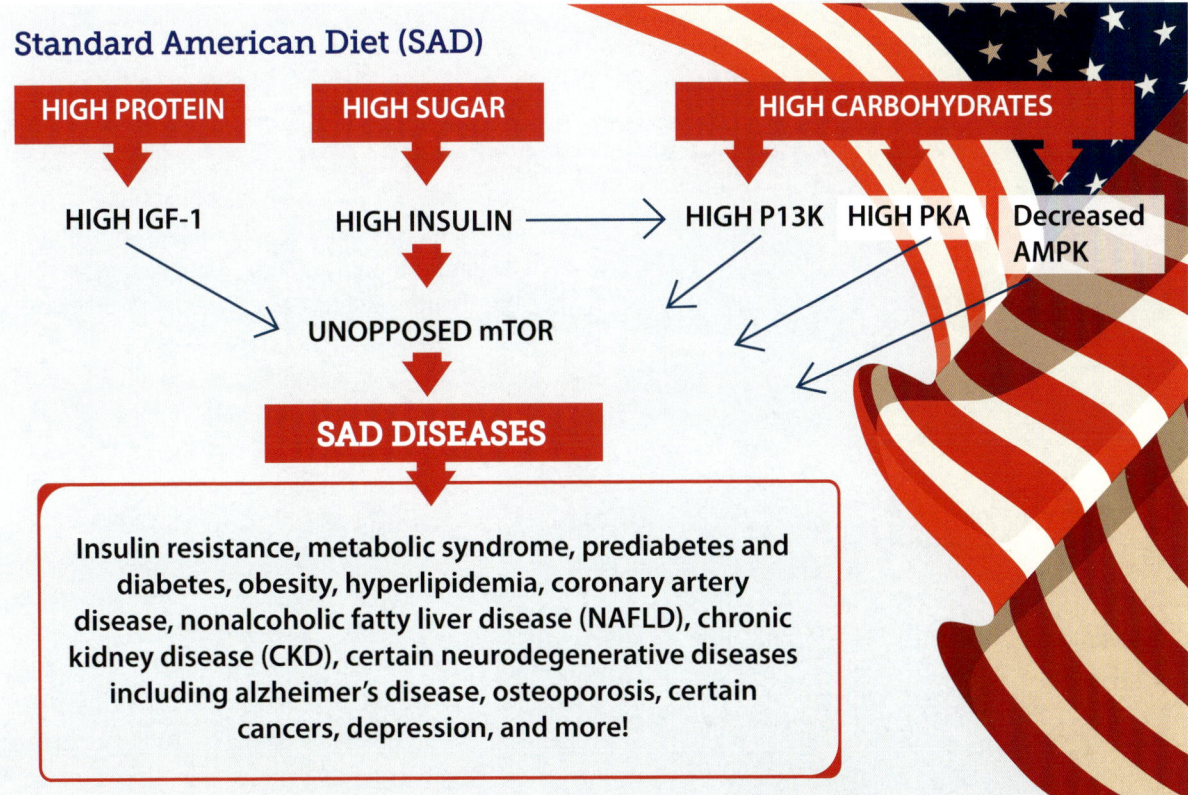

FIGURE 16.1 | Standard American Diet

Glucose and mTOR

Glucose is the single biggest factor driving the mTOR pathway. If we reduce our intake of sugar and highly refined carbohydrates, which will lower our insulin levels, we downregulate the constant-on mTOR and extend both our healthspan and our lifespan. This can't be done with a drug—it needs to be done by changing our diet.

The changes needed go beyond simply reducing sugar and refined carbohydrate consumption. To reduce insulin resistance, we need to decrease the endocrine disrupting chemicals in our environment so that our insulin receptors can once again become sensitized.

Finally, we need to increase the amount of fiber we eat and improve our gut microbiome. Again, this cannot be achieved just with a drug—improving our environment, diet and lifestyle are, once again, key.

And we cannot do it alone. Food companies and better farming methods are needed to upgrade the quality of our food while simultaneously eradicating multiple toxic chemicals in our environment in order to enhance the health of our planet.

Let us explain a little more biochemistry.
At the molecular level in your body, a finely tuned symphony of metabolic pathways balance aging and illness. These metabolic pathways sense the nutrients you give your body. They have balance points, or checkpoints, which act like traffic lights and allow the nutrients to flow one way or the other. These checkpoint systems are made up of special enzymes called kinases. In all, you have at least 538 different kinases that control all aspects of your metabolism. The key metabolic kinases—the ones that give direction to others both upstream and downstream—are mTOR, AMP kinase (AMPK), and PI3 kinase.

AMPK

When we cut calories, we alter the balance between mTOR and another kinase called AMPK (adenosine monophosphate (AMP)-activated protein kinase). When nutrients are reduced, the mTOR pathway senses that food is scarce and slows down or even shuts off the anabolic pathways. At the same time, the AMPK pathway senses the reduction in nutrient levels and energy production and triggers a number of catabolic changes that tell your cells to conserve energy. The signals tells your cells to make more mitochondria (the energy-producing structures in your cells) in order to produce more energy and improve insulin sensitivity so more glucose flows in. Under the influence of AMPK, your cells become more fuel-efficient and stress-resistant. However, in the presence of glucose, AMPK function is impaired.

AMPK also activates autophagy (literally, "self-eating"). In this process, your cells break down old proteins and recycle their amino acids into new ones. As part of recycling, autophagy also removes cellular debris, such as damaged proteins, that clog up the cells. In other words, autophagy is one your body's most important take-out-the-trash mechanisms. It plays a key role in preventing cancer and autoim-

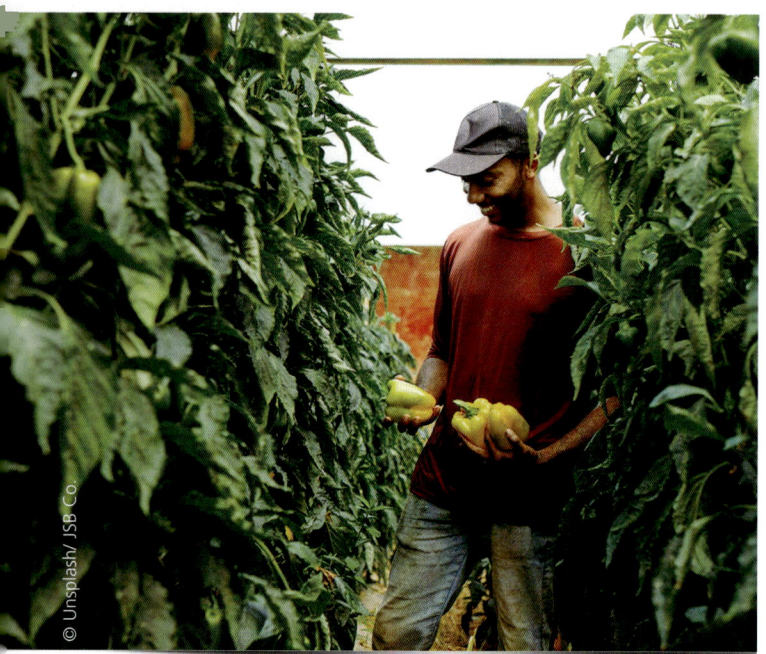

mune diseases by removing damaged or aberrant cells.

We know that one consistent way to make animals live longer is to reduce their calorie intake. The lower glucose, carbohydrate, and protein levels increase AMPK and drive autophagy. During the fasting state, the body burns fat and decreases oxidative stress and inflammation.

PI3 Kinase

A third kinase called PI3K (phosphoinositide 3-kinase) plays an important role in insulin pathway signaling. It allows glucose to enter your cells and be burned for energy. Once the glucose is in the cell, AMPK decides what happens next. If the cell needs energy, AMPK signals the mitochondria to burn more glucose. But if the cell doesn't need to produce energy, AMPK gets turned off, and the mTOR pathway takes over. Depending on the energy level in the cell, mTOR tells it to divide, stay put, or allows it to self-destruct through autophagy.

PI3K is found in elevated levels in cancer cells and fetal cells. Yet blocking PI3K doesn't improve cancer outcomes. The reason here is that insulin drives glucose into the cancer cell, fueling its growth, even when PI3K is inhibited. Once again, we see why insulin resistance is such a problem, and why it is so important to lower insulin levels.

Balancing the Pathways

We were designed by evolution to have times of food abundance and feasting, with resultant switching on of mTOR, alternating with periods of lower food intake or even famine, which stimulate AMPK. However, as sugar and refined carbohydrates have become an increasing part of our diet, many of us have chronic high levels of insulin. As a result is constant-on of mTOR, which stimulates PKB and PI3K and switches off AMPK. On top of this, the high protein in SAD switches on growth hormone or IGF-1. The result: the accelerator pedal on mTOR is constantly pressed. And when mTOR is constantly on, we see a host of seemingly unrelated diseases occurring together, which we call the SAD diseases.

When our diet is rich in nutrients but low in glucose, the intricate balance among the PI3K, AMPK, and mTOR pathways results in normal growth and normal energy production. When we bombard our cells with glucose, however, we disrupt the balance, leading to the metabolic syndrome, early aging, cell death, and low-level inflammation. We become more likely to get SAD diseases.

Caloric restriction, intermittent fasting, fasting mimicking diets, ketogenic diets, curcumin, resveratrol, EGCG (epigallocatechin gallate, found in green tea), genistein (soy), 3.3-diindolylmethane (found in cruciferous vegetables), caffeine, and drugs like rapamycin (including rapalogs, which are similar) and possibly metformin, can all either increase AMPK or suppress the mTOR pathway, thus reversing aging and illness.

Valter Longo, PhD, a longevity researcher and author of *The Longevity Diet*, is the Edna Jones Professor in Gerontology and Professor in Biological Science at USC. He is also the Director of the USC Longevity Institute and is the developer of the acclaimed and popular PROLON Diet. This five-day fasting-mimicking diet works by stimulating AMPK and lowering mTOR. Scientific studies have shown this diet can reverse type 2 diabetes as well as slow aging, promote multisystem regeneration, enhance cognitive performance, and improve healthspan. It helps mitigate the damaging effect of a high-fat diet on cardiometabolic risk, autoimmune disease, and lifespan. It will promote intestinal regeneration and reduce inflammatory bowel disease pathology. In animals with cancer, fasting during chemotherapy improves outcomes and reduces pathology. Studies are ongoing in humans. This is just a brief look of what we can do when we learn to balance these pathways.

What Is Rapamycin?

Rapamycin is a drug discovered on Easter Island as an antibiotic produced by a specific strain of Streptomyces bacteria. It's named for the island's indigenous name, Rapa Nui, and is also known as sirolimus. Rapamycin inhibits the mTOR pathway, specifically the mTOR subtype, mTOR Complex 1 (mTORC1). Its primary use is as an immunosuppressant for organ transplant patients; it's also used to coat the stents that keep clogged coronary arteries open, as a cancer treatment, and as an antifungal.

Because rapamycin is a cell growth inhibitor and immunosuppressant and because studies in mice have shown that rapamycin can delay age-related diseases, such as cognitive decline, tumors, heart disease, and immune dysfunction, today there is a great deal of interest in rapamycin as an anti-aging drug. Rapamycin activates increased autophagy by inhibiting mTOR, which is why it has potential for extending lifespan. When used continuously as an immunosuppressant, it doesn't improve lifespan in animal models, but used intermittently and in low doses, it appears to do so.

Note that mTOR overstimulation does not cause SAD diseases – it simply accelerates a natural tendency toward them!

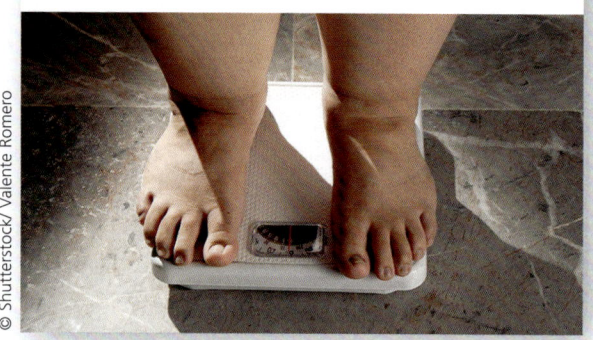

But Wait, There's More!

As if poor nutrition from SAD were not enough, our environment is further complicating our problems. Microbiome disruption and environmental toxins are resulting in an alarming increase of what we term environmentally induced autoimmune diseases. In addition, we are seeing an ever-increasing upswing in GI-related issues, ranging from functional disorders like irritable bowel syndrome and SIBO to a rise in inflammatory bowel disease and even an increase in colon cancer in young adults. We feel much of this rise in gut-related disease is caused by the heavy use of antibiotics in our animal foods and by the widespread use of pesticides, herbicides, and other toxins in agriculture.

We need to be concerned about human-caused illness. Although we are seeing that much of our human-caused illness is getting worse, we also now know it can be reversed. We'll discuss this further in Chapter 21.

CHAPTER 17

Understanding Pain

Your Body As Your Biography: How Pain Can Give You a Different Perspective on Yourself and Your Life

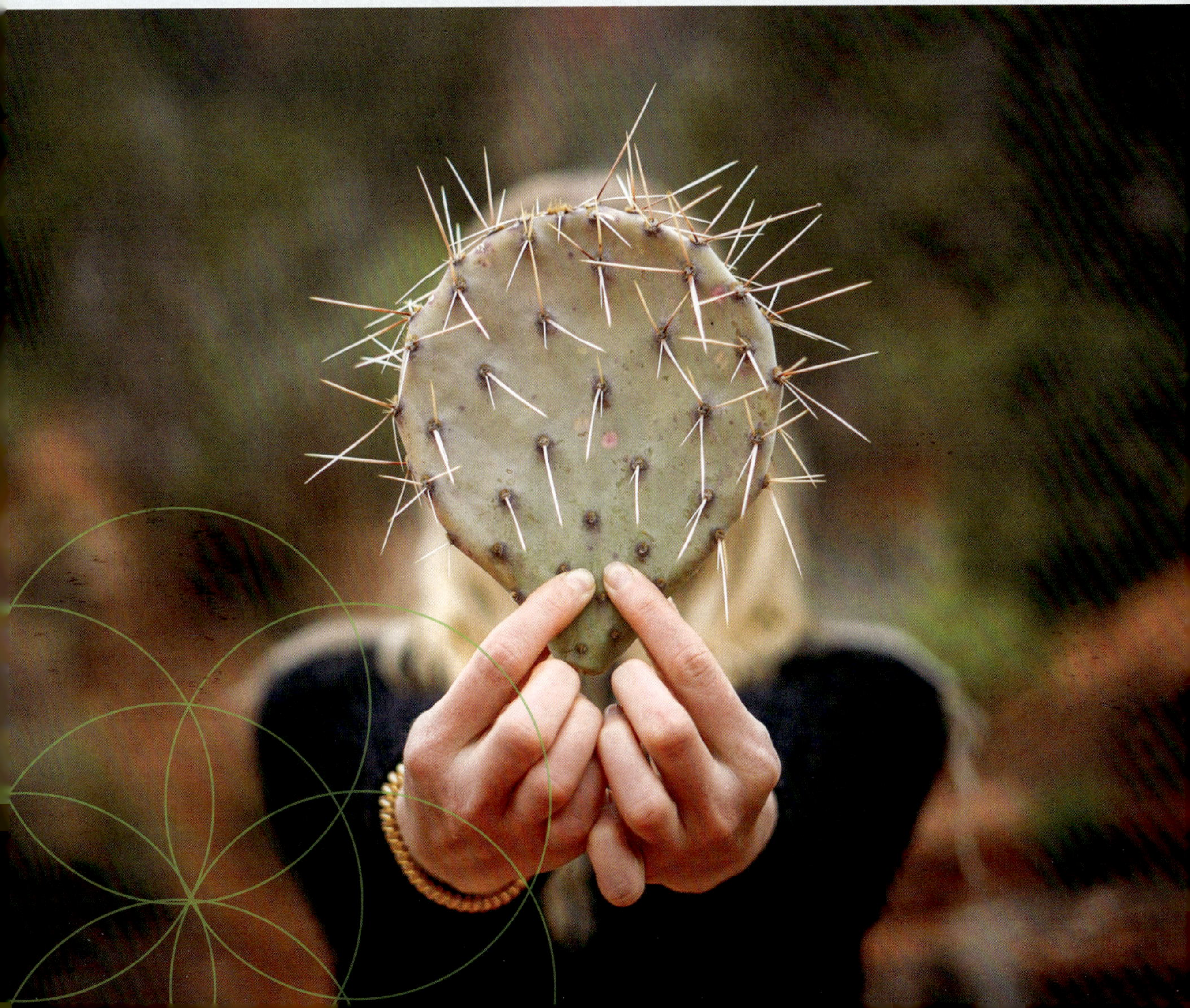

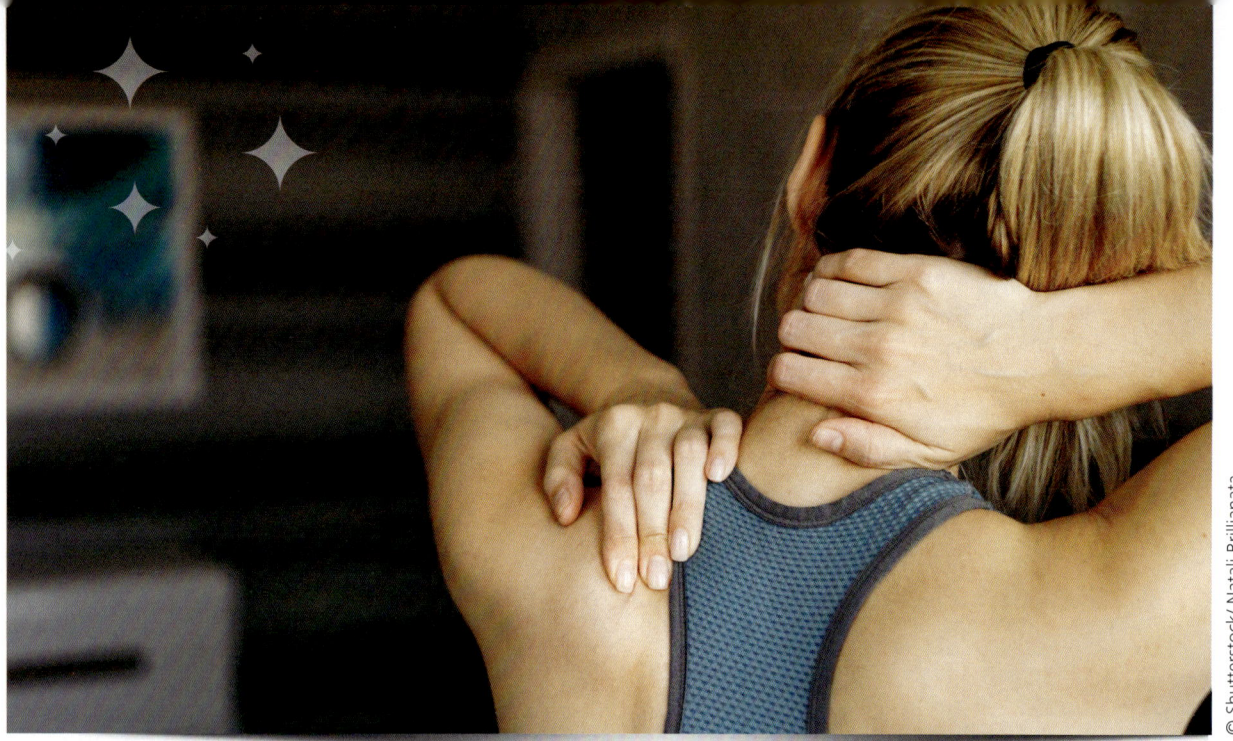

Although acute pain can put us in agony in an instant, it is also a highly effective protective mechanism. If we accidentally put our hand too close to a fire, we abruptly feel pain. This normal physiologic response is tied to saving our lives. We respond quickly by pulling our hand away from the fire. Modern medicine is good at using highly effective drugs to relieve acute pain. However, the overuse of opioids has led to widespread issues relating to narcotic dependency, addiction, and abuse. For these and other reasons we like to use integrative medicine.

The Reality of Chronic Pain

Chronic pain is defined as discomfort that persists for either three months or for longer beyond what is expected following normal healing. It is very different from acute pain.

Chronic pain may affect as many as 20 percent of all Americans and up to one-third of the world's population at any given time, but few receive effective treatment for it. Usually, the body has a pain generator somewhere, an underlying factor that is causing the problem. The pain may be the result of an injury or the secondary effect of some other condition present in the body, such as cancer, osteoarthritis, myalgic encephalomyelitis/chronic fatigue syndrome (ME/CFS), or endometriosis. It could be generated by a chronically inflamed disc or joint, or it might be coming from a knotted spasm in a muscle—a trigger point. In any case, the body often interprets that signal as a chronic problem.

Reverberating Pain Signals

Often, chronic pain is like a persistent warning light on your car's dashboard. You call the dealership, and they tell you not to worry. "It's just a minor malfunction—come in when you can and we'll fix it," they say. Despite this, the warning light continues to bother you. Eventually, you refuse to drive the car, convinced that something bad is going to happen.

Chronic pain is similar. The warning light is constantly on. Instead of saying, "OK, I know what's going on. You can switch off now," the body remains in a hyperalert state, constantly trying to figure out the source of the pain. This hypervigilant state becomes another source of stress, further inflaming muscles and nerves and draining the body of energy.

In hypervigilance, the central nervous system (CNS, meaning the brain and spinal cord) and the peripheral nervous system (meaning all the other nerves in your body) become sensitized and involved in a never-ending loop of chronic pain.

Whatever the original source of the discomfort, the pain is sending a message up to the brain. Once it senses pain, the brain should send a "switch-off" message: an inhibitory signal that travels back down the spinal cord and turns off the pain. In other words, the body should recognize chronic pain and respond, "Oh, I know what that is, it's the site of my old injury, but I don't need to worry about it. It's not going to break, it's just hurting."

The "switch-off" or inhibitory signal is affected by your levels of serotonin and other neurotransmitters, such as norepinephrine. Chronic stress depletes these neurotransmitters. When serotonin and norepinephrine levels get too low, the body can't switch off the pain, leading to more stress and perpetuating a vicious cycle of pain.

The ACTTION Pain Taxonomy

The American Pain Society has created a standardized system for classifying pain. The ACTTION (Analgesic, Anesthetic, and Addiction Clinical Trial Translations, Innovations, Opportunities, and Networks) Pain Taxonomy breaks pain down into these types (https://www.acttion.org/):

1. Peripheral and central nervous system
2. Musculoskeletal pain
   a. Osteoarthritis
   b. Systemic arthritides, such as rheumatoid arthritis and gout
   c. Low back pain
   d. Myofascial pain, chronic widespread pain, ME/CFS
3. Orofacial and head pain disorders
4. Visceral, pelvic, and urogenital pain
5. Disease-associated pain not classified elsewhere, such as cancer or Parkinson's disease

These pain patterns and diseases are not mutually exclusive. A patient may have rheumatoid arthritis, which requires an anti-inflammatory approach, as well as myalgic encephalomyelitis/chronic fatigue syndrome (ME/CFS), also known as fibromyalgia, which requires an approach for central sensitization. Similarly, about 40 percent of patients with chronic low back or neck pain will also have ME/CFS.

Vicious Cycle #1: Pain → Depression, Sleep Problems, Fatigue → More Pain

Here's how the cycle works. It starts when stress leads to pain. Then the pain leads to depression and sleep problems, which amplify pain, which leads to more stress and depression. Get the picture?

If you have chronic pain, you're probably not sleeping well, which means you're not regenerating neurotransmitters such as serotonin very efficiently. You understandably become focused on the pain, which means you sleep less and suffer more. You quickly slip into the "inflamed and exhausted" mode of the stress curve (see Chapter 2 to see the stress curve chart). As your inflammation levels rise, the inflammatory cascade is turned on, releasing cytokines and a whole array of other signaling chemicals that amp up the immune response and the pain. This pain is due to central nervous system sensitization. Central pain is associated with hyperalgesia (an increased sensitivity to feeling pain and an extreme response to pain). Peripheral pain is associated with allodynia (experiencing pain from stimuli that aren't normally painful, such as cold temperatures or hair brushing).

Chronic Pain and the Brain

Glutamate, serotonin, and norepinephrine are all neurotransmitters involved in chronic pain. That's why drugs that alter how neurotransmitters are used in the brain, such as gabapentin, pregabalin (Lyrica), and duloxetine (Cymbalta), are sometimes used to treat chronic pain.

Other biochemical mediators of pain include calcitonin gene-related peptide (CGRP), brain-derived neurotrophic factor (BDNP), and nerve growth factor (NGF). Genetic variants associated with chronic pain include catechol-O-methyltransferase, the serotonin transporter gene (5-HTTLPR), adrenergic receptor genes (5-HT2 receptor), and mu-opioid genes.

MRIs of the brain in patients with chronic pain show structural changes. Functional MRIs (fMRIs) can also show typical pain patterns. For example, an fMRI can show increased brain connectivity between the default mode network (DMN) and the left mid/posterior insula, a region of the brain involved in pain perception.

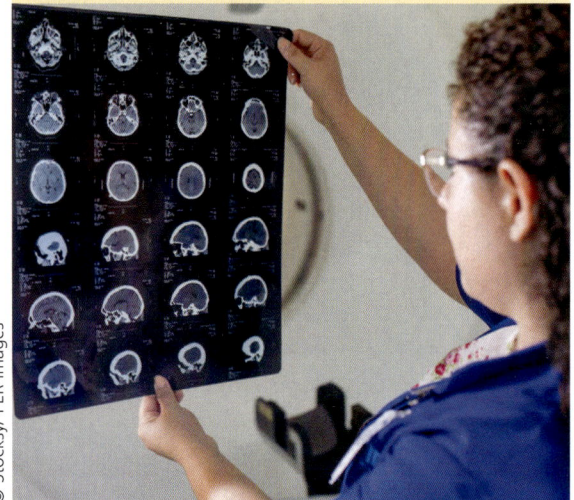

> *Pain is just another form of information.*
> —Don Delillo, **Underworld**

Vicious Cycle #2: Pain → Spasm → More Pain

The body responds to pain by trying not to use the painful area. This causes you to move differently (you limp on your sprained ankle, for example) and may also cause muscle spasms around the injured area to protect it. Most of the time, pain and muscle spasms diminish as the injury heals, and we resume our normal movement. But sometimes, muscle memory keeps us moving differently even though the injury has healed. The changes in movement can lead to changes in other parts of the body. If you're limping on your right ankle, other joints in your legs and hips might start to hurt from the extra strain.

Vicious Cycle #3: Pain → Fear Avoidance → Disuse → More Pain

Fear-avoidance beliefs, or concerns and fears that physical activity will be painful and do additional damage to the affected area, can lead to spasms in the injured area that never really go away. This type of pain is often found in myofascial disorders but also in chronic neck or low back pain caused by degenerative joint disease. In these cases, the pain causes you to catastrophize your fear that moving will cause more pain in the injured area, and the fear makes you magnify the pain and feel helpless and depressed about it. Fear avoidance leads to disuse of the area, which leads to more pain and possibly disability.

Vicious Cycle #4: Pain Due to Peripheral Sensitization

When someone has damaged discs in the spine or damaged joints from degenerative disease (usually osteoarthritis), their body releases chemicals that sensitize the peripheral nerves. The result is chronic pain. Instead of becoming resistant to the input of these chemicals, the body becomes sensitized, and increased activity causes further pain.

Peripheral sensitization further sensitizes the central nervous system, and vicious cycle 1, Pain → Depression, Sleep Problems, Fatigue → More Pain starts again.

Conventional Medicine and Pain

Conventional medicine has succeeded in its approach to acute pain. Anesthesiologists are experts at relieving pain after surgery. Epidural steroids, nerve blocks, and drugs have allowed physicians to master acute painful conditions. Unfortunately, chronic pain is different.

In our experience, when it comes to conventional medicine, chronic pain suffers the same fate as most chronic medical conditions. The longer the pain persists, the less likely conventional medicine will cure it. If a patient has two or more areas of chronic pain, there is even less likelihood that there will be a cure. In addition, chronic pain is often medically undertreated for fear of addicting patients to opioid medications.

This is where an integrative approach can be helpful. All over the country, health systems are realizing that we need to approach pain differently. They are incorporating low-cost, high-touch, personalized approaches that incorporate integrative modalities as a routine part of their treatment approach. In 2019, the US Department of Health and Human Services published Pain Management—Best Practices. The report emphasizes the importance of individualized patient-centered care in the diagnosis and treatment of acute and chronic pain and outlines ways to include integrative therapies in pain management. The report is a blueprint for moving forward with a better approach to pain management—one we hope will be widely adopted.

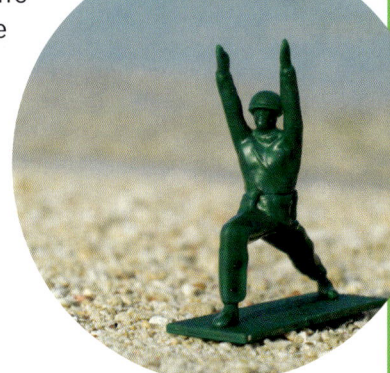

Risk Factors for Chronic Pain

Some people have a higher risk for chronic pain than others. These include those with genetic or familial tendencies to chronic pain, underlying immune or inflammatory diseases, or repetitive strain injuries. People who are obese, who have depression, or who tend toward inadequate coping or catastrophizing are also at a higher risk for chronic pain. We work with these patients to find safe, effective ways to treat their pain while also working to discover and treat the underlying causes of the pain.

We're particularly concerned about helping younger patients, people who are unemployed because of pain, people receiving compensation for pain or other illnesses, and people with mood disturbances and poorer quality of life. These patients are at greater risk of developing chronic pain that seriously affects their quality of life.

Patients who already have widespread pain prior to an injury or surgery, such as a joint replacement, are more likely to have increased opioid use and worse outcomes.

A Shift in Perspective

If you're living with persistent pain or discomfort, it is useful to look at the body as a whole—as a structural marvel and not just as a series of problematic parts. While patients and doctors alike focus on the painful part of the body, understanding the whole body will deepen your understanding of why you have pain and will help move you toward a solution.

Tensegrity: The Body's Elegant Balance

An idea common to both engineering and biology is tensegrity, the elegant balance between the continuous "pull" of muscles and connective tissue and the "push" of our bones. This balancing process is ongoing, synergistic, and dynamic. Like everything else in the body, it is a drive toward the overall balance we call homeostasis. The word tensegrity was introduced by the architect R. Buckminster Fuller, who coined it from the phrase "tensional integrity." Initially, it was used in architecture and engineering, but physiologists, anatomists, and physicians soon realized they could apply the terminology to the most wondrous of all structures: the human body.

Consider the miracle of how our bodies work. Basically, we're just a stack of bones held together by ropes we call muscles, ligaments, and tendons.

Our bones connect at our joints. In our legs, for example, the thigh bone, or femur, fits into the hip using a ball-and-socket arrangement. The femur is elegantly poised above a multifaceted hinge joint (the knee) that connects it with the two bones of the lower leg, the tibia and the fibula. Our knees are an ingenious feat of engineering. They remain stable while still allowing us to perform all kinds of subtle, complex movements, like twisting, squatting, kneeling, and climbing. This is accomplished by the ligaments, which hold the bony parts of the knees in place, while the muscles of the legs act as pulleys to enable us to move and bend. The muscles that surround the joints pull on them like levers, allowing us to move. Muscles are attached to bones via ropes called tendons. The cartilage, or meniscus, acts as a shock absorber, while guiding our femur and tibia to act as cantilevers that enable us to step, lean, stretch, reach, and balance.

Muscles are surrounded by a white, sinewy connective material called fascia, which wraps around the muscles throughout the body. It also surrounds, supports, and penetrates all our muscles, nerves, and organs. A clear example of the fascia can be seen in a chicken drumstick or salmon fillet—it's the white membrane that surrounds the muscles. In fact, the fascia forms a structure that connects and envelops every major muscle and every organ in our bodies, extending uninterrupted from the tops of our heads to the tips of our toes! Fascia binds us together, much as plastic wrap around a sandwich holds it together.

The fascia is made up largely of collagen fibers that can resist great forces pulling from different directions. Ordinarily, the fascia is free, flexible, and moves easily. If it is bound or stuck in places, pain and functional problems can develop.

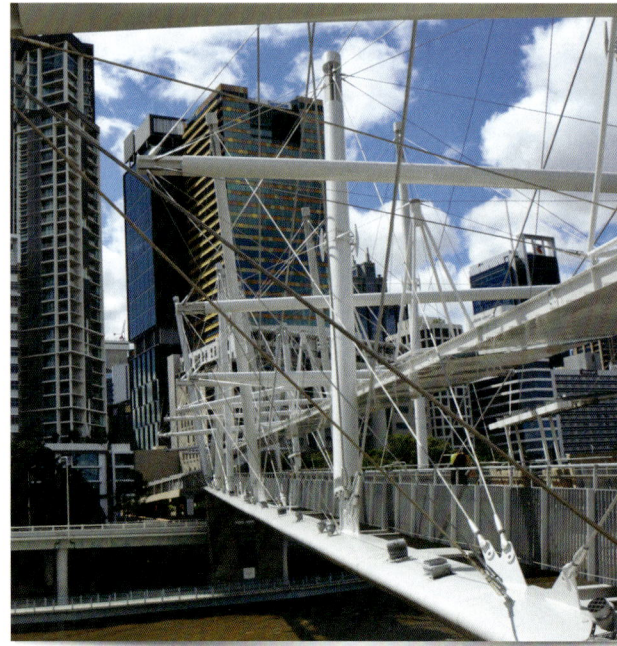

© Shutterstock/ 365 Focus Photography

Another way to look at the fascia is as our body's internet. It wraps around all the muscles and nerves, acting as a massive unseen network of connectivity. This is important because acupuncture and bodywork, such as massage or Rolfing, work in part by freeing the fascia or by sending messages through it. The fascia itself is part of the interstitium, a network of fluid-filled spaces supported by a mesh of connective tissue.

Kinetic Chains

Kinetic chains are groups of muscles and joints working together to perform movements. They all connect through the spine. The upper kinetic chain consists of the fingers, wrists, forearms, elbows, upper arms, shoulders, and shoulder blades, where it connects to the spine. The lower kinetic chain consists of the toes, feet, lower legs, knees, upper legs, hips, and pelvis, where it connects to the spine.

When we treat chronic pain or use regenerative medicine in healing, we're working with both tensegrity and kinetic chains. We need to treat not just the area directly involved, but also the links in the kinetic chain to restore the tensegrity balance.

The Domino Effect of Injury

Once you begin to think about the body in terms of tensegrity—this constant pull–push that interacts with the nervous system—it is easy to see that when the body goes out of balance after an injury or overexertion, that imbalance can ricochet throughout the system. The body compensates by attempting to balance the imbalance. A right ankle injury may throw the left hip out of balance. This can affect the right side of the chest, and ultimately the left shoulder.

While pain may be in one area of the body, it is always important to also understand pain as an expression of the body as a whole. Once

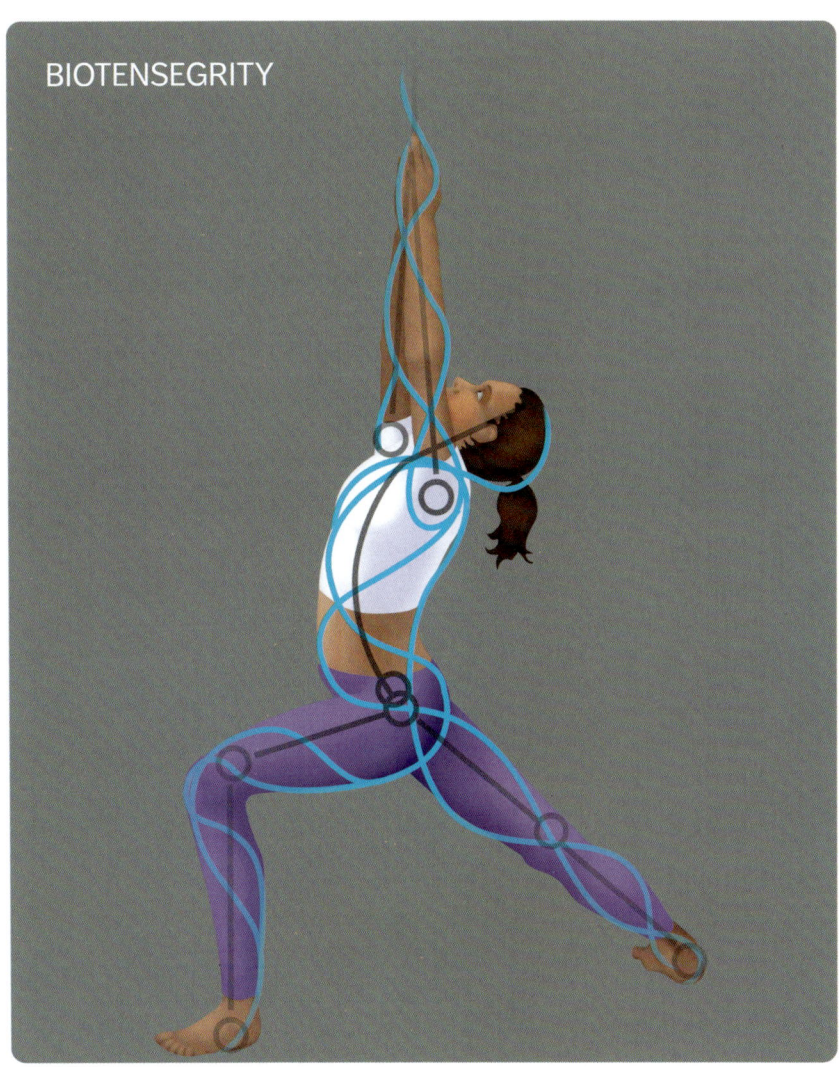

FIGURE 17.1 |
Biotensegrity

again, we need to view the body from a systems perspective. Pain is a complex interaction between these systems. It is affected by tensegrity; stress and neurotransmitters; metabolic, inflammatory, and immune problems; and even hormonal imbalances. ==To treat chronic pain, we need to view the whole person.==

The Integrative Diagnosis of Pain

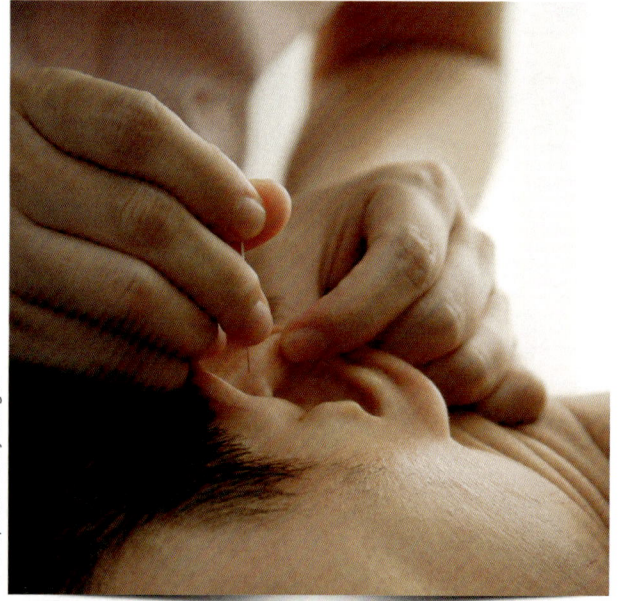

Pain is one of the top three complaints people bring to their doctor. It is likely you yourself have been in pain for a while and you may not have found anything that relieves it. Identifying the source of the pain is often difficult. However, once you understand more about how pain is generated, your options for treatment will expand significantly. Diagnosing the source of your pain and finding the best treatments is a stepwise process.

A Stepwise Approach to Understanding Your Pain

Step 1. A Medical Neuromusculoskeletal Evaluation

Step 2. Identifying Pain Generators: Muscles, Ligaments, Tendons, Bones and Nerves

Step 3. Understanding Body Mechanics, Structure, and Function

Step 4. Central Sensitization: Evaluating Depression, Sleep, and Fatigue

Step 5. Immunity Evaluation: Identifying an Upregulated Immune System

Step 6. An Acupuncture Evaluation

Step 7. Understanding Your Biopsychotype: How Your Body Affects Your Mind

Step 8. How Your Mind Affects Your Body: Evaluating Depression, Catastrophization, and Coping Mechanisms

Step 9. A Lifestyle Analysis: Finding the Causes and the Solutions

Step 10. An Integrative Diagnosis and a Transformational Treatment Plan

Step 1. A Medical Neuromusculoskeletal Evaluation

A medical neuromusculoskeletal evaluation is a typical examination done by physicians, such as a primary care doctor, orthopedist, physical medicine and rehabilitation physician, sports medicine physician, neurologist, or neurosurgeon. In conventional medicine, it is essential to find the exact neuromusculoskeletal reason for the pain. This is what medical doctors are trained to do.

Standard examinations require a thorough knowledge of anatomy, neurology, and the musculoskeletal system. Testing typically employed in these conventional workups includes x-rays, MRIs, CT scans, ultrasounds, and electromyograms (EMGs), which show nerve conduction problems in the muscle and can be very helpful for finding the source of the pain.

An abnormal test result, however, does not necessarily mean that the test has revealed the source of the pain. Studies have shown that most people have one or two bulging discs in the spine that do not cause pain. On the other hand, 50 percent of people with back pain have normal MRIs, with no apparent evidence of an abnormal disc. We always say, "We need to treat the patient, not the test!"

In some cases, by moving the body in a certain way or prodding the correct area, the doctor can reproduce the pain. This lets them know they are treating the right problem.

A doctor's diagnosis needs to correlate with the patient's symptoms. If not, the resulting treatment may not be what they want. A good example is a patient who has back surgery when he should have had a hip replacement, or vice versa.

Musculoskeletal Ultrasound

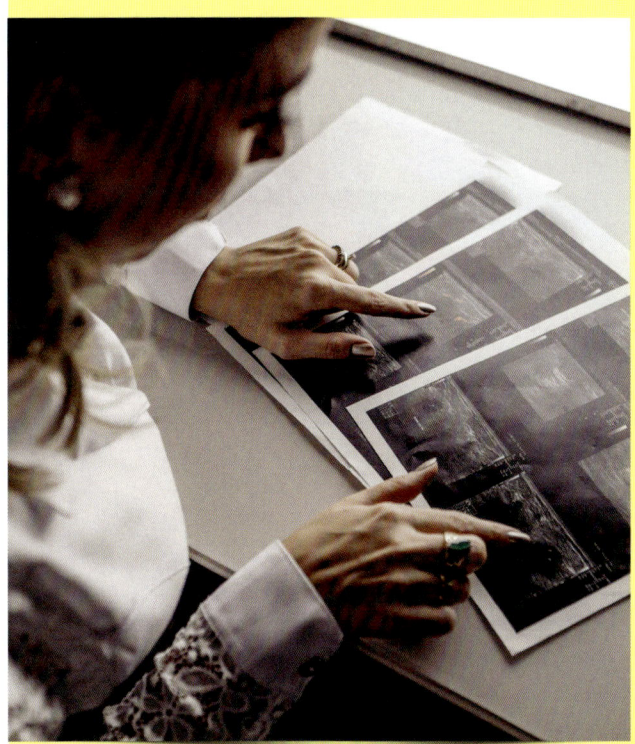

© Unsplash/ JSB Co.

As ultrasound machines have become smaller and cheaper, their use as a diagnostic tool is becoming invaluable. We now think of ultrasound as the pain practitioner's new stethoscope—the one tool we can't do without. Rather than send a patient to a radiology center for an MRI that might take days to schedule, we can instead use the ultrasound machine to look for musculoskeletal, joint, and nerve problems in the office quickly and easily. Then, also under ultrasound guidance, it is possible to precisely inject painful areas with medication, prolotherapy solution, or stem cells exactly where they are needed. As a bonus, with ultrasound we can see what happens in a joint as it moves.

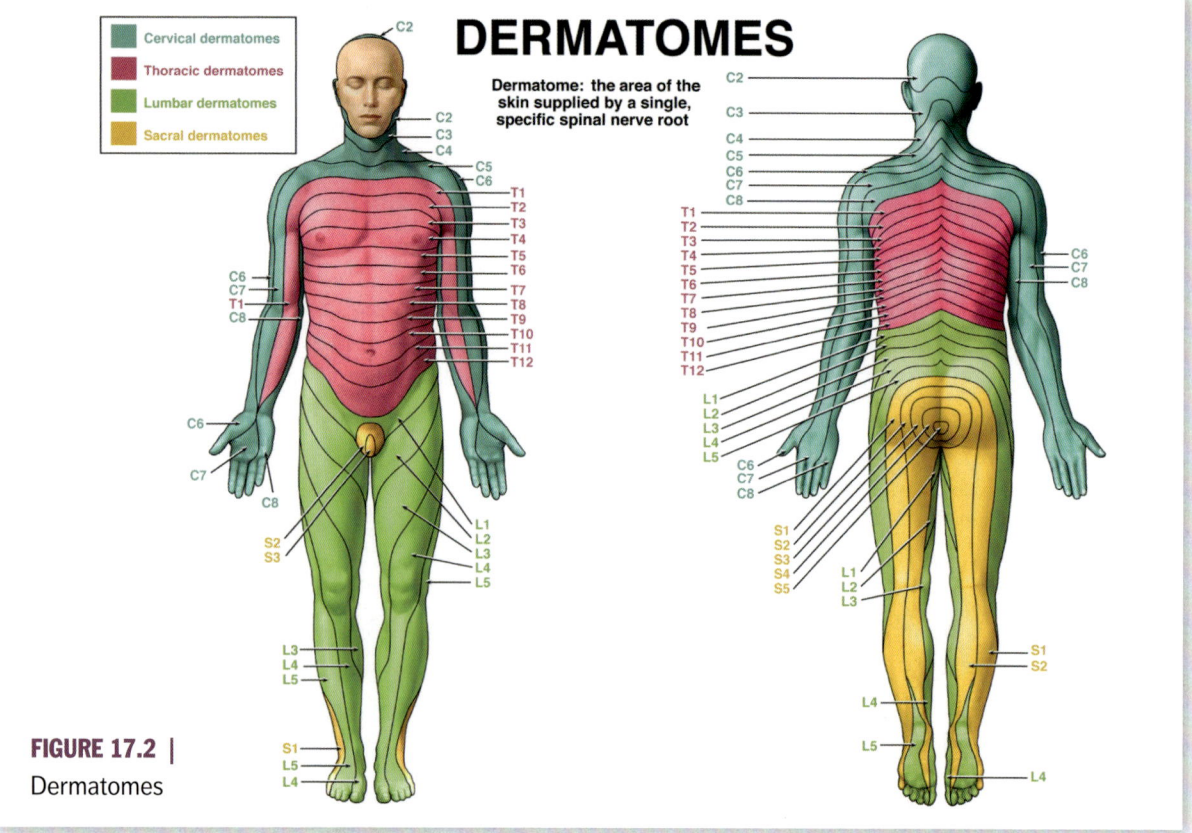

FIGURE 17.2 | Dermatomes

Excluding Other Causes of Pain

We need to understand where the pain is coming from and why it's there. We need to rule out other possible causes, such as autoimmune disease, cancer, and a variety of other illnesses. Hormonal issues such as hyperparathyroidism can cause pain, and hypothyroidism can cause fatigue. Nutritional deficiencies may aggravate pain. Vitamin D deficiency can lead to pain, while vitamin B1, B2, B6, B9 (folic acid), and B12 deficiencies are all associated with nervous system problems.

Patients who have headaches should have a thorough neurological exam. Interestingly, while patients who have headaches are often concerned about brain tumors, headaches are rarely a brain tumor symptom. Much more common are neurological symptoms such as weakness, blurred vision, or slurred speech, usually accompanied by weight loss, nausea, and vomiting. What is more concerning is the sudden severe headache, where you feel as if you've been hit on the head with a baseball bat. Here, an aneurysm or brain bleed needs to be excluded immediately.

Step 2: Identifying Pain Generators

Once we've ruled out other possible sources of your pain, we are left with the muscles, ligaments, cartilage, tendons, joints, bones, and nerves—alone or in combination.

Nerve Pain: Dermatome Pain Patterns

As each nerve emerges from the spine, it supplies sensation to certain specific areas of the body known as dermatomes. Damage to a nerve that comes from the thoracic (chest) part of the spine, for instance, can cause pain that wraps around the chest and goes into the abdomen, to the point where it can be confused with gallbladder pain.

The pain sensation is sometimes felt in

Herniated Disc in His Neck Causes Radiating Pain Down His Arm.

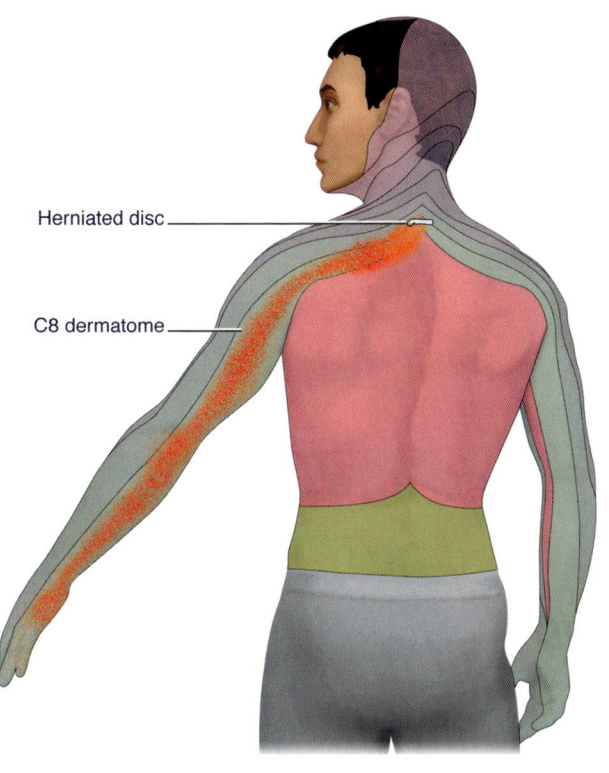

FIGURE 17.3 | A Herniated Disc

an area that is far away from the actual source. Doctors call this referred or radicular pain. A bulging or herniated disc or a bone spur may impinge upon or "pinch" a nerve as it exits the spinal cord and goes into a small canal called the foramen. For example, a pinched nerve in the lower back may cause leg pain; likewise, a pinched nerve in the neck can result in arm pain. By identifying the distribution of your pain, tingling, or numbness, your physician can work backward to understand which disc is herniated and which nerve is being pinched. Similarly, the pain from angina, a heart problem, can be confused with neck pain. Also, leg pain from peripheral vascular disease (e.g., blocked blood vessels) in the leg can be confused with the pain from spinal stenosis in the lumbar, or lower back, region.

Nerve Pain in a Headache

Migraine headaches are generally associated with both inflammation of the blood vessels and nerve irritation, resulting in a chemical cascade that ultimately becomes a migraine headache. Tension headaches are usually just from tight muscles around the head and neck, which can irritate nerves and cause a headache. Either way, we can treat the nerve pain with a nerve block, usually an injection of the local anesthetic lidocaine. We can also try injections of a dextrose solution around the trigger points, or tender areas, in the scalp. Often this is a cheap, safe, and fast way to get rid of a severe or long-lasting headache. If these techniques don't relieve the headache, it immediately alerts us that we need to look for another source of the pain.

Identifying Trigger Points and Myofascial Pain

Trigger points are especially sensitive areas in skeletal muscle that often have palpable nodules (knots) or taut bands (tightness). Trigger points can often be seen on ultrasound. Clearly, trigger points hurt. They also create referred pain patterns, meaning they can cause pain elsewhere in the body that doesn't seem directly linked to the painful point. We call this type of pain myofascial pain, meaning it comes from the fascia surrounding the muscles (myo = muscle). By injecting trigger points with local anesthetic, placing acupuncture needles into them, or even massaging them deeply, we can usually eliminate not only the pain in that area but also any referred pain. Deep massage can further help by freeing blockages in the fascial planes, allowing the muscles to glide freely over each other again. Perineural injections treat locally inflamed subcutaneous nerves irritated by chronic constriction injuries nearby.

Nerve Pain or Muscle Pain?

Nerve pain (sometimes called radicular pain) is caused by an irritated or pinched nerve, while muscle pain comes from an irritated trigger point. Sometimes differentiating between the two can be difficult. What makes this even more challenging is that both problems may occur simultaneously. To help differentiate this, we often recommend two tests: an EMG and an MRI.

EMG is helpful for detecting altered nerve function. An MRI, in contrast, can show the painful area in detail, letting us see all the structures, such as a bulging disc in the spine that is pinching a nerve. We have no good tests to detect trigger points, however. Instead, we check for them the old-fashioned way: with a physical examination.

Instinctively, we all know about trigger points, because most of us develop an inflamed trigger point at some time in our lives. Our instinctive response to the pain from a trigger point is to rub it hard, which can give an "ooh" sensation of relief.

Complex Regional Pain Syndrome

Complex regional pain syndrome (CRPS, also known as reflex sympathetic dystrophy or RSD) is one of the conditions a doctor will look for in a standard medical workup for chronic pain. Millions of people in the United States are living with CRPS. The main symptoms are various degrees of severe pain, swelling, and hypersensitivity to touch, usually in an arm or leg. CRPS usually happens after a triggering event, such as an injury, surgery, stroke, or heart attack that causes nerve irritation and pain in the affected area. The pain persists longer than expected and is often out of proportion to the severity of the initial injury. A patient may feel burning, muscle or joint stiffness, rapid hair and nail growth, and constriction of blood vessels at the site. The pain then becomes more severe, often associated with osteoporosis, muscle weakness, and further stiffening of the joints—sometimes until the joints become fixed in a contracted position. Although CRPS usually follows an injury or surgery, sometimes no cause can be found. If you have unusually intense, persistent pain, discuss the possibility of CRPS with your doctor. There's sometimes an unfortunate tendency for doctors to dismiss the debilitating pain of CRPS as "all in your head." If you're having this sort of pain, even if you haven't had an injury or surgery, insist on being heard and taken seriously by your medical team.

© Stocksy/ Marta Lebek

Pain

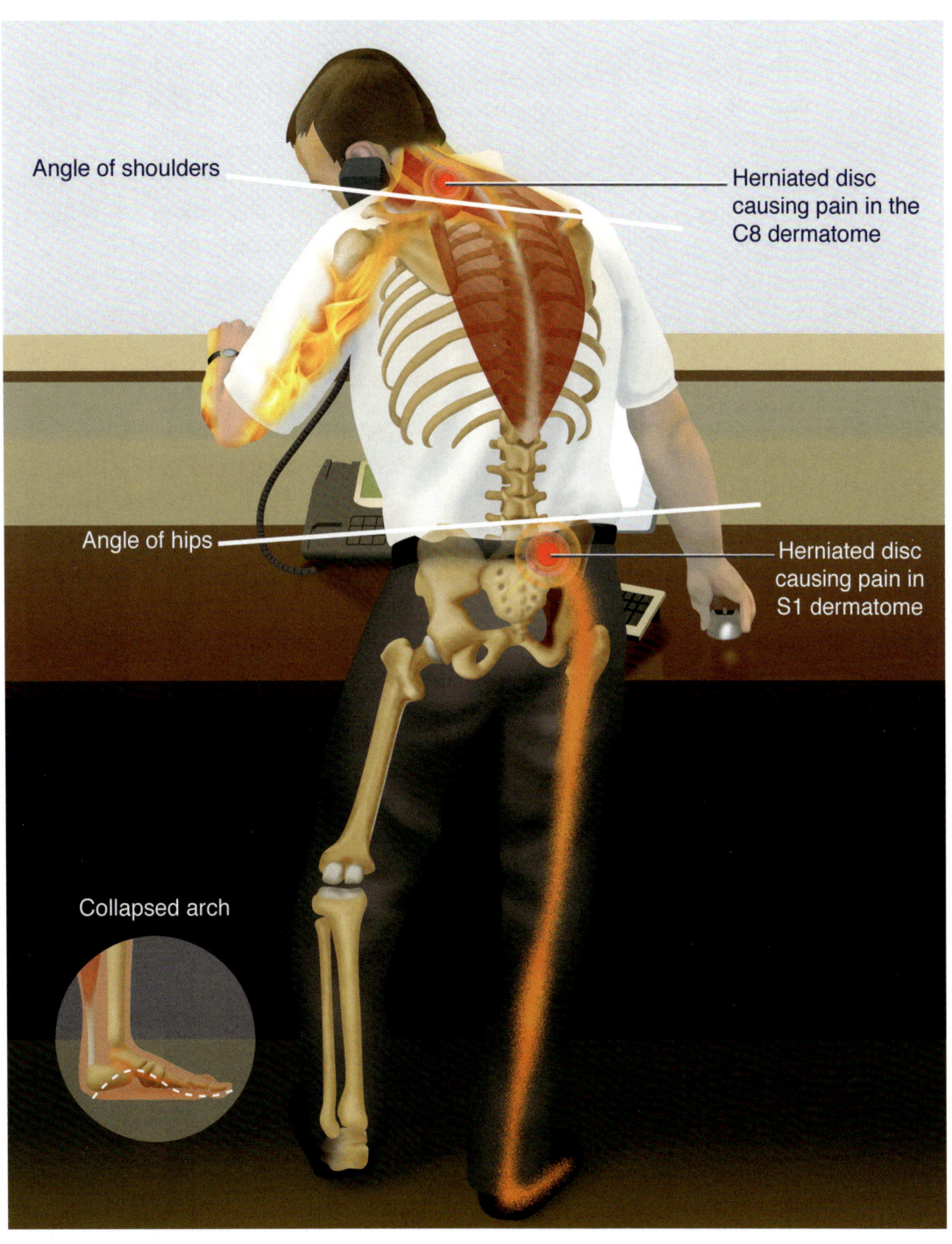

FIGURE 17.4 | Pain

Step 3: Understanding Body Mechanics, Structure, and Function

A biomechanical approach to diagnosing and treating chronic pain is based on the concept of tensegrity—the pull and push that is always being exerted on the bones, muscles, ligaments, and tendons.

Chronic imbalance sets us up for injury. When one muscle group is always pulling harder than the opposing group, it creates tension in the system. If muscles are pulling too hard in a particular area around the spine, the excessive stress in that area puts us at risk for injury. The spine needs to move fluidly, with each vertebra moving just a little as we twist or bend. When there is spasm in a particular area, that segment of the spine will "lock up." A healthy disc in the adjacent segment must compensate, taking on some of the biomechanical stress of the spine and extending the range of motion beyond normal limitations.

Another tipping point. When an area of the body is in a state of chronic stress or weakness, it doesn't take much to tip it into crisis. If, for instance, there is a weakened disc in the lower back, falling or bending the wrong way may be enough to cause that disc to herniate.

Another vicious cycle. Chronic muscle spasms are the body's basic response to injury and pain. If a disc in the spine is injured, however, spasms only irritate it further. This triggers the vicious cycle of spasm–pain–spasm.

Evaluating Body Mechanics, Structure, and Function

When we work with a patient in pain, we do a complete exam to evaluate the person's body mechanics, structure, and function. We start by looking at the most painful part of the body. We want to know how well that area of the body moves. Is it stiff and sore, implying that it is in spasm, or is it red and hot, suggesting inflammation? Can we make the pain return by moving or palpating that area in a certain way? If we can reproduce the pain, we have a better idea of what's causing it. Is the area tender? If so, the pain is originating from that area. If not, it is being referred from somewhere else.

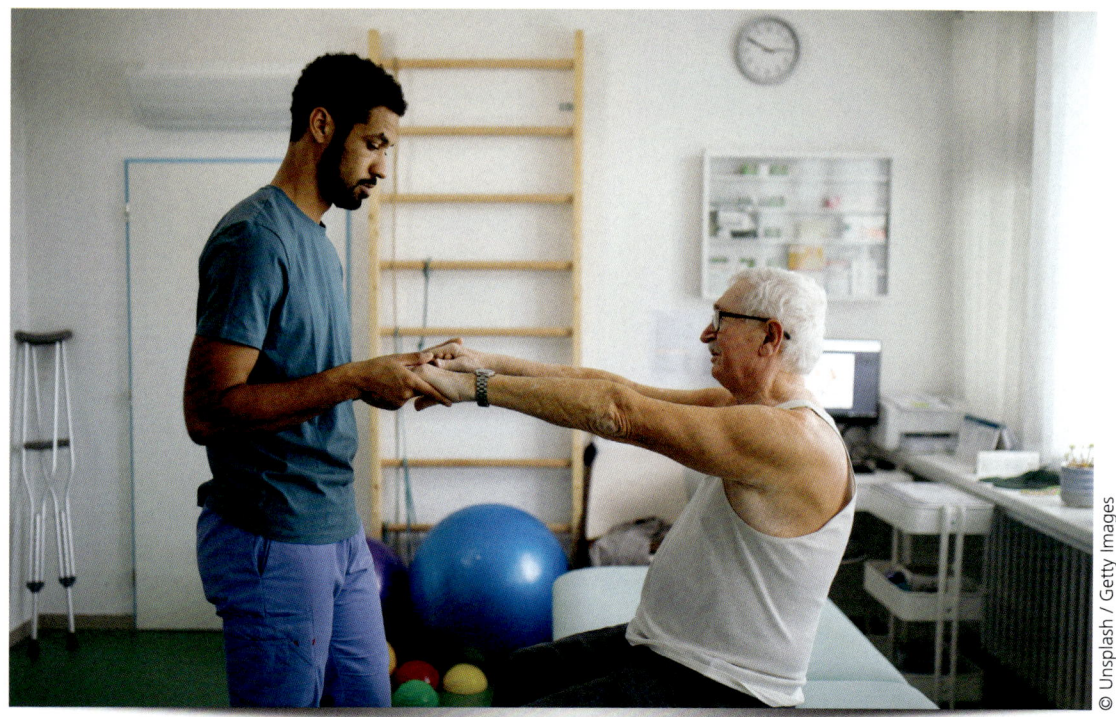

Understanding Pain from a Tensegrity Perspective

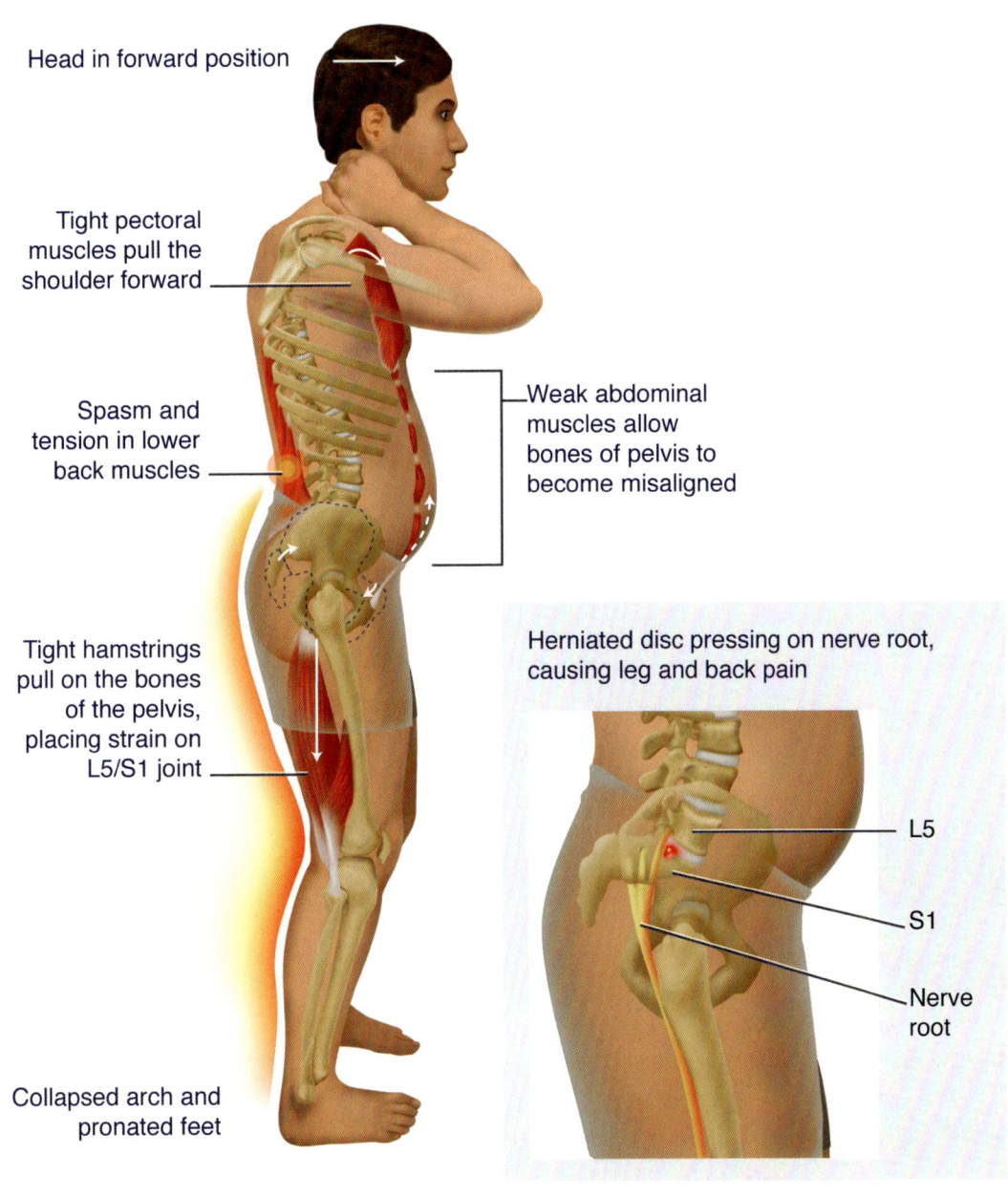

FIGURE 17.5 | Body Mechanics

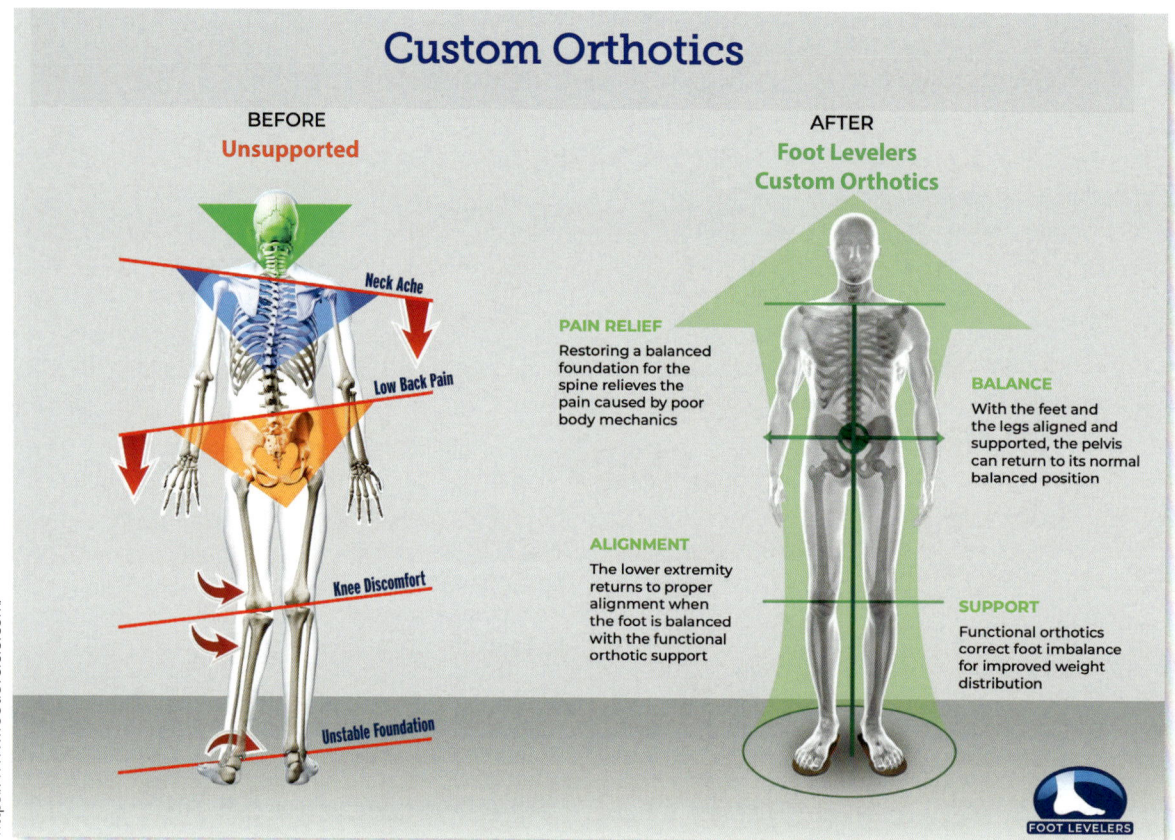

FIGURE 17.6 | Custom Orthotics. Image credit property of Foot Levelers, Inc.

Next, we evaluate the spine. We apply gentle pressure to the spine to find areas of tenderness. We also look at how each vertebra moves to learn if there is any dysfunction in that area.

After that, we look at the whole structure of the person's body to see how it could be affecting or causing chronic pain. We check to see if the hips and shoulders are level and if they move well. Sometimes the problem is caused by a misaligned kneecap. Do the arches of the feet drop?

We view the patient's profile from the side, looking for posture problems. Is the head in a "head-forward" position? Are the shoulders directly above the ankles? If not, what kind of pressure is this placing on the system?

We look at the status of the person's muscles, ligaments, and tendons. How do all the parts move together? Does the person have chronic tension in the muscles? What does the person look like when sitting, standing, walking, or running?

And finally, we ask, "What is the easiest, safest, most cost-effective way to get you better?"

Using Orthotics to Correct Posture

The diagram helps you understand how a problem in the foot can result in widespread interference in kinetic chains and tensegrity of the entire body. In treating chronic pain, we always look at the feet. We often recommend custom foot orthotics—shoe inserts that help correct a variety of foot problems by relieving pressure or realigning the feet.

When Pain Becomes Self-Perpetuating

Pain can breed pain. A good example is pain that develops after a motor vehicle accident. Right after a car accident that causes a whiplash-type injury to the neck, the person usually has only mild pain. At that point, x-rays and neurological exams are usually normal. Hours later, however, the injured muscles often go into spasm, causing pain. Typically, the muscles in spasm then recruit adjacent muscles, which also go into spasm as the body attempts to immobilize and stabilize the area. Within a few weeks, the injured person may be experiencing pain throughout the entire body. Pain can interfere with sleep and neurotransmitter regeneration, especially if the person was already stressed. This pain can continue for months or even years if not properly treated.

Myalgic Encephalomyelitis/Chronic Fatigue Syndrome (ME/CFS)

Myalgic encephalomyelitis/chronic fatigue syndrome (ME/CFS), also called fibromyalgia, is a complex illness that is characterized by long-term, body-wide pain and fatigue, often accompanied by problems with sleep, memory, and mood. It is also associated with other syndromes such as irritable bowel syndrome, migraines, tension headaches, TMJ syndrome, mitral valve prolapse, and interstitial cystitis.

We don't have a lab test or scan that can definitively diagnose ME/CFS. Instead, we do a thorough physical exam, then run blood tests and sometimes other tests to rule out other conditions. (It's important to remember that someone can have ME/CFS along with another condition.) During the physical exam, we ask about your energy level, fatigue, brain fog, memory problems, and sleep patterns. We also ask a lot of questions about your pain. In ME/CFS, pain that isn't caused by an injury is very common—and quite variable. The type of pain,

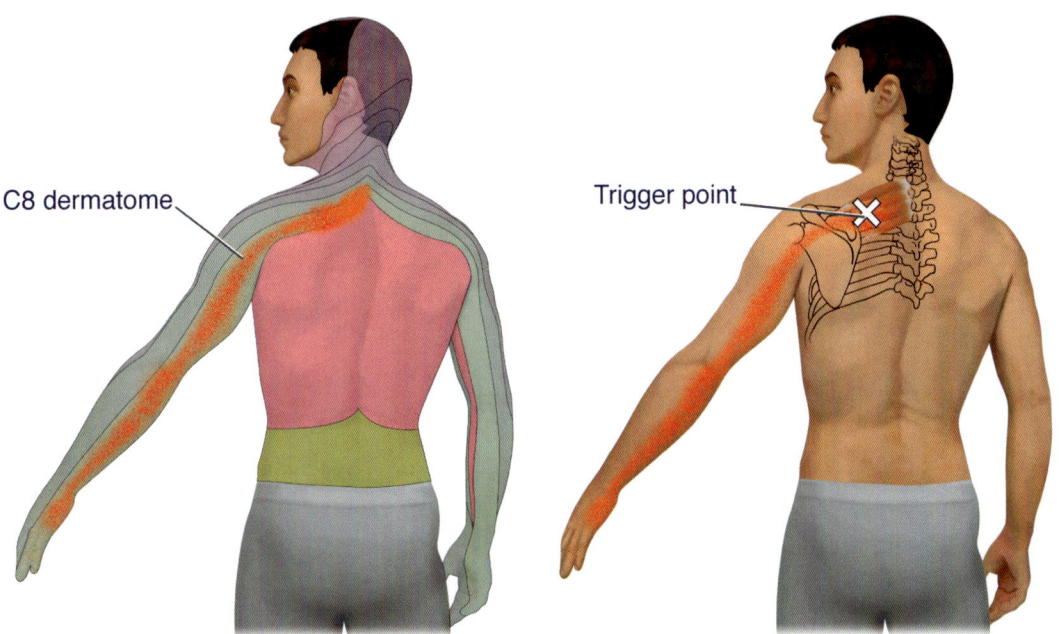

Is It a Pinched Nerve, Or an Irritable Trigger Point?
Referred myofascial pain and radicular pain (from a pinched nerve) can look and feel similar, but the treatment is different.

Dermatomal pain caused by a pinched nerve.   Myofascial pain caused by a trigger point.

FIGURE 17.7 | Referred Myofascial Pain

Trigger Points and Referred Pain

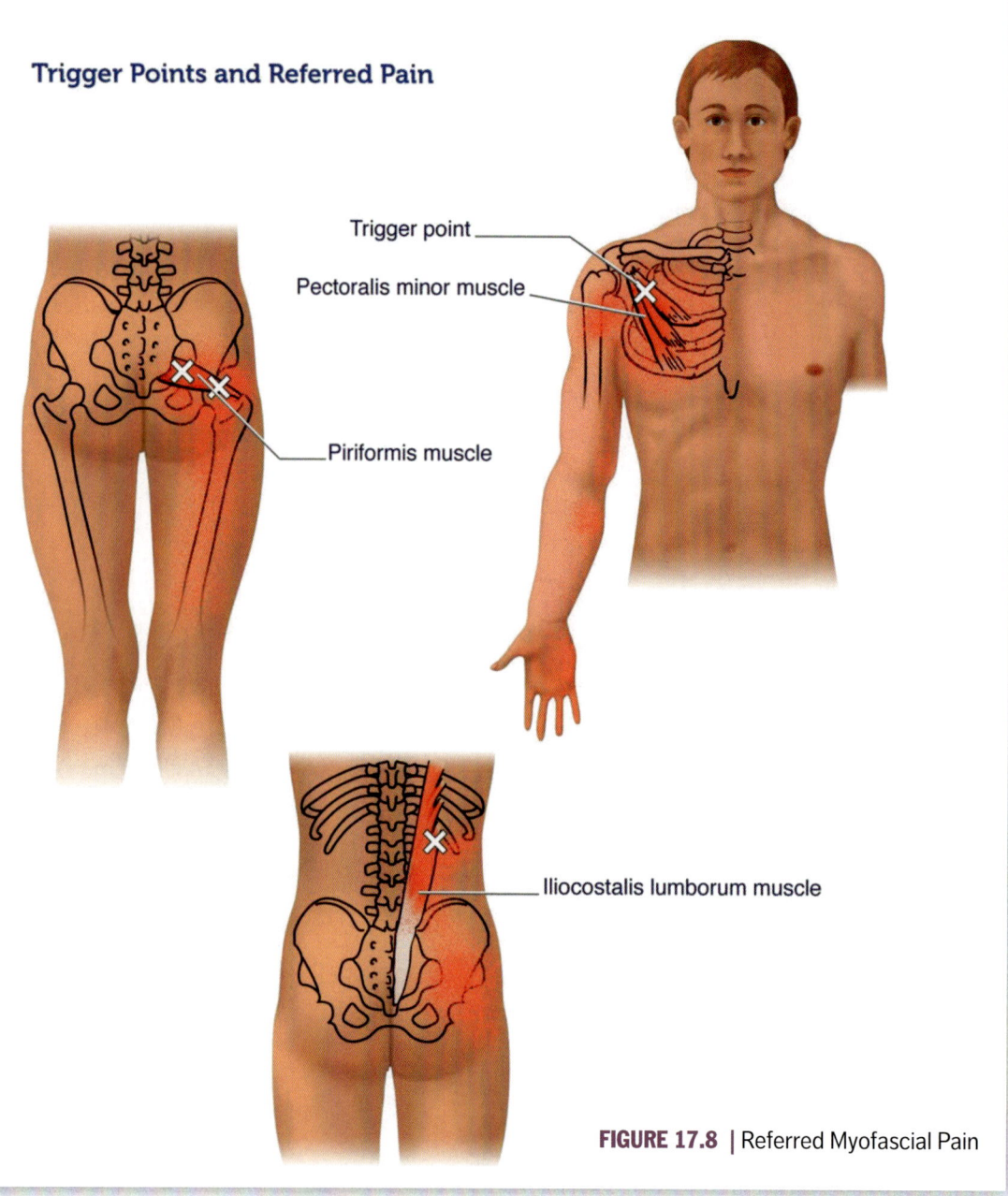

FIGURE 17.8 | Referred Myofascial Pain

where you feel it, and how severe it is can fluctuate a lot over time. We most commonly see muscle aches and pains, joint pains without swelling or redness, and headaches.

The tender points characteristic of ME/CFS are found all over the body, from the back of the head to the inner knees. Tender points are small spots on the body that are painful when pressed on firmly. They resemble trigger points, but the tender points of ME/CFS are associated with body-wide pain, while trigger points usually cause pain that is focused in just one area of the body.

We look at all your symptoms when making a diagnosis—not just your pain. Although there's no cure for ME/CFS, many of the gentle techniques we use for other forms of pain, such as massage and acupuncture, can be very helpful. We help you find ways to get better sleep, which helps improve energy levels and reduce pain.

Step 4: Central Sensitization: Evaluating Depression, Sleep, and Fatigue

Your brain and spinal cord make up your central nervous system, which controls all voluntary movement (such as walking and talking) and all involuntary movement (such as breathing). Your central nervous system is also where your thoughts and perceptions arise.

Central sensitization occurs when you become particularly sensitive to things that are processed by the central nervous system. That includes things you feel, such as pressure, itchiness, cold, heat, and pain. When your central nervous system is sensitized, you feel these sensations more strongly in two ways.

In hyperalgesia, something that is ordinarily painful to the average person is extraordinarily painful to you—it's like the volume on the pain is turned up. When you have hyperalgesia, something that causes chronic pain, such as an arthritic knee, can be very debilitating to you. When people with hyperalgesia are prescribed opioid painkillers, they can develop opioid-induced hyperalgesia, where the drug makes them become even more sensitive to pain.

A second form of central sensitization is allodynia, where you feel pain from things that ordinarily don't hurt, like cold temperatures, the feel of clothing against your skin, or even being hugged.

The causes of central sensitization vary from person to person and often involve one of three things: an underlying problem with inflammation; a problem in the autonomic nervous system (the part of your nervous system that controls involuntary actions; such as your heartbeat or blood pressure); or a problem with the body's stress response. We feel it is very important to track the sensitization to its source, not just prescribe drugs to treat the pain (and possibly make the pain worse).

Step 5: Immunity Evaluation: Identifying an Upregulated Immune System

When your immune system is chronically upregulated, it's sending out too many chemical messengers that cause inflammation, kill off healthy cells, create oxidative stress, and make your blood more likely to clot. Your joints hurt, you have aches and pains in other places, and you feel tired all the time. Such upregulation can lead to autoimmune and neurodegenerative diseases, which bring their own chronic pain.

Understanding Pain from Autoimmune Disorders

Autoimmune diseases affect the collagen-based connective tissue of several organs and systems. In autoimmune conditions, the body makes antibodies that attack its own tissues instead of attacking a foreign substance. Autoimmune disorders involving the musculoskeletal tissue include conditions such as rheumatic fever, scleroderma, rheumatoid arthritis, systemic lupus erythematosus, periarteritis, and serum sickness.

Autoimmune disorders almost always affect multiple systems of the body, so the pain they cause may be due to multiple reasons. For example, Crohn's disease may cause arthritis; other autoimmune diseases may cause myofascial pain and ME/CFS. Autoimmune diseases may also be associated with stress and depression, nutritional problems, inflammation, oxidative stress, gut disorders, and hormonal problems. (For more on autoimmune diseases and their treatment, refer to Chapters 10 and 11.)

Step 6: An Acupuncture Evaluation

Acupuncture—treating health problems by inserting and manipulating very fine needles into selected points on the skin—has been around for about three thousand years. The World Health Organization has cited acupuncture as a legitimate therapy for more than a hundred conditions, including many

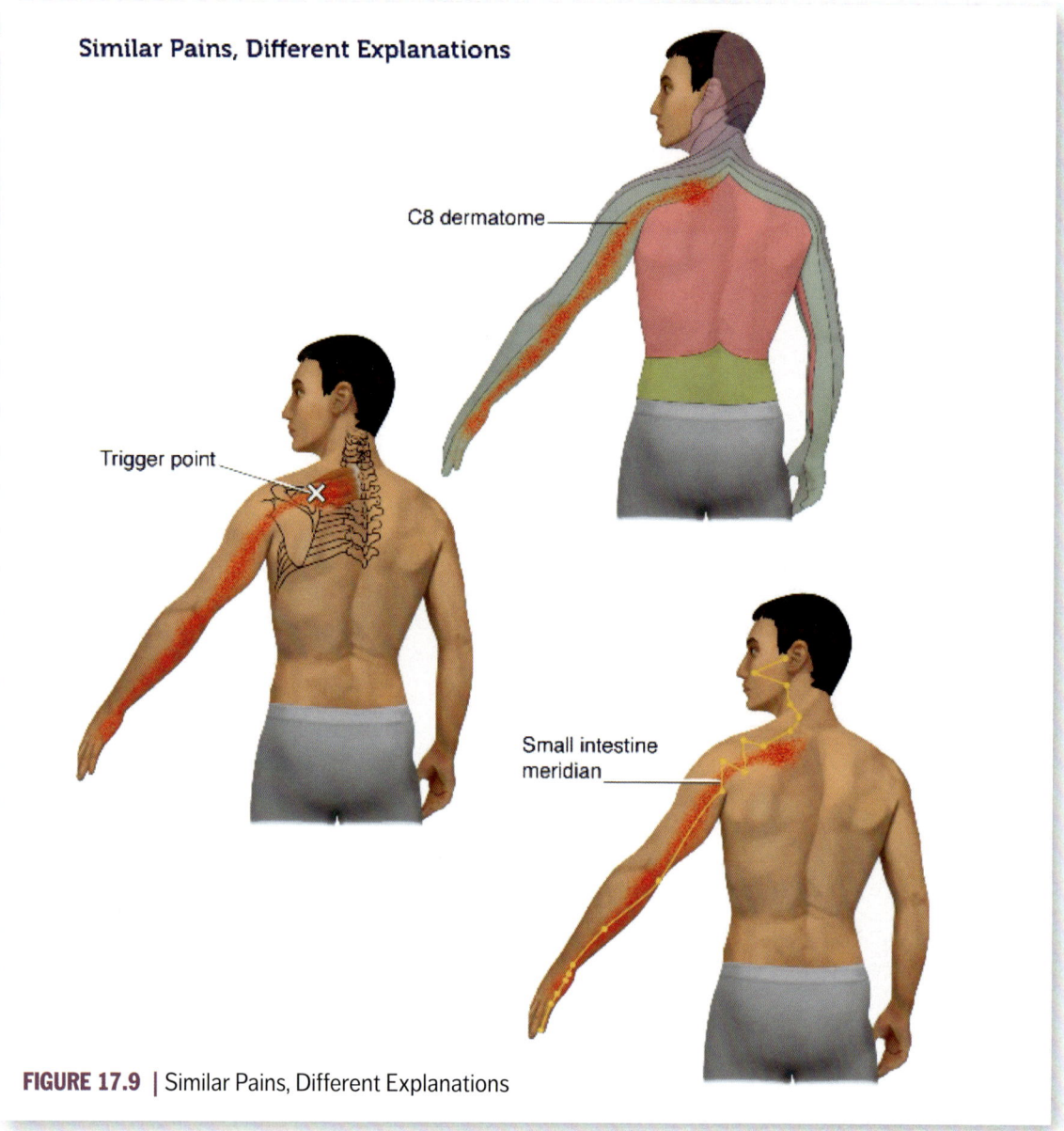

FIGURE 17.9 | Similar Pains, Different Explanations

related to chronic pain, such as low back pain, facial pain, and CRPS. Acupuncture isn't just a treatment, though—it's also a valuable diagnostic tool in dealing with chronic pain.

Acupuncture to Diagnose Pain and Discomfort

Traditional acupuncturists weren't taught to diagnose pain from a conventional, Western-based medical point of view. Rather, they saw pain as an expression of blocked chi. In traditional Chinese medicine, chi (also spelled qi) refers to an invisible electrical-type energy that flows around the body through meridians, or channels. Inserting acupuncture needles into the meridians at the right points unblocks areas of stagnant chi and restores the proper flow of energy. Unblocking chi is often helpful for relieving chronic pain.

Medical acupuncture builds on traditional acupuncture but takes a more scientific view of how acupuncture can achieve pain reduction. Acupuncture relieves spasms by deactivating trigger points, influences nerve and nervous system function, and seems to communicate with the whole body through the fascia.

Acupuncture is a wonderful tool to use for diagnosing chronic pain. There is a striking similarity between the location of acupuncture points and common trigger points. In fact, over 90 percent of these points overlap. Placing an acupuncture needle into a trigger point is somewhat like injecting it with a local anesthetic, although the pain relief is not immediate. In acupuncture, these points are referred to as ashi (pronounced "ah-shee") points, meaning "ow," which implies a sensitive spot.

Acupuncture meridians also correlate with the fascial planes of the body. In fact, injecting acupuncture points with a harmless radioactive dye shows the dye traveling down the fascial plane/meridian pathway. If the fascia is the body's internet, then the meridians are the electrical cables on which the information travels around the body.

One important series of points along the acupuncture meridians are the command points, located on the arms between the elbows and the fingers, and on the legs from the knees to the toes. Most of these points overlie large nerves. Inserting a needle at these points is a way of manually promoting changes in the nervous system—it can be compared to reprogramming the body's software.

Overlapping Systems

Acupuncture meridians, trigger points, fascia, and dermatome (nerve) pathways all have a

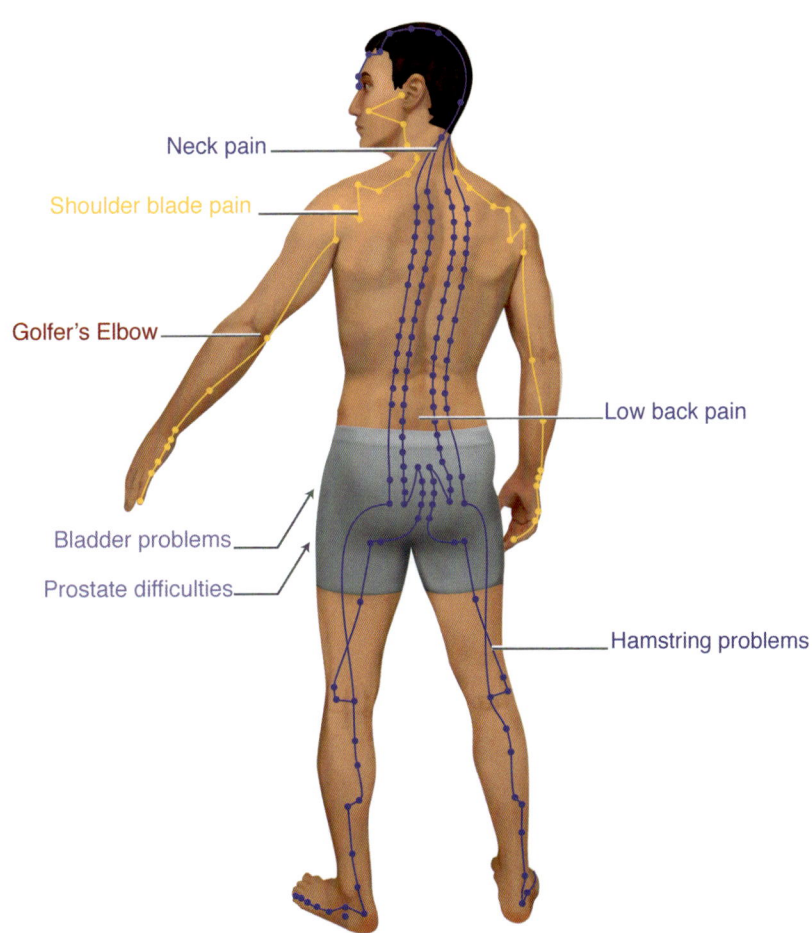

FIGURE 17.10 | Understanding Medical Problems from an Acupuncture Viewpoint

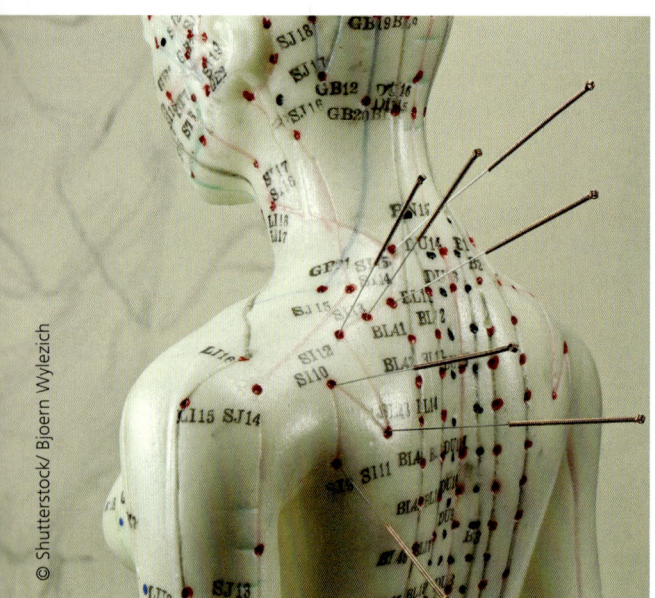

significant degree of overlap. As Figure 17.9 on page 258 shows, a pinched nerve at one of the vertebrae in the neck (C8), a trigger point in the shoulder, and an affected acupuncture (Small Intestine) meridian all involve the same area. After decades of experience of working with patients, we have come to see these systems as complementary. They are simply different dimensions of the body that provide a greater understanding of pain conditions. (We'll go deeper into how acupuncture works in the next chapter.)

Step 7: Understanding Your Biopsychotype: How Your Body Affects Your Mind

The propensity to develop certain illnesses—or to be healthy—is called a biopsychotype. Each biopsychotype is predisposed to certain physical and psychological problems. Understanding a person's biopsychotype is like understanding a computer's operating system—it teaches us a person's strengths and weaknesses, attributes, qualities, and tendencies to dysfunction or disease. When we learn how to correct this software program, we can correct multiple problems at the same time.

Understanding Biopsychotypes

The term biopsychotype was coined by Joseph Helms, MD, a wonderful teacher of ours. Dr. Helms has distilled his knowledge of acupuncture from Chinese, Japanese, Vietnamese, and French techniques. (French missionaries were some of the earliest Western practitioners of acupuncture.) Dr. Helms goes into detail in explaining these concepts in his excellent book, *Getting to Know You*.

Dr. Helms teaches how in everyone, four acupuncture meridians group together to form an archetype that is a predilection for both health and disease in that person. There are three main archetypes:

- **The Vision/Action Biopsychotype**
- **The Nurture/Duty Biopsychotype**
- **The Will/Spirit Biopsychotype**

Each biopsychotype is made up of four of the twelve traditional acupuncture meridians. When something goes wrong along any one of the four meridians, it is likely that there will be problems related to the other three as well. So, when patients learn they have problems occurring along their meridians, they can begin to see themselves in a different way. Instead of seeing multiple problems, they see that they have one global dysfunction, and they feel an immediate sense of empowerment just by knowing this.

The real benefit, though, is that when we start using acupuncture to treat problems along the meridian complexes, other problems go away—simultaneously and effortlessly. In acupuncture, the body and mind are seen as interconnected. Because the meridians deal with both psychological and physical problems, acupuncture treatment does not differentiate between mind and body dysfunction. Treating a meridian complex or biopsychotype helps both.

understanding

Understanding Your Biopsychotype

Most of our patients readily recognize important aspects of themselves in one of the three fundamental biopsychotypes. Not every characteristic of the biopsychotype will match each of your characteristics. In fact, some may even appear to contradict each other. They actually do. They represent the yin and yang values of each biopsychotype. In real life, we usually fall mainly in one category but have smatterings of other qualities and disturbances. A good acupuncturist will treat your current symptoms while balancing the rest of the energetic system, with the goal of preventing future problems.

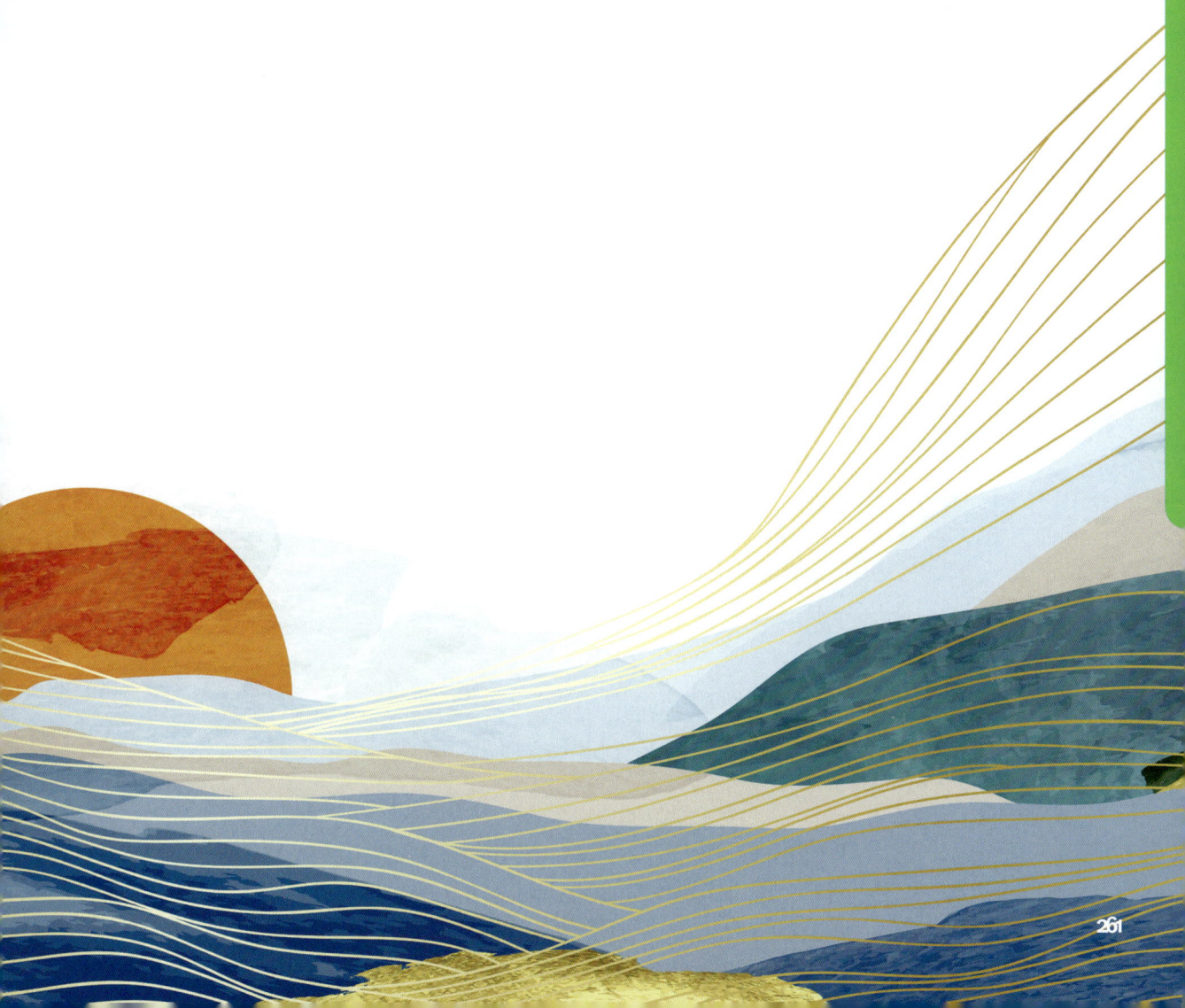

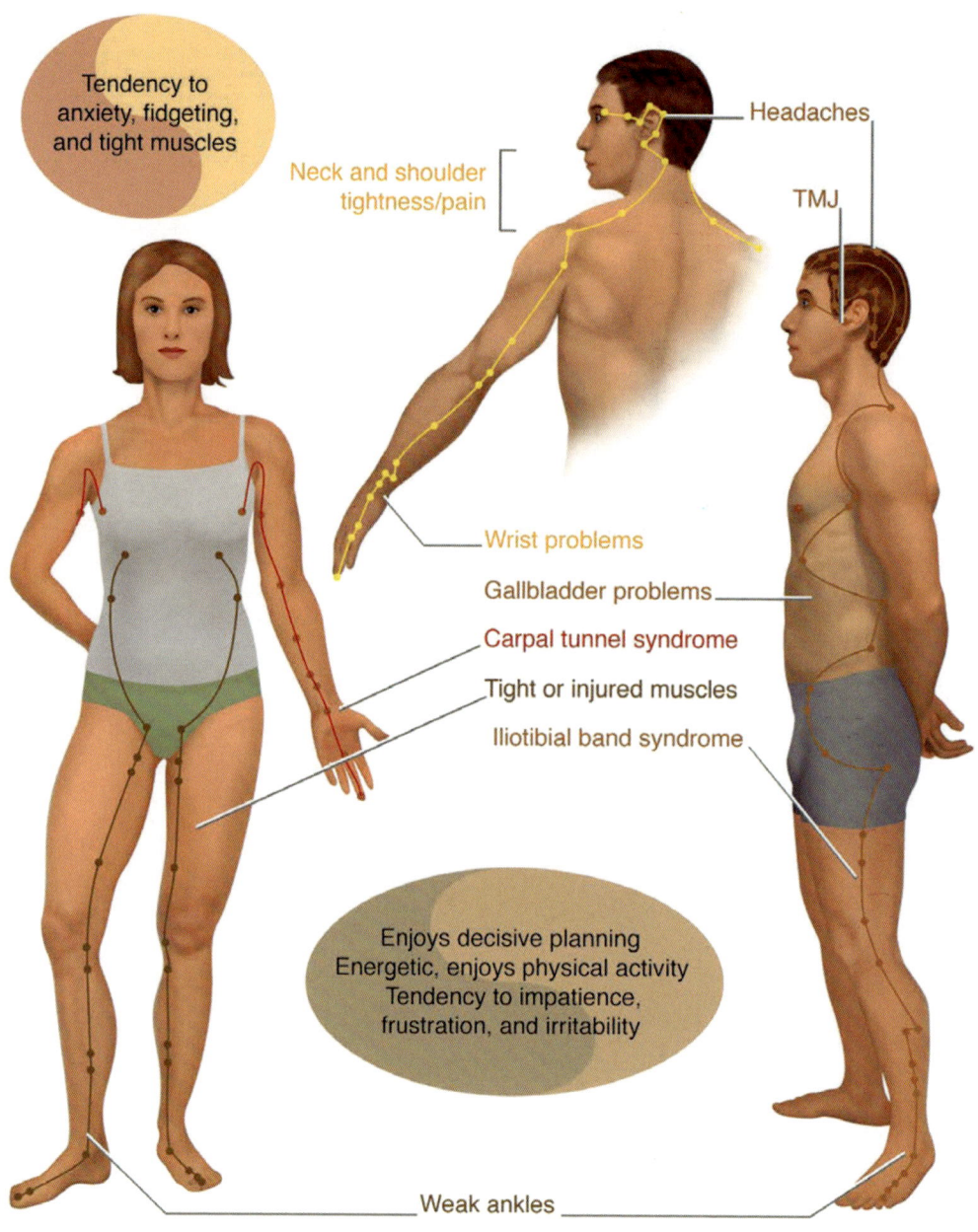

FIGURE 17.11 | The Vision/Action Biopsychotype

The Vision/Action Biopsychotype

Ask yourself if any of these characteristics of the vision/action biopsychotype apply to you:

- Are you ambitious and driven?
- Do you have a tendency to impatience and irritability?
- Do you find that you really need to exercise?
- If you get stressed, do you find you tend to get very anxious, fidgety, and even hypochondriacal?
- Do you crave caffeinated beverages, coffee, or dark chocolate?
- Do you use alcohol to calm you when you get anxious?
- Do you experience problems along the Liver, Gallbladder, Master of the Heart, or Triple Warmer meridians? Common problems are headaches, neck and shoulder pain or tightness, carpal tunnel syndrome, wrist problems, tight or injured muscles, dry eyes or vision problems, gallbladder problems, iliotibial band (ITB) syndrome, and weak ankles.

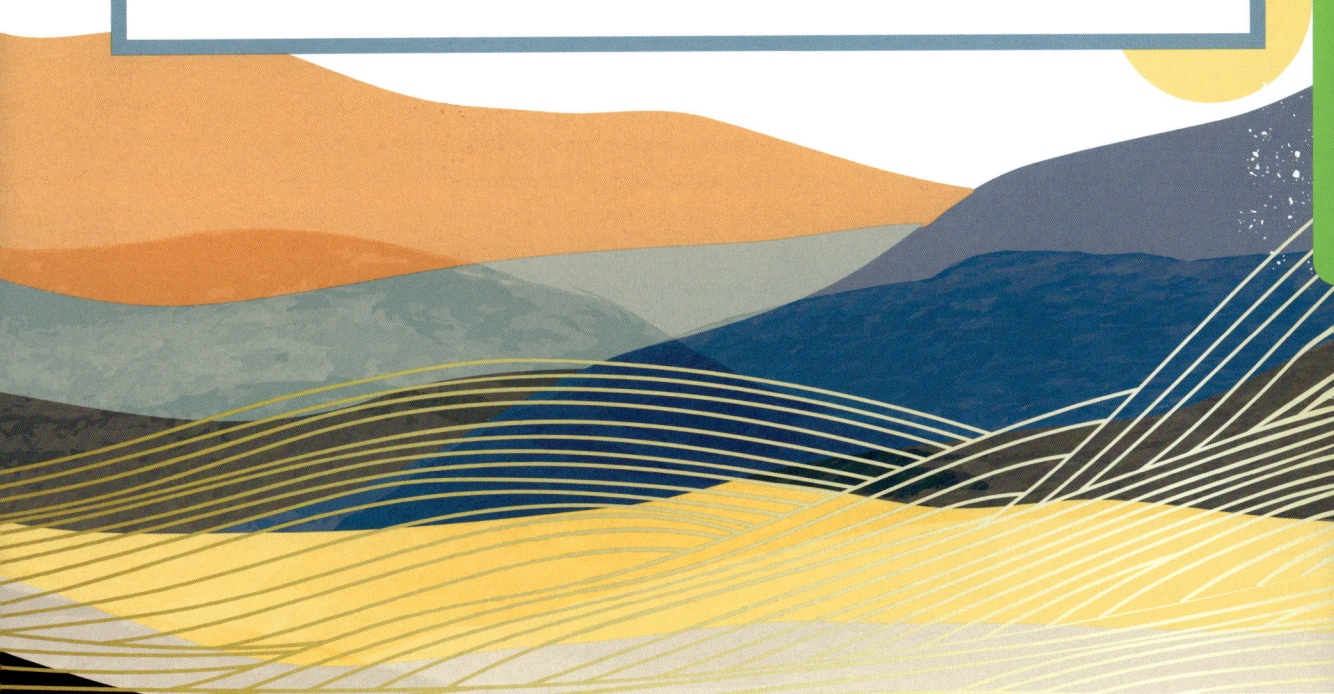

The Nurture/Duty Biopsychotype

Ask yourself if any of these characteristics of the nurture/duty biopsychotype apply to you:

- Are you organized and neat?
- Are you disciplined and responsible?
- Are you over-nurturing? Do you sometimes feel the need to take care of everybody you know?
- Do you put on weight easily?
- Are you calm and easygoing?
- Do you tend to get colds easily?
- Do you have a melodic or soothing voice?
- Are you a perfectionist? Do you tend to be self-critical?
- Do you sometimes go overboard with the good things in life, like overeating or overdrinking?
- Do you have a build that is quite thin?
- Did you gray early?
- Do you tend to have problems with belching, heartburn, cramping, or diarrhea?
- Do you have painful or irregular periods?
- Do you tend to worry or easily become melancholic?
- Do you have any of the following physical problems found along the Spleen, Lung, Large Intestine, and Stomach meridians? Common problems include chronic respiratory problems, difficulty getting pregnant, fibroids, a feeling of heaviness in your legs, hemorrhoids, varicose veins, diabetes, anemia, and De Quervain's tenosynovitis.

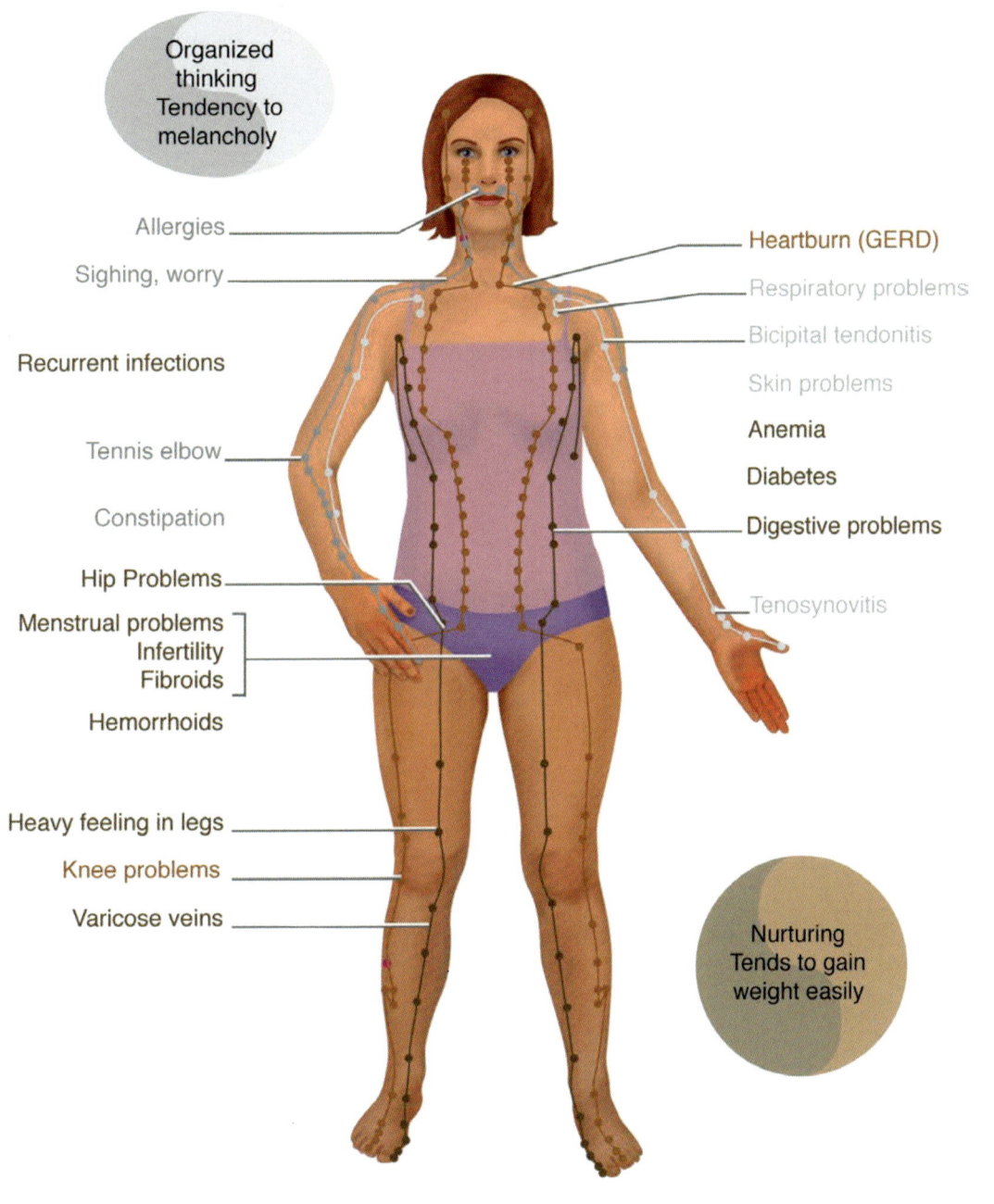

FIGURE 17.12 | The Nurture/Duty Biopsychotype

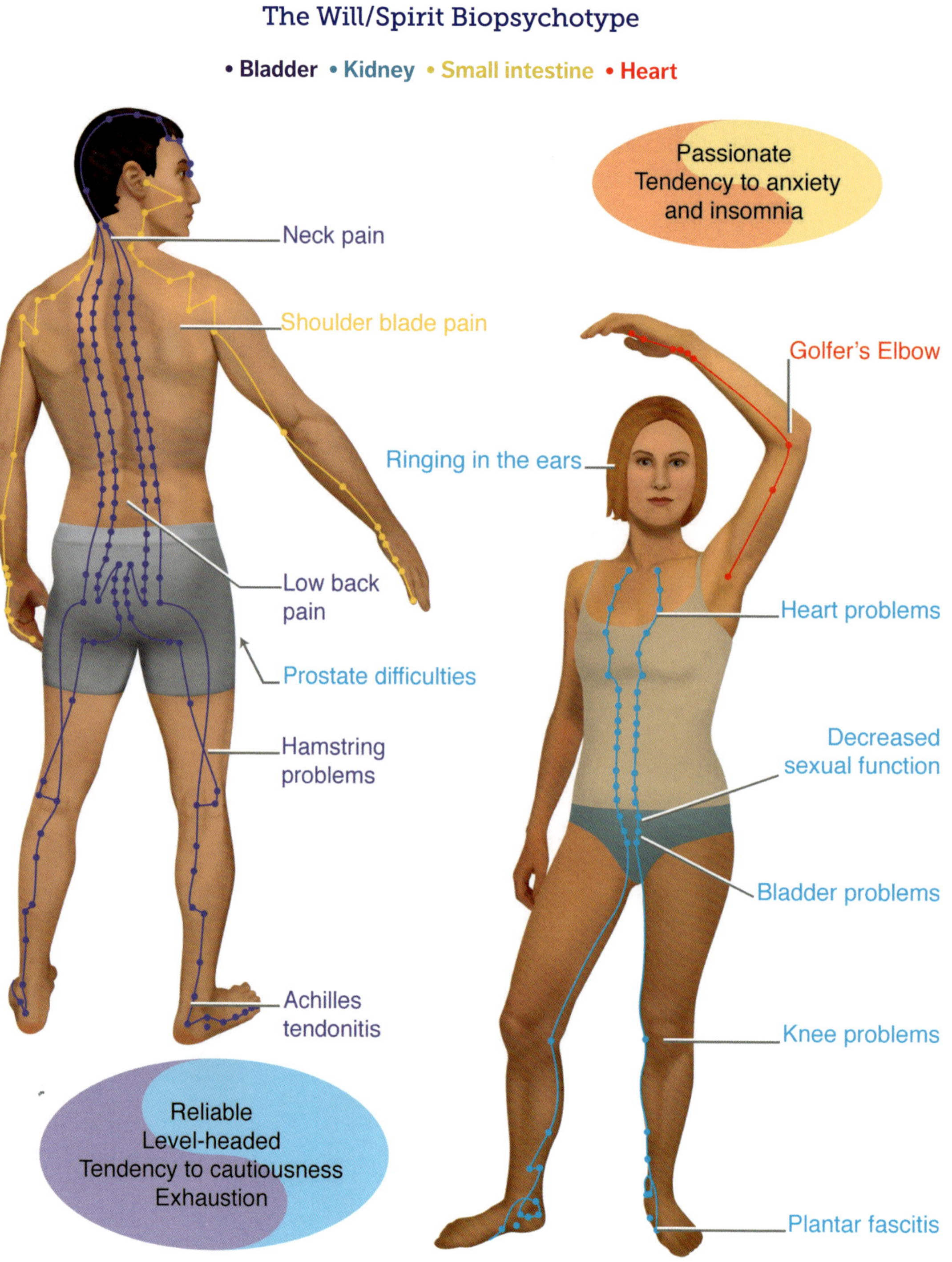

The Will/Spirit Biopsychotype

• **Bladder** • **Kidney** • **Small intestine** • **Heart**

- Neck pain
- Shoulder blade pain
- Low back pain
- Prostate difficulties
- Hamstring problems
- Achilles tendonitis
- Ringing in the ears
- Golfer's Elbow
- Heart problems
- Decreased sexual function
- Bladder problems
- Knee problems
- Plantar fascitis

Passionate
Tendency to anxiety and insomnia

Reliable
Level-headed
Tendency to cautiousness
Exhaustion

FIGURE 17.13 | The Will/Spirit Biopsychotype

The Will/Spirit Biopsychotype

Ask yourself if any of these characteristics of the will/spirit biopsychotype apply to you:

- Are you reliable and level-headed?
- Are you a good leader or an ardent follower?
- Are you usually in good health and hard-working?
- Are you full of doubt or lacking confidence at times?
- Are you passionate, sexual, and creative?
- Did you start balding early?
- Do you suffer from back problems or joint stiffness?
- Do you have chronic sleep difficulties?
- Do you have physical problems along the Kidney, Heart, Small Intestine, or Bladder meridians? Common problems include plantar fasciitis, Achilles tendonitis, prostate difficulties, bladder problems, low back pain, neck pain, ringing in the ears, golfer's elbow (medial epicondylitis), pain in your shoulder blades, and hamstring problems.

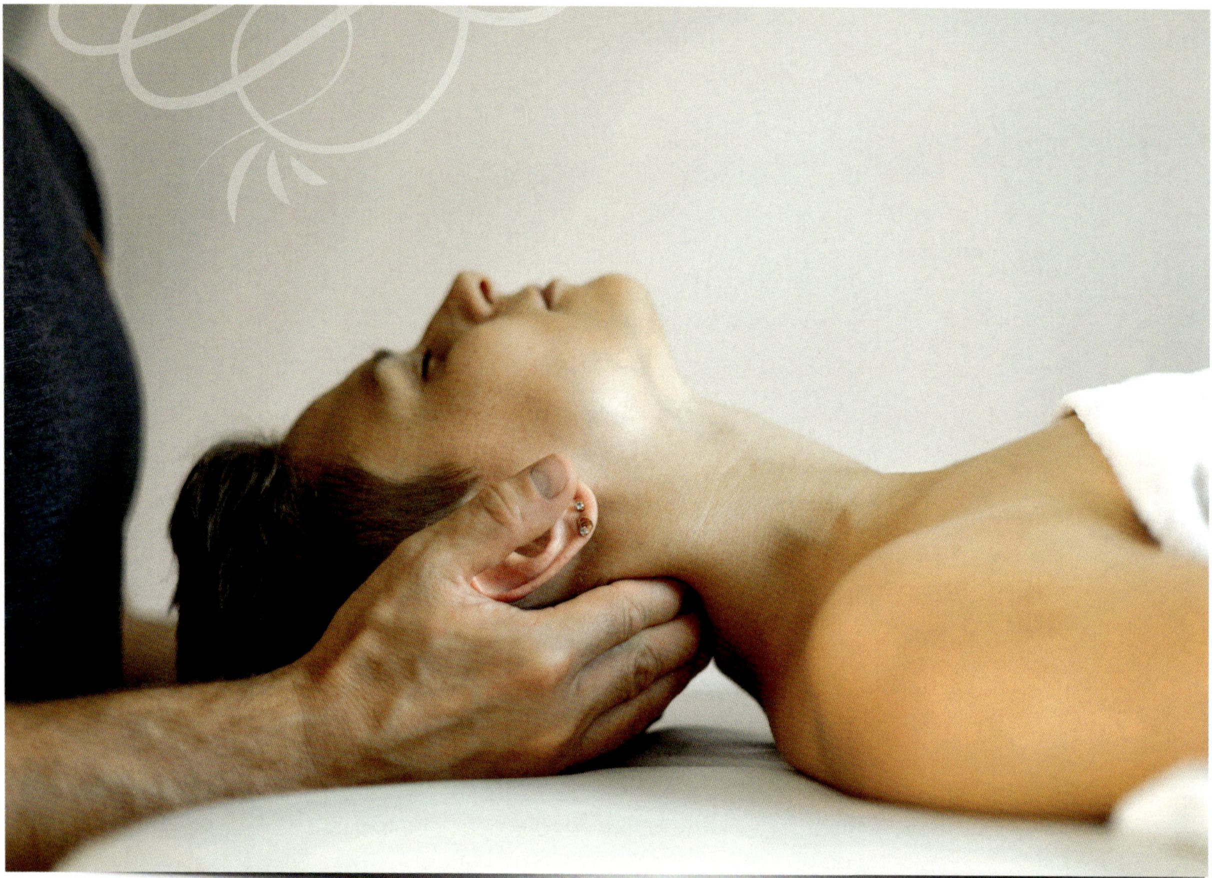

Bodywork and Suppressed Emotions

The biopsychotype is a helpful concept for understanding the mind-body connection. Physical problems are often associated with emotional issues and vice versa. A legitimate but uncommon concern for massage therapists, yoga instructors, and other therapists who touch their clients is that a patient may sometimes become very uncomfortable or upset during the session. An example is a woman who starts suddenly sobbing uncontrollably when her thighs are massaged. The action of the massage therapist has possibly triggered a forgotten or suppressed memory of being sexually molested as a child. Similarly, physical pain may be related to traumatic events, such as a car accident or seeing a pet get run over by a truck. Some bodywork therapies allow the patient to release hidden emotional issues and then process them in a safe way. Therapies combining touch and talk include Rubenfeld Synergy, the Rosen Method, and the Trager Approach.

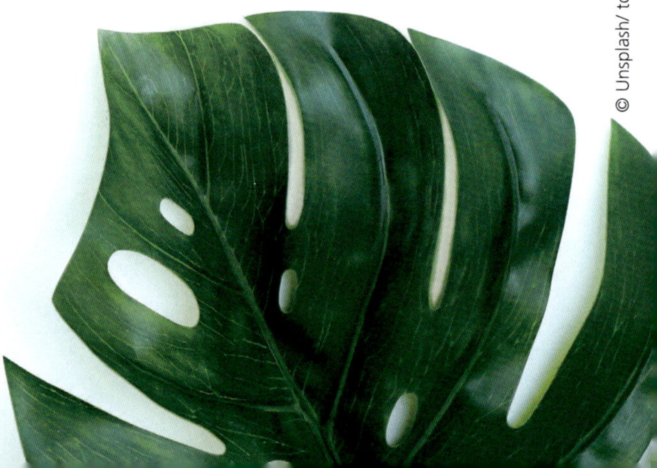

Energy in the Eastern Traditions

In every traditional healing system, working on the bioenergetic system of the body is integral to treatment. In China, the energy is referred to as *chi* or *qi*; in Japan it is called *ki*, and in India it is referred to as *prana*. In fact, almost every traditional culture has a word for the body's bioenergetic system. It denotes an energetic force or vitality—a force that underlies and supports health. Each system differs slightly in how it achieves this. Acupuncture masters insert acupuncture needles to improve the level and flow of this energy in the body, while others suggest *tai chi, chi gong* (*qigong*), or acupressure. Ayurvedic physicians of India often suggest yoga. Practitioners of martial arts cultivate their chi to become stronger, move better, and remain healthier.

Does this concept have a place in contemporary medicine?

We have a great deal of electrical activity in our bodies, much of which can be measured. An electrocardiogram (EKG) captures the electrical activity as it moves through the heart. An electroencephalogram (EEG) reads electrical brain wave activity, while an electromyogram (EMG) measures electrical activity produced by skeletal muscles. Magnetic resonance imaging (MRI) uses a magnet that creates a spin in our electrons, which is then translated into useful images of the inside of the body. On the other hand, the electrical activity in a cell wall that occurs each time a nerve fires still can't be measured. Measurable or not, any electrical impulse in the body creates an electromagnetic field—and every living object is surrounded by an electromagnetic field.

Today, no one would refuse to turn on the radio just because they can't observe radio waves, and no one would stop using the microwave oven because they can't perceive microwaves. After a century of breakthroughs in modern physics, we take these principles of electromagnetism for granted, even though we can't see them and don't even really understand how they work. Is it possible that we just haven't yet developed a technology sophisticated enough to properly assess the bioenergetic systems described in Ayurvedic and traditional Chinese medicine?

Bioenergetic distortions in traditional healing systems reflect physical, emotional, and spiritual imbalances. In other words, the electromagnetic field seems to be an interface between physiology, psychology, and spirituality. In India, yogic theory suggests that this power is concentrated or stored at nerve nodules along the spine, described as chakras. The chakras serve as power grids, sending energy out to the extremities where smaller transducers around the joints, called nadis, then help transfer bioenergy to the tissues. If traditional Indian philosophy refers to the power grids of bioenergy or chakras, traditional Oriental medicine has been more concerned with the flow of energy between them. These are the meridian systems, which act as power lines, or the network on which the software of the body runs. The entirety of the bioenergetic field that exists in and around the body is thus called *prana* or *chi* (*qi*). This subtle physical energy is also referred to as the aura of the body.

Energy Healing

Energy healing refers to a group of therapies such as healing touch, therapeutic touch, and Reiki. Energy healers train to increase their perception of the aura, the subtle physical energy of the body. They are taught to sense imbalances in the body and then correct them on a bioenergetic level. In our experience, the ability to do this can vary greatly. However, in a study we did at our center, we found that trained energy healers were able to perceive areas of pain on patients without even asking them where the pain was. In our study, we recruited patients who had reported back pain and had recently had an MRI. We asked the patients to draw their pain on an anatomical chart. Two energy healers drew their perceptions of the patients' pain on a similar anatomical chart, without any input from the patient. We compared both charts to the results of a third chart, an MRI-generated image which showed a typical nerve-generated pain pathway. The healers' drawings resembled the subjects' drawings more closely than the MRI-generated images. In other words, they were able to perceive where the patient felt pain much as the patient did.

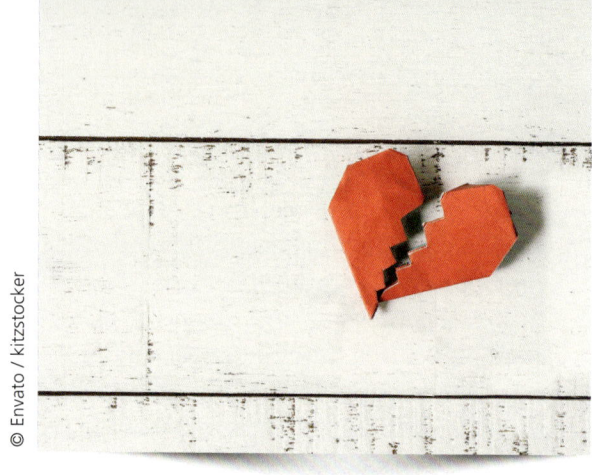

© Envato / kitzstocker

Step 8. How the Mind Affects the Body

We often come across patients who give us metaphorical clues to what is going on in their minds and in their lives. Thoughts are a window to the subconscious. A patient with heartburn may confide that he "can't stomach" a certain situation. People with neck pain may tell us about the "pain in the neck" in their lives. Patients with back pain may fear their support system is crumbling and may talk about feeling forced to "back down." Very subtly, they are giving us insight into the interrelationship between their minds and their bodies.

This idea was long dismissed by scientists. However, a very real syndrome that mirrors this is called the broken heart syndrome or Takotsubo cardiomyopathy, originally described by Japanese cardiologists in 1991. In this syndrome, the apex of the heart, located on its lower tip, enlarges shortly after a stressful situation, such as the death of a loved one. Patients feel sudden chest pain, often thinking they are suffering a heart attack. Fortunately, the syndrome, though frightening, only rarely causes any permanent heart damage or death.

There are many links between mind and body. One of the major connections is the interaction between neurotransmitters, stress hormones, and the pain generators that exist in our bodies.

Every time we have a thought or an emotion, our nervous system is flooded with neurotransmitters. Some, like serotonin and GABA, produce a sense of calm and well-being. Others can cause anxiety, fear, or anger. When we have the same repetitive negative thoughts or feelings, we bathe our bodies in stress hormones, depleting neurotransmitters such as serotonin. Since one of serotonin's jobs is to switch off pain, a patient depleted of serotonin will end up in the pain–depression–pain cycle.

Sometimes, adding an antidepressant medication is all that's needed to break the cycle. For other patients, the addition of an antiseizure medication such as gabapentin (Neurontin), pregabalin (Lyrica), valproic acid (Depakote), carbamazepine (Tegretol), or topiramate (Topamax) will help to calm down the nervous system and relieve pain. The pain fibers of people with chronic pain are switched on all the time. These medications help to soothe them and relieve the pain. Yet there are other times when even the best medication doesn't seem to help, or its side effects become intolerable.

In these cases, we need to do more. This is where we find that looking at other systems can help. For example, rebalancing the adrenals or reducing inflammation might be what's needed to help improve a patient's mood and pain.

Previous Trauma and Pain

Imagine someone who has lived through a highly traumatic situation such as a rape, an accident, a disaster, or a war experience. Often, these people suffer from post-traumatic stress disorder (PTSD), an anxiety disorder that is triggered by experiencing an event that causes intense fear, helplessness, or horror. Every time something happens that reminds the victim of the original experience, the body is triggered into a highly reactive state—a flashback—that recreates the neurochemicals and the emotions associated with the original event. Emotionally, the person feels as if the traumatic event were occurring all over again. For example, someone who was traumatized by war may find that any loud noise can set in motion a biochemical and emotional cascade—a stress response in which the nightmare of the original war trauma will be replayed.

Although not everyone who has experienced a horrific event suffers from PTSD, most of us have suffered events involving emotional trauma or even abuse. High-intensity pain or emotion, sexual abuse, or a change in consciousness due to trauma or even an anesthetic can be indelibly engraved into our minds.

Previous stress can trigger a state of chronic hypervigilance, with resultant anxiety, mood swings, and depression. This state of stress can lead to the domino effect of emotional trauma: inflammation, exhaustion, and depression. For someone who has lived through trauma or intense stress, sometimes even a minor event can easily topple them into a chronic pain condition.

A skilled mind-body therapist can play an important role in helping patients who are struggling to cope with their pain and grapple with post-traumatic stress. Diagnosing mind-body problems is not always easy. Some disorders are obvious, such as mental suffering that clearly begins after an emotional trauma, while others are not. Emotional trauma should always be considered for unexplained cases of pain.

Step 9. Lifestyle Analysis: Finding the Causes and the Solutions

To treat pain disorders properly, we need to know if the patient has counterproductive lifestyle habits that can reactivate the pain. Sometimes the causes are obvious, but in other cases, they are elusive. The solution is for the patient to have a good observer and coach and to become more self-aware. We look carefully at habits and activities that can affect body mechanics and recovery.

Habits that Affect Body Mechanics

• **Repetitive motion.** Performing the same movement repeatedly can cause an injury. Knitting, typing, hammering, digging, or even texting on a phone can be culprits here.

• **Posture.** Are you slumping forward, slouching, or hunching your shoulders? Do you hold your phone between your neck and your shoulder? What is your posture like when you sit at a desk? Are your shoulders close to your ears when you're on the computer? Do you use an ergonomic rest pad for your wrists? All of these factors can affect the physical stress you place on your body.

• **Clothing or accessories that affect the body.** Are you sitting on a fat wallet in your back pocket? This can irritate your sciatic nerve. Knee-high socks can pinch the peroneal nerve, causing leg pain. Heavy purses, bags, and backpacks can cause neck, shoulder, and back pain. Pay attention to your areas of discomfort and see if any of these factors are irritating you.

• **Under- or over-exercising.** Both lifestyles can cause problems. Too little exercise leads to under-conditioning. Too much exercise leads to overuse and repetitive stress injuries.

- **Lack of stretching or lack of strengthening.** Both can affect the balance and tensegrity of the body, making injury more likely.

- **Sleep position and sleep deficiency.** People who sleep lying on their stomachs with their neck twisted to the side place a significant amount of stress on the neck. In addition, sleep deficiency can lead to poor recovery from pain.

Habits that Affect Recovery

- **Smoking.** Decades of research has shown that smoking leads to constriction of arteries and blood flow and, as a result, to poor healing. Smokers who have back surgery do much worse than nonsmokers. Similarly, smokers take longer to recover from injuries in general.

- **Alcohol or substance abuse.** While one to two drinks a day seems to be beneficial to most people, alcohol abuse results in problems throughout the body. In addition to causing bodily damage, alcohol abuse can cause depression, leading to more pain. Street drugs can aggravate pain conditions in myriad ways.

- **Excess caffeine or overuse of other stimulants.** Stimulant use can be associated with poor sleep and an adrenalized "wired and tired" state, leading to the need for more stimulants.

- **Stress excess and stress addiction**. Ever notice how some people are drawn to drama? We all tend to be sucked into drama, whether we are watching it in the movies or on the evening news—or feel as if we are involved in our own personal reality show. In our world full of information, technology, and action, we need to learn to switch off at times. The drama will always continue. We don't need to remain attached to it!

- **Negative self-talk.** Every time you find yourself doing this, make a conscious decision to get well, be well, live well, and stay well!

- **Nutritional deficiency.** Poor diet can lead to a lack of the nutrients necessary to repair our ligaments, tendons, muscles, and organs. (For ideas on how to nourish your body, see Chapter 9.)

- **Many other habits that can influence your recovery.** Pay attention to what is going on in your life and see how it is affecting you!

Step 10. An Integrative Diagnosis and a Transformational Treatment Plan

Getting sick is a process. Getting well is a process too.

In a stepwise fashion, we just took a brief look at how chronic pain develops. The next step is to apply a systems approach to help you get better.

Here are some of the most important elements to focus on as you consider this:

- Your body is your biography. It can give you—and us—insight into many of the conditions you are suffering from.

- A physical examination and palpation of the body can give us an idea of your makeup, your lifestyle, your hormonal balance, and your previous injuries. It can show us structural changes, as well as clues to underlying emotional states. We can then use this information to figure out impending problems. From there, you can take steps to avoid future illness.

- Draw on the knowledge of several disciplines. Learn to access information from different diagnostic and healing modalities. Use what is safe and effective—and what makes sense to you. They need to make sense to you. They need to be safe and effective.

- Access new tools for diagnosis. As you explore this stepwise approach to diagnosis, you will gain access to the tools you need to resolve your health issues. This multidimensional understanding will give you the insight and tools to enable you to play a greater role in your own healing.

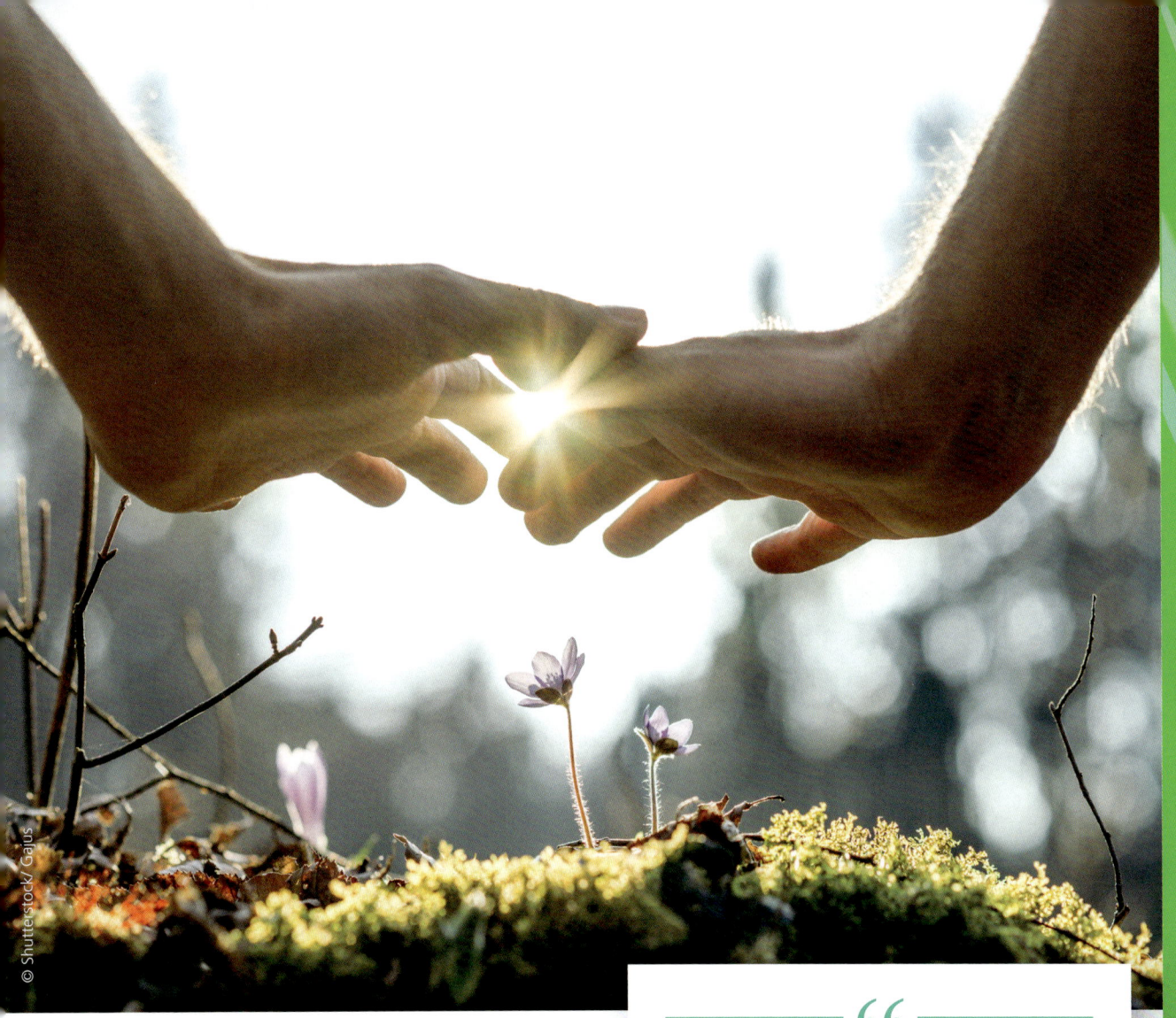

- Tap the resources of a healthcare team. In addition to medical diagnostics, an integrative team typically includes resources for evaluating biomechanical issues, nutritional problems, psychological concerns, and more. Working with more than one provider expands your treatment options and can have a synergistic effect on healing.

- Remain open to a range of reasonable solutions. There is no one way to achieve health and healing. You will need to assess safety, cost, and benefit before you decide what to do.

> When we change our daily lives – the way we think, speak and act – we change the world.
>
> –Thich Nhat Hanh

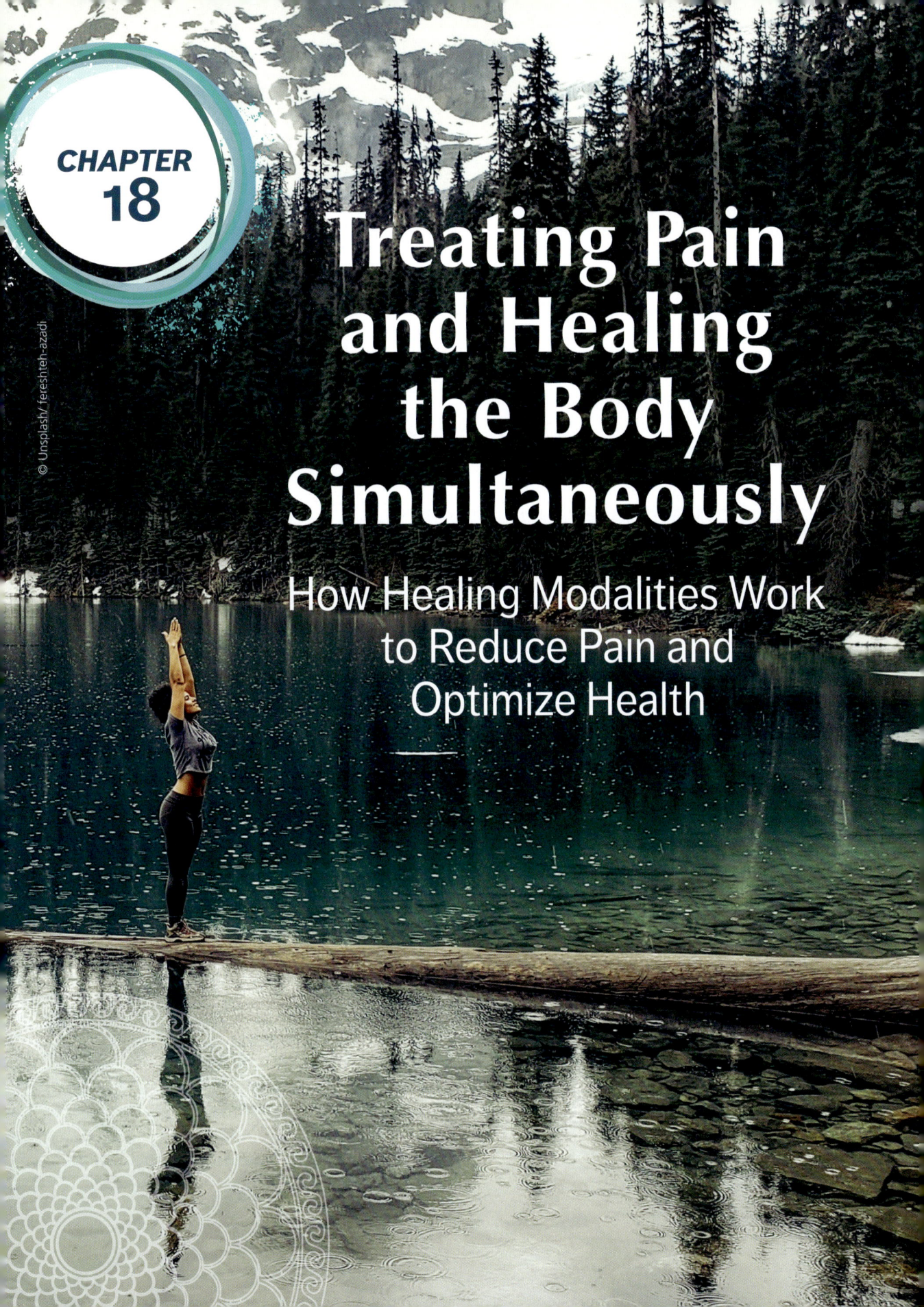

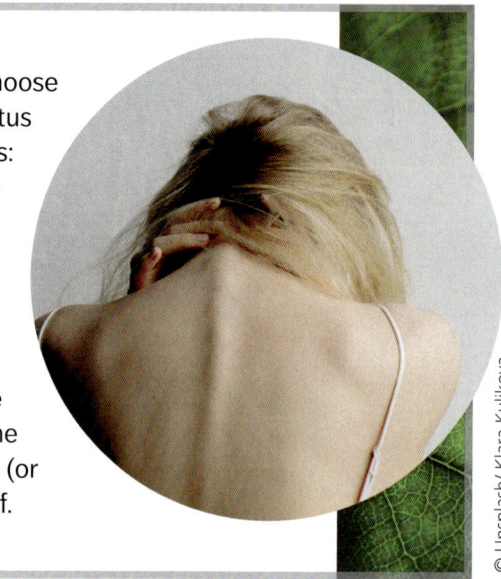

Pain is that initial awareness that we need to choose another path. Chronic pain is often the impetus to help us make changes. The big question is: Which changes? What will it take to make the pain go away? Obviously, if you already knew what you should be doing, you would have been doing it. Pain is the impetus to seek help.

That is why patients with chronic pain come to us. Patients want a quick fix. But, as we always say, getting better is a process. As health care providers, we want to partner with you. We want to find out what the best options are for you. We want to find out what we (or others) can do for you and what you can do for yourself.

© Unsplash/ Klara Kulikova

Our Stepwise **Approach to Chronic Pain**

We begin by thoroughly assessing the patient from a medical standpoint. We like to know everything about their pain. We look at x-rays, ultrasounds, magnetic resonance images (MRIs), electromyograms (EMGs), and standard lab blood work including vitamin D, high-sensitivity C-reactive protein (hs-CRP), and thyroid levels. We use standard medications and refer for physical rehabilitation, epidurals, and surgery where appropriate. After that, we follow these steps:

1. **We assess and treat what are called comorbid medical conditions.** In other words, what else may be contributing to the pain?

2. **We assess and treat depression.** As we have seen already, neurotransmitters can play havoc with pain.

3. **We like to know what the patient's stress level is and how it is being dealt with.** Certain people tend to somatize their pain. In other words, they take emotional pain and put it into their body. Other patients may be hypervigilant, which makes them anxious and unusually responsive to pain. We try to teach patients to observe rather than react to their symptoms. If necessary, we recommend psychological counseling in various forms for this.

4. **We examine all our patients carefully, looking for "pain generators."** We especially want to find the source of "invisible" or myofascial pain. Often we can press on a trigger point and reproduce the very pain they are having. We treat this using massage, acupuncture, Rolfing, and occasionally muscle relaxant herbs or medications.

5. **We look for and treat dysautonomia.** This is especially important in patients who have a chronic regional pain syndrome (CRPS) or reflex sympathetic dystrophy. CRPS can sometimes be aggravated initially by direct therapy, so if it is severe, we will use energy healing modalities or acupuncture at different sites in the body. (Refer back to Chapter 15 for a discussion of CRPS.)

6. **We assess patients from a structural standpoint.** We look at the area of pain as well as the reciprocal area. For

instance, if a patient has neck pain, we look at the front of their neck, as well as their shoulders, lower back, pelvis, legs, and feet. We look for a "march of symptoms." Did the pain start in the right ankle, then move to the right knee, low back, shoulder, and finally to the neck? Treatment includes manipulative therapies, acupuncture, Rolfing, and massage.

7. **We assess what is known as the biological terrain.** In other words, we try to assess what kind of physiology a patient has. We use functional labs to further evaluate nutrient deficiencies, oxidative stress levels, mitochondrial dysfunction, dysbiosis in the gut, and hormone and neurotransmitter levels. We treat this appropriately with supplements and/or medication.

8. **We assess bioenergetic imbalance.** We treat this using acupuncture, energy healing, and frequency specific microcurrent.

9. **Finally, we like to understand the patient from a social and spiritual perspective.** We want to know about family, work, and community life, and whether aspects of these are increasing or decreasing stress and coping levels. Treatment for this aspect is obviously delicate, and it is of utmost importance that the therapist acts only as a guide and a reflector for the patient. It is important not to impose opinions or spiritual beliefs on a patient. We do know that when people are engaged in their own communities and feel a part of something larger than themselves, they do better. Our job is simply to facilitate this.

10. **Then, as patients get better, we want to see if regenerative medicine may have value for them.** Are they at an early stage of joint disease where their cartilage is fraying, ligaments are loose, or they have early joint degeneration? This is now all treatable with prolotherapy and stem cell therapy.

The good thing about today's information age is that all of us can quickly learn about the various treatments that are available. On the other hand, claims sometimes abound with little validating evidence. That is why you need to be a key player on your own healthcare team. You will want to consider outcomes, safety, and cost and then decide what you want to do.

As you embark on your transformational treatment plan, remember that chronic pain doesn't just suddenly disappear. Typically, you will pass through several healing stages on the way to recovery.

Stage 1: Relief and Repair

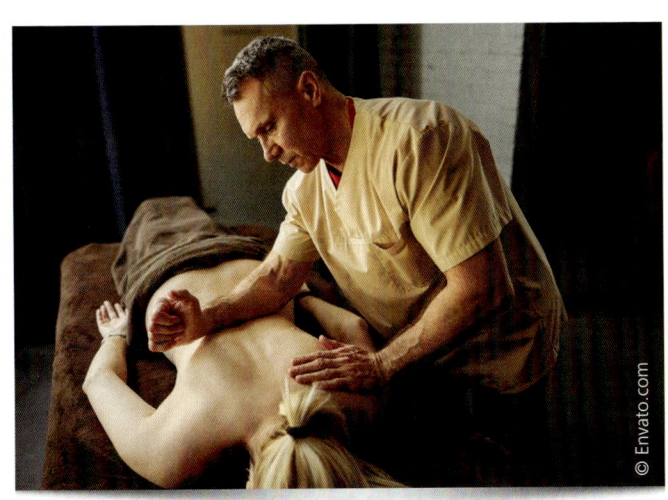

In Stage 1, people with chronic pain usually need consistent and relatively frequent care. At this point, if you are in enough pain, you may need rest to let your body heal. Your treatments will start to give you relief, but the process takes time, and you still need to take it easy. Depending on the type, cost, and availability of the treatment modalities you have chosen, you may need to be seen by multiple practitioners more than once each week.

In general, we like our patients to have about 40 to 50 percent pain relief within four to five treatments. Range of motion should begin improving, and inflammation should start to subside. We create what we call a trajectory of improvement. Rapid improvement is usually an encouraging sign, while slower improvement signifies that your condition may be more involved than anticipated.

Most patients take longer to get better than they expect. Occasionally, someone needs up to ten treatments before we see any improvement. It's important to be open. If one type of therapy isn't helping, a different one may.

Stage 2: Restoration and Regeneration

In Stage 2, your body has started to heal, and you can start to restore normal function and resume your usual daily activities. We want to return you to your previous, pain-free status. The aim here is to restore balance to the body's mechanics, with the emphasis on bringing you as close to a normal anatomical pattern as possible. By this point, you should be feeling somewhat better. Both you and your provider should get a sense that your body is healing. When you get to this point, your soft tissue begins to feel more pliant and responsive. Muscles become stronger and ligaments feel more elasticized. Similarly, the joints and extremities regain smooth movement and function. Your body's biotensegrity is starting to return to normal, without extra strains and stresses throwing it out of balance.

Stage 3: Realignment and Revitalization

In this stage, you're feeling good again. For you to keep feeling that way, it's important to remember that optimum health is a dynamic process. Ongoing maintenance is required to keep the body functioning well.

We have learned this through years of experience with our patients. At first, when patients recovered from an injury and were pain-free, we would simply say, "Come and see us when you need us." When they did come back, they would be in severe pain again, and we would have to start over in Stage 1 of treatment. We realized that if patients saw us regularly, we would notice little cues that indicated a problem was developing, and we could treat it before it got worse. In some cases, a segment of the spine would be a little stiff. In others, the person might not be able to rotate the neck as well. Many patients would have niggling aches and pains that meant they were likely to have an injury soon.

Today we take a proactive approach to prevention. By working initially with manipulative therapies, acupuncture, energy healing, and massage and bodywork therapies, we can support health in several areas simultaneously: relieving current symptoms, preventing future problems, and working on healing past problems. To this, we add prolotherapy and stem cell treatments. These allow us to get the body to rejuvenate itself and heal from many injuries that previously either required surgery or could not get better at all.

How Do You Know a Therapy Is Working?

With hands-on therapies such as massage or acupuncture, the benefit is often a direct reflection of the skill of the practitioner. A treatment with a good practitioner can be profoundly different from the same treatment provided by someone who isn't as skilled. How do you know? The simple answer is that you should feel better. However, keep in mind that it is not uncommon for aches and pains to get a little worse after a treatment. This should be temporary—just a day or so—and should never be severe.

When you have a profoundly relaxing treatment that places you in a state of deep

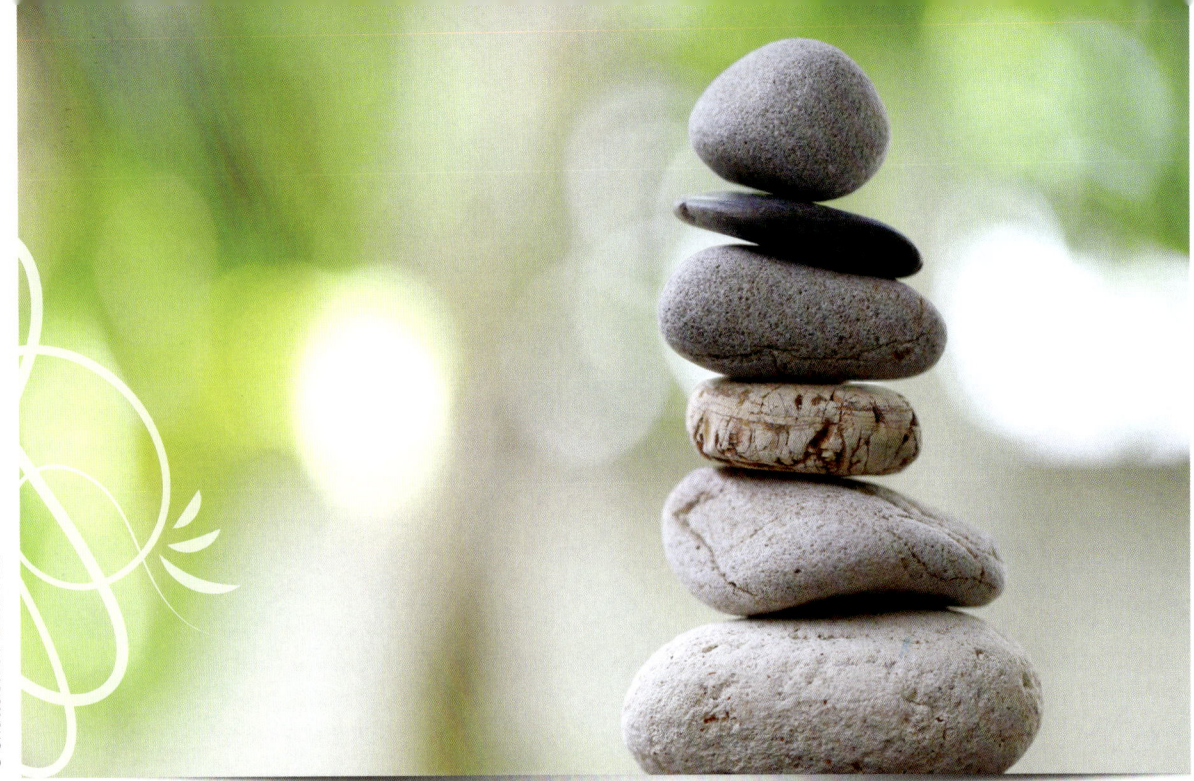

rest, your body will be able to do what it needs to do in order to heal. After a treatment, you may find yourself needing to sleep. This effect usually carries over—you will probably find that you sleep deeply that night and possibly for days afterward. Your body needs that deep rest to heal. We always tell our patients not to fight the effect with caffeine or other stimulants.

Finding a Good Healthcare Provider

To find a good healthcare provider with experience in treating chronic pain, start by looking in your area. You will need to do a little homework here. Ask for referrals from your physicians and from friends who have been seen by the type of provider you are seeking. Look initially for training, licensing, and certification. Ideally, your practitioner (a massage therapist, for example) will have attended an accredited training program, meaning one that meets the established standards for the field set by an independent agency or association. Your practitioner should also be certified, meaning they have met a recognized professional standard from an objective certifying agency. Although requirements vary from state to state, most non-physician practitioners also need to be licensed by whatever government agency regulates the profession. Licensing assures that the practitioner has a high degree of competency.

The next step is to look for skill, experience, and a good fit. How long has the provider been doing this? Have they seen a lot of people with your kind of problem? How successful have their results been? Bear in mind that every patient is different, and how one patient responded isn't necessarily how you will respond. Finally, do you feel comfortable with this provider? Do they listen and respond to your concerns, adjusting treatment as necessary?

To find practitioners near you, ask for recommendations from your doctor, other practitioners, and from friends and family. You can also check the websites for the national accrediting organizations. For example, the American Chiropractic Association has a searchable online directory at handsdownbetter.org. To find a qualified medical acupuncturist, search at medicalacupuncture.org. Licensed acupuncturists can be found on websites such as acufinder.com.

Effective Pain Therapies

Chronic pain can almost always be helped—it's usually just a matter of finding the right therapy or combination of therapies that's best for you. We always suggest starting with conventional medicine. Your primary care doctor or a specialist such as an orthopedist, physical medicine and rehabilitation physician, sports medicine doctor, neurologist, or neurosurgeon will usually have several good options for treating you.

If you have a severely arthritic hip joint, for example, integrative therapies may help to relieve the pain for a time, but there may come a point when hip replacement surgery is the best option. If you have a large, herniated disc causing pain or weakness in your arms or legs, then back surgery is a good option. However, if you have spinal stenosis or several small, herniated discs with chronic pain, surgery may not be the most effective treatment. Sometimes getting a second opinion can be extremely helpful for understanding your options—or confirming that surgery is needed.

Using a team approach from the perspective of several disciplines, we can provide earlier resolution of chronic pain and deeper, more effective, and more permanent healing. Ultimately, we are looking for a synergy of treatments to put you back in balance so healing can happen. The core idea is to restore function to the body's structure as much as possible so you can then return to a dynamic physical balance.

Therapies for Wellbeing

The therapies we offer are not just to treat pain. Our goal is to ensure that you feel comfortable in your own body. We like to see dynamic balance in the body, so whenever possible, we try to recreate the kind of fluid movement that one might see in a world-class athlete. This is a sense of equipoise—a balance between contraction and relaxation—that transcends the purely physical.

Manipulative Therapies

Manipulative therapies can be performed by chiropractors, osteopaths, and physical therapists. They are effective for acute and chronic low back pain, neck pain, spinal stenosis, headaches, shoulder pain, and hip and knee osteoarthritis. Manipulative therapies work well with sports injuries like ankle sprains and appear to work with certain non-musculoskeletal disorders such as vertigo and even colic in babies.

Adjusting the Spine

In chiropractic thinking, spine problems radiate throughout the body by affecting the entire nervous system. Adjusting the spine can help relieve pain and other symptoms. Chiropractic is widely recognized as one of the safest nondrug, noninvasive forms of healthcare for treatment of neuromusculoskeletal complaints. Numerous research articles have shown the value and safety of chiropractic treatment. This therapy has been evaluated in hundreds of clinical trials that show it is efficacious and cost-effective, particularly for treating low back pain.

Compared to other treatments for back pain, neck pain, headache, and joint pain, chiropractic is very safe. The risks associated with both over-the-counter and prescription nonsteroidal anti-inflammatory drugs (NSAIDs) and prescription painkillers are significantly greater than those of chiropractic manipulation. Chiropractic treatment may also help prevent opioid dependence and abuse by helping to relieve both acute and chronic pain enough that patients don't feel the need for these drugs. Chiropractic patients often learn that just tapping into their natural healing processes will help them feel better—and that drugs aren't always necessary to treat pain.

A spinal adjustment can be performed

in several different ways, but it is usually done by a quick, deft thrust or high-velocity, low-amplitude manipulation. During this type of spinal adjustment, you may hear a cracking or popping noise called a cavitation. This is normal and safe. Research has shown that small pockets of air or bubbles are found in the fluid surrounding a joint capsule. When the joint tissues are stretched during an adjustment, the gas pockets "pop," creating this cracking sound.

The adjustment appears to increase the amount of joint fluid. This improves both range of motion and the ease of movement of surrounding tissue; it also decreases pain. People who are concerned this technique may cause further injury may prefer a quick, low-force impulse from a small handheld tool called an Activator. Another option is a low-velocity adjustment, such as the osteopathic counterstrain technique, in which the patient is simply held in a specific comfortable position for 90 seconds. A physical therapist may achieve results similar to manipulation using a technique called mobilization, where parts of the spine are gently moved up and down to help improve range of motion and function.

Research supports the idea that proper alignment of the spine not only improves nerve function through the peripheral nerves, but also through signals sent to the brain. The central nervous system (the brain and spinal cord) shows improved function with chiropractic manipulative treatments. Cognitive and emotional function may also improve.

Chiropractic treatment uses manipulation to correct and realign joints that are out of position. The manipulation doesn't always hold in the corrected position, however. Home rehabilitation helps adjustments stay in place longer. A good chiropractor will teach you some simple exercises to help you maintain the adjustment and suggest ways to reduce the repetitive stress you've been placing on your body. In some cases, proper alignment can be better achieved and sustained when prolotherapy is combined with chiropractic manipulation. The cumulative effect of both therapies improves outcomes.

The most common side effect of manipulative therapy is temporary soreness of the surrounding muscles, which typically fades within 48 hours. Occasionally, a patient may have a flare-up following a treatment. In this case, symptoms appear to be worse for a few days. In our experience, this can be a good sign and often heralds a movement toward healing. Manipulative therapy can have severe but very rare side effects, such as stroke, disc herniation, or fractures of the vertebrae or ribs. One big concern is about arterial dissection and rupture following a chiropractic manipulation. This typically involves the carotid or vertebral artery and may lead to neurologic deficits or stroke. Fortunately, this is extremely rare. We always recommend discussing cervical manipulation with your chiropractor if you are concerned about this, especially if you have rheumatoid arthritis, which can affect the stability of the upper cervical vertebrae. This is where your chiropractor may choose to do a low-velocity manipulation.

Acupuncture

Acupuncture involves inserting very fine needles at specific points, or acupoints, on the skin surface, following traditional acupuncture meridians. Typically, the patient feels nothing or feels only a slight pinch as the needles are inserted. During the session, patients usually feel very relaxed, and it is not uncommon for them to fall into a deep, comfortable sleep. They typically awaken feeling refreshed and rested, with a greater sense of wellbeing. Sometimes the needles are stimulated with a transcutaneous electrical nerve stimulation (TENS) unit. This is a well-researched practice called electroacupuncture that shows excellent outcomes. Acupuncture points are sometimes stimulated with low level laser therapy, a technique called needleless acupuncture or painless acupuncture. Unfortunately, we have not seen good clinical results from this technique.

We strongly recommend working with a well-trained and experienced acupuncturist with good credentials. Results can vary among practitioners. There are many different styles, techniques, and backgrounds. If you find that acupuncture isn't helping, you may benefit from treatment by a different practitioner.

Both acute and chronic pain, ranging from acute injuries and sprains to chronic neck and low back pain, often respond well to acupuncture. Arthritis, bursitis, fibromyalgia, frozen shoulder, and tennis elbow are just some of the pain conditions that can benefit from acupuncture. Post-surgical pain can be alleviated as well.

Acupuncture is sometimes thought of as a technique to treat only pain and musculoskeletal problems. This isn't true. Acupuncture is effective for a variety of problems, including:

- Neurological disorders, such as strokes, migraine headaches, tension headaches, chronic daily headaches, and Ménière's disease. It is also helpful for neuralgias and neuropathies, including trigeminal neuralgia, carpal tunnel syndrome, postherpetic neuralgia (shingles), and Bell's palsy
- Infections, allergies, and respiratory problems
- Immune support: studies show that acupuncture can improve the function of T cells in the immune system, which helps fight infection and inflammation.
- Stress, anxiety, depression, and insomnia
- Drug addiction and smoking cessation (as an adjunct treatment)
- Chronic fatigue: it is used for long COVID, as well as chronic Lyme disease symptoms.
- Sexual health in both men and women – libido, prostate and infertility issues
- Menopausal symptoms, menstrual problems, and premenstrual syndrome
- Nausea due to morning sickness, chemotherapy, and anesthesia
- Interstitial cystitis

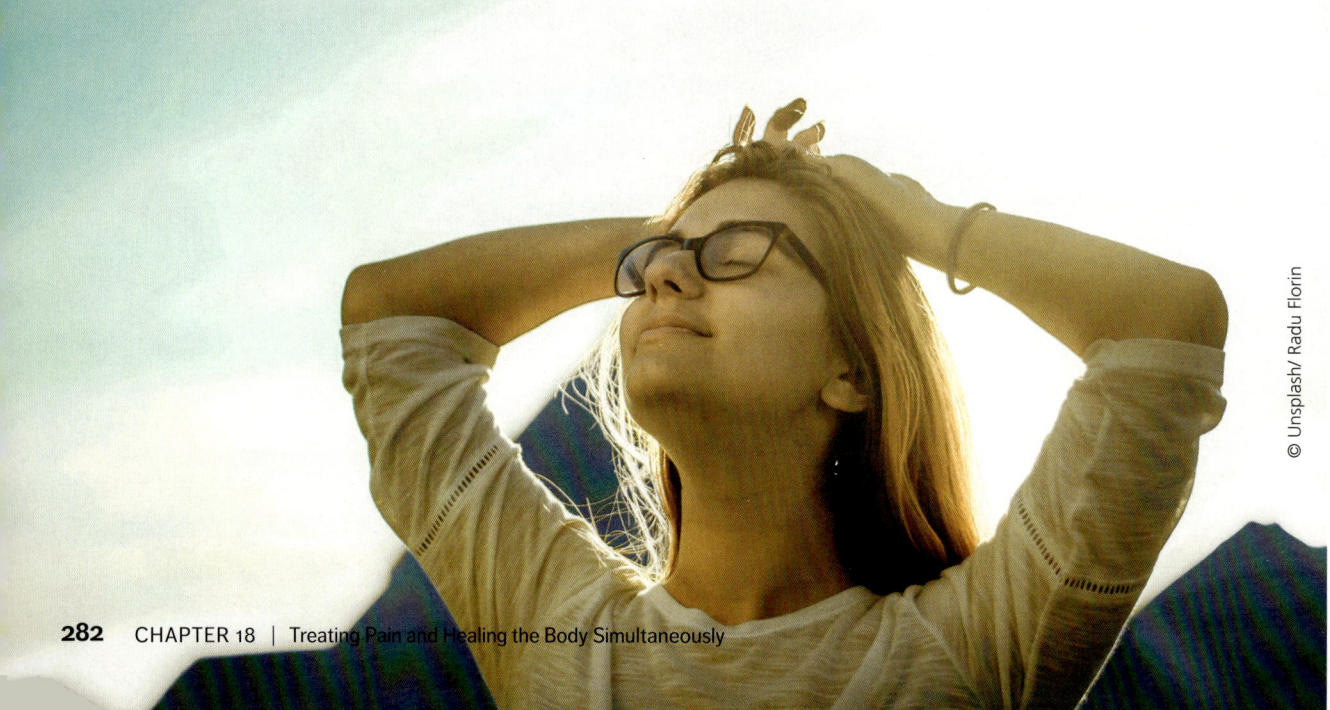

© Unsplash/ Radu Florin

- Gastrointestinal disorders such as gastroesophageal reflux disease, irritable bowel syndrome, and constipation

Done well, acupuncture should treat current issues and help heal previous problems, while simultaneously preventing new ones. It will often leave a patient with a profound sense of wellbeing. This is why we use it as a tool for Transformational Medicine.

Acupuncture in Our Practice

Over the past two decades and more, our physicians have averaged over ten thousand acupuncture treatments per year. In doing so, we have amassed significant experience regarding acupuncture. We have also met with, worked with, and observed acupuncture masters all over the world. As members of the American Academy of Medical Acupuncture, we have remained open to different professional perspectives on this approach to illness. We have seen seemingly miraculous turnarounds in situations ranging from asthma and allergies to strokes and pain.

However, in general, acupuncture really shines when used either early in an illness or with what we call functional illness. Good examples include myofascial pain, migraine headaches, and irritable bowel syndrome. What's more, acupuncture has almost no side effects.

Acupuncture excels in its ability to predict how certain people are predisposed to certain problems based on their biopsychotypes. (Refer to Chapter 15 for information on biopsychotypes.) Using this approach, we can individualize treatments to address several existing problems simultaneously while also addressing older issues and preventing future problems. In this way, we can treat, for example, allergies, heartburn, and knee pain simultaneously. The same treatment will also boost the immune system and make the patient feel better and be more resistant to illness.

How Does Acupuncture Work?

Patients often ask us, "How does acupuncture work?" The ancient Chinese theory of qi flowing through meridians is one way to explain it, but we believe there is a more scientific, Western-based answer using modern medical knowledge. Here is a glimpse of what we now know, based on thousands of research studies:

- Acupuncture creates a tiny injury at the site of the needle insertion. The body responds by sending healing chemicals to that area. Local release of chemicals (such as adenosine, bradykinin, and histamine) at the site of needle insertion appears to be involved in the healing process. Often the skin will turn red at this site, indicating that a healing process is occurring.

- Acupuncture has been found to reduce pain signals as they travel to and from the brain; it also modulates these signals in the brain.

- Functional MRI (fMRI) studies of blood flow in the brain show that when major acupuncture points such as those on the hand are stimulated, blood flow is improved in the brain. The influence of acupuncture on cerebral circulation helps explain why acupuncture relieves chronic pain.

- Acupuncture promotes the release of endorphins (pain-relieving chemicals) in both the brain and the spine.

- Acupuncture calms the sympathetic nervous system and improves activity in the parasympathetic nervous system. By balancing the autonomic nervous system, acupuncture helps switch the body out of the stress response into the relaxation response, a mode of healing.

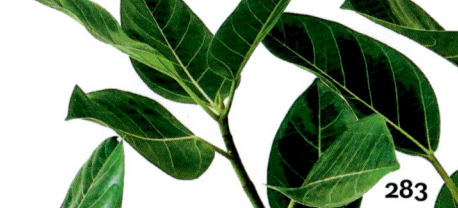

Unsplah/ Josh Calabrese

- Placing a needle in a muscle in chronic spasm causes the muscle to relax and stops the pain almost at once.
- Research by Helene Langevin, MD, has shown that the fascial network, or as we call it, "the internet of the body," is one of the ways in which different areas of the body communicate. Most major acupuncture meridians are now believed to run along planes of the fascia, the white sinewy material that surrounds and separates muscle groups and organs. Acupuncture seems to enhance this communication network, reprogramming the body's software.
- Many important acupuncture points turn out to overlie major nerves. Stimulating these points sends a message into the nervous system, telling it to behave differently.
- Acupuncture has been shown to alter gene expression. In other words, acupuncture can regulate the activity of your genes.
- Studies using fMRIs show that the same acupuncture point can have different effects on the same patient at different times. This helps to explain why an acupuncturist's ability to find the correct acupoint is so important and why acupuncture is difficult to research.

Professional Acupuncturists

Professionals trained to provide acupuncture include medical acupuncturists (MDs or DOs with additional training), licensed acupuncturists (L.Acs), and, in some states, physical therapists and chiropractic physicians who have had additional acupuncture training. When choosing a practitioner, inquire about training and see if the practitioner has had good results in treating the kind of problem you have.

Many physical therapists and chiropractors have been trained in a form of acupuncture called dry needling. In this technique, a fine needle is inserted into a trigger point to decrease tightness, increase blood flow to the area, and reduce local and referred pain. Dry needling is effective only for local pain—and can be painful to experience. Discuss it with your practitioner before you decide to try it.

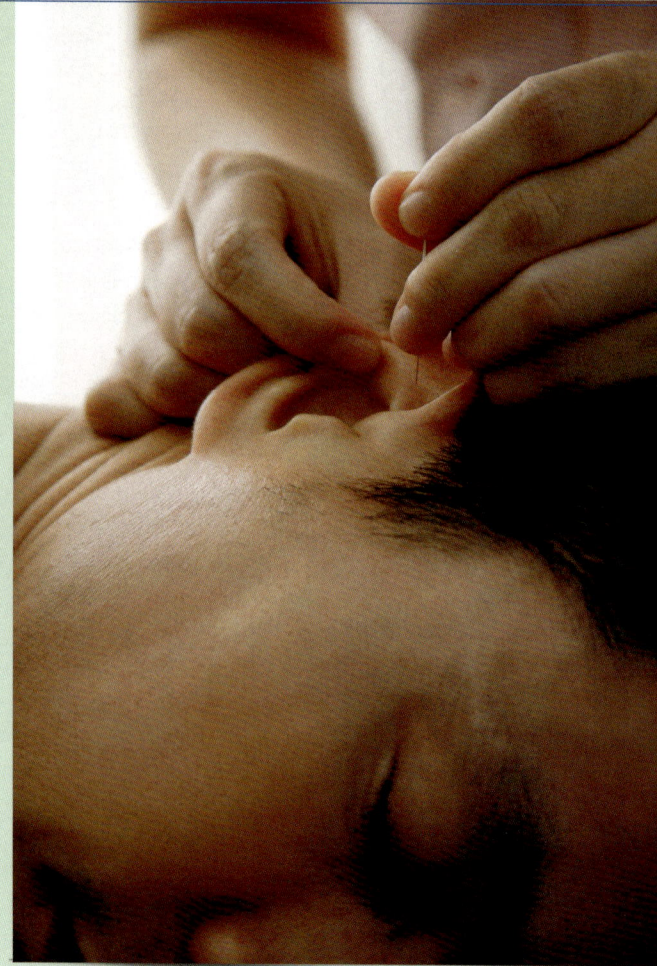
© Unsplash/ Getty Images

Risks of Acupuncture

In general, the risks of acupuncture are minimal. Infection from needles is very rare because disposable, single-use sterilized needles are the standard in treatment. The most common response is occasional bruising or redness at the needle insertion points. As with other manual therapies, a flare-up of pain may occasionally occur after treatment. Very rarely, patients experience lightheadedness and sweatiness, especially during the first treatment. This is usually not a problem and goes away as soon as the needles are removed. An extremely rare complication is a puncture of an underlying organ such as the lung. However, extensive reviews conducted in the United Kingdom, Sweden, and Japan of records on more than 140,000 treatments did not find even one major adverse event.

Integrative Therapies for Myofascial Conditions

Integrative therapies can be very effective for myofascial conditions—those affecting the muscles and the fascia that surrounds them. Acupuncture, for instance, directly treats the myofascial network. Rolfing and other touch therapies can also be very helpful. Other alternative, complementary therapies that affect the fascia include osteopathy, massage, the Feldenkrais Method, the Alexander Technique, and energy healing.

Prolotherapy: Safe Regenerative Therapy

Prolotherapy is a form of regenerative therapy—a treatment that triggers damaged tissues to repair themselves. It uses injections around joints to strengthen ligaments and tendons after injury or overuse. Prolotherapy injections contain a combination of dilute dextrose (sugar water) and 1 percent lidocaine (a short-acting, local anesthetic).

The injection solution is a mild irritant that creates a temporary, acute inflammatory response in the injured area. In response, your body sends in white blood cells and growth factors, stimulating a natural healing response. The response can also help halt the progressive joint degeneration in osteoarthritis and tendinopathies such as tennis elbow.

Even though prolotherapy irritates the injured area, it almost always causes only minor discomfort that usually goes away within 24 to 48 hours. Most patients need two to four treatments to the affected area, each about a month apart. The injections lead to steady improvement and by the time they finish the treatment, patients usually experience significant, long-lasting pain relief.

Prolotherapy can be very helpful for treating joint problems from arthritis, sports injuries, and other causes. We've found that it works very well for:

- Elbow problems, including tennis elbow (lateral epicondylitis) and golfer's elbow (medial epicondylitis)
- Foot and ankle problems, including chronic ankle weakness, recurrent sprains, plantar fasciitis, and heel spurs
- Knee problems, including patellofemoral syndrome (PFS), iliotibial band syndrome (ITBS), chondromalacia, chronic sprains/strains, and osteoarthritis
- Low back problems, including lower back pain from osteoarthritis, disc herniation, facet atrophy, and sacroiliac joint instability
- Neck and head problems, including whiplash, osteoarthritis, disc/facet issues, and temporomandibular joint (TMJ) pain
- Shoulder problems, including rotator cuff injuries, impingement syndrome, and recurrent dislocations

Prolotherapy works because joint problems such as osteoarthritis often begin with instability or laxity in the ligaments that hold the bones of a joint together. This laxity lets the joint move too freely, creating inflammation and pain. Rather than using drugs to relieve the inflammation, prolotherapy gets to the source of the problem. The injection helps tighten up the ligaments and reduces the laxity and instability causing the pain. Since prolotherapy works by causing local inflammation, it is important to avoid anti-inflammatory drugs and supplements for a week before a treatment and for one month after treatments are finished.

Perineural Injection Therapy (PIT)

Also known as neuroprolotherapy, PIT works on the same principle as prolotherapy for joints. It's a safe, effective treatment for nerve-related (neuropathic) pain and disability. A 5 percent dextrose solution is injected around the sensory nerves just under the skin of the painful area. Randomized clinical trials of PIT have shown it can be helpful for chronic low back pain, Achilles tendinitis, total knee arthroplasty, and carpal tunnel syndrome. A three-year study of people with Achilles tendinitis, for example, showed a 92 percent success rate a year later. We have seen excellent results in Morton's neuroma (a painful foot condition), sports injuries, trauma, arthritis, postsurgical pain, and overuse conditions.

> PIT may be used in conjunction with other therapies such as prolotherapy or acupuncture. While it is important to avoid NSAIDs during prolotherapy, this is not necessary if having PIT alone. PIT targets transient receptor potential vanilloid 1 (TRPV1) receptors in the nerves, thereby reducing the inflammatory chemicals CGRP and substance P.

Stem Cell Therapy:
Can We Make Ourselves Young Again?

Stem cells are undifferentiated cells in your body that have the potential to develop into many different types of cells. In other words, stem cells are the raw material from which all other cells originate. In adults, stem cells have the potential to generate replacement cells for those lost to normal wear and tear, injury, or disease.

Today, stem cells are being studied for their potential to treat many sources of chronic pain, such as osteoarthritis, by regenerating the damaged area. Stem cells injected into an arthritic knee, for instance, can potentially stimulate the growth of new cartilage cells to replace those that are damaged or worn away. The new cells provide the support and cushioning that the joint needs to function smoothly and without pain.

The stem cells can be harvested from your bone marrow or blood or sometimes from your body fat. Because the harvested stem cells are your own, your body accepts them, and rejection isn't a concern. The process can help slow cartilage loss, repair damaged cartilage, and reduce the inflammation and pain in the joint. The side effects are minimal, although some people may have temporary increased pain and swelling in the area.

Several solid studies have shown that stem cell therapy can be helpful for joint pain, particularly that caused by knee osteoarthritis, but it is still considered investigative by the FDA. It's far from a miracle cure—in fact, it doesn't always work. The pain relief isn't immediate, and you may need more than one injection to get the healing process started. The pain relief generally takes about two to three months to be felt, and it isn't permanent. Its benefit usually lasts anywhere from six months to several years. For many people, however, stem cell therapy is helpful for relieving debilitating chronic pain without the need for powerful anti-inflammatory drugs, opioid painkillers, or surgery. In our experience, success with stem cell therapy depends upon correct patient selection. Patients who have advanced arthritis or who are very sick with another illness don't typically do well. On the other hand, for patients with labral (cartilage) tears, tendon damage, ligament damage, or early arthritis, this form of treatment can make all the difference.

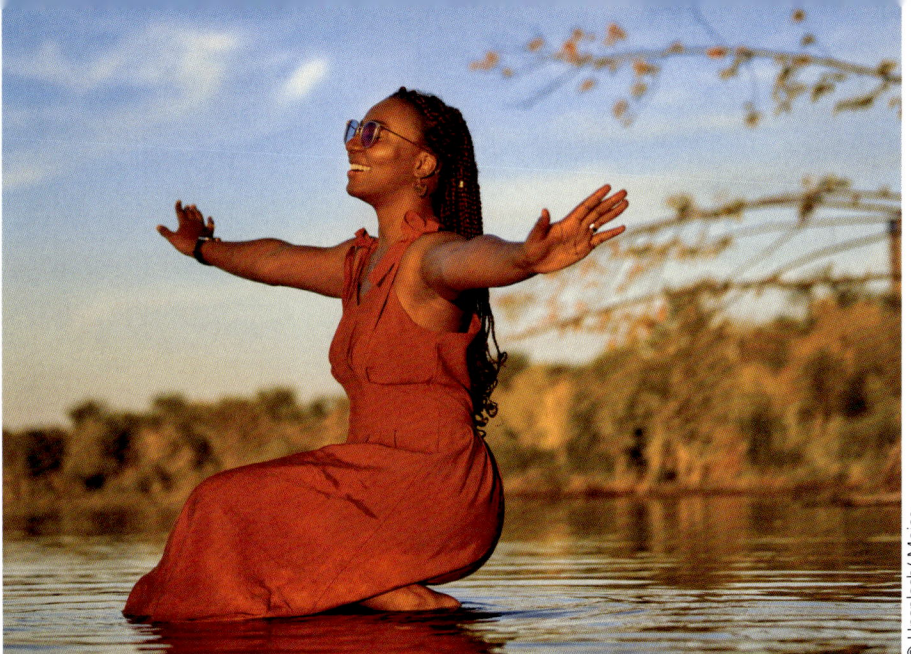

© Unsplash/ Moise

Platelet-Rich Plasma

Platelet-rich plasma (PRP) therapy is another way to use regenerative medicine to treat disorders of the joints and muscles. Platelets are tiny particles in your blood that are needed for clotting. In PRP therapy, we draw a small amount of blood from you (up to three tubes) and then use a centrifuge to concentrate the platelets and keep the plasma (the liquid part of your blood). The concentrated platelets and the plasma are then injected into the painful area. Ultrasound is often used to guide the needle. The platelets and the various growth factors in the plasma stimulate healing in the area and may also help relieve pain.

Because the PRP is created from your own blood, there is very little risk of rejection. PRP is a low-risk treatment that has a lot of potential to improve or speed healing. It works best when it is administered soon after the injury, when inflammation and cell proliferation are at their most active.

Massage, Trigger Point Therapy, and Bodywork

There are literally hundreds of forms of massage and bodywork, including deep tissue massage, medical massage, myofascial release, postural integration, Rolfing, shiatsu, Swedish massage, Thai massage, Trager Approach, trigger point therapy, and Watsu (a form of aquatic bodywork).

Massage and bodywork can be very helpful for relieving chronic pain. Touch is a basic aspect of human experience that can have a profound impact on health. Studies done by Tiffany Field, PhD on premature babies showed that those who received massage gained weight much more quickly than those who were not massaged. Studies of massage for patients with back pain show they have less pain, depression, and anxiety, as well as improved serotonin and dopamine levels. Other studies have reported that massage helps normalize cortisol levels in patients with fibromyalgia, depression, and post-traumatic stress disorder. Patients with cerebral palsy and Down syndrome receiving massage have shown enhanced flexibility and muscle tone. Massage research has also documented reduced pain in cases of carpal tunnel syndrome and juvenile rheumatoid arthritis and improved range of motion and strength in patients with spinal cord injuries. The healing benefits of touch have also been shown to boost general immune function and promote sleep. Massage has also been shown to improve our general sense of wellbeing.

Massage therapy is one of the safest and oldest forms of all the healing therapies. In hiring bodyworkers for our practice, we look for therapists who have both an innate sense of the body and a natural, intuitive gift of touch, as well as excellent clinical results.

Alliance Integrative Medicine has been a pioneer in the effort to bring the healing benefits of therapeutic massage into the arena of conventional medicine. While many of us think of massage as a spa-based luxury, more and more research supports the vision AIM has held for many years: massage helps us heal.

Massage is also a way to help you feel more relaxed and less anxious; it can help reduce many kinds of pain. At AIM, our massage therapists work closely with our medical doctors, chiropractors, and other therapists to select the massage technique that is best for each individual patient.

> *I'm a massage therapist. I solve problems you don't know you have in ways you can't understand.*
>
> **—Unknown**

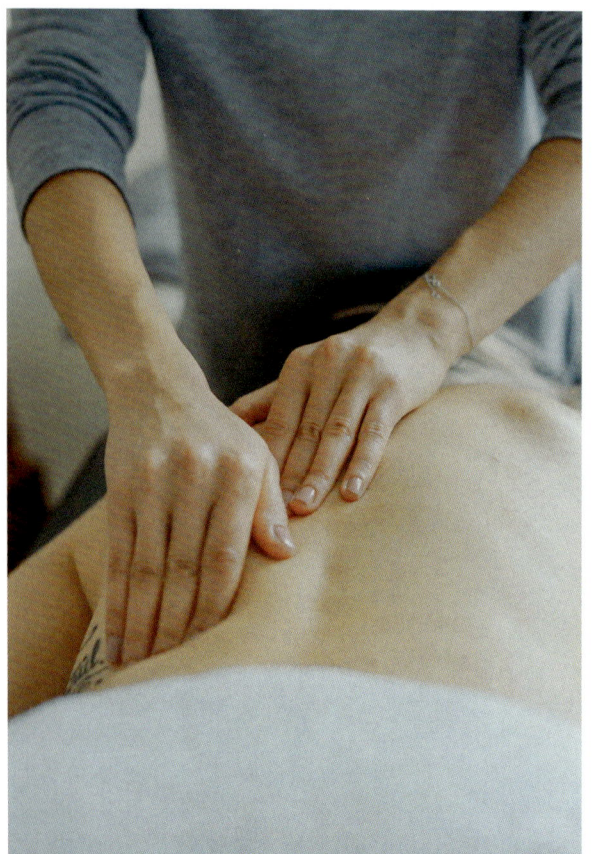

Craniosacral Therapy

Craniosacral therapy (CST) is a gentle, hands-on technique usually performed by a chiropractor or licensed massage therapist. Craniosacral therapy is a soft-touch manipulation using gentle force (no greater than the weight of a nickel) that addresses the alignment of the head, spinal column, and sacrum. The technique is thought to improve the fluid movement of the craniosacral system—the membranes and fluid that surround and protect the brain and spinal cord, as well as the attached bones, including the bones of the skull (the cranium), face, and mouth and down the spine to the sacrum. Improving the fluid movement may enhance and complement the body's natural healing mechanisms.

Conditions Treated by Craniosacral Therapy

Craniosacral therapy can benefit anyone who wants to achieve an optimal and balanced state, where the body's systems are working in harmony with each other. Craniosacral therapy can enhance the body's resistance to disease and is effective for a wide range of medical problems associated with pain and dysfunction, including migraine headaches, chronic neck and back pain, motor coordination impairments, colic in infants, and several other musculoskeletal and neurological conditions.

How Does Craniosacral Therapy Work?

Craniosacral therapy is said to improve fluid movement in the systems throughout the body. Improved fluid movement can enhance many body functions: the provision of nutrients to cells; the removal of toxins and waste products from tissues; the circulation of immune cells; the delivery of fresh blood to organs and tissues; and the movement of cerebrospinal fluid.

For a craniosacral treatment, the patient lies fully clothed on a padded table. The therapist begins by placing hands on the body. The cranium (skull) and the sacrum are very often where most of the touch occurs; other body parts may be gently contacted.

During a session, the central nervous system calms down and a deep sense of relaxation occurs. As the mind becomes more still, the patient can often sense movements of energy or releases in specific areas of the body. Each session is further individualized according to patient response.

Rolfing Structural Integration

Rolfing Structural Integration is a holistic system of soft tissue manipulation and movement education, organizing the whole body in gravity. Rolfing was developed by biochemist Ida P. Rolf more than 50 years ago. It remains a valuable bodywork therapy that can:

- Improve posture and promote fluid, graceful movement
- Ease chronic pain or discomfort resulting from injury or repetitive motion stress
- Improve overall functioning through stress reduction and increased awareness of self as a whole being

How Does Rolfing Work?

Rolfing creates more efficient use of the muscles, helps reduce chronic stress, and can change the body's structure. Most Rolfing practitioners believe that it balances the body in all directions, from head to toe, integrating layers of connective tissue. In the process, the body can return to a state of balance, which helps to maximize its functions.

Rolfing is a hands-on practice that includes mild and deep myofascial structural work, soft tissue manipulation, and motion enhancement. Because movement education is an essential component of the practice, Rolfing addresses more efficient transitions while lying down, sitting, standing, walking, and performing daily activities. Patients often experience an improved sense of body awareness.

Although Rolfing isn't painful, deep massage may cause some temporary discomfort. The hands-on treatment varies in intensity, depending on your needs. A Rolfing therapist may apply sustained pressure to release "stuck" patterns. This "good" pain can lead to increased mobility, creating a deeply satisfying, healing, and transformative experience.

At AIM, our goal is to effect greater ease of motion and freedom for our patients—not to increase their pain and discomfort! All our certified Rolfing therapists are trained at The Rolf Institute of Structural Integration's headquarters in Boulder, Colorado—the only school in the United States that certifies Rolfers.

Infant Massage

This gentle therapy is useful for relieving gas pains, constipation, and colic. It is also helpful for stimulating weight gain and boosting our youngest patients' immune systems.

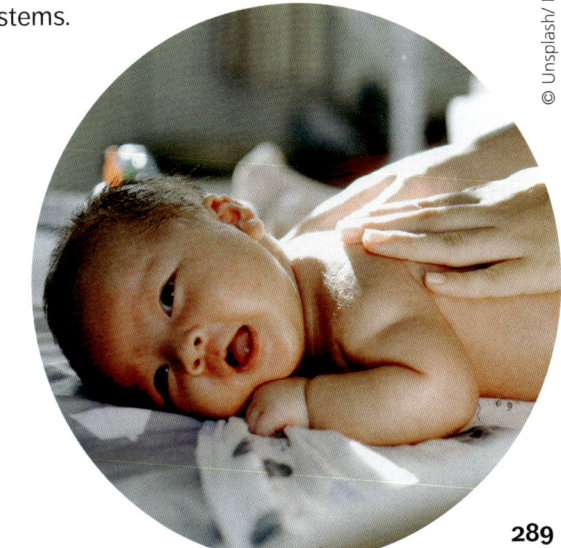

© Unsplash/ Moise

Manual Lymphatic Drainage

The lymphatic system in your body helps move cellular waste back into the circulatory system to then be removed by your liver. When this system becomes sluggish, you may experience pain and swelling. The massage practitioner uses light pressure and rhythmic, circular massage to stimulate movement in the lymphatic system. This treatment is often recommended to help resolve an acute problem that involves swelling, such as a sprained ankle. It may also be used to treat general joint swelling, to reduce scar formation, and to boost energy. Patients diagnosed with fibromyalgia and lymphedema (especially after a mastectomy) can benefit significantly from this type of massage.

Myoneural Release for TMJ syndrome

Myoneural release relaxes the medial and lateral pterygoid muscles (the muscles at the hinge of the upper and lower jaw) to reduce pain associated with headaches, TMJ, and extensive dental work. The massage therapist or chiropractor performing myoneural release wears sterile gloves and works inside the patient's mouth to relax the muscles.

Precision Neuromuscular Therapy

Often recommended for any part of the musculoskeletal system that is in pain, to treat headaches, or to increase range of motion and mobility, this form of massage is a very muscle-specific treatment. The patient and practitioner work together, communicating assessments while the practitioner shares insights about how the affected muscles work together.

Prenatal Massage

Massage therapy can be incorporated into routine prenatal care to support both physical and emotional health. Prenatal massage helps relieve many of the usual discomforts experienced during pregnancy, including backaches, neck stiffness, leg cramps, headaches, and swelling. Studies show that massage therapy during pregnancy can reduce anxiety, decrease symptoms of depression, relieve muscle aches and joint pains, and improve labor outcomes and newborn health.

Energy Healing Techniques

When provided by a gifted practitioner, energy healing induces a state of deep relaxation. These therapies appear to enhance and complement the body's natural healing mechanisms.

There is currently no regulation or licensing of these therapies. Practitioners have a wide range of skill levels and natural talent.

Patients receiving energy healing often find that they melt into a state of wellbeing in which pain and anxiety are quickly relieved. These therapies also seem to boost the immune system and have myriad other benefits.

In our experience, energy healing techniques are helpful in dealing with acute and chronic pain. Numerous conditions frequently associated with pain, such as connective tissue disorders and autoimmune conditions, and stress-related issues such as anxiety and depression, chronic fatigue, central nervous system dysfunction, and post-traumatic stress disorder can all respond well to energy healing—if it is done by a skilled and experienced practitioner.

Understanding Energy Healing

One of the oldest forms of healing in the world, energy healing is the art of correcting imbalances in the body's flow of energy. The human body generates an electromagnetic field. Measurements of this field are often used in conventional medicine to diagnose illness and disease. For example, we commonly use electroencephalograms to measure brain activity, electrocardiograms to chart heart activity, and MRIs to get detailed looks inside the body.

This electromagnetic field or aura around the body can also be detected without instruments by a trained energy therapist. In fact, research at AIM has shown that some individuals are able to see beyond the normal visual spectrum and into this field. An imbalance in the aura can eventually lead to physical disease. Restoring balance in this field aids in healing the physical body.

Conditions Treated by Energy Healing

At Alliance Integrative Medicine, we have integrated several different types of energy work, including therapeutic touch, healing touch, and principles from the Japanese art of reiki. During an energy healing treatment, the therapist assesses the body's energy field and attempts to correct any imbalances detected by placing their hands on the patient. They are then taught how to gently influence this field. Because energy healing practitioners can sense electromagnetic field imbalances before they affect the physical body, individuals can benefit from energy treatments to help prevent illness. This includes anxiety and pain of all types. At AIM, we have found energy healing to be a useful adjunct in the treatment of all diseases.

During an energy healing treatment, the therapist first assesses the patient's energy field and determines if there are any imbalances. They will then discuss these imbalances with the patient and have the patient lie down on a padded table as they initiate treatment to balance the energy field.

The patient may feel a warm sensation and sometimes even a tingling or vibration. It is very common for a patient to feel relaxed, comforted, and even fall asleep during a treatment.

After the treatment, patients may feel a little sleepy and should rest until they are able to resume normal activities. We suggest that you drink lots of water and refrain from strenuous activity and heavy exercise for 6 to 24 hours following a treatment.

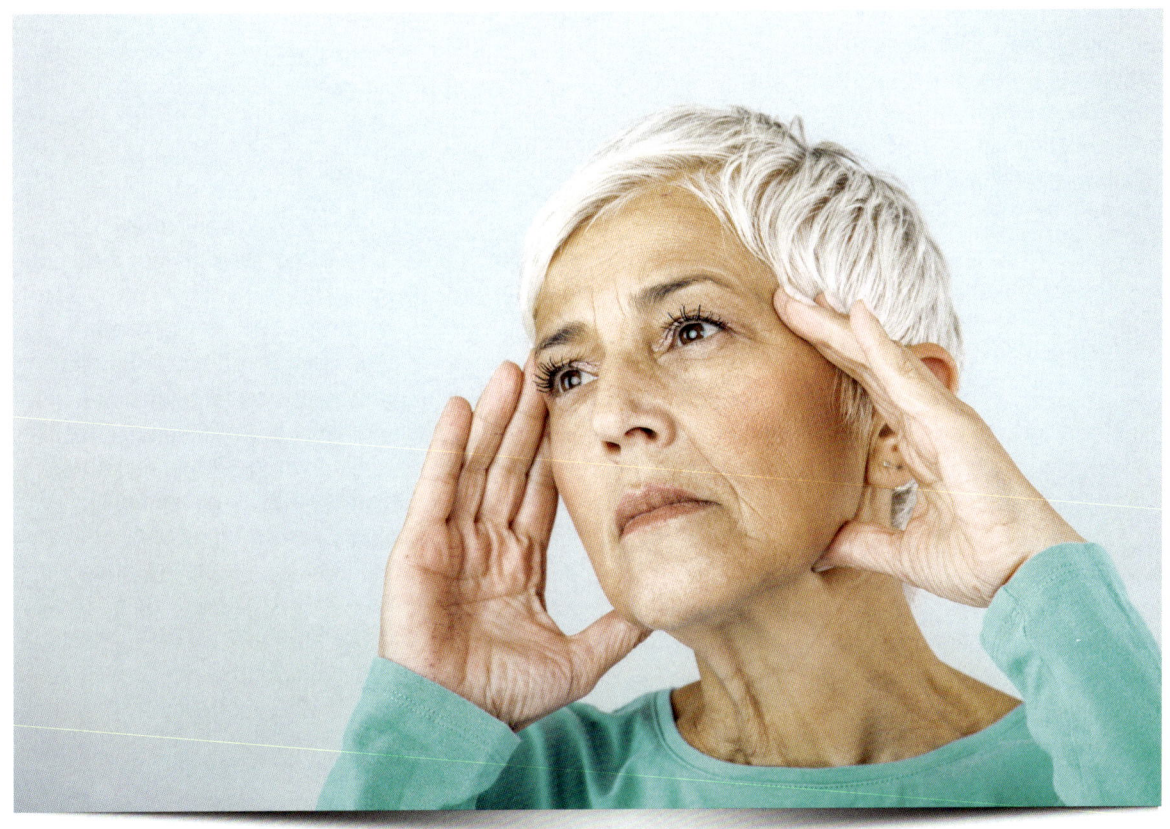

© Unsplash/ Getty Images

ACE Healing Treatment

A unique combination of Acupuncture, Chiropractic, and Energy healing, the ACE Healing Treatment™ is our most popular and highly regarded wellness offering. When a healing partnership is established and integrative therapies are used together, the cumulative effect can far exceed the benefit of any one of these therapies on its own.

The synergistic effects of this treatment combination are designed to activate and accelerate the body's natural healing process. When we use integrative therapies together, the cumulative result can far exceed the benefit of any one individual therapy on its own. ACE is highly effective for relieving symptoms of chronic illness, speeding recovery, and maintaining wellness.

ACE Healing Treatment can provide outstanding relief for many ailments by helping restore your overall health and sense of balanced wellbeing. Having an ACE Healing Treatment regularly is an excellent way to maintain your health and only takes 60 to 90 minutes. Most importantly, an ACE Healing Treatment puts you firmly on the path of getting well, being well, and staying well.

Studies show that the healing benefit of combining the ACE therapies in one treatment session outweighs that of each of its components as stand-alone treatments. As we explain to patients: Imagine your body as a water pipe.

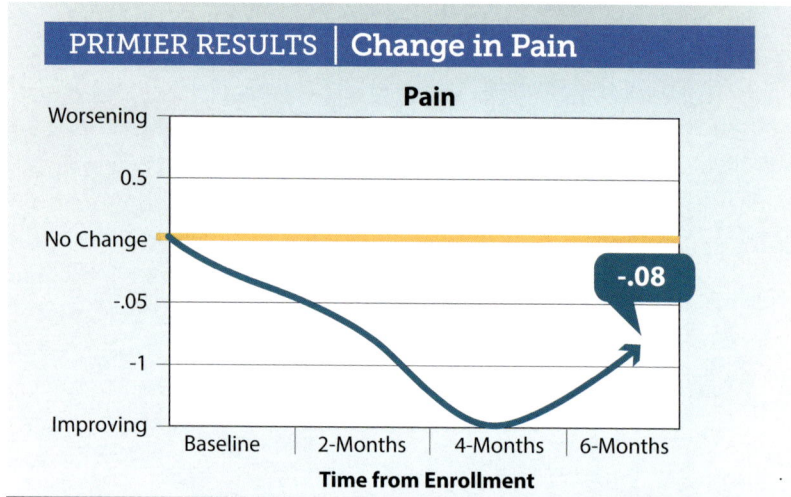
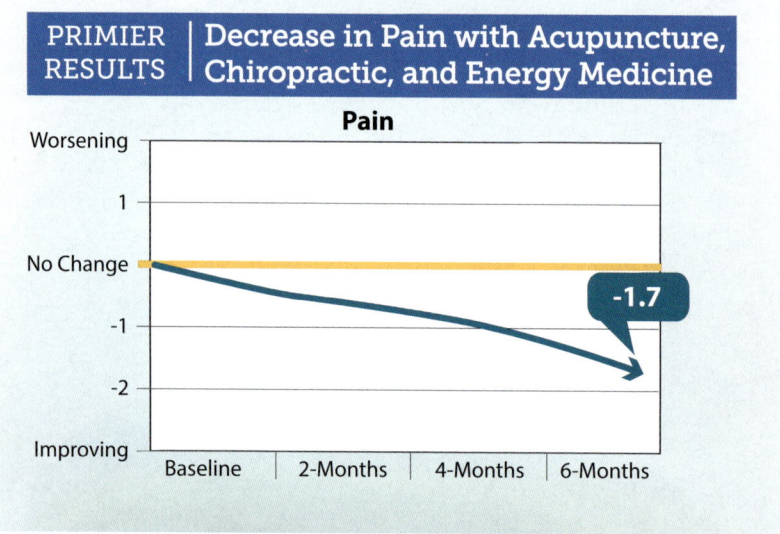

FIGURE 18.1 | Primier Results

Chiropractic fixes the kinks. Acupuncture directs and pressurizes the water. Energy is the water.

In 2015, the Bravewell Collaborative published an initial overview of the PRIMIER study (Patients Receiving Integrative Medicine Interventions Effectiveness Registry). In this study, patients from 14 clinical centers, including Alliance Integrative Medicine, were asked for patient-reported outcomes on the effect that integrative medicine had on their pain.

Interestingly, pain scores tended to decrease for the first four months of treatment,

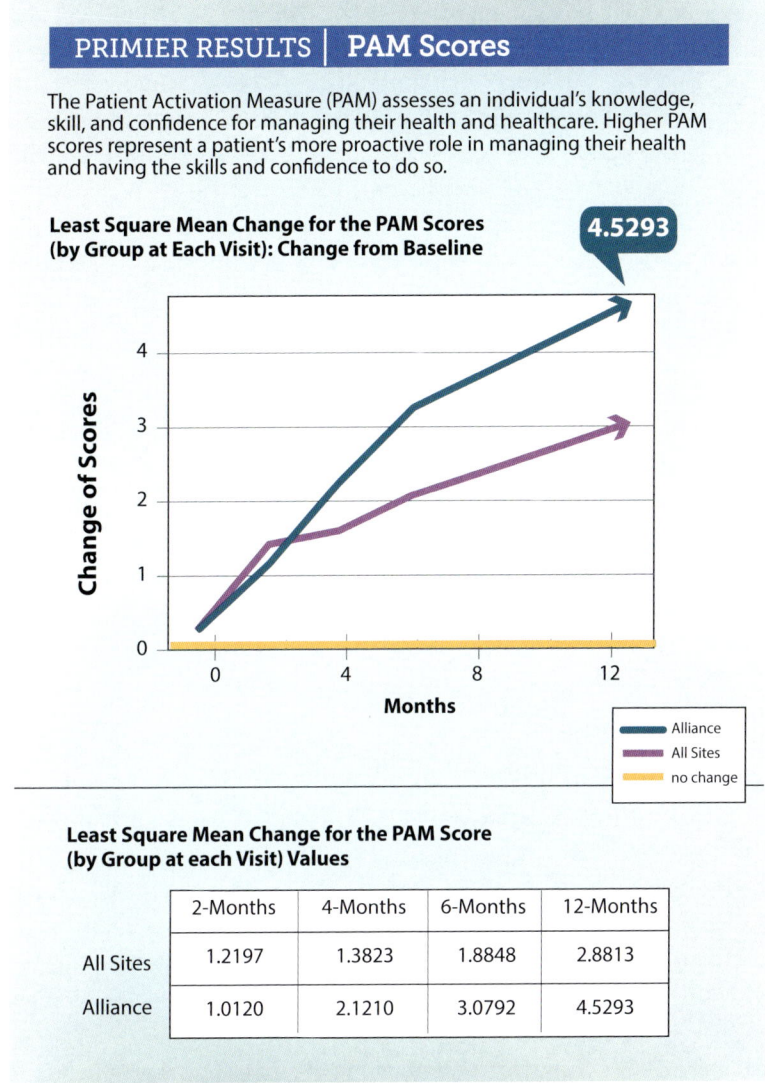

FIGURE 18.2 | Primier Results

but then trended up again. However, in patients who had ACE treatments, pain continued on a downward trend for the full six months they reported. The combination of pain treatments was more successful in bringing pain down!

Interestingly, the longer patients participated in this study, the higher their patient activation measure (PAM) scores. PAM is a measure of the knowledge, skills, and confidence essential to managing your own health and healthcare. In other words, the participating centers in this study were educating patients and helping them improve their skills and increase their confidence in managing their health. As a result, they were able to maintain behavioral changes over time.

Supplemental Therapies

Additional therapies for pain include mechanical and electrical units that can be used on their own or as a supplement to other therapies. These include transcutaneous electrical nerve stimulation (TENS), interferential and horizontal microcurrent, low-level laser therapy, ultrasound, and frequency specific microcurrent.

In general, these therapies are nontoxic, noninvasive, and safe. They have minimal side effects, but their effectiveness varies. Depending on the type of therapy, they can improve blood flow, speed localized healing, reduce muscle spasms, prevent blood clots, train muscles to increase strength, prevent tissue and muscle degeneration, and stimulate peripheral nerves to help reduce pain or improve function.

Once again, work with a practitioner who is properly trained in the modality you are receiving. While these modalities are generally safe, be sure you are getting the results you have been promised.

Frequency Specific Microcurrent (FSM)

FSM is a system of treatment using microamperage electric current and the resonance effects of different frequencies on tissues and conditions to create beneficial changes to symptoms and health.

Microamperage current is the same kind of electric current your body produces on its own within each cell. Because the current used in FSM is in millionths of an amp, it's so low that it doesn't stimulate sensory nerves. Although the current can't be felt as it is applied, the healing effects are powerful and immediate. The changes FSM produces in damaged tissue make it an indispensable tool in treating pain and many other health concerns. Scientific studies have shown that it reduces inflammation by 62 percent, increases ATP (energy production) by 500 percent, and increases protein synthesis by 70 percent.

Years ago, we treated one of the top tennis players in the world after he suffered a severely sprained ankle at the Association of Tennis Professionals Tennis Tournament. His MRI showed three torn ligaments and a large bone bruise, an injury which normally takes three to six months to heal. We used gentle manipulative treatments, acupuncture, and FSM when he came to our office soon after the injury. He then used a home FSM device for a few hours every day. One week later, his repeat MRI showed a normal ankle and 12 days later he played in the US Open in New York!

FSM Treatment

FSM is applied to the affected area by special gloves worn by the practitioner, by damp towels placed over the affected area, or by acupuncture needles. The practitioner selects the frequency (the rate at which the electronic pulse is produced) based on the type of injury or condition and the part of the body or type of tissue affected. Specific frequencies are selected to encourage the body to heal itself and to reduce pain.

The wide range of frequencies offered by FSM makes it a versatile tool able to help a variety of clinical conditions. FSM is especially good at treating nerve and muscle pain, inflammation, and scar tissue. It works well for lower back pain, upper back pain, and neck pain due to sports injuries, bursitis, arthritis, tendinitis, and even fibromyalgia.

Other clinical problems where FSM is helpful include:

- Allergies and sinus problems
- Bronchitis, asthma, and chronic obstructive pulmonary disease
- Colitis and irritable bowel syndrome
- Endometriosis, fibroids, and pelvic pain
- Kidney stones
- Shingles, postherpetic neuralgia, and neurogenic pain

Extracorporeal Shockwave Therapy (ESWT)

Shockwave therapy has been around in Europe for quite a while and is now starting to become popular in the US. Shockwave therapy works in a way similar to lithotripsy, a treatment that uses soundwaves to painlessly break up kidney stones into particles that can pass from the body easily.

Extracorporeal (meaning "from outside the body") shockwave therapy promotes regeneration and reparative processes in the bones, tendons, ligaments, and other soft tissues. It can also be used to help repair nerve function, reduce pain, and speed healing.

Shockwaves used in this therapy help reverse chronic inflammation by initially increasing, then decreasing, mast cell stimulation. They also stimulate the production of new collagen fibers, which helps tendons regain strength and structure; promote new blood vessel formation; dissolve calcium buildup in areas of tendon and muscle microtears; release trigger points; and disperse substance P, a natural peptide linked to increased pain and inflammation in injured areas. Pain relief is often immediate, but chronic pain often takes six to ten treatments.

ESWT has two forms:

Radial pressure wave (RPW) therapy. The tip of a handheld sound applicator is held to the skin above the affected area and vibrates rapidly up and down, transmitting a subdermal sound shockwave. It is often used in conjunction with Focused Shockwave Therapy, as there is a degree of overlap between these two treatments.

Focused shockwave therapy (FST). This technique uses a high-energy acoustic wave aimed at the painful spot. FST can penetrate up to 5 inches, so it is used for deeper and more chronic conditions. FST is FDA-approved for treating chronic plantar fasciitis.

Shockwave is used for a range of conditions, including chronic neck and low back pain, tennis elbow, golfer's elbow, painful shoulder (including calcific tendinitis and frozen shoulder), jumper's knee, chronic tendinopathy, medial stress syndrome of the leg, hip pain, osteoarthritis of all joints, patella and achilles tendinitis, plantar fasciitis, bone spurs, bursitis, sexual dysfunction and erectile problems, non-union of fractures, and neuropathy.

The choice of Radial vs Focused shockwave depends on the skill and choice of the practitioner.

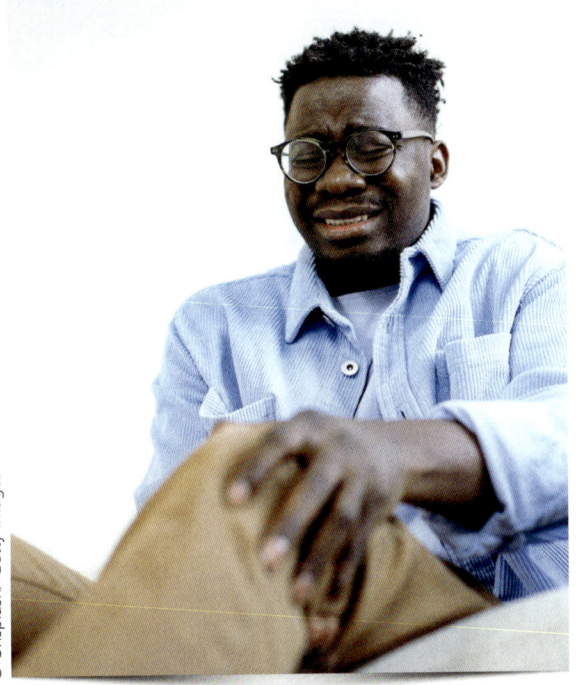

Extracorporeal Magnetotransduction Therapy (EMTT)

EMTT is a noninvasive, safe form of magnetic therapy used for a wide range of musculoskeletal diseases, especially chronic wear-and-tear conditions, overuse injuries, degenerative arthritis, sports injuries, and rehabilitation. A looplike magnet is placed near the painful area and a series of short, painless, high-energy magnetic pulses are then transmitted to your body. A single treatment session lasts between 5 and 20 minutes. Depending on the severity of the condition and the response to the therapy, six to eight sessions are usually required over several weeks.

Low Level Laser Therapy (LLLT)

LLLT, also known as photobiomodulation, uses nonthermal laser light at specific wavelengths to treat pain and inflammation, enhance tissue healing, and increase circulation. The process works because the light photons emitted by the laser modulate mitochondrial function at a cellular level. LLLT is safe and painless, and treatment is very quick.

For acute injuries, LLLT is used daily for two to three days, then every other day for a week, and finally twice a week until the injury is better. For chronic injuries, we recommend treatment twice weekly initially, then weekly until improvement reaches a plateau.

Nutritional Supplements for Pain

Nutritional supplements may be very helpful for pain. Unlike medications, they usually take a while to work. To see if a supplement is helpful, we usually suggest trying it for six to eight weeks. By that point, if the supplement is helping, you should feel a significant decrease in pain. But if after a few weeks you find yourself vacillating as to whether you should keep taking it, then the supplement probably isn't working for you. When a supplement works, you know it!

Many supplements have been marketed for pain relief. Most are ineffective, and some could have dangerous side effects and drug interactions. Discuss any pain supplements you want to use with your doctor before you try them. We have found a handful of pain supplements that are genuinely helpful.

Specialized Pro-Resolving Mediators (SPMs), or Resolvins, for Chronic Inflammation and Pain

Resolving inflammation and the pain it causes is a complex and highly active process. In most cases—a sprained ankle, for instance—the resolution process happens normally. The pain, redness, and swelling from the initial injury gradually go away, and the joint returns to normal, pain-free function. To switch off the inflammatory response, your immune system uses chemical messengers called specialized pro-resolving mediators (SPMs). Sometimes, however, your body can't produce enough SPMs to shut down the final phase of inflammation. Instead, the inflammation and the pain it causes lingers on long after the acute phase of the injury or illness is past. The body never truly returns to homeostasis, and the pain becomes chronic.

SPMs are the result of a multistep conversion process in the body that begins with dietary omega-3 fatty acids. Unfortunately, the complex conversion process is slow and inefficient, even in the healthiest individuals. When we see pain from an injury or illness continuing longer than usual, we recommend SPM supplements to help the body complete the healing process.

Turmeric and Boswellia

The natural anti-inflammatory compounds in turmeric (*Curcuma longa*), especially curcumin, can help reduce pain and inflammation symptoms such as aching joints. Turmeric has also been shown to help decrease the damage from a cytokine storm, caused when the immune system overreacts to a pathogen. Turmeric works by blocking the LOX and COX inflammatory pathways. Another plant, Boswellia serrata, also known as Indian frankincense, works in a similar manner. We find that combining both supplements is very helpful for chronic inflammation, especially for people who can't tolerate NSAIDs.

PEA

PEA (palmitoylethanolamide) is a chemical derived from fat. It is found in the human body in small amounts; supplements are derived from foods that contain palmitic oil, such as palm oil. PEA is very safe and can be very helpful in reducing pain from swelling and inflammation, particularly from osteoarthritis.

Cannabidiol (CBD)

CBD is one of the many cannabinoids, or chemicals derived from the cannabis plant. Unlike tetrahydrocannabinol (THC), a cannabinoid that makes you high, CBD has no psychoactive effects (as long as it's not contaminated with THC). CBD helps relieve pain through its effect on the endocannabinoid receptor system (ECS), a huge network of chemical signals and cellular receptors found throughout the body. Cannabinoid receptors in the brain regulate many other neurotransmitters and modulate their activity. Molecules called endocannabinoids stimulate the cannabinoid receptors. These molecules, including CBD, are very similar to molecules in the cannabis plant. The endocannabinoid stimulation releases anti-inflammatory and pain-relieving chemicals. Using CBD has a similar stimulating effect on the ECS and may be helpful for people with chronic pain from osteoarthritis and other problems.

CBD comes in different forms—tinctures, oils, gummies, capsules, creams, gels, and patches. Because products vary in potency and quality, it is important to do some background research and find a reliable dispensary. The hemp plant tends to absorb toxins in the environment easily, so choosing organic products is vital. CBD is safe to use, with very few side effects. Topical products such as gels don't enter the bloodstream.

Medical marijuana contains both CBD and THC, as well as several other cannabinoids. While marijuana seems to help relieve pain, the potency of products varies quite a bit, which has an impact on their efficacy. Our concern is that long-term marijuana use may cause mood disorders, exacerbation of psychotic symptoms in vulnerable people, cyclic vomiting, cognitive impairments, and even an increase in cardiovascular and respiratory disease. Like all drugs, marijuana appears to have both benefits and side effects. If you are thinking of using it for pain, we strongly advise you to discuss this thoroughly with a physician who prescribes medical marijuana.

At the federal level, CBD is legal if it doesn't contain more than 0.3 percent THC. In some states, however, sales of CBD are restricted. At the federal level, marijuana is considered a dangerous drug and is illegal. Some states have legalized marijuana for recreational and medicinal use, while others restrict it to medicinal use with a doctor's prescription. Of course, in some states, no marijuana use is legal.

Low Dose Naltrexone (LDN)

LDN can sometimes be very helpful in treating chronic pain. High dose naltrexone (at doses from 50 to 200 mg) is used to treat heroin addiction and alcoholism, but low dose naltrexone (given at doses from 1 to 4.5 mg) works differently. LDN is made in a compounding pharmacy and works by temporarily binding and blocking a mechanism called the mu receptor, which is linked to chronic pain. When the receptor is blocked, it makes your body think it's not producing enough endorphins, our natural pain relievers. Blocking the receptor stimulates the release of more endorphins. In addition, because the receptor is temporarily blocked, the body responds by upregulating, or increasing the amount of these receptors. *The result is that chronic pain goes down.* We often use LDN in a "cocktail" with CBD and PEA. It's a wonderful, safe, cheap trifecta for patients who have tried everything else.

Your Role in Your Treatment

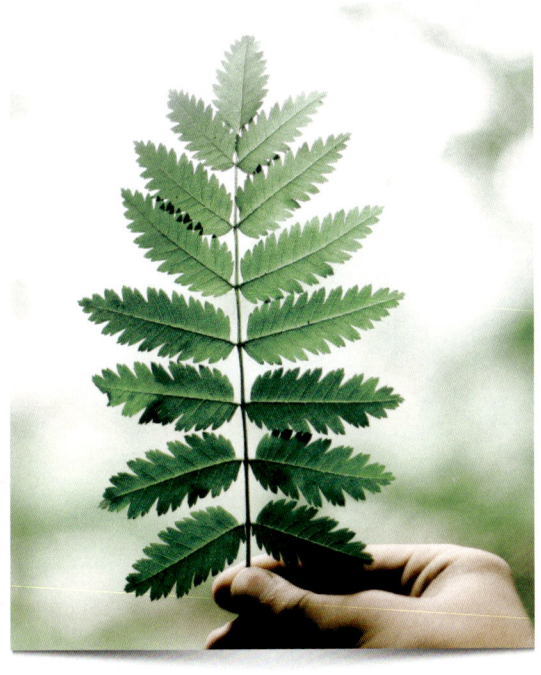

Do you have to believe in these treatments for them to work? In other words, is their effectiveness just a placebo? The answer is no. They work on rats and animals, and they work even on the most skeptical of patients. However, we have always seen that some patients seem to have an enhanced response. They do so because they create a state of physical and mental receptivity that encourages the body's own healing processes. This is very different from lying there passively while treatment is done to them. So, we encourage our patients to engage in this healing process: we encourage them to tune in and see how their bodies are feeling at that moment. We call this a state of willing openness. In this state of receptivity, patents report a heightened awareness of what is happening within their bodies and in their environments. They report

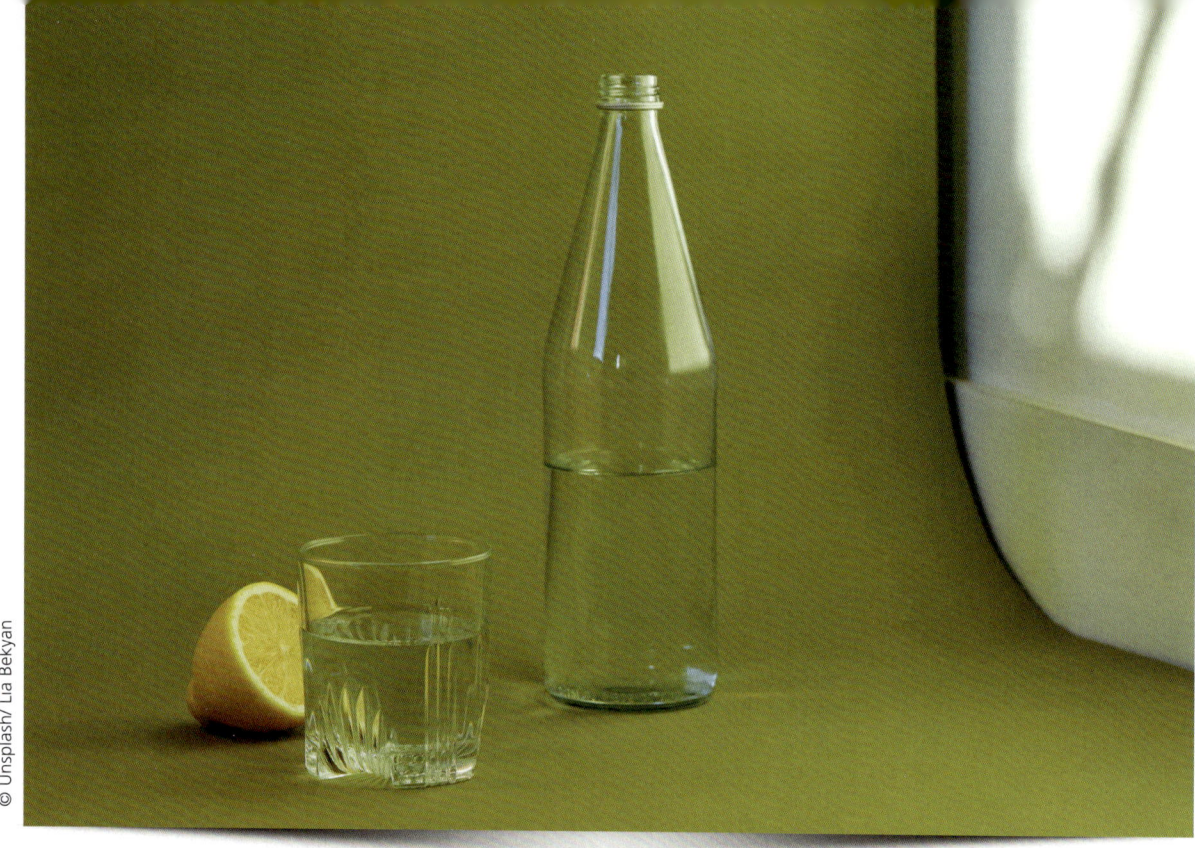

experiencing a sense of balance and equanimity, something that has been missing from their lives because of their conditions or chronic pain. In this restfully alert state, they begin to appreciate the healing process and are better able to assist it. This heightened awareness also gives them greater control over their healing and vitality—helping them become themselves once again.

After a treatment, we advise patients to drink plenty of water and get plenty of rest. The body seems to want to balance itself after a treatment. If, for instance, you have been in a sleep-deprived state, you may want to sleep. If you have been feeling sluggish and depleted, you may find yourself filled with energy as the body repletes itself. In any case, you should experience a sense of improvement after the treatment. Pain usually will diminish after a treatment, but symptoms may worsen slightly right after the treatment and then diminish within about twelve hours.

When the body's natural healing processes are stimulated, it will shunt healing chemicals to the areas where they are needed. In order not to interfere with this process, we suggest going into your treatment well hydrated. Afterward, eat lightly; avoid heavy meals and food that is very hot, spicy, or cold. Drink lots of room-temperature water. Avoid alcohol, heavy exercise, or sexual activity for about six to twelve hours, because all of these activities shunt the body's attention elsewhere.

At our center, patients often tell us that healing starts the moment they walk through the door. We have tried to create a total therapeutic environment, with soft colors, soft music, and aromatic scents, rather than a sterile, hospital-type environment. As integrative physicians, we go out of our way to find staff who are warm and friendly.

Taking Care of Ourselves

Sometimes amid our busy lives, we forget to make time for ourselves. If we want to get well and stop getting sick or being in pain, however, we need to take the time for self-care. Forgetting to do so becomes self-defeating. If we don't look after ourselves, we ultimately cannot help those around us. As we often remind our patients, you can't pour from an empty cup. Self-care is not selfish. Think of the mom on the airplane who is told to put on her oxygen mask first before giving it to her children. Likewise, self-care with a mindset that nurtures and nourishes us is the first step to us look after others in our lives.

We first learned about self-care when we first visited Hong Kong and Taiwan in the 1980s. We were amazed to see hundreds of people practicing the slow, circular, rhythmic movements of tai chi each morning in public parks. When we asked tai chi masters about why they did this practice, they typically explained to us that when they reached their 40s and 50s, they found themselves lacking in vitality and stamina. Their bellies and libido had begun to sag, and they tended to develop problems with their blood pressure and general health. After practicing tai chi for a few months, their health problems disappeared, and their vitality returned. As they continued the practice over decades, they found themselves doing better and better. Their bodies felt better, and their minds were clearer and sharper.

Adherents to yoga practice often report a similar return to health. These practices help reduce pain and improve stamina, mood, and vitality. Tai chi or yoga are not the only answers. Any type of regular, gentle exercise has broad and lasting benefits. You may want to start with walking, gentle stretching, lifting light weights or even Pilates.

The question is: What are you going to do to help yourself regain a positive sense of vitality? How can you restore your sense of abundant well-being? Are there ways you can restore your health without medication? We believe that a practical, balanced lifestyle, individualized to your condition, provides the foundation for almost any form of treatment.

Using Pain as a Guide

Our culture wants us to switch off pain as fast as we can, but pain isn't always a bad thing. If you have chronic pain, we encourage you to change your viewpoint and see your pain as something to work with, not against. We would like you to listen to your body as you learn to heal. If a certain exercise hurts, you might be doing it wrong, so don't do it!

There is a difference between what we call an "oooh" pain and an "owww!" pain. An "oooh" pain is one that says, "Go deeper." This is a typical sensation you may feel when a massage therapist works out a knot in your muscle or when you are enjoying a stretch. An "owww!" pain is an important message from your body that says, "Stop now." Patients often tell us about little "owww!" pains that precede a much bigger one. These occur in golf games, yoga classes, and even bending down to put on socks. Learning to pay attention to the little pains—and then finding a way to get rid of them—can prevent much bigger problems later.

Healing Your Feelings

In some cases, the body can help us understand suppressed emotions. Sometimes, chronic pain can mask underlying issues caused by physical or emotional trauma that has been overlooked. When there is no physical cause of your pain that makes sense, you need to consider this as a possibility. In Chapter 4, we suggested ways to learn to become mindful of underlying emotions.

Often, the first stage in learning to heal emotions is by becoming aware of intense emotions that surface as you have bodywork done. You might say, "I've had headaches and neck pain ever since my parents divorced" or "Ever since I

© Unsplash/ Madison Lavern

started my present job, my neck and shoulders are tight when I get stressed." In addition, by paying attention to what you're thinking and feeling every time your stomach hurts or your shoulders ache, you will begin to realize how your job, relationships, or other stresses are affecting you. You can become attuned to the way your body's responses serve as a barometer of your emotions. It is often the early warning radar system that is telling you about stress long before your mind consciously realizes it.

Finding Help

When it comes to self-help, there are so many different practitioners and philosophies that it can be difficult to know where to start. If you are in pain or in poor physical shape, you may want to look for a physical therapist or personal trainer with expertise in this area. If you just want to improve your health, we suggest exploring the more popular gyms, personal trainers, exercise studios, yoga centers, and self-care practitioners in your area. No matter what the modality, you want to leave the class or session feeling alive, invigorated, inspired, and empowered. A good teacher should encourage you and stimulate your personal growth.

If going in person to the gym or other exercise classes isn't a good option for you, there are many online ways to explore helpful modalities. The internet is full of free exercise videos, yoga classes, and ways to learn tai chi and other forms of exercise at home. If you're over 65 and on Medicare, you may qualify for the SilverSneakers program, which provides free gym membership and many free online exercise videos in a range of modalities.

How Much Exercise?

How much exercise is right for you depends on where you are on the stress curve. (Check back to page 58 to see this diagram.) If you are on the left side of the curve (feeling wired and tired), heavy exercise can be beneficial. It helps to burn off excess adrenaline and calm you down. As you head toward the right side of the curve (feeling exhausted, inflamed, and depleted), heavy exercise can make you feel worse. How do you know? Go exercise and see how you feel. If you feel worse after you exercise or need more than a day off to recuperate, then your body is more run down than you think, and you need to use a gentler form of exercise.

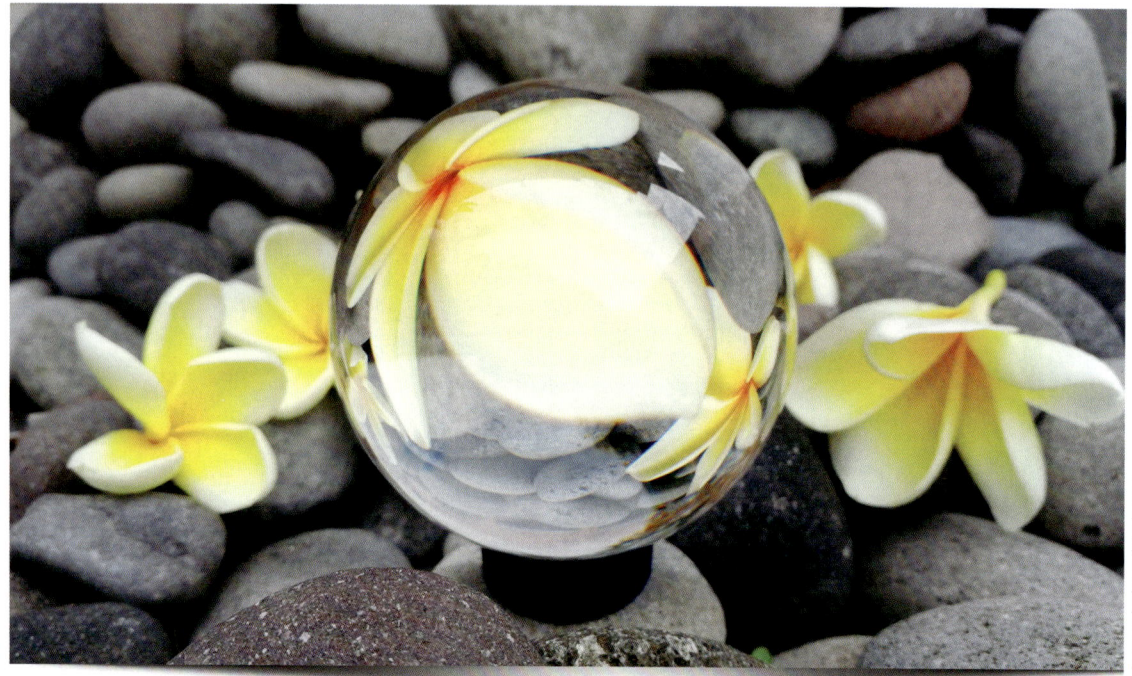

Pain and Discomfort as a Door to Transformation

At the beginning of this book, we asked you how you really feel about your health. Some of you may have reported all kinds of problems, while others may have blissfully denied anything wrong, content to live in denial that something could be a problem. The truth is that we all have health issues to deal with. Wellness is a state we need to work at and live for. Pain and discomfort nudge us to change. As you go forward into your life, embrace this philosophy. Allow your body to give you feedback that you willingly act upon, making yourself healthier every day.

There is **Hope!**

Transformational Medicine is about turning your life around. We see people get better every day. We see people improve their health every day. You can do the same. Envision yourself as already well. The body is a homeostatic organism—that is, it tends toward balance. To allow it to heal, we need to tip the balance to favor factors that promote healing.

As you read on, you will learn how to create a plan that will enable you to do this.

Remember, we don't just want your problem to go away. We want you to use the problem to help you make your health and your life better. This for us is Transformational Medicine—the same treatment that treats a problem also prevents future problems before they happen!

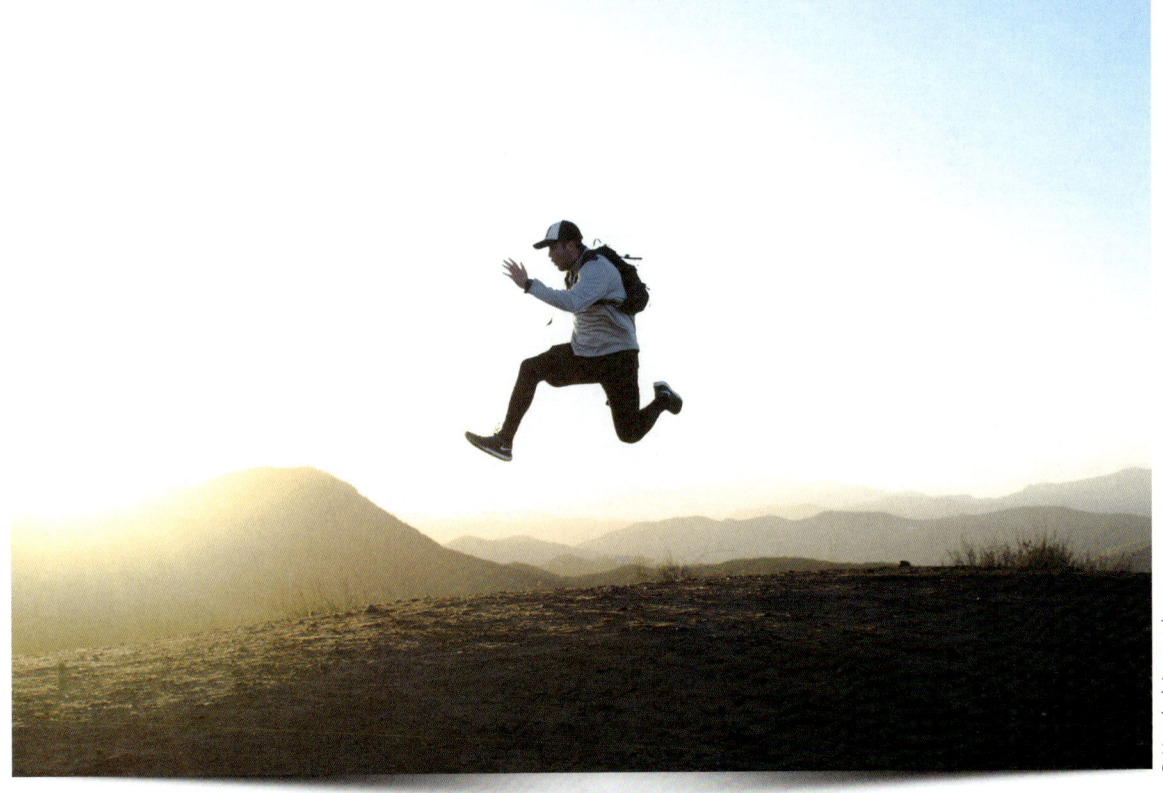

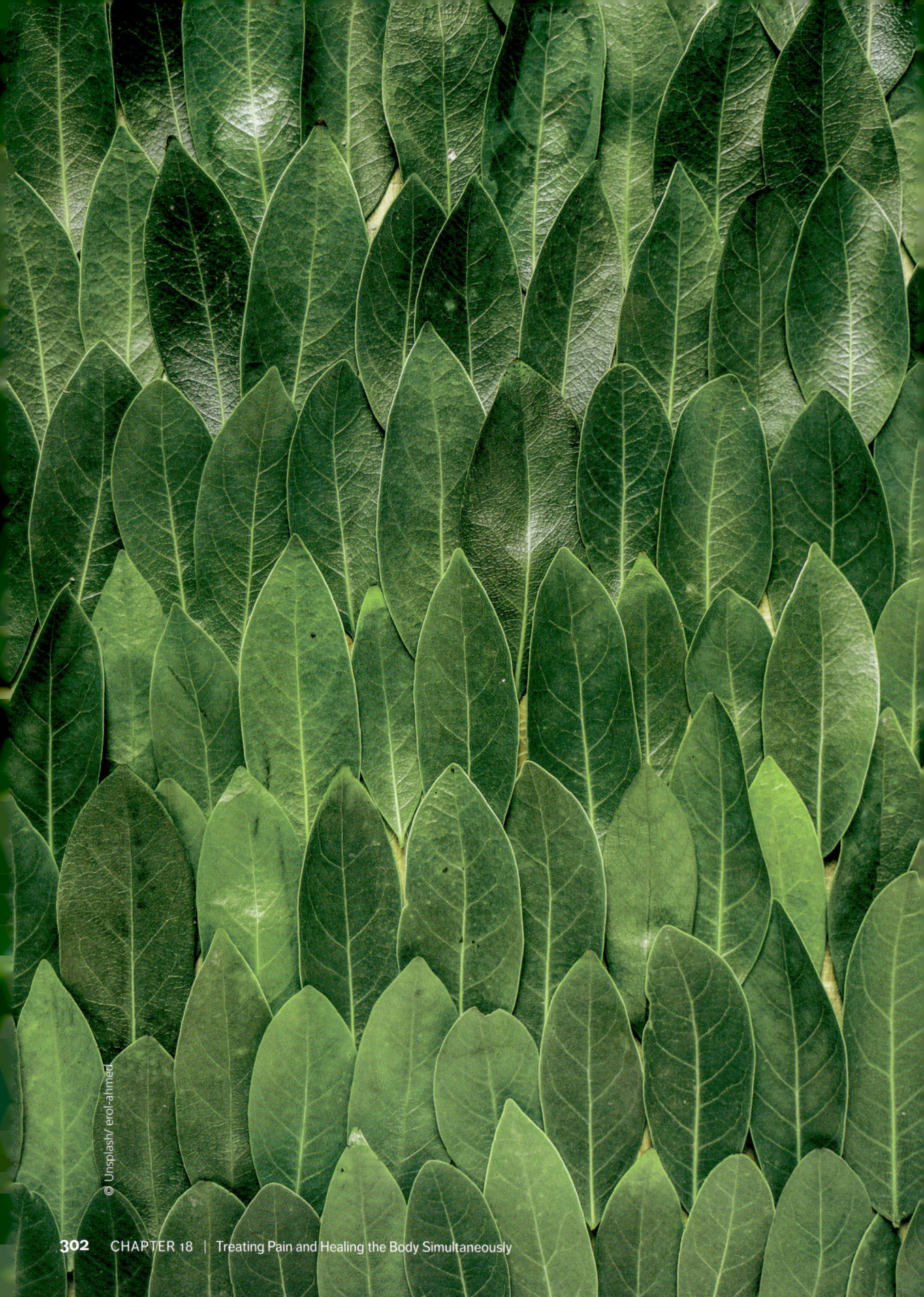

CHAPTER 19
Reversing Cardiovascular Risk

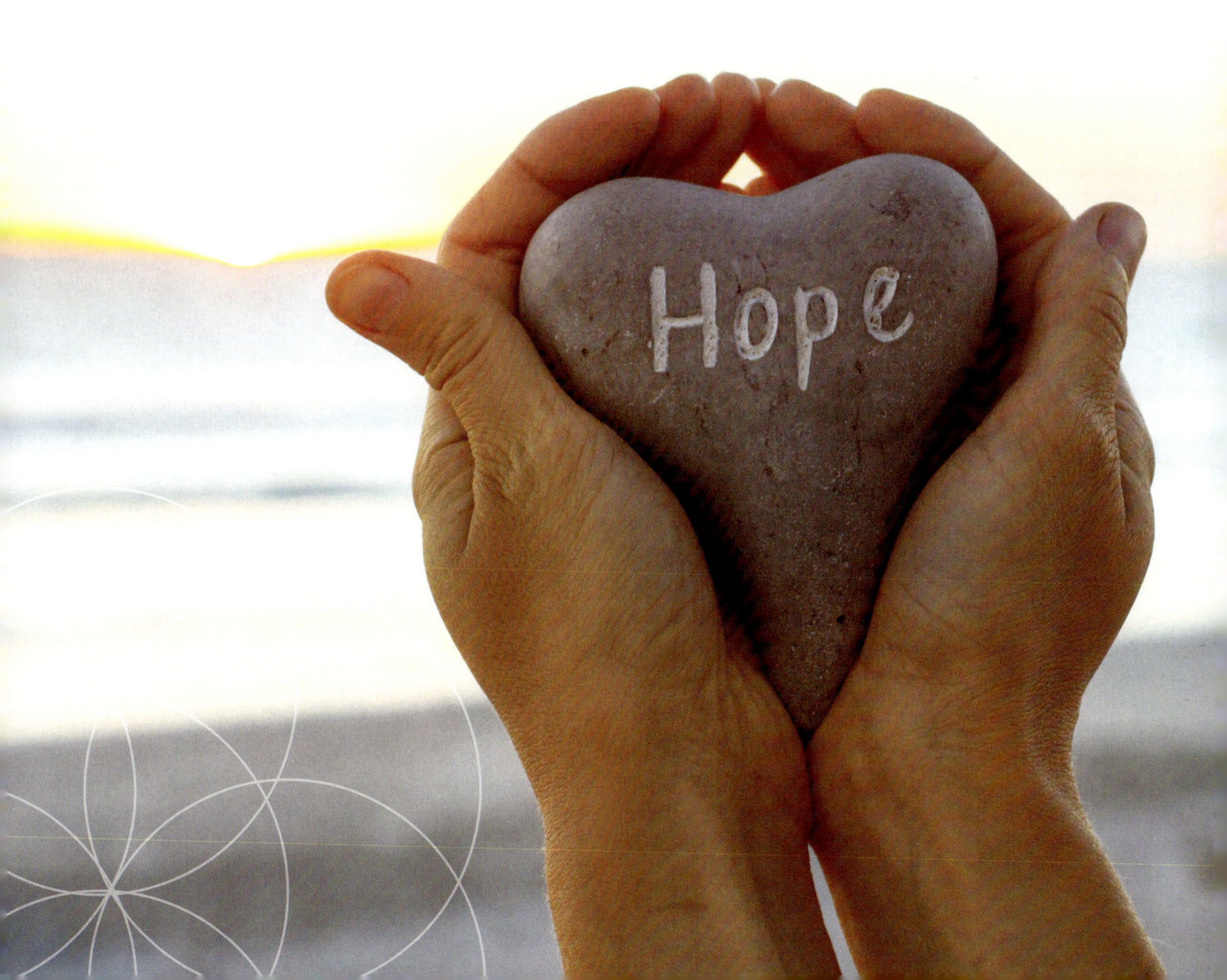

The health of your arteries—especially the arteries that nourish your heart—is vital to your overall wellbeing. By improving the health of your arteries, we can do a lot to reverse your risk of a heart attack. Arterial health is an area that showcases the benefits of an integrative medicine approach. Diet, lifestyle, stress reduction, nutritional supplements, and medications can all be used wisely to optimize arterial health and reduce cardiovascular risk.

Your blood vessels are the roads and highways of your body, busy transporting life-giving blood from your brain to your toes. Your blood carries vital nutrients and oxygen to every cell in your body and then carries their waste products to your liver, kidneys, and lungs to be eliminated from the body. In this chapter, we'll talk about your cardiovascular (heart and associated blood vessels) risk, particularly the risk of a heart attack or stroke, but it's important to remember that we want to keep all your blood vessels healthy so they can nourish every part of your body, including your kidneys, eyes, nerves, peripheral arteries, the male penis and more!

Heart disease is the leading cause of death for both men and women in the U.S. About 659,000 people die from heart disease every year—about one in every four deaths. Understanding cardiac risk can help you look into your own crystal ball, understand your personal risk, and then understand what you can do to lower your risk of cardiac disease.

Coronary Arteries and **Heart Risk**

When the flow of oxygen-rich blood in one or more of the coronary arteries, which supply the heart muscle, is suddenly severely restricted or blocked, you have a heart attack, also known as a myocardial infarction (MI). The affected section of the heart muscle can't get enough oxygen and starts to die. A heart attack can be followed by changes in the heart's beating rhythm, leading to sudden cardiac death. If you survive a heart attack, you're at high risk for another—and also for complications such as dangerous arrhythmias or heart failure.

Most heart attacks are caused by coronary artery disease, or a build-up of cholesterol-containing deposits called plaque inside one or more of the coronary arteries. Plaque can narrow the arteries, restricting the blood flow to the heart. If a plaque deposit ruptures, it spills its contents into the artery, causing a blood clot that partially or completely blocks the blood flow. If blood flow isn't restored quickly, either by a medicine that dissolves the blockage or a catheter placed within the artery that physically opens the blockage, that area of heart muscle begins to die.

Each year, more than a million Americans have a heart attack, and about half of them die. Half of those who die do so within an hour of the start of symptoms and before reaching a hospital.

Although a heart attack seems to be a sudden, catastrophic event, in most cases it really isn't. The warning signs were present for hours, days, weeks, or even months but weren't recognized or were ignored. (This is even more common in women, unfortunately, as they often don't suspect heart disease, believing it to be a "man's illness.")

We want to keep you from having a heart attack by detecting and treating problems with your coronary arteries long before a blockage develops. We can reduce your risk even if your arteries are already clogged with plaque, and even if you've already had a heart attack.

Artery Health

We start by looking at the condition of your coronary arteries. If you're trying to grow flowers and they're not blooming well, you don't just look at the plants. You also look at the environment that the flowers are growing in: the soil and its nutrients, the water or lack of it, the light and shade, the temperature and humidity, bugs and plant diseases, and all the other factors influencing their growth. Similarly, when we look at an artery, we want to look at all the factors that influence its health.

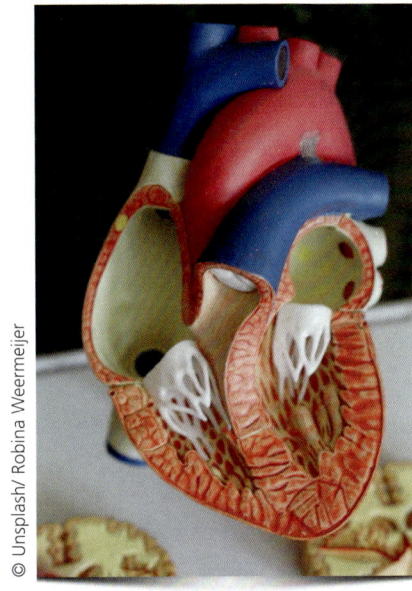

Your arteries carry blood away from the heart to the rest of the body. (Veins return the blood to the heart.) Arteries are strong, flexible tubes made up of three layers. The inner lining of the artery is called the endothelium; this is the part of the vessel that is in direct contact with the blood that flows through it. The next layer, the media, is made of muscle fibers. The media allows the artery to expand and contract to handle changes in your blood pressure. The outer layer is the adventitia, the connective tissue that surrounds the media and anchors the artery to surrounding tissues.

The blood that flows through your arteries contains components that can affect the artery wall. The three components that can damage your arteries are cholesterol, inflammatory molecules, and clotting factors.

Cholesterol

Cholesterol is a waxy, yellow, fat-like substance your body needs for good health. Cholesterol is the primary building block of steroid hormones, for instance, and is also crucial to strong cell membranes. Most of the cholesterol in your body is manufactured in your liver; most of the rest comes from animal foods in your diet. A normal amount of cholesterol in your blood is necessary for maintaining your body, but unhealthy levels can lead to hypercholesterolemia, better known as high cholesterol.

Because fats and water don't mix, molecules of cholesterol are coated with a protein to form a tiny particle—a lipoprotein—so they can travel through your watery bloodstream to where they're needed. The particles come in two main forms: low-density lipoproteins (LDL) and high-density lipoproteins (HDL). We call LDL bad cholesterol because this is the form that clogs arteries. HDL is called good cholesterol, because it transports excess LDL particles back to the liver to be eliminated from the body. You can think of LDL as garbage and HDL as the garbage truck that takes it away.

LDL Patterns

LDL particles are much smaller than a red blood cell. They range in size from large to very small. Think of the larger LDL particles as big beach balls that bounce around in your arteries. They're too large to penetrate the lining of the arterial wall, so they can't cause problems. Smaller LDL particles are more like beach sand, getting into any little crack or crevice in the arterial wall. If the wall is already roughened by inflammation, smaller LDL particles are even more likely to get into it.

To get a better idea of your heart risk from LDL cholesterol, we do a blood test that directly measures the size, distribution, and number of the lipoproteins. The test tells us if you have LDL pattern A or LDL pattern B. LDL pattern A means your LDL particles are mostly large and "fluffy." LDL pattern B means you have a substantial proportion of abnormally small, dense LDL particles. If you have pattern B, you should discuss taking a statin drug with your doctor. If you have pattern A and your total cholesterol is high, you should still discuss taking a statin drug with your doctor. High cholesterol, no matter what the pattern, is undesirable.

Inflammatory Factors

If your body is inflamed, you have high circulating levels of numerous blood factors that can make the walls of your coronary arteries rough instead of smooth. We like to describe the endothelium as the carpet over which the blood flows. If the carpet is rough, thick, or shaggy, it's easy for the small cholesterol particles to stick to it, penetrate into the arterial wall, and start the development of plaque.

Clotting Factors

Inflammation raises the amount of clotting factors such as fibrinogen in your bloodstream. When the level is abnormal, you are more likely to form a clot near an area of a plaque-clogged artery. The clot can partially or completely block the flow of blood downstream and cause a heart attack. Similarly, if an area of soft plaque ruptures and spills cholesterol into the artery, it stimulates the formation of a clot in the area, blocking blood flow.

Plaque

Plaque, the buildup of cholesterol in an artery wall, usually begins in the intima, the inner lining of the artery, and then extends into the media and adventitia. Plaque begins when cholesterol molecules stick to an area of the intima that is injured or inflamed—and penetrate into it, causing an area of local inflammation and making the intima thicker. To fight back, your immune system sends white blood cells and other substances to trap the cholesterol. Unfortunately, this makes things worse, because the white blood cells mix with the cholesterol and cause more inflammation. Now you have a small area of soft plaque that can penetrate into the media. This triggers muscle cells in the adventitia to multiply and form a fibrous cap over the plaque as a way to isolate it. The cap is thin and fragile, however, and it can easily rupture or wear away—if your blood pressure suddenly spikes, for example. The pocket of soft plaque then breaks open and spills out into the artery; a clot forms on it, and you have a heart attack. Roughly three out of four heart attacks are caused by ruptured plaque.

In time, soft plaques become larger and get harder as they accumulate cellular products, calcium, and more cholesterol. Hard plaques have been packed down over time, but they can narrow and stiffen the arteries and block blood flow. They're typically covered by thicker fibrous caps that are less likely to break. Hard plaques that block an artery can be treated by inserting a wire mesh tube called a stent near the blockage to prop the artery open.

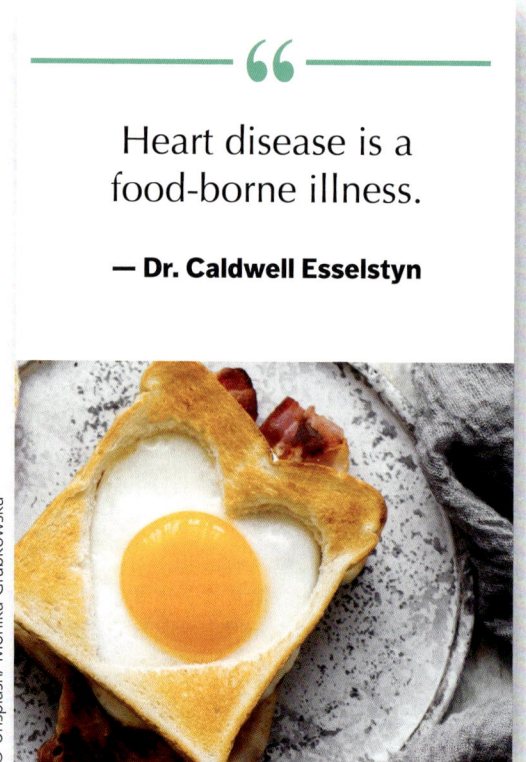

> "
>
> Heart disease is a food-borne illness.
>
> — Dr. Caldwell Esselstyn

© Unsplash/ Monika Grabkowska

How Inflammation Relates to Heart and Blood Vessel Disease

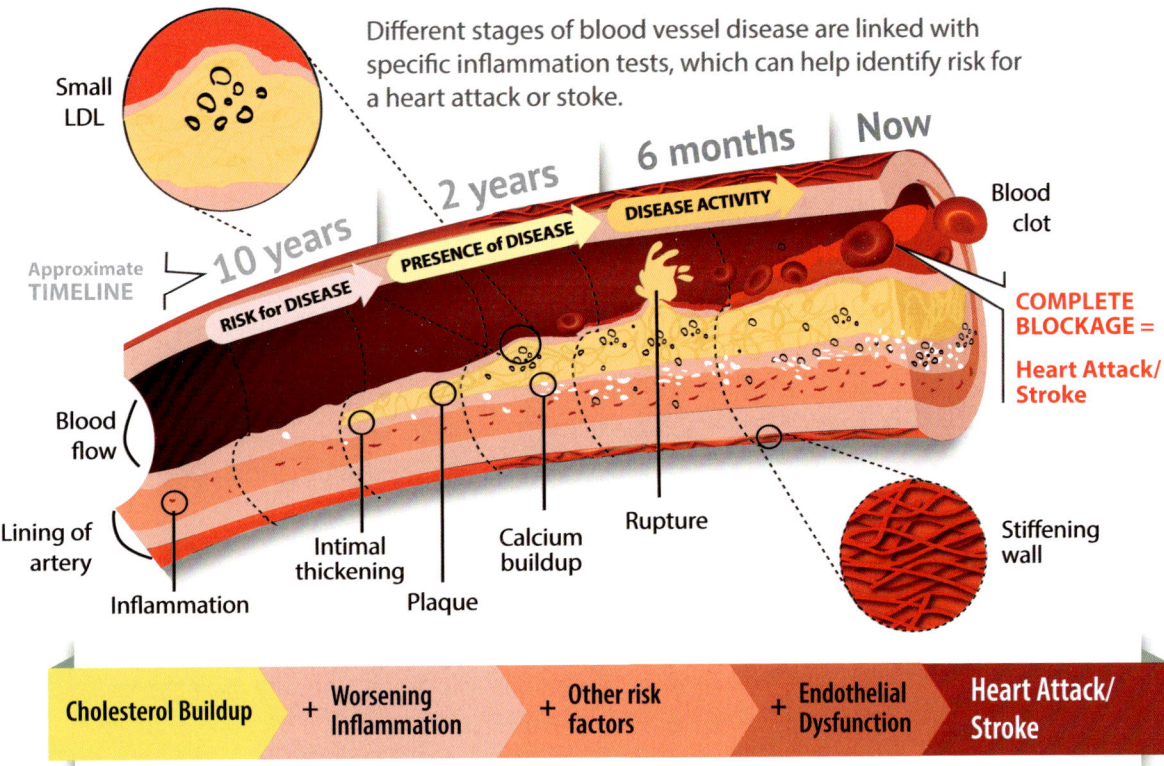

FIGURE 19.1 | How Inflammation Relates to Heart and Blood Vessel Disease

Assessing Your Risk

In general, cardiovascular risk can be divided into two categories:

1. **Progressive arterial blockage that happens over years.** This sort of plaque can begin accumulating while you're still in your 20s. It slowly builds up over decades into arterial blockages that result in cardiovascular disease that appears when you're in your 50s, 60s, or older. It is this process that we must detect early on, because it is REVERSIBLE! Yes! You read that right. You can reverse this process and make your arteries look and behave younger!

2. **The other category of cardiac risk is the sudden catastrophic event.** We often hear about these as tragedies of a relatively young person, previously well, who had a massive heart attack, sudden arrhythmia, aortic rupture, or fatal stroke. Thankfully, sudden catastrophic events are relatively rare compared to the slowly progressive group. These events are hard to predict, although we now have some blood and genetic testing that is better able to forecast them.

Causes of Cardiovascular Disease

The three primary causes of cardiovascular disease are high blood pressure, smoking, and high cholesterol. However, there are many factors to consider:

- **Family history:** Your genetic makeup is important. We can now do complete genetic testing to see the science behind your family history.
- **High blood pressure:** Think of the heart and arteries as a pump and pipes. Your blood pressure is the pressure the blood exerts on the pipes. When the heart pumps (systolic pressure), the pressure rises. When the heart rests (diastolic pressure), the pressure decreases. If either pressure is too high, it can damage the pipes (arterial dysfunction) or the pump (heart failure).
- **High cholesterol:** Plaques in the arteries narrow them and can cause a heart attack.
- **Gender:** Heart disease is thought of as a male problem, but that's far from the truth. Men are about twice as likely as women to have a heart attack, but a heart attack is only one form of heart disease. Among men, the prevalence of heart disease is about 12.6 percent; among women, it's 10.1 percent. Heart disease causes about 24 percent of all male deaths; it causes 22.3 percent of all female deaths. Today atherosclerotic heart disease is the leading killer of women.
- **Age:** Although increasing age is associated with increasing heart disease, ageing itself doesn't have to cause heart disease. If we address all of the other risk factors involved, we can mitigate the effects of age.
- **Diabetes:** High blood sugar levels cause inflammation and can damage both large and small blood vessel walls. We need to get blood sugar levels down and under control.
- **Inflammation:** Inflammation often involves blood vessels throughout the body, damaging the inner lining of arteries and allowing for deposition of cholesterol into plaque. Vascular inflammation is associated with heart attack and stroke.
- **Autoimmune diseases:** System lupus erythematosus, rheumatoid arthritis, and other autoimmune diseases are often associated with inflammation but can also directly affect the arterial wall.
- **Hormones:** Estrogen, birth control pills, and testosterone supplements may negatively influence blood pressure, cholesterol, and blood clotting factors.
- **Obesity:** Obesity is often associated with high blood pressure, high cholesterol, prediabetes, and diabetes. Obesity is also associated with elevated levels of inflammation.
- **Oral hygiene:** Poor oral hygiene, particularly gum disease (gingivitis), is associated with inflammation and heart disease
- **Stress:** Stress has both direct and indirect effects on coronary artery disease. Directly, it causes an outpouring of adrenaline and cortisol, which raises blood pressure and blood sugar levels, causing potential damage to the arteries. Stress is also often associated with lifestyle factors such as poor sleep, bad diet, and no exercise, all of which indirectly adversely affect the arteries.
- **Smoking:** Smoking releases free radicals, which are toxic to the lining of the arteries. It also increases levels of carbon monoxide in the blood, which decreases oxygen delivery to the tissues, including the heart.
- **Poor sleep:** Altered circadian rhythms (sleep-wake cycles) can also negatively affect the heart.

Tests for Heart Disease

We can detect the signs of heart disease and determine how bad it is using a wide range of tests.

To find early disease, we start with very basic testing. The first is the simplest of all: check your blood pressure. You can do this at home with an inexpensive blood pressure monitor, or you can check it using the free machine found in many pharmacies. Your doctor will routinely check your blood pressure at every visit, no matter why you're there.

We then move on to simple blood tests that look at your cholesterol levels (lipid panel). We check your total cholesterol, LDL, HDL, triglycerides and the cholesterol/HDL ratio as well as non-HDL cholesterol. We also usually test for other metabolic markers, like blood glucose and calcium (comprehensive metabolic panel). The information we get from these tests is a good start, but if we suspect heart disease, we like to expand on it.

Newer technology lets us look at subfractions within the LDL and HDL molecules and see their size. In general, the smaller a cholesterol molecule, the more atherogenic (plaque-creating) it is. To continue with our garbage and garbage truck metaphor, we call the small LDL "smelly garbage." Similarly, within the HDL (good cholesterol) molecules, the bigger the better. Smaller HDL molecules don't work very well. They're like garbage trucks that should be in the shop.

We like to measure inflammatory markers that help us ascertain risk. In general, high cholesterol is a marker of cardiovascular risk, but it's really the inflammation it causes that makes your risk go up. We measure inflammation in the arteries using a test called hs-CRP (highly sensitive C-reactive protein). The risk for cardiovascular disease goes up as LDL and hs-CRP go up together.

Heart Imaging

For detecting blockages in the coronary arteries, an EKG (electrocardiogram) is helpful only if you are actually having a heart attack. We want to detect a blockage before you have a heart attack, so we use a variety of imaging tests to visualize the arteries.

The most common test is an exercise stress test. By making your heart work harder as you walk on a treadmill, and by recording your heartbeats on an EKG and taking your blood pressure, we can detect low blood flow in the arteries. The problem with the exercise stress test is that it only detects a blockage if the artery is at least 70 percent clogged. In addition, this test isn't very sensitive. It only detects about 70 percent of the people with arteries that are severely clogged, and it doesn't work as well on women and people with diabetes.

When we add an echocardiogram (sound wave pictures of the heart) to an exercise stress test, also known as a stress echo, the sensitivity increases to between 79 and 85 percent, and it works well on everyone. Similarly, myocardial perfusion imaging, also called nuclear stress

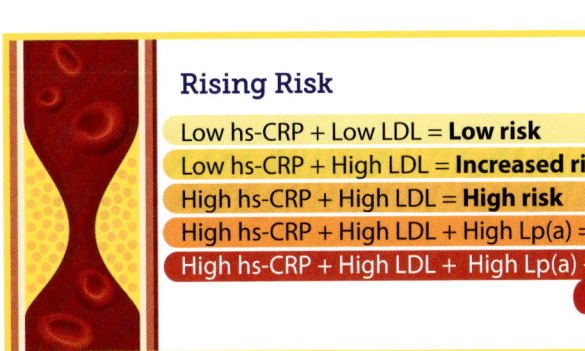

FIGURE 19. 2 | Heart Risk

testing, has a sensitivity of 83 to 85 percent.

Stress positron emission tomography (sPET) scanning with rubidium has increased sensitivity and specificity (accuracy) for detecting blockages when compared to traditional nuclear stress testing. As such, sPET has been incorporated into recent clinical guidelines for the evaluation of patients with chest pain or with high-risk characteristics that rule out an exercise stress test. We don't use it routinely for other patients.

Cardiac Score

Cardiac calcium scoring, also called a heart scan or calcium score, is a noninvasive computed tomography (CT) scan of the heart. It measures the amount of calcified (hardened) plaque in your coronary arteries. The total calcium score reflects your risk for developing cardiovascular events such as a heart attack, stroke, or the need to have a coronary bypass or angioplasty, but it doesn't tell you if any specific artery is significantly narrowed or blocked. Calcium scores are helpful for stratifying your risk. This test is attractive in that it is fairly cheap (although health insurance may not cover it), easily accessible, and uses low-dose radiation. This test picks up only calcium deposits, which represent hard plaque (the less dangerous kind). It can be misleading because it doesn't detect the more dangerous soft plaque. We want to know about both kinds.

When patients have been on high-dose statins, their cardiac calcium score will increase. This is because statins remove cholesterol and "pack" the soft plaque down so it becomes hard plaque. We stop following cardiac scores for these patients because the results become unreliable.

Coronary Catheter Angiogram

The gold standard for detecting blockages is the invasive coronary catheter angiogram, where a thin catheter is inserted through the wrist or groin and snaked up to the heart. Then dye is injected into the coronary arteries while X-rays are taken. This shows where the blockages are and lets the cardiologist decide whether medication, stents, or surgery (or some combination) is the best way to treat the arteries.

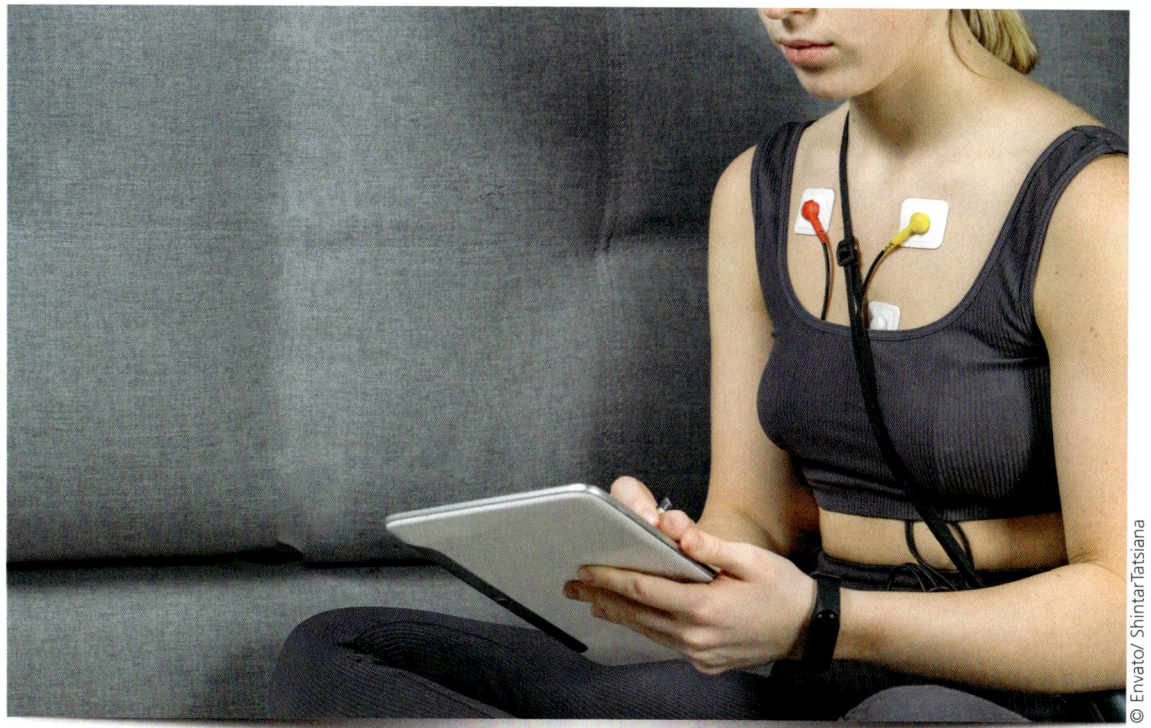

Coronary Computed Tomography Angiography

Coronary computed tomography angiography (CCTA) uses an injection of iodine-containing contrast material and CT scanning to examine the coronary arteries. The test can reveal if and where the arteries are narrowed or blocked and how badly they are blocked. A CCTA will detect both hard and soft plaque.

This test can see problems in all three layers of the artery wall. CCTA can also characterize atherosclerotic plaque by its level of calcification, which is valuable for risk stratification and appropriate treatment. The drawback is it exposes you to a lot of radiation and may not be covered by health insurance. Unlike standard coronary angiography, which is performed by an interventional cardiologist, CCTA is done by a technician. If a stent is needed, it can't be done on the spot.

Measuring Carotid Atherosclerosis

The carotid arteries carry blood to the brain. Like the coronary arteries, they can get clogged with plaque, which could lead to a stroke (brain attack). We can use Doppler ultrasound to check for clogging in these crucial arteries. The process is noninvasive, quick, and painless. It's sometimes offered by healthcare centers as part of an inexpensive package that also includes an EKG and an abdominal ultrasound to check for aortic aneurysm (a bulge at a weak spot in the aorta).

The carotid Doppler test may be useful in older adults, stroke patients, and people at risk of stroke. This test shows the severity of carotid blockage, which helps you and your doctor decide on the best course of treatment. Finding a blockage in the carotid artery also alerts us to check for atherosclerosis elsewhere. If you have a blockage in the 50 to 70 percent range, we usually recommend repeat scanning every six months. If a blockage exceeds 70 percent, your doctor may recommend inserting a stent to open the artery or surgical endarterectomy to remove the plaque.

A carotid intima-media thickness test (CIMT) uses ultrasound imaging to measure the thickness of the two inner layers (the intima and media) of the carotid artery and determine the extent of plaque build-up. If a CIMT shows increased thickness, you may be at greater risk for cardiovascular disease and stroke. CIMT is used mainly for research and usually far less often than a typical carotid ultrasound

Testing for Endothelial Function

Endothelial function testing looks at the endothelium, the thin layer of cells that lines the interior of your blood vessels. Endothelial cells control the relaxation and contraction of the blood vessels. When the endothelial function isn't working well, you may have non-obstructive coronary artery disease, also called microvascular disease. You don't have any blockages in your coronary arteries, but they're stiff and narrowed so they can't dilate (open up) enough to let more blood through when your heart needs it—when you exercise or are under stress, for example. This condition tends to affect women more than men. Symptoms include chronic chest pain (angina), shortness of breath, and constant tiredness and loss of energy.

A loss of endothelial function is a warning sign that atherosclerotic plaques are probably in your future. It's also a warning of future heart failure. It is possible to have macrovascular disease (where plaque is seen) as well as microvascular disease (where no plaque is seen) together with endothelial dysfunction – all happening simultaneously!

Endothelial dysfunction is often underdiagnosed because the symptoms can be vague and are easy to attribute to something else. In medicine there is also an unfortunate tendency to minimize women's symptoms and just dismiss them as stress—even though non-obstructive heart disease is more common in women. A further obstacle to diagnosis is that until recently, we didn't have a good test for endothelial dysfunction.

The EndoPAT test is the only FDA-cleared test for the non-invasive assessment of endothelial dysfunction. This is a safe, noninvasive, office-based test that uses sensors placed on two fingers to assess artery health. The test gives us a score we can use to detect and monitor changes in endothelial function over time.

We can treat endothelial dysfunction to relieve symptoms and keep it from getting worse with medications to lower blood pressure and blood cholesterol. In severe cases, we can use nitrate therapy to relieve chest pain.

ED = ED

Endothelial dysfunction can equal erectile dysfunction. When endothelial function is poor, the small arteries don't open up well. Men start noticing their erections are not as strong. This can be an indicator that other small arteries are also not working as well. Arteries in the brain can get blocked, causing cerebral microinfarcts that can lead to dementia. In the kidneys, endothelial dysfunction can cause loss of kidney function; in the eyes, it can cause vision loss. In fact, any part of the body can be damaged by endothelial dysfunction in the small arteries.

A Healthy Glycocalyx: The Key to Endothelial Function

It now seems apparent that the key to healthy endothelial function is a healthy glycocalyx, the inner lining of the endothelium. The glycocalyx is a micron-thin, carbohydrate-rich layer that coats the endothelial cells of the intima, the inner lining of arteries. It forms a permeable barrier between the blood that flows through the artery and the endothelium. The glycocalyx acts as a control center for this microenvironment. In healthy vessels, the endothelial glycocalyx influences vascular permeability, minimizes dysfunction between blood cells and vessel walls, and senses sheer pressure, which can cause tears in the vessel wall. The glycocalyx keep cholesterol molecules from sticking to the endothelium and penetrating into the intima. It also stops the build-up of blood clots, reacts with nitrous oxide (NO) to dilate the arteries, and decreases vascular permeability, or leaky blood vessels. Clearly, the glycocalyx is highly protective of the artery walls. If it's disrupted or dysfunctional, the protection is decreased or lost. Damage to the glycocalyx is associated with coronary artery disease, stroke, peripheral artery disease, kidney disease, diabetic neuropathy, and erectile dysfunction.

The same things that damage other parts of your body also damage the glycocalyx: high blood sugar, a high-carb diet, air pollution, smoking, alcohol, aging, inflammation, hypertension, and stress.

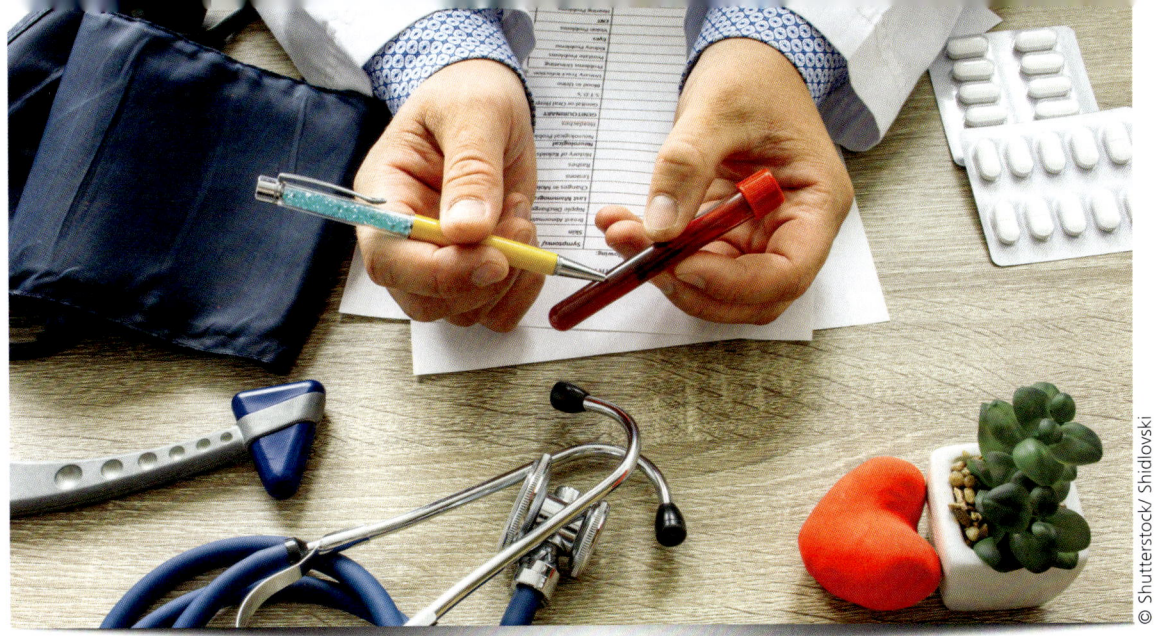

In-Depth Testing: Looking for Progressive Arterial Damage

We can make the crystal ball of diagnosis clearer with in-depth testing that investigates specific markers and warning signs of cardiovascular disease and helps us know what to do to reverse them. Not everyone needs this level of testing, and not every test is appropriate. We work with our patients to decide which tests to do and help them understand the results.

Atherogenic Factors

Cholesterol isn't the only blood factor that can cause or contribute to atherosclerosis and plaque formation. We like to look at apolipoprotein B (Apo-B). This protein is found on the surface of LDL particles. It allows the LDL to attach to receptors on the surface of cells, especially in the liver. It tends to track with your LDL level. High levels of Apo-B dramatically increase your risk of coronary artery disease. To lower your risk, we need to lower your overall LDL level using diet, red rice yeast extract, or medications.

Lipoprotein(a), or Lp(a), is an LDL particle containing a protein called apolipoprotein(a). This particle forms a sticky globule that tends to clog up small arteries, not only in the heart but also in the brain, where it can cause a stroke, and in the hip, where it can cause a breakdown of the bone called avascular necrosis. Unfortunately, there are no good treatments for Lp(a) lowering. Instead, we reduce your other risk factors, especially your LDL.

Inflammatory Markers

Inflammatory blood markers help us assess your risk of blood clots and oxidative stress that can lead to endothelial dysfunction:

- **Hs-CRP is a marker of inflammation in the blood vessels.** The ideal level is 1 mg/L or less; moderate levels are between 1 and 3mg/L. Between 3 and 10 mg/L is concerning for high inflammation in the blood vessels. Higher than 10 mg/L is usually associated with a viral or bacterial illness or an autoimmune disease.

- **Fibrinogen antigen shows an increased risk of blood clots**. Myeloperoxidase and oxidized LDL

(OxLDL) show high oxidative stress, which triggers inflammation and the risk of future plaque build-up. Changing diet and lifestyle habits is helpful to correct this.

- **The F2-isoprostane/creatinine ratio is also used to measure oxidative stress.** ADMA (asymmetric dimethylarginine) is helpful for looking at endothelial function.

- **SDMA (symmetric dimethylarginine) is a helpful marker to look at both chronic arterial disease and also chronic kidney disease.**

- **Lp-PLA2 helps evaluate the risk of developing coronary heart disease (CHD) and the risk of having an ischemic stroke.** Lp-PLA2 increases with active cholesterol buildup in the arterial wall and therefore should be taken seriously.

- **Myeloperoxidase (MPO) is an enzyme that is associated with an increased risk of plaque rupture causing a heart attack.** If MPO and Lp-PLA2 levels are both high, this implies active coronary artery disease. We need to take immediate steps to reduce the risk.

Metabolic Markers

Your risk of coronary artery disease—and other diseases such as diabetes—is higher if some metabolic markers, such as insulin, are high. We look at several of these to get a total insulin resistance score. The score is helpful for telling us if you have prediabetes and, if so, how far along in the progression to type 2 diabetes you are.

- Fasting glucose levels tell us what your blood sugar is after a 12-hour fast. Ideally, it will be around 100 and no higher than 129.

- HbA1C is a blood marker that tells us the three-month average of your glucose levels. Ideally, it will be 5.7 percent or below. The higher it is above that number, the greater your risk for developing or already having type 2 diabetes.

- Intact insulin, C-peptide, and total insulin levels are markers that tell us how well your body is using the hormone insulin.

Other Markers

The next things we look at are a range of other markers that give us a better picture of your overall health.

- **Homocysteine:** a marker of the chemical process known as methylation. Methylation problems have been implicated in heart disease, strokes, cancer, and a host of other medical problems

- **Vitamin D levels:** Low blood levels of vitamin D are associated with an increased risk of heart attacks and strokes and with worsening heart failure.

- **TMAO levels:** TMAO is a metabolite produced by your gut bacteria when you digest red meat. It can be used as a surrogate marker for dysbiosis in the gut.

- **Omega-3 fatty acids in the blood:** Omega-3 fatty acid supplements, typically from fish oil, have been shown to reduce cardiovascular events in people who already have cardiovascular disease. We can check your levels with a blood test using the omega-3 index. We prefer to get a better idea by looking at your three-month average using the OmegaCheck blood test.

PULS Testing: Assessing Risk for an Acute Coronary Event

Is it possible to predict the rupture of an unstable plaque lesion before it happens? Or, in other words, is it possible to predict and prevent a heart attack? Until recently, this was very difficult. Studies have shown that more than half of the people who have a first heart attack have at most only one risk factor, as defined by the usual guidelines. What we want is a test that looks deeper into multiple biomarkers and tells us if someone at apparently low risk is actually in more danger. The PULS Cardiac Test is a sophisticated blood test that measures multiple biomarkers of the body's immune system response to endothelial damage and inflammation, which can ultimately lead to unstable plaque. The test uses an algorithm of age, sex, diabetes, and family history of heart attack, combined with serum levels of seven biomarkers (CTACK, eotaxin, Fas ligand, HGF, IL-16, MCP-3, and sFas) to come up with a score that shows the risk for an acute cardiac event within the next five years. This improved accuracy in cardiovascular risk classification could lead to improved preventive care and fewer deaths.

Treating Coronary Artery Disease

The most important factor when treating cardiovascular disease is a good diagnosis. Once you have this, you can tailor your treatment regimen to treat the problem, reverse the atherogenic process, and prevent future problems.

We feel it is imperative that you work with an excellent cardiologist. We are fortunate to have access to a world-renowned cardiac care team available to us in Cincinnati at The Christ Hospital, led by Dr. Dean Kereiakes.

But before we move to drugs and invasive treatments, we need to look at the bigger picture for you as an individual.

Do we need to treat? Some patients have elevated cholesterol but zero other risk factors. They may not need any treatment at all. Conversely, we see many patients who have fairly normal cholesterol levels but have other risk factors that need very aggressive treatment.

What about diet and lifestyle? We cannot overstate the benefits of a good diet. We have seen patients with severe heart disease who could not tolerate medication reverse their cardiovascular disease with diet, exercise, and stress reduction. In fact, this is the basis of the Ornish Program, where Dr. Dean Ornish uses a vegetarian diet, fish oil, exercise, and stress reduction. For most of our patients we recommend a modified Mediterranean diet as described in chapter 9.

Supplements for Heart Health

What about supplements? Many, many dietary supplements are said to help prevent or treat heart disease. The reality is that while some help, most are ineffective. Taking a handful of supplements each day isn't a substitute for lifestyle changes and medical treatment.

Those supplements we have found to be helpful include:

- **Red rice yeast extract (RRYE):** This is the nutritional supplement from which the original statin, lovastatin (Mevacor) was derived. In fact, RRYE is so similar to a statin that drug companies have made it very difficult for supplement companies to use high-grade RRYE. We suggest RRYE for patients who can't tolerate the side effects of statin drugs.

- **Fish oil:** Fish oil is well recognized for its heart-healthy benefits. Two main omega-3 fatty acids, eicosapentaenoic acid (EPA) and docosahexaenoic acid (DHA), are found mainly in fish and fish oil. Omega-3s from fish and fish oil have been recommended by the American Heart Association (AHA) for the past 20 years to reduce cardiovascular events, like heart attack or stroke, in people who already have cardiovascular disease (CVD). Fish oil is also excellent at lowering triglycerides. We prefer patients to get nutritional supplements through food, but it's difficult to get enough omega-3 fatty acids simply by eating fatty fish. We recommend eating fish at least twice a week and taking a daily high-quality, mercury-free fish oil supplement. It's possible that fish oil could increase the risk of atrial fibrillation, so we don't recommend this supplement for people who have been diagnosed with this condition. Fish oil may also prolong bleeding, so patients on blood thinners should discuss this topic further with their physicians.

- **B vitamins and magnesium to treat high homocysteine:** This is controversial, because studies show that treating high homocysteine doesn't necessarily improve cardiovascular outcomes. However, high homocysteine shows that you're not methylating well, which confers a higher risk for many illnesses, including stroke, cancer, and depression.

- **Niacin:** Niacin can help lower triglycerides–Lp(a) to a small extent, and LDL–but this is controversial. Niacin in general is very cheap, but it can cause flushing, raised liver enzymes, and even gout. Low-flush niacin or niacinamide is a little more expensive but causes fewer problems. Niacin and niacinamide are no longer as popular as studies have not shown long-term benefits.

- **Treating the glycocalyx:** A supplement called Arterosil is probably the only one on the market that does this well. It is a patented seaweed extract that can stabilize and regress vulnerable plaque.

- **Coenzyme Q10 (CoQ10):** This is a substance similar to a vitamin, in that it's found in every cell in your body and is needed to produce energy. Because it's all over, or ubiquitous, it's also called ubiquinone. CoQ10 is said to help heart failure and boost energy, but most of our patients take it because statin drugs tend to leach CoQ10 from the body. It's possible that low levels of CoQ10 cause some of the fatigue and muscle pain associated with these drugs. We suggest taking 100 mg to 300 mg daily.

- **Fiber:** Fiber lowers cholesterol and improves both gut and heart health (see chapter 10). The best way to get fiber is from your food. If you don't get enough this way, a daily fiber supplement will help.

- **Magnesium:** Low magnesium levels are linked to hypertension and plaque buildup and can be a predictor of heart disease. The best way to get more magnesium is by eating foods such as nuts, beans, and dark-green leafy vegetables. If you want to take a supplement, magnesium glycinate and reacted magnesium are absorbed and tolerated well. Do not take magnesium citrate, which causes diarrhea and should be limited to the treatment of constipation.

- **L–carnitine:** Studies using the amino acid L-carnitine have shown an improvement in heart function and a reduction in symptoms for people who have angina or heart failure. Taking L-carnitine may also help reduce damage and complications following a heart attack.

- **Resveratrol:** This antioxidant is found in red wine and appears to have a protective effect on arteries. Unfortunately (or perhaps fortunately), if you want to get enough resveratrol to help, you need to drink about two thousand bottles of red wine a day. Supplements are a better choice.
- **Green tea:** Green tea is a good antioxidant that appears to have a mild cholesterol-lowering effect.
- **Garlic:** Garlic in various forms is used to lower blood pressure and cholesterol, although we have never found this to be true. Allicin, one of its components, is very helpful in treating SIBO. We recommend garlic as a food.
- **Nattokinase:** An enzyme derived from fermented soybeans, nattokinase appears to lower fibrinogen and is helpful for preventing blood clots in patients with high levels of fibrinogen antigen.
- **Vitamin D:** Vitamin D has multiple benefits in the body, including improving the way the immune system functions.

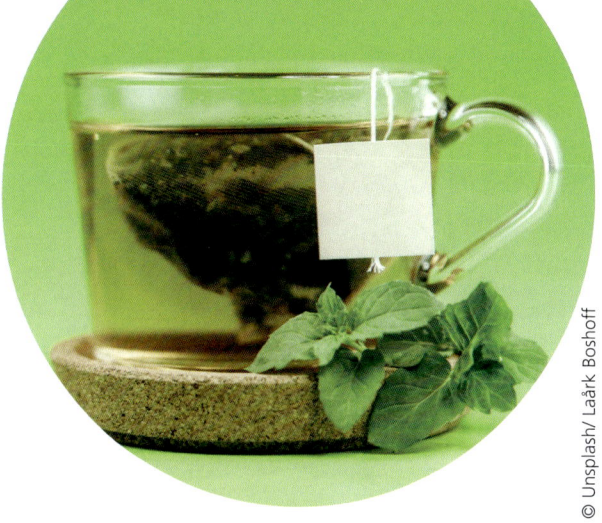

It is also very important for the integrity of the blood vessel wall.

Supplement Cautions

Research all supplements thoroughly using reliable sources before you start taking them. Do not rely on the advice of the sales clerk in the health food store! Tell your doctor about all supplements you take, even a multivitamin. Supplements can have side effects and may trigger interactions with your prescription and nonprescription drugs.

Cholesterol-Lowering Drugs

Two types of drugs—statins and PCSK9 inhibitors—are very effective for lowering blood cholesterol and helping to stabilize plaque. The first statin drug was introduced in 1987. Since then, statins have become the mainstay of drug treatment for atherosclerosis. These drugs work in three main ways:

1. They block an enzyme called HMG-CoA reductase that your liver needs to make cholesterol. This lowers cholesterol in your bloodstream.
2. Statins help reabsorb existing cholesterol. By lowering the amount of cholesterol your liver can make, statins make you reabsorb cholesterol that has built up as plaques containing LDL in your arteries. This is one of the ways it helps to remodel plaque formation and reopen clogged arteries.
3. Statins lower inflammation.

Statin drugs do have some side effects, such as muscle pain and raised liver enzymes. Most people can easily tolerate the side effects, and they often diminish within a few months. Often patients on statins develop insulin resistance and we see their glucose levels rise. Some people, however, have more severe side effects, and some people with very severe high cholesterol don't get enough help from the drugs. For these people, we suggest PCSK9 inhibitors alirocumab (Praluent) and evolocumab (Repatha). These drugs block PCSK9, a protein that limits the effectiveness of cholesterol receptors in the liver. By blocking the protein, the receptors are better able to remove cholesterol from your bloodstream. These drugs are remarkably effective, slashing LDL cholesterol levels by an average of 47 percent and reducing the risk of a heart attack by 27 percent. When combined with a statin, a PCSK9 inhibitor can lower LDL levels by more than half.

If statins or PCSK9 inhibitors are not an option, there are other types of drugs such as fibrates, bile acid resins, selective cholesterol absorption inhibitors, and adenosine triphosphate-citrate lyase (ACL) inhibitors.

Can You Lower Cholesterol Too Much?

This is a question we're often asked by patients. Since cholesterol is needed in the body, especially to make hormones, doesn't lowering LDL result in long- term harm? For most people the answer appears to be no. Studies have not shown significant detrimental effects on hormones, mood, or a variety of other issues. This doesn't mean these drugs are free of side effects. We recommend you always research recommended drugs and discuss the pros and cons with your doctor.

Opening Up Arteries: Stents and Bypass Grafts

Prior to the advent of statin drugs, we remember patients who would have one bypass graft after the other, usually succumbing to a heart attack or heart failure because the grafts clogged with cholesterol. Stents and cholesterol-lowering medications have literally revolutionized the ability to open up arteries and restore blood flow (revascularize), not only in the heart, but the neck, kidneys, and lower extremities. This has saved and restored healthy lives to countless patients.

The **Bottom Line**

It is now possible to reopen arteries and restore a healthy blood flow all over the body. While drugs and stents do an excellent job to reopen and remodel the artery wall, it is imperative we don't rely just on them.

When we correct all the surrounding factors that are associated with cardiovascular disease, something interesting happens:

- Health in other areas of the body improves.
- Vitality is restored.
- We can transform lives!

Cardiovascular disease is an area where we see Transformational Medicine work extremely well. We see people all the time who have had a heart attack then use the experience to transform their lives in the most meaningful ways. But the best time to improve the heath of your arteries is before you get sick. Using the diagnostic tools we have shown you, you too can start working on your arteries today.

You, too, can Get Well, Be Well and Stay Well!

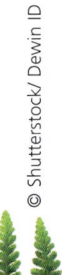
© Shutterstock/ Dewin ID

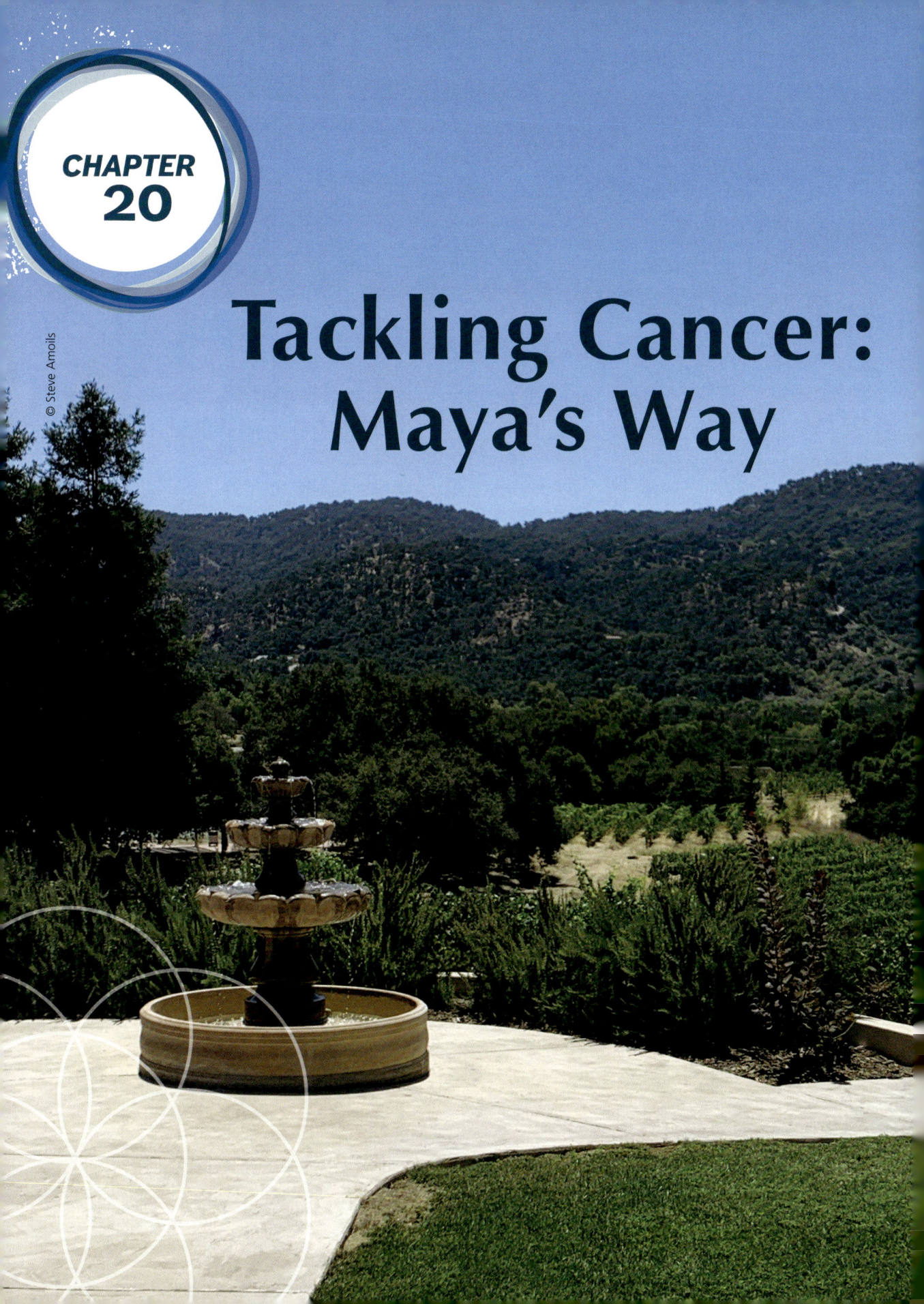

CHAPTER 20

Tackling Cancer: Maya's Way

> Your experience has been an extraordinary one.
>
> **Let it undo you.**
>
> **Let it break you and make you whole again.**
>
> Walk away from it bigger, brighter and filled with what you need to live like your soul is on fire.
>
> —Maya Amoils

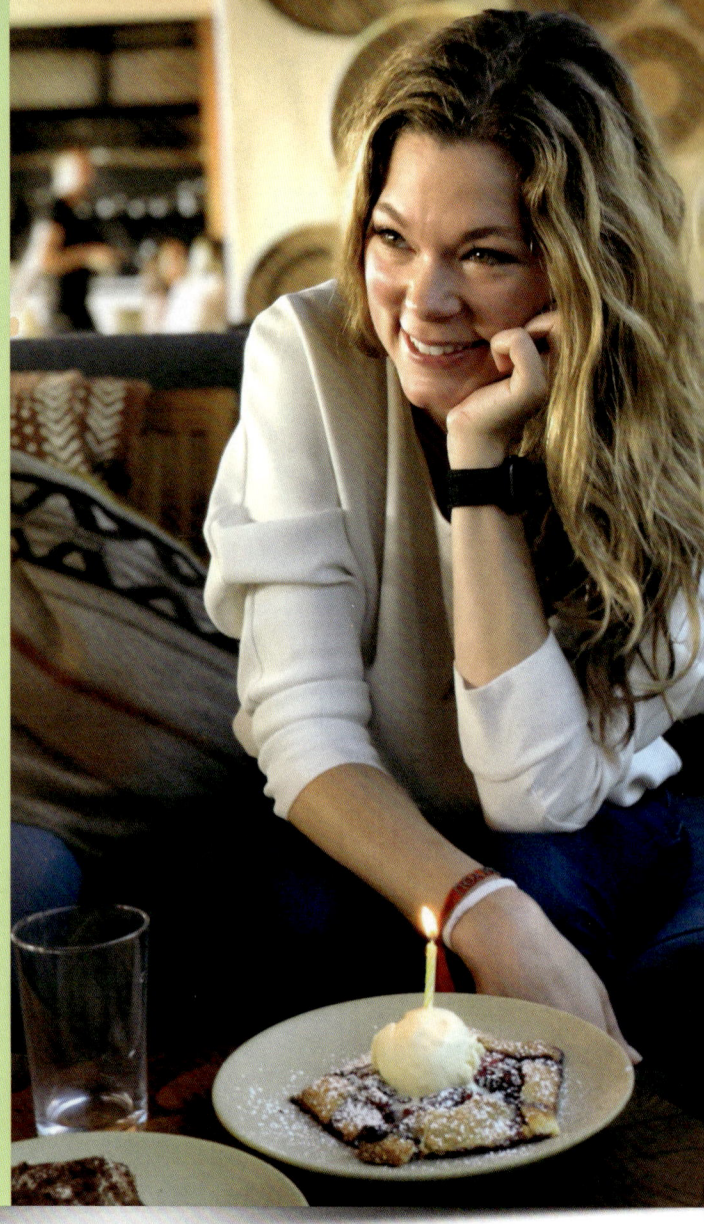

On November 13, 2018, we received a call that no parent ever wants to hear: Our twenty-eight-year-old daughter, Maya, had been diagnosed with stage 4 ovarian cancer. She was the epitome of health and vibrancy but now faced a cancer that is almost universally fatal. We were shocked! Maya was our energizer bunny. Her work took her all over the world every month. She had just run a half-marathon. She ate a fantastic diet, exercised daily, meditated, never smoked, had no family history, and no risk factors! We knew we were dealing with a formidable adversary.

The world of oncology is rapidly changing. Treatments are improving, achieving better outcomes with fewer side effects. Maya's oncology team directed her treatment using evidence-based medicine, while we focused on giving Maya the ancillary tools to cope with her new reality. We also knew that if we could help her see the cancer differently, we could empower her to take control of aspects of her life that would improve her quality of life, help her reduce side effects, and aim to enhance her clinical outcomes. She needed to learn to lower her stress levels, ensure adequate sleep, focus on daily movement, use supplements and integrative therapies to reduce side effects, and increase her energy level. We wanted her to utilize everything she could—mind, body, and spirit—to help her face this daunting challenge.

We regularly see patients who seek help with integrative medical options for a cancer diagnosis. Despite continually looking at claims that alternative therapies can cure cancer, we have never found this to be true. We do think that integrative medicine offers an extremely valuable approach to cancer, but that it should be used as adjunctive care. In other words, integrative medicine does not replace conventional oncological care, but it is incredibly helpful in a supportive role.

Patients sometimes don't want to hear this. Getting a diagnosis of cancer is very traumatic. They feel they can't or don't want to go through chemo, radiation, or surgery because they have heard so many horror stories about these treatments. Because conventional chemotherapy kills both healthy and cancer cells, both conventional and older chemo drugs may cause lots of side effects: hair loss, peripheral neuropathy, rashes, bone marrow suppression and resultant infections (often severe), anemia, bleeding, and systemic symptoms such as nausea, vomiting, and fatigue. This is because chemotherapy works like chemical warfare. It acts as a large bomb against cancer cells but in the process of killing them causes a lot of collateral damage. For all the side effects, chemo may not even succeed in killing all the cancer cells, either in the immediate or long-term, allowing the cancer to recur or metastasize.

Unsurprisingly, many patients want to know if we can offer some gentler integrative therapeutic option. Isn't there a way to magically take the cancer away? Our answer is: *"We wish!"* We have been looking for a magical cure since the 1970s, and we simply haven't found it.

What do we suggest to our patients? Firstly, it is important to learn the language your oncologist is speaking and to begin to understand medical terminology. This will help you have a clear grasp of your treatment plan, its goals, and your long-term outlook. Then, look at where and how the integrative options we discuss in this chapter can help.

In Maya's case, her initial treatment included three rounds of chemo, followed by huge pelvic and abdominal surgery. After a difficult recovery, she once again resumed cycles of heavy chemotherapy every three weeks. To say this was an extremely difficult time is a complete understatement. Over the course of three years, she completed sixty rounds of chemotherapy, took oral hormone blockers, and even tried an anti-cancer vaccine. This sounds horrendous, and in many ways it was. But Maya never once bemoaned her fate, whined about her diagnosis, or mired herself in self-pity. She was never a victim! She was, in fact, the healthiest sick person we had ever seen. She laughed, inspired others, went to work, traveled, Facetimed and Zoomed, and even officiated a wedding for her good friends!

When Maya was diagnosed, she wanted to focus on living her best life despite the cancer. She didn't want to read about statistics on the internet without having the medical knowledge to interpret them. So our family became her "Iron Dome," a shield from the potential negative barrage of information, filtering what she needed to hear, and helping her decide on and get through the arduous course of treatment. Thanks to integrative medicine therapies, she didn't lose her hair or suffer from peripheral neuropathy. Using a mix of conventional and alternative therapies, we were able to largely mitigate her abdominal symptoms and pain. (We'll discuss some of these later in this chapter.) To someone who didn't know Maya, she would not have appeared to have cancer or any sort of illness.

Typically a cancer is staged at the time of diagnosis to help doctors understand the extent and decide on the appropriate treatment. The most common staging system is known as TMN (some cancers, such as blood cancers, use different systems). In the TNM system:

- The T refers to the size and extent of the main tumor. The main tumor is usually called the primary tumor.

- The N refers to the number of nearby lymph nodes that have cancer.

- The M refers to whether the cancer has metastasized. This means that the cancer has spread from the primary tumor to other parts of the body.

Additional information about the cancer, such as the size of the tumor or the number of lymph nodes involved, is usually added. The TNM system helps describe cancer in great detail, but healthcare providers usually use a simplified staging system when talking about your cancer. In this system, the stages are numbered:

Stage 0: Abnormal cells are present but have not spread to nearby tissue. This is also called carcinoma in situ, or CIS. CIS is not cancer, but it may become cancer.

Stage I: This is early stage. Cancer may be locally invasive, but has not spread to surrounding lymph nodes.

Stage II: Cancer has grown, or may have spread to surrounding lymph nodes.

Stage III: Cancer has spread regionally.

Stage IV: Cancer has spread (metastasized) to distant parts of the body.

In general, early-stage cancers are often treated with surgery or radiation, while later stage cancers are treated with chemotherapy, targeted drug therapy, or immunotherapy.

As we have worked with cancer patients, we have tried to help them factor various options into their decision making. What are their underlying health conditions? What are the likely treatment outcomes, and what will they need to go through in order to get to the other side of the treatment? What does the latest research show? Are there any promising clinical trials? Finally, what are their wishes? We need to empower them to understand they have some control of this process. It has been our experience that once patients can feel more empowered by their decisions, they cope better.

The Evolution of Cancer Therapies

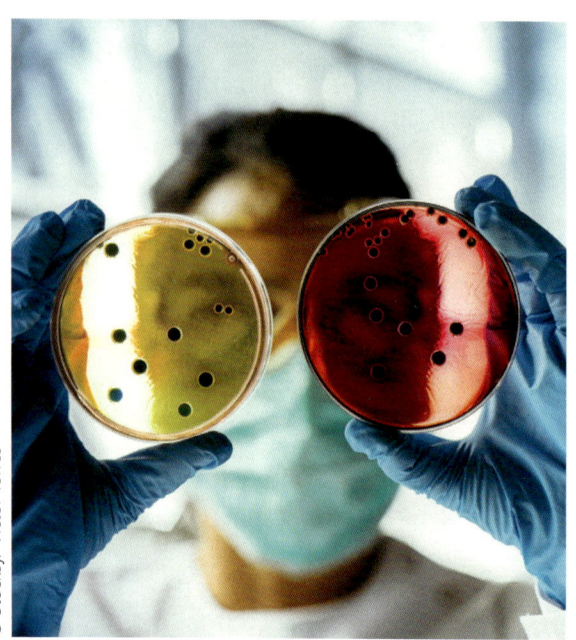

Cancer treatments are being developed in new and exciting ways and at what seems like breakneck speed compared to prior glacial progress. If we compare traditional chemotherapy to large indiscriminating bombs, the new treatments are more like smart bombs, able to seek and destroy cancer cells specifically—and with relatively little collateral damage. We have to remember, however, that cancer is not a uniform disease. Cancers with identical staging may respond to treatment very differently in different patients. That's why we want to personalize the treatment for each individual. This is what we call precision or personalized medicine.

As our understanding of cancer improves, we need to consider some important points when deciding on treatment.

The Genetics of the Cancer

When scientists first started to study the genetic changes that cause cancer, many hoped to find the single gene that was the culprit. This approach turned out to be wrong. They soon realized that cancers have multiple potentially causative genes, as well as a host of environmental or epigenetic contributors. This is why two patients with apparently identical cancers (stage 3 invasive ductal carcinoma breast cancer, for example) may actually have completely different genomic profiles. **Different underlying genes are contributing to what looks like the same cancer.** These seemingly identical cancers will respond differently to treatment, such as chemotherapy, because of their different underlying genetics. If a cancer recurs, it may have the same genes that were found in the original primary cancer, or the genes may have mutated to become different.

What this means is that oncologists have to pay attention to not only the staging of the cancer, but also to the underlying genetics of the patient and the cancer itself. It also means that drugs originally designed to work in one type of cancer may work really well for a different type. Genetic variations such as BRCA, which predispose some people to breast or prostate cancer, have become a good target for new medications called PARP inhibitors. BRCA genes can also play a role in other tumors. For instance, we have a patient who tested positive for a BRCA gene when being treated for a sarcoma, a type of muscle tumor, in his leg. PARP inhibitor drugs have been able to shrink his leg tumor, as well as the metastases in his liver. This demonstrates the power of genomic testing to guide treatment options.

Oncologists increasingly order genetic analyses when treating cancer patients. Advanced as this is, genetic analysis still isn't to the point where it can guide all treatment or predict the response. Not **all cancers** are driven by their genetic makeup. In addition, we get so much information from full **genome testing** that it **can be hard to interpret.** We foresee a time when this information will be used to maximize and personalize outcomes for each cancer patient, but we're not there yet.

In Maya's case, we were fortunate to obtain sophisticated genetic analyses, but the answer they provided was that genes didn't seem to play much of a role in her cancer. Unfortunately, there were no markers that we could easily target.

Treating the Cancer Microenvironment

Cancer cells create a microenvironment around themselves that lets them grow with little oxygen. They also produce chemical signals that message **the adjacent normal cells and get them to turn into cancer cells. The neighboring cells begin growing new blood vessels to feed the cancer,** a process called angiogenesis, and the cancer begins to spread. Today numerous drugs are being repurposed or developed to target the tumor microenvironment and the cells around it, as well as to stop the development of new vessels and reduce inflammation around the cancer.

Looking at New Therapies

New treatments known as ADCs, or antibody-drug conjugates, are very exciting. They work by loading an anticancer drug into a "caboose" that's chemically linked to a monoclonal antibody. The antibody binds to its **matching antigen** on the surface of the cancer cell and gets absorbed. **The ADC then acts like a smart bomb, de**positing **the drug right into the cancer cell and avoiding healthy cells.**

New cancer therapies are constantly being researched and developed. Immune checkpoint inhibitors are drugs that make the cancer visible to the immune system, so that your own immune cells can attack it. Adoptive cell transfer (ACT) is a transfusion of immune cells with the aim of controlling or eradicating tumors. Flash radiation concentrates weeks of radiation therapy into a few days. New imaging technologies light up cancer cells during surgery to help surgeons better see and remove them. We are hopeful that the future will bring new and better ways to detect cancer early and treat it effectively.

New methods are also being developed to supercharge the body's immune system and help it target cancer cells. Anticancer vaccines are also showing promise. Biologic agents, immune stimulants, and other innovative therapies are all in the pipeline. The treatment of cancer is progressing faster than ever. Patients should seek out cancer specialists who are aware of all the changes going on in the field, as well as ongoing clinical trials.

Early Detection

Cancers that are detected at an early stage are easier to treat, so we try to discover them sooner. This is the reason regular Pap smears (cervical cancer), mammograms (breast cancer), colonoscopies (colon cancer), and PSA tests (prostate cancer) are recommended. We don't have effective screening tests for other cancers, however. Patients often ask us what else they can do. Whole-body MRI scans have been suggested, but these aren't really helpful. The scans often detect unusual but not pathological abnormalities, such as cysts or atypical masses. While these may not cause disease or even have any impact at all, detecting them can cause patients and their physicians a lot of unnecessary anxiety. Newer blood tests called liquid biopsies are promising. These can detect multiple types of cancer by looking for fragments of DNA from the cancer floating in the blood. Unfortunately, these tests currently have many false positives. Newer blood tests looking at methylation can show the amount of mitotic (dividing) cells in the body. Because a hallmark of cancer is rapid, uncontrolled cell division, further investigation is definitely recommended if a patient scores above the 90th percentile. Whole-body MRIs and liquid biopsies can be very useful at this point.

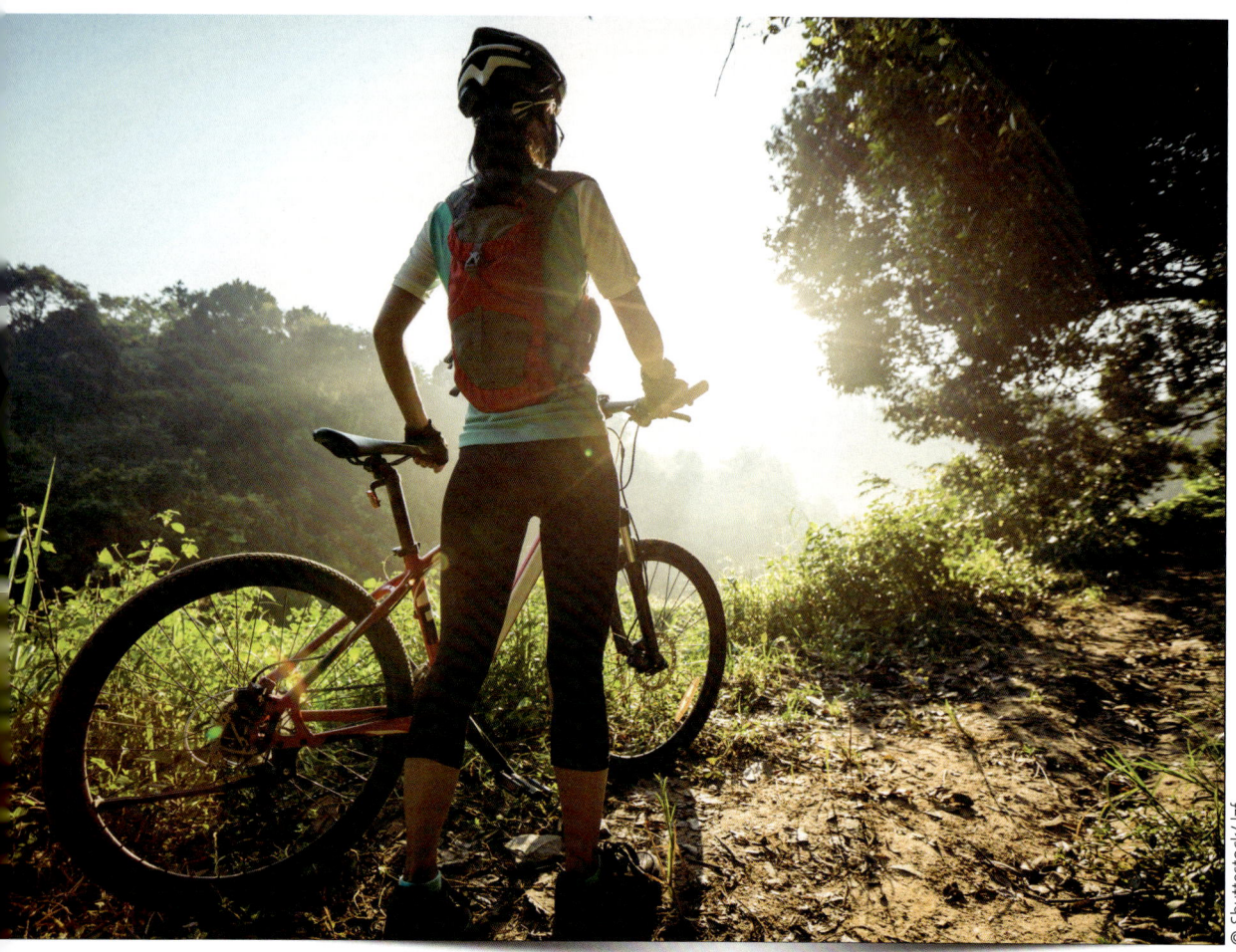

Treating the Macro Environment:
The Human Host

Too often in cancer care, the patient becomes a number, an end point to be treated. This depersonalizing process is also incredibly demoralizing and disempowering for the patient. They begin to feel as if they don't really matter. In our experience, patients who feel this way experience worse outcomes. It becomes a self-fulfilling prophecy. This is where integrative medicine plays a shining role. We find that when we add integrative therapies into the mix, patients feel better and do better, and their outcomes are usually better as well. These therapies help patients reduce side effects and improve quality of life. In addition, they help patients overcome their perceived powerlessness in the face of a supreme foe.

When patients learn to dig deeply to reassess their lives and find a profound feeling of spiritual alignment—to make something good out of a terrible diagnosis—we find their outcomes often improve. We have been clear that in systems biology there is always a multidirectional input between systems. As patients work on themselves, their immune systems seem to listen.

The lens of Maya's journey illustrates where and how integrative therapies can help patients. Maya embodied an internal sense of philosophical strength, and an outlook and approach that we feel could benefit many cancer patients. *We call this Maya's Way!*

Maya really taught us how best to help her navigate the cancer journey. While her experience was unique to her, we learned lessons that will benefit most patients with cancer. Most patients see integrative therapies, diet, and supplements as the treatments to look for first. But because we want cancer patients to understand how important their outlook is, we're going to start with that.

Create an attitude of accepting what you cannot change, while actively working on what you can. Maya knew from the beginning that she had a terrible cancer, and that she needed to go through an arduous process of treating it. She knew she needed to deal with the side effects and focus on her quality of life. Many patients are in a different situation. Their cancer may be completely curable, but the treatment is still difficult and many uncertainties remain. Maya's pragmatic approach allows for a realistic understanding of what it takes to live optimally every day.

Look forward, not back. Maya never allowed herself to delve into the what ifs: What if my doctor had picked this up earlier when I went to see her for my annual visit? What if I could have started treatment earlier? Instead, she looked forward every day.

Self-empowerment. Maya always wanted to know what lifestyle factors she could use to mitigate side effects and to optimize her well-being. Here are some of the lifestyle factors she focused on:

1. Each day she would make sure to meditate at least once.
2. She used visualization techniques to help her reduce pain, cope with side effects, and see herself doing well.
3. She exercised daily, whether by walking, doing yoga, or attending classes when she could.
4. She made sure to get sufficient sleep.

Self-development. Cancer is an incredible driver toward self-development. It is often a time when patients realize that they need to

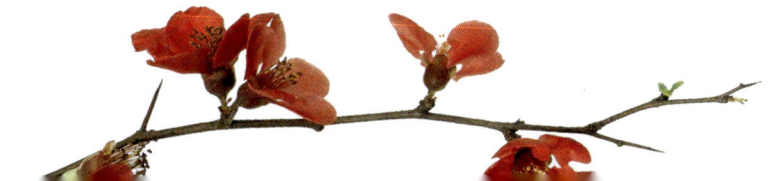

change their worldview. Money, careers, and looks become less important. Love, relationships, self-appreciation, and self-love become more important. Maya took advantage of this by doing extensive reading, undergoing regular therapy, and participating in self-development workshops.

Gratitude. Gratitude is often a difficult emotion to feel when facing a terminal or horrible diagnosis. Yet Maya made sure the last thing she did before going to bed every night was to write down three gratitudes in her journal. This now has translated into a family ritual, where we each say what we are grateful for every night at the dinner table. We highly recommend this to everyone. It engenders a sense of humility and kindness into your day.

Actively create a supportive care team. Doctors, nurses and medical staff are often overworked and stressed. Being kind and clear with them helps them to do their job better, and helps them see you not as a cancer patient but as a real person with a life, who also happens to have cancer. Friends, family, and colleagues all become an invaluable part of the care team by bringing friendship, love, and nutritional and emotional sustenance.

Create a nurturing and healing home environment. Maya turned her condo into a sanctuary by focusing on everything from a garden roof deck to candles to an inspirational quote wall. She also became a dog-mom to a miniature goldendoodle who she named Honey. (Maya felt that the bee symbolized much of what she represented. Aerodynamically, bumble bees should not be able to fly, as their body is too large for their wingspan, yet they do. Their pollination is also vital to our survival as a species. She wanted to pollinate everyone with wisdom, love, and friendship.)

Find humor. Maya had an infectious laugh, and finding humor in difficult situations was often the easiest way to diffuse stress. Laughter and fun became an important pursuit for us all. Humor has many benefits, including assisting in pain management, reducing anxiety and depression, modulating the stress response, and aiding the immune system by increasing the natural killer T cell response.

Music therapy. Music therapy has been shown to have benefits in many chronic illnesses. Music was very important to Maya. Not only did she make extensive playlists, but she enjoyed exploring a wide diversity of musical tastes. She had psych-up playlists, pre-chemo playlists to help her relax prior to chemo, playlists for fun, for exercising, and more.

Looking good helped her feel good. Maya felt that if she looked better, she felt better. She was unapologetic about it. This was not vanity but a genuine understanding of who she was. She took advantage of free hair-care and extensions supplied by a hospital nonprofit, took good care of her skin with a daily routine, and loved good clothes (which during COVID became an exceptional athleisurewear wardrobe)!

Create rituals. Subconsciously, many of us create rituals to bring order to our day. When in the shower, we may shave first. then wash our hair, or vice versa. Some people may lay out clothes the night before bed. Rituals help. Maya created a ritual when going to chemo, always taking comforting items with her. These included:

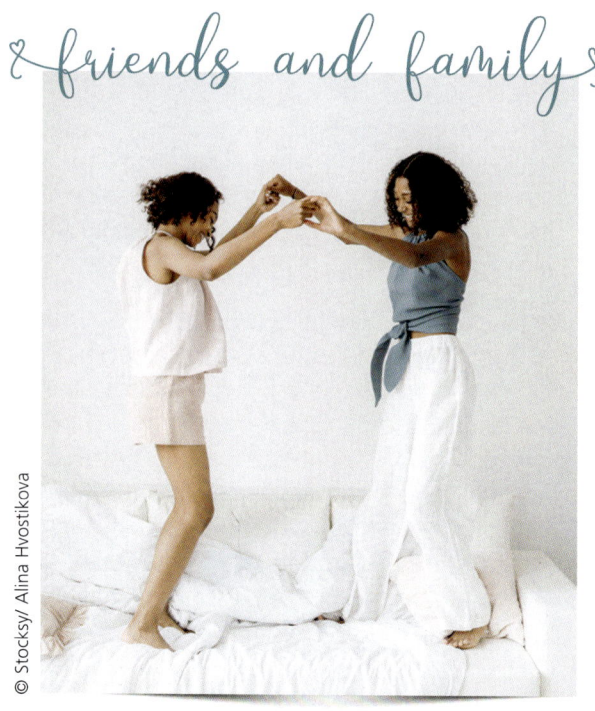

friends and family

1. An ultrasoft pillow and blanket
2. A comfy robe and warm socks
3. Playlists and earphones
4. Reading material and the crossword/spelling bee
5. Guided meditations, mainly as chemo began
6. An attitude of gratitude and kindness to all around her
7. And when possible, friends and family to keep her company.

Diet and good nutrition. Maya ate a diet filled with abundant fruit and vegetable dishes. Maya loved food and food preparation, so she spent a lot of time doing this. She also used intermittent fasting as a way to improve the effectiveness of chemotherapy. For a couple of days before her first few rounds of chemo, she used the Prolon low-calorie, ketogenic diet. This approach is being studied in women who are receiving chemo for breast and ovarian cancer, and initial results look positive.

The anti-inflammatory, low glycemic load, nutrient-dense diet we've discussed earlier in this book is filled with anticancer phytonutrients. We suggest a plant-based diet that avoids refined foods and added sugar and limits alcohol. Tomatoes, especially tomato sauce, contains lycopene, which decreases the risk of prostate and breast cancer. Broccoli contains sulforophane, and cruciferous vegetables contain indole-3-carbinol, which all help prevent breast cancer. Apple peels contain phenolic compounds which stop cancer from dividing. Garlic and onions both help with detoxification and decrease cancer cell activity. Turmeric contains curcumin, which has anti-inflammatory and anticancer activities.

To be sure of getting a large daily dose of anticancer plant nutrients, we recommend our Supernutrition Smoothie. The basic recipe is in chapter 9. If increased calories are needed, add some avocado or a couple spoonfuls of nut butter. Additional ingredients can include green tea powder, mushroom powders such as reishi or turkey tail, and probiotics.

The ketogenic diet may be beneficial in cancer. This approach keeps blood sugar levels low. The theory is that glucose may feed the tumor, while the keto diet will starve it.

Integrative Therapies

Integrative medicine includes the best of both conventional therapies, behavioral approaches, and a host of alternative therapies. Maya used a number of integrative therapies:

1. ***Acupuncture*** can be used to promote a sense of wellbeing but also to prevent and treat side effects such as peripheral neuropathy, nausea, fatigue, and pain.
2. ***Energy healing*** can be used for similar reasons to acupuncture. It really works well for anxiety, fatigue, and overall wellbeing.
3. ***Manipulative therapies*** can be used for back pain and discomfort.
4. ***Massage*** can be used regularly, and especially the day before chemo.
5. ***FSM*** (Frequency Specific Microcurrent) is a modality that was particularly helpful in reversing her peripheral neuropathy.
6. ***Supplements*** can be used; these will be discussed in more detail below.

We generally recommend using these therapies in the days prior to chemo, as that is when immune cell counts are usually highest. You can also use them during or even after chemo, but at that point immune cell counts may be dropping and the risk of infection is slightly higher. As always, we suggest discussing these with your treating physician before using them.

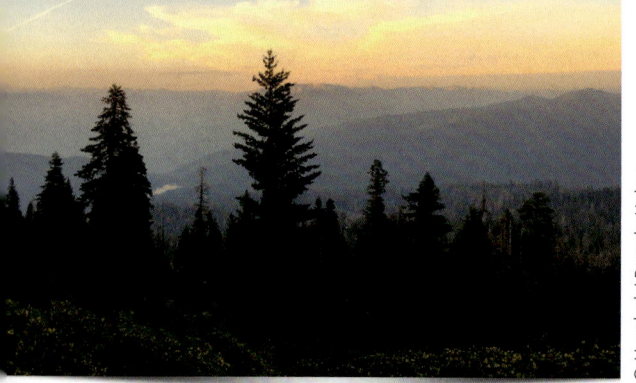

Supplements

Many dietary supplements are beneficial for cancer patients. These need to be personalized according to each patient, the type of cancer they have, and the type of treatments they are receiving. Here are some examples:

- **Supplements to augment general nutrition:** These include vitamin D, methylated B vitamins, highly absorbable magnesium (reacted magnesium, or magnesium glycinate), and fish oil.

- **Supplements to augment the immune response to cancer:** These include mushroom extracts such as turkey tail or reishi, green tea powder or concentrate in the form of EGCG, and turmeric. Other supplements are astragalus, omega 3 fatty acids, vitamin C, vitamin D, and full-spectrum vitamin E with gamma and delta tocopherols (not just alpha tocopherol), or tocotrienols.

- **Supplements to treat side effects:** Many different supplements are helpful here.
  - **Peripheral neuropathy:** L-glutamine (also helps gut issues) and B vitamins
  - **Nausea:** Ginger
  - **Loss of taste.** Zinc
  - **Constipation:** Probiotics, flax seed, fiber, magnesium citrate
  - **Diarrhea:** Probiotics, activated charcoal, fiber
  - **Fatigue:** CoQ10; L-carnitine
  - **Mouth sores:** Dabbing a drop of lavender aromatherapy oil on the ulcer stings for a moment but then helps it heal.
  - **Brain fog:** Ginkgo biloba (this can thin blood, so be cautious when on blood thinners); glutathione

Many other supplements can be safely used to help relieve side effects. They should be prescribed by an experienced healthcare professional who understands the type of cancer the patient has and knows about potential drug-supplement interactions.

Learning More

Cancer is a complex, often confusing disease, and every patient is different. Much of the information online is inaccurate, biased, misleading, or outdated—and there are many cancer scams. Be especially careful with information you find through online discussion groups and social media.

A good starting point for comprehensive, reliable cancer information is cancer.net, a website from the American Society of Clinical Oncology (ASCO).

Websites and Apps we recommend:

- **cancerchoices.org**

  Evidence-based information regarding the use of integrative oncology approaches, advice on whole-person healing, informed therapy choices, self-care and more

- **anticancerlifestyle.org**

  A credible, empowering website with good resources, such as recipes and blogs, it delivers advice on decreasing inflammation, boosting the immune system, and lowering the risk of cancer, cancer recurrence, and chronic illness.

- **bcpp.org** (breast cancer prevention partners)

  This is a good resource regarding potential carcinogenic chemicals and how to eliminate them. Their goal is to save lives and prevent disease before it happens.

- **Google the Dirty Dozen Clean Fifteen list**

    EWG (Environmental Working Group) provides lists of produce with the highest and least amounts of insecticides. This is worth knowing and updated regularly.

- ***Yuka App***

    A guide to help improve the purchase of healthier processed foods and cosmetics

- ***Insight Timer, Headspace*** and ***Calm Apps***

    Good resources to help with meditation, relaxation and personal growth

Maya's Journey

© Steve Amoils

Despite all Maya did, nothing could stop the insidious spread of cancer throughout her body. Maya passed away on January 18, 2022 after a valiant fight. There is no doubt in our minds that the way she dealt with her cancer improved her quality of life and likely also prolonged her life significantly. When she realized that there was nothing more that anyone could do, she faced her impending passing with great courage, showing more concern for her friends and family than for herself. In her final days, she asked us to set up a nonprofit organization to help men and women under 40 with cancer. This we have done. It's called *Maya's Way*. The aim is to empower these patients with cancer to live (health)fully, despite their diagnosis. We are working with men and women in the Cincinnati area and hope to show that this process translates into better outcomes and better lives.

More information is at:

https://aimforwellbeing.org/mayasway

Donations: Maya's Way is managed by The Christ Hospital Foundation. You can contribute by clicking below and **choosing "Maya's Way" in the Gift Designation drop down.**

https://www.thechristhospital.com/about-the-network/foundation/donate-online

> That is how you live a vibrant life in the face of death, darling.
>
> ## You stare it down & blind it with compassion & laughter & love & human connection.
>
> You defeat it with the conviction to make it better.
>
> —Maya Amoils

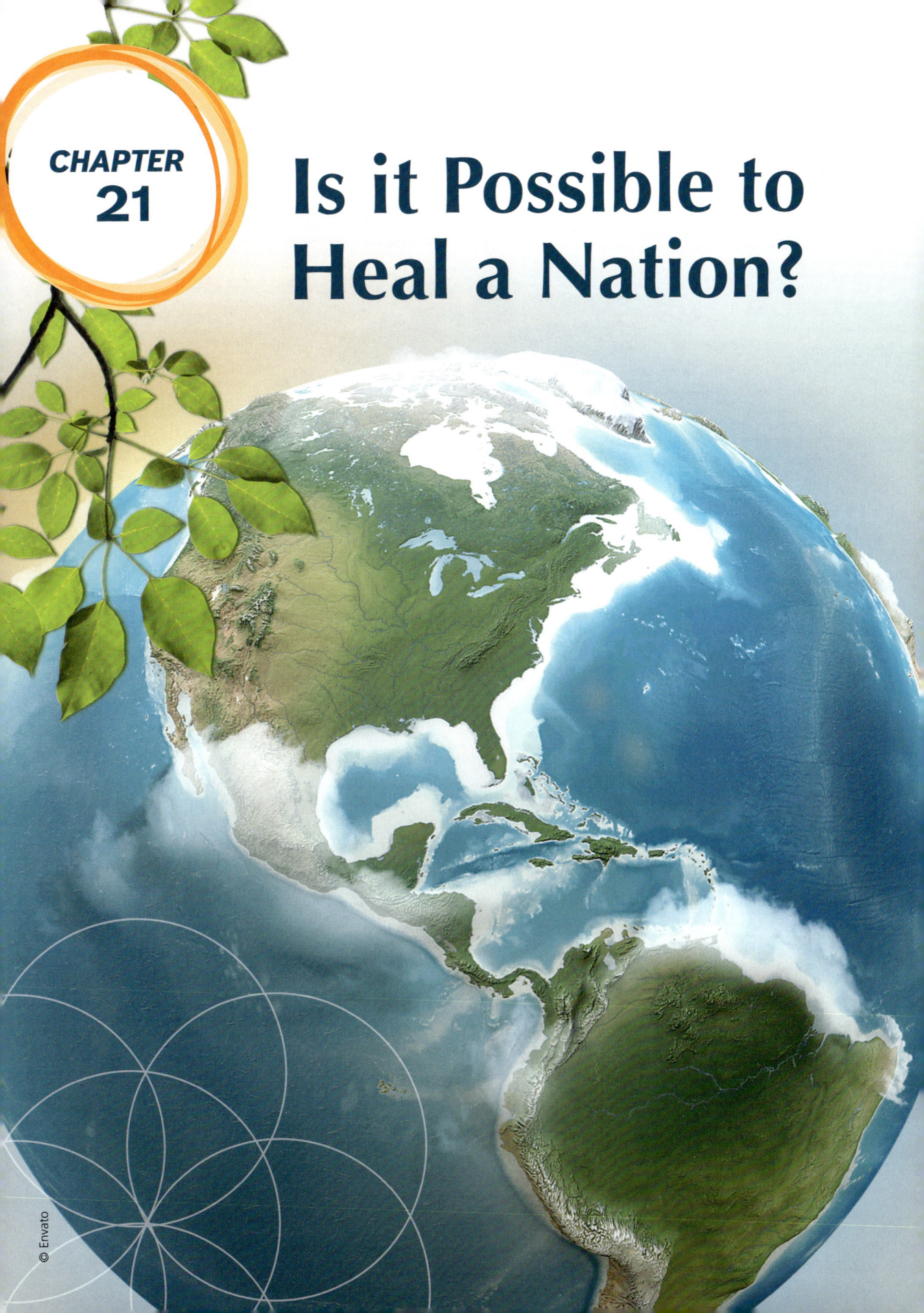

CHAPTER 21
Is it Possible to Heal a Nation?

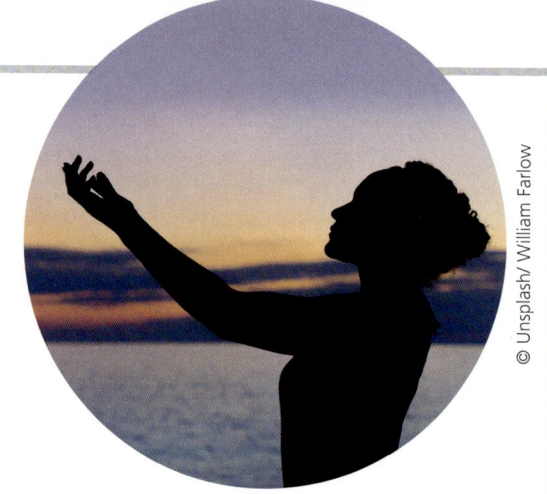

Many years ago, our extremely wise Japanese master acupuncture teacher interviewed us to become his students. As happens sometimes with Japanese teachers, the master will lob a difficult question to his students, not to get an answer but to see how they answer. One of the questions he asked was, "How would you diagnose the disease of a nation, and how would you heal it?"

We were completely thrown off by the question at the time but have been pondering the answer for the past forty years. How could a nation have a single disease? If so, how would you even go about healing it? In this book, we have discussed the underpinning of a systems biology approach. Rather than diseases existing as separate entities, we see that they are somehow all connected. Dr. Jeff Bland, the father of functional medicine, and Dr. Robert Lustig, a prominent physician and author, have influenced us greatly in coming to this conclusion. We finally think we have an answer.

A Sad Situation + SAD Diseases =
The SAD SYNDROME

Our nation and most of the developed world is suffering from a number of ailments: rising illness and obesity, pollution, worsening food quality and supplies, political divisions, huge areas of poverty amid pockets of huge wealth. Can such a powerful nation have a disease and, if so how would you heal it?

In Chapter 6, we discussed what we see as a Sad situation. We discussed how the perpetuating effects of physical and emotional trauma could leave a lasting effect on a person's psyche. The same might hold for a nation.

Then, in Chapter 15, we discussed the SAD diseases, a constellation of common diseases related to the Standard American Diet, especially sugar and ultraprocessed foods.

Aha! We realized we have a mind-body problem. This is exactly the kind of medicine we practice.

By definition, a syndrome is a set of medical signs and symptoms that are correlated with each other and often associated with a particular disease or disorder.

We put the two together and we realized we have THE SAD SYNDROME.

In thinking this through, we can now place most of the common maladies of our nation into a better systems biology way of both comprehending and approaching them.

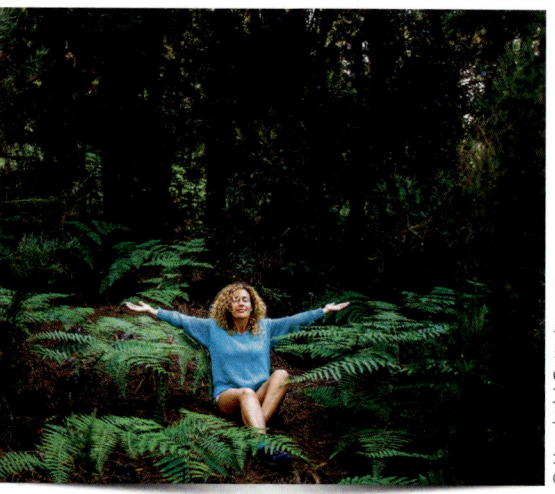

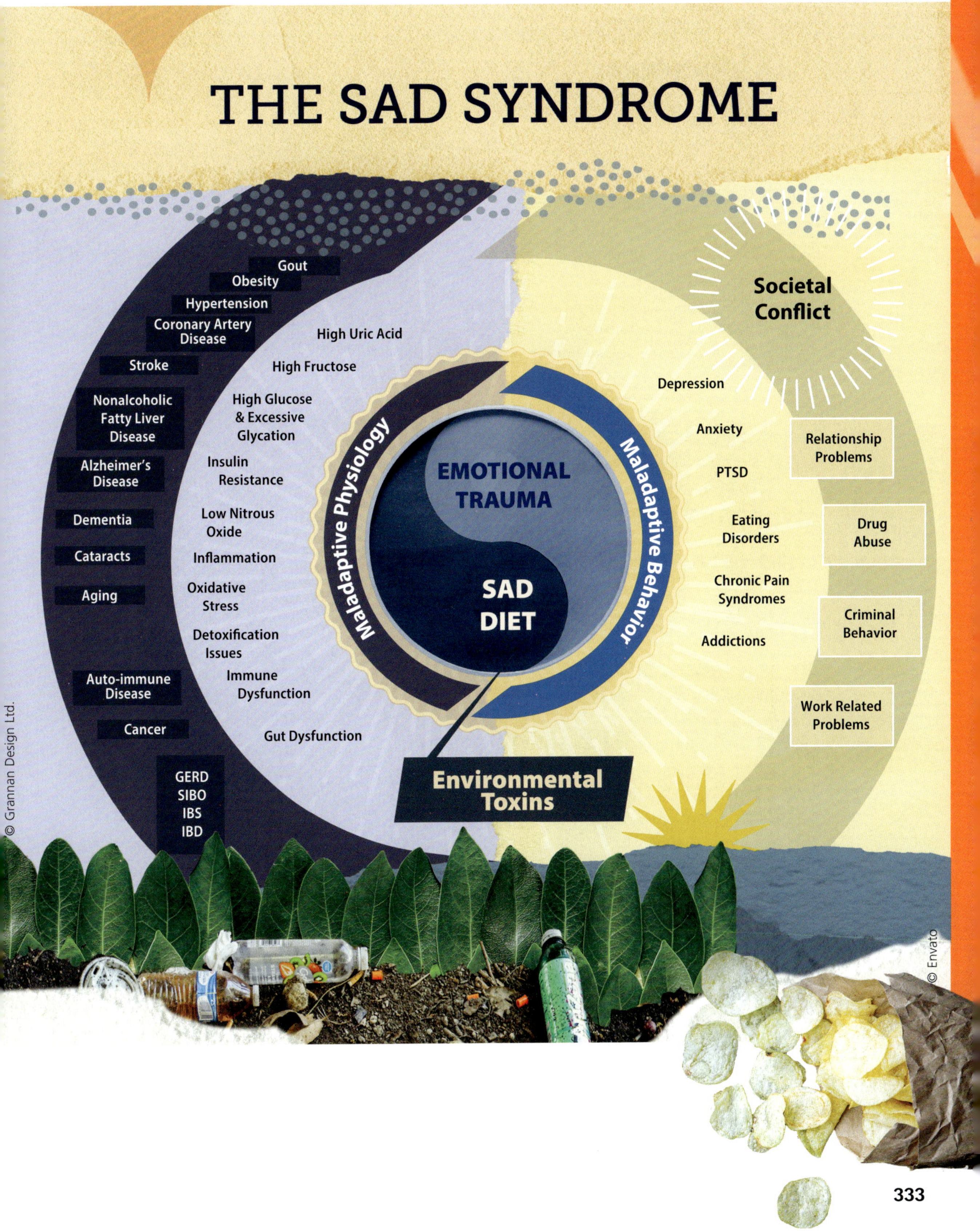

THE SAD SYNDROME

Maladaptive Physiology

- Gout
- Obesity
- Hypertension
- Coronary Artery Disease
- Stroke
- Nonalcoholic Fatty Liver Disease
- Alzheimer's Disease
- Dementia
- Cataracts
- Aging
- Auto-immune Disease
- Cancer
- GERD
- SIBO
- IBS
- IBD
- High Uric Acid
- High Fructose
- High Glucose & Excessive Glycation
- Insulin Resistance
- Low Nitrous Oxide
- Inflammation
- Oxidative Stress
- Detoxification Issues
- Immune Dysfunction
- Gut Dysfunction

EMOTIONAL TRAUMA

SAD DIET

Maladaptive Behavior

- Depression
- Anxiety
- PTSD
- Eating Disorders
- Chronic Pain Syndromes
- Addictions

Societal Conflict

- Relationship Problems
- Drug Abuse
- Criminal Behavior
- Work Related Problems

Environmental Toxins

How Do We Heal **The SAD Syndrome**?

THE SAD SYNDROME

SAD DISEASES - Fueled by Diet/Environmental Toxicity

- Obesity/Type 2 Diabetes
- Cardiovascular Disease
- Non-alcoholic Fatty Liver Disease
- Chronic Kidney Disease
- Certain cancers
- Osteoporosis
- Alzheimer's Disease
- And more ...

A SAD SITUATION - Fueled by (Recycled) Trauma

- Aggression/Greed
- Abuse/Neglect
- Addictions/PTSD
- Depression
- Anxiety
- And more

At its core, we need to heal the interlocking basic elements of the SAD Syndrome: diet and trauma. We need some guiding principles to point us in the right direction.

Here are our principles:

Principle 1: Less Sugar, More Love

To remember what we need to do, we need a basic or keystone principle. (A keystone is the central part of an arch that locks the structure together.) This is our keystone principle: less sugar, more love.

We need to know how to mend the body and how to mend the psyche. This is a true yin-yang principle. We cannot do one without the other.

Healing the Body: Less Sugar

The Standard American Diet is laden with sugar, ultraprocessed foods, too much protein, and bad fats. It appears to be the driving force of many of the illnesses we see today. At its core appears to be high sugar and refined carbohydrates intake and their disruptive effect on glucose metabolism. Reducing our intake of these foods will help take the foot off the constant-on accelerator of mTOR.

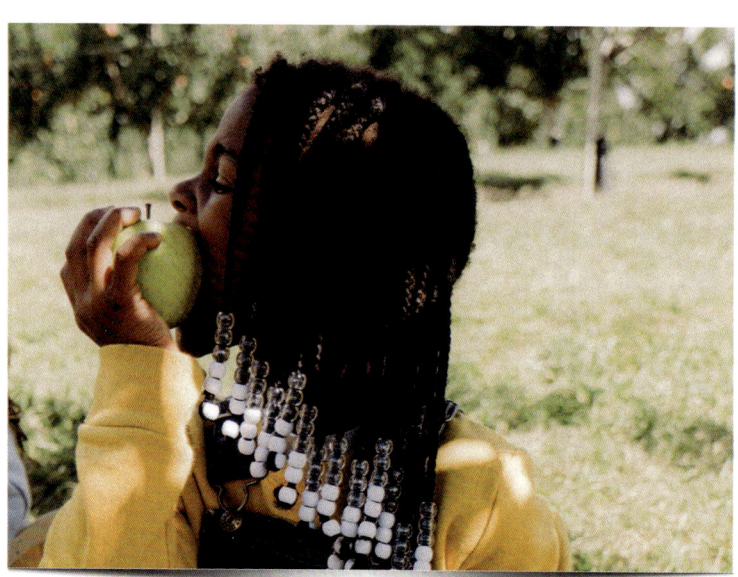

To lower blood glucose, we need to dramatically reduce consumption of glucose, sucrose (cane sugar), high-fructose corn syrup, and fructose (purified fruit sugar in the form of fruit juices and additives). We need to cut out refined sugary foods and beverages and move toward eating real food. This is a sea change critical to our healing. It is no good to have zero-calorie drinks full of chemicals and flavorings. Cutting calories doesn't solve the problem of a diet made up mainly of sugar and ultraprocessed foods. We need good, wholesome food again, food our ancestors would recognize. We shouldn't have to read ingredients labels to see if a food is good for us. We should inherently know by its smell, taste, color, and texture, not by the chemicals it contains.

We also need to improve our agriculture to be less damaging and more sustainable. We need to look at techniques such as regenerative agriculture, where farming mimics the cycles found in nature. Regenerative agriculture utilizes biodiversity of crops and livestock, with intensive rotational grazing. By using cover crops to restore the soil, it aims for a closed-loop system where nutrients are recycled and utilized, rather than the land being stripped bare. Regenerative agriculture also promotes wildlife habitat and uses integrated pest management, which means minimal uses of herbicides and insecticides.

When we improve our diet and our agricultural practices, we will automatically have healthier microbiomes, with all the health benefits that provides.

Finally, we need to find healthier alternatives to the plastics and toxic chemicals that are filling up our planet. Not only will this be good for the planet, but it will be good for our livers, which are struggling to detoxify the overload of chemicals in our environment. That, in turn, will help stop insulin resistance. It's a positive feedback cycle. And as William James famously said when asked if life is worth living, *"It all depends on the liver."*

Healing the Mind: More Love

Love is the universally healing emotion. In its highest (agape) form, we can never have enough. It is the solution to much of the pain we suffer from. And it is that pain that underlies the greed, corruption, anger, guilt, and fear principles on which much of the world runs.

Love can be taught. It is taught by modelling and not by lecturing or reading about it. This is why it is so problematic. We need to teach love by first learning how to feel true love. In this way, we become light bulbs or miniature suns who can further spread it.

Adults who have been brought up in pain have lots of inner work to do. This can be done through self-reflection, therapy, and loving-kindness meditation. The new resurgence in psychedelic drugs may be a harbinger of new ways to experience love. People who use these drugs report they experience enormous love and relief of old pain. We can teach people to overcome addictions and replace this with more self-love. More self-love will lead to more of an inner sense of peace. More peace will lead to more healthy prosperity, less conflict, and more love!

What if we change our negative addictions to being addicted to living positively and doing good? If we can do this, we can addict ourselves to a positive feedback loop. We can become healthier, live longer, feel happier, do better. It's a win-win! Our guiding principle for decisions should be: how do we create optimal health and wellbeing for all? If we keep asking that question

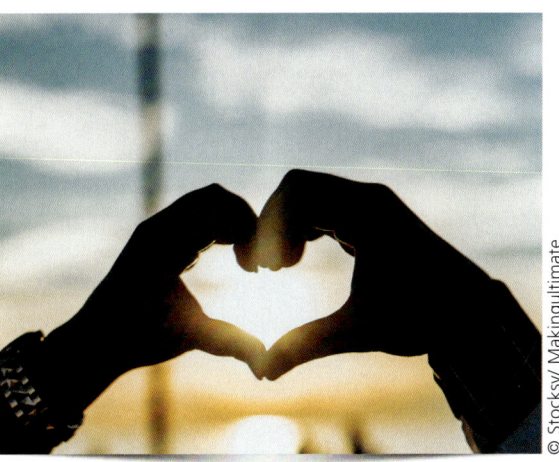

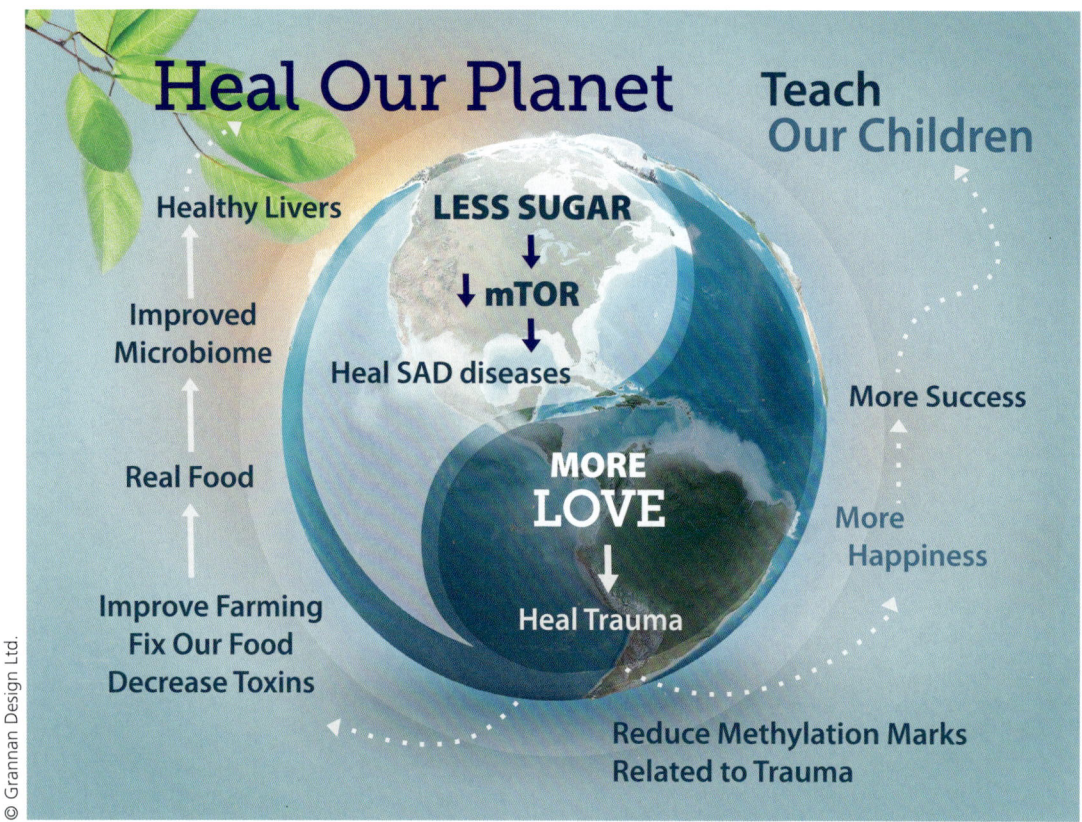

as we make our decisions, we can only move toward a healthier and better planet.

Ultimately, we will have more happiness, which is what everyone wants. We will develop a greater sense of unity and self-fulfillment. This is the solution to greed, avarice, and war.

In systems biology we learn that all the interacting parts affect the whole. We need to see this in more global terms. As soon as we realize globally that our common health and highest good are completely interconnected, we will become a better planet.

Principle 2: Educate Our Children (Correctly)

Right now, we are leaving a mess of a planet for our children—one choked by pollution, marked by intolerance, threatened with pandemics, wracked by planetary climactic upheaval, menaced by war and the potential of international nuclear war, and worried about artificial intelligence-gone-wrong on the horizon. The potential for mass extinction, and destruction of cities, infrastructure, and the environment has never been greater. Yet never has human society held in its hands the ability to transform itself for the better to this degree.

We believe the solution is to constantly teach children to strive for better.

We need to teach them principles of better and healthier eating and the value of nutrition on health. This is not just a do-good issue. It has huge implications for the health of our nation and our planet. The public school system in the US is the largest purveyor of fast food in the country. We need to help it move away from refined and ultraprocessed foods to those that supply better nutrition, all at a lower cost. This is already being done in some places through programs such as EatReal.org. We need more organizations like this.

We need to teach children how to build companies focused on doing good and making money at the same time. We can't rely on past leadership to do this—they don't know how.

Our children will grow up with access to more knowledge, better computing, and uses of artificial intelligence than we could ever dream of. It is our children who will help us solve this SAD SYNDROME problem. And it is important that they do solve it. The alternative is dire. In our daughter Maya's honor, we are working with her alma mater to create a five-year middle school and high school curriculum to do just this. The goal is to build a curriculum that can be used in schools across the country. We want schools to educate our children to learn about mental health, self-worth, resilience, and how to solve problems by really listening to the opposing side and then coming up with win-win solutions that will benefit both sides, as well as the planet.

If we can teach our children about eating right and about true love, we can create a different planet. We can create profitable, sustainable ways of feeding the entire planet. We can even create ways to eradicate poverty. And if we teach them how to love properly, without avarice, malice, or greed, we can teach them to eradicate war. We can reduce the epigenetic marks that promulgate the SAD SYNDROME.

It is possible to heal our nation! NOW is the time!

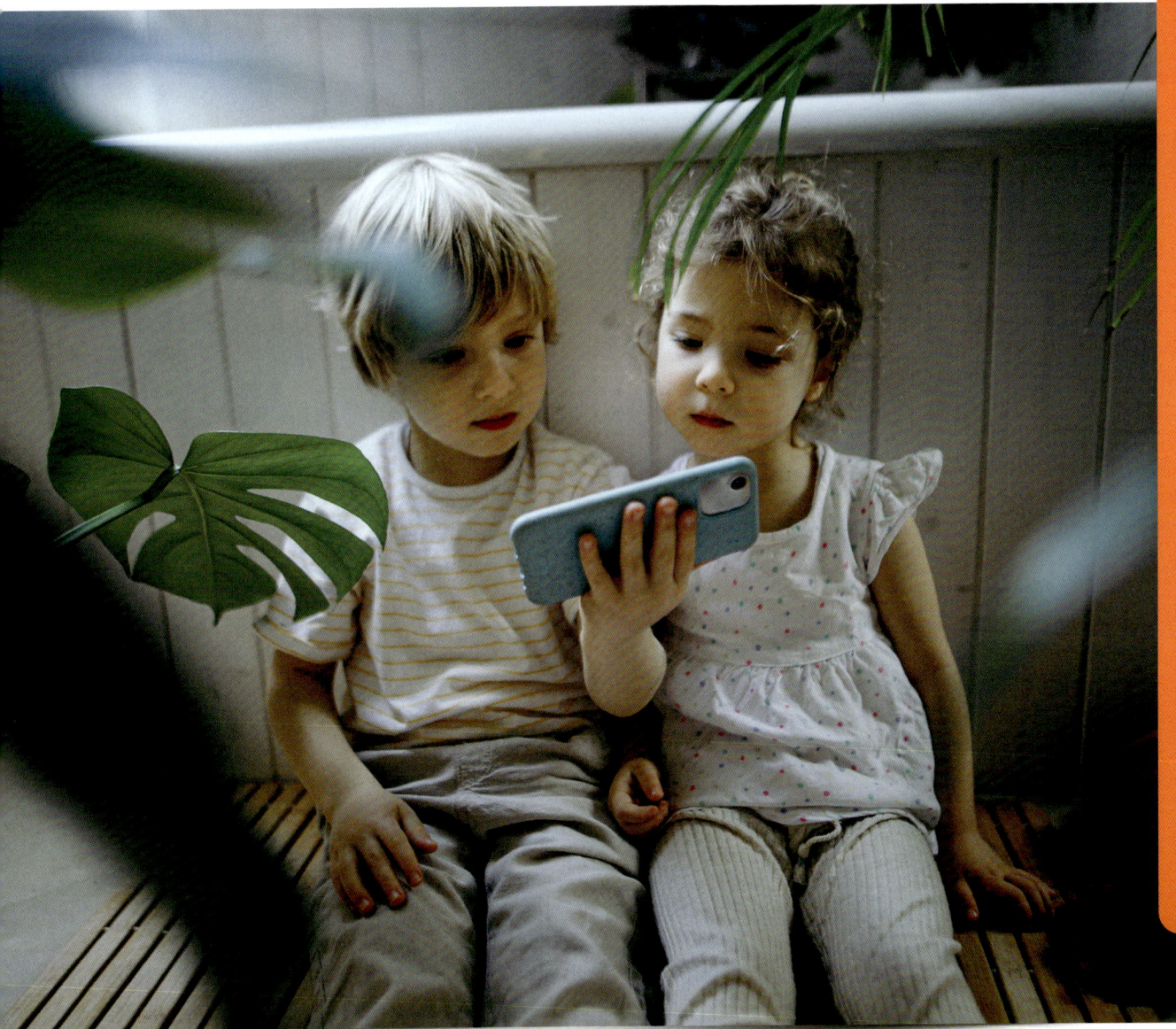

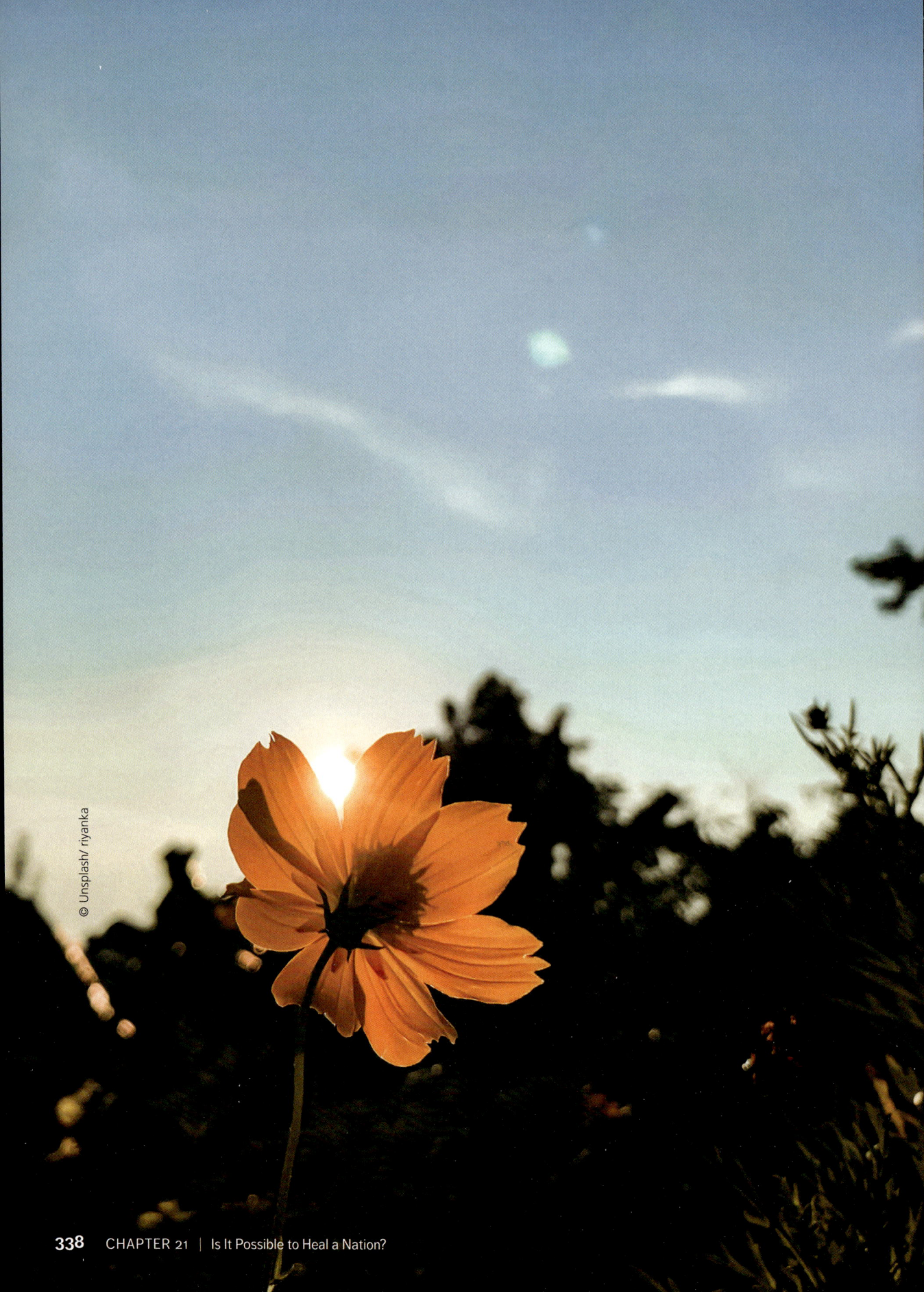

CHAPTER 22

Aging As You Know It Is About to Change

... the Allure of Modern Wellness

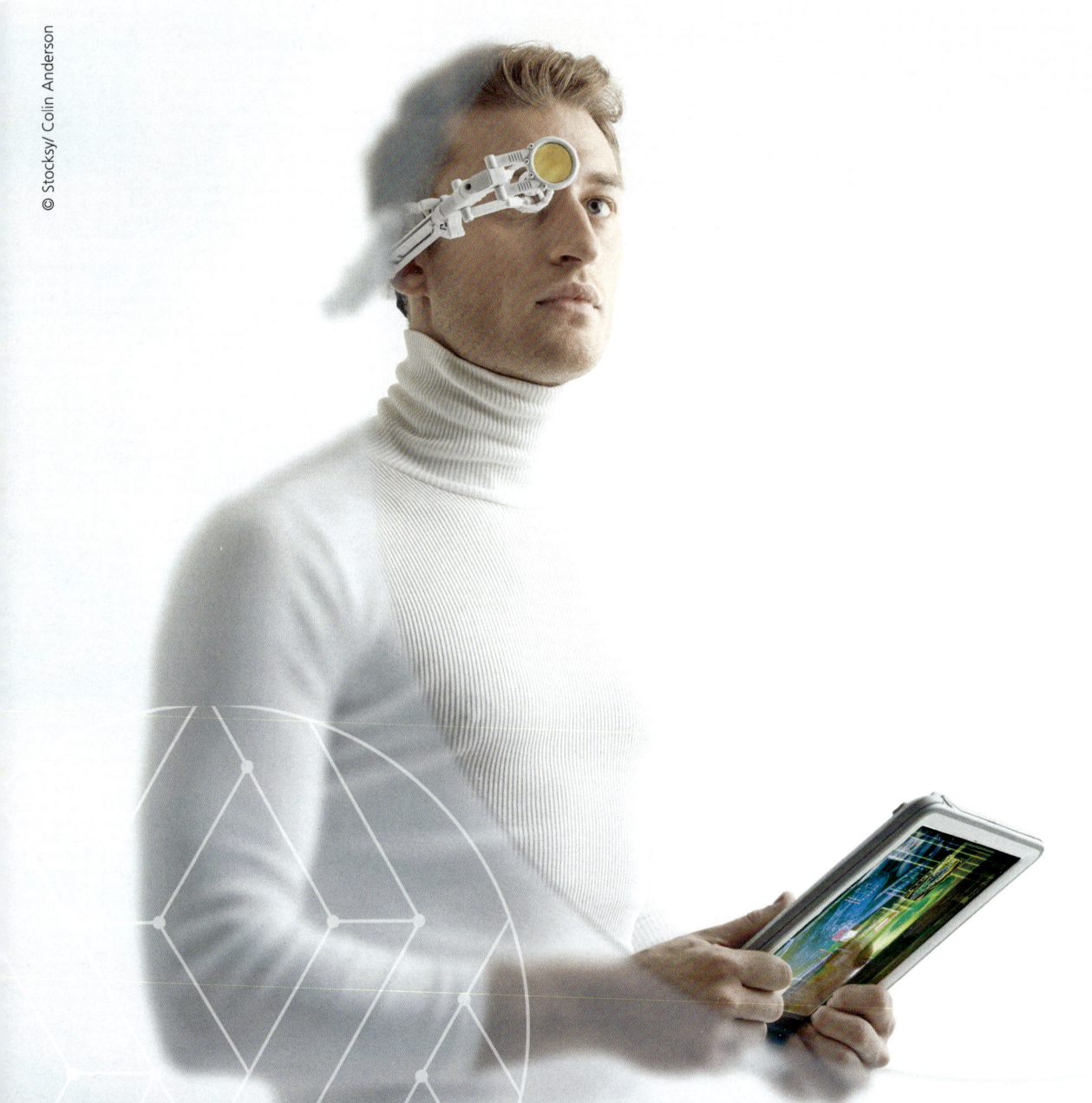

The Promise of **Modern Wellness**

Throughout this book, we have alluded to exciting new options for all of us, with the potential to reverse our biological clocks. We have also discussed that our biological age is not necessarily the same as our chronological age.

At the end of chapter 2, we discussed how tech mogul Bryan Johnson is attempting to reverse his biological age with a multimillion-dollar, all-encompassing program. Obviously, that kind of money or intensity isn't available for the average person. What if we could do something cheaper and easier? What if you could feel, look, and be younger, lengthen your lifespan, and improve your healthspan?

Is aging a normal phenomenon or an "Uber-illness," an umbrella under which all other diseases fall?

We have always considered aging to be a normal phenomenon. Some people seem to age faster, while others do so at a slower rate. We used to think aging was something out of our control. Not true! It's clear that factors such as stress, smoking, alcohol, poor nutrition, and lifestyle all affect the rate of aging. Most realize this too late.

Today, aging-in-place and even reverse-aging are genuine prospects, likely to be realized in the next decade or two. Aging-in-place refers to freezing the biological age where you are at, while continuing to age in chronological years. Reverse-aging takes this further, attempting to reverse your biological age somewhere to your mid-twenties. (This is being done in animals, and does not seem possible or even desirable to go beyond this.) Companies such as Google, Amazon, and Pfizer have bet large amounts of money on this. Promising the elixir of youth may in fact turn out to be the best business of all!

David Sinclair, A.O., Ph.D. is a tenured Professor in the Department of Genetics at the Paul F. Glenn Center for Biology of Aging Research at Harvard Medical School and serves as President of the Academy for Health and Lifespan Research. He is best known for his work on understanding why we age and how to slow its effects. Dr. Sinclair's research is fascinating. He has discovered that every cell in the body has within itself a perfect copy, which we can access later in life. He has shown that it is possible to age a mouse forward and give it dementia, then take that same mouse and reverse the dementia. This discovery has enormous implications. If we can age a person backward, we might be able to restore them to a state before they ever got sick. Wow!

We have already discussed how mTOR, AMPK, sirtuins, and insulin resistance have all been implicated in aging. It appears that these enzymes and pathways can be switched on or off with protein transcription factors called

Yamanaka factors. In 2006, Drs. Kazutoshi and Shinya Yamanaka showed that it is possible to reprogram cells using just four master genes: Oct3/4, Sox2, Klf4, and c-Myc (OSKM). These are all important for creating induced pluripotent stem cells, almost-immortal cells that have the ability to become any cell in the body. The Yamanaka transcription factors could be used to reprogram cells in some cancers and neurodegenerative diseases and could also be used for rejuvenation. Sinclair has utilized the Yamanaka factors to reverse aging and improve memory in mice. He has also been able to restore vision in mice that had mechanically damaged optic nerves, a feat never before even imagined!

Dr. Sinclair said in an article in Nature, "We set out with a question: if epigenetic changes are a driver of ageing, can you reset the epigenome?" In other words, "Can we reverse the clock?" The answer appears to be a resounding yes.

In the future, it might be possible to insert Yamanaka factors early in life and then activate them later with a course of the antibiotic doxycycline. This brings up the possibility of reverse-aging to our pre-illness state and restoring the "perfect copy" of the cell prior to the onset of illness!

Many questions about Yamanaka factors remain and much research must still be done before we can use them safely and effectively in humans. Still, the future looks bright. With the rapid progress of medical technology and AI, we now have the ability to speed up research and do in months what previously would have taken decades to accomplish. The possibility of a normal healthspan until you are 120 years old or even more is no longer a dream.

You don't need to wait . . .

Reverse Your Age
Five Years in Eight Weeks

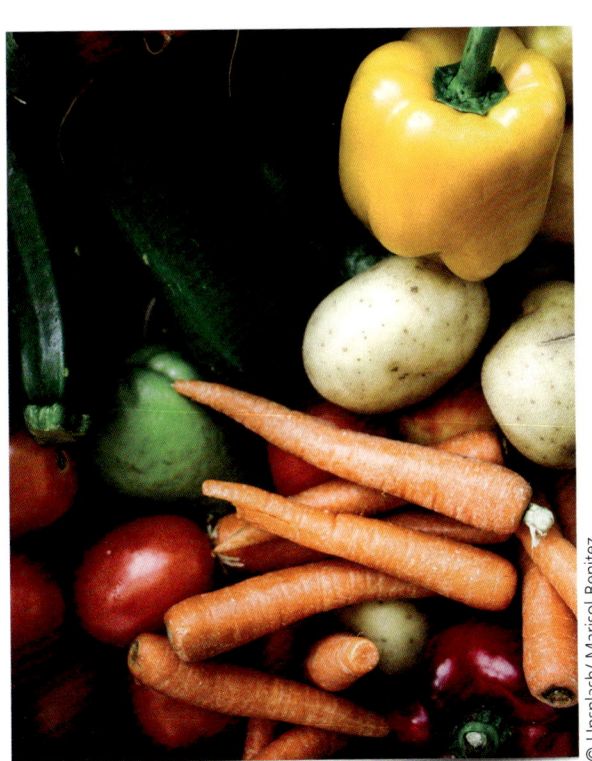
© Unsplash/ Marisol Benitez

Kara Fitzgerald, ND, author of *Younger You: Reduce Your Bio Age and Live Longer, Better* and did an exciting pilot study on reversal of aging in six women between the ages of 46 and 65. They all underwent an eight-week intensive program that included alterations to diet, sleep, and exercise. They were also given relaxation guidance, probiotic and phytonutrient supplements, and nutritional coaching.

Blood tests showed a reduction in biological age of up to 11 years in five of the six women, with the average participant experiencing a 4.6-year decrease, according to the study published in March 2023 in the prestigious journal *Aging*.

Participants had an average chronological age of 58 years at the beginning of the study. At the end, all but one had a younger biological age. Because of this, it's unlikely that the reduction in biological age most participants experienced during the study was due to disease improvement. Instead, the improvement "might be attributed to underlying age mechanisms," the authors surmised. In other words, the lifestyle changes they made appeared to reverse aging.

As part of the study, participants were asked to consume the following foods daily:

- 2 cups dark leafy greens
- 2 cups cruciferous vegetables
- 3 cups colorful vegetables
- ¼ cup pumpkin seeds
- ¼ cup sunflower seeds
- 1 to 2 beets
- Liver or liver supplement (three 3-ounce servings per week)
- 1 egg (a total of 5 to 10 per week)

They were also asked to eat two servings daily of methylation adaptogens—foods that support DNA methylation, a process that controls gene expression.

These foods included:

- ½ cup berries, preferably wild
- 2 medium garlic cloves
- 2 cups green tea, brewed 10 minutes
- 3 cups oolong tea, brewed 10 minutes
- ½ teaspoon rosemary
- ½ teaspoon turmeric

Participants also made the following daily lifestyle adaptations:

- Take 2 probiotic capsules
- Take 2 servings of green powder
- Drink 8 cups of water
- Exercise for at least 30 minutes
- Practice breathing exercises twice
- Sleep at least 7 hours
- Fast 12 hours after their last meal of the day

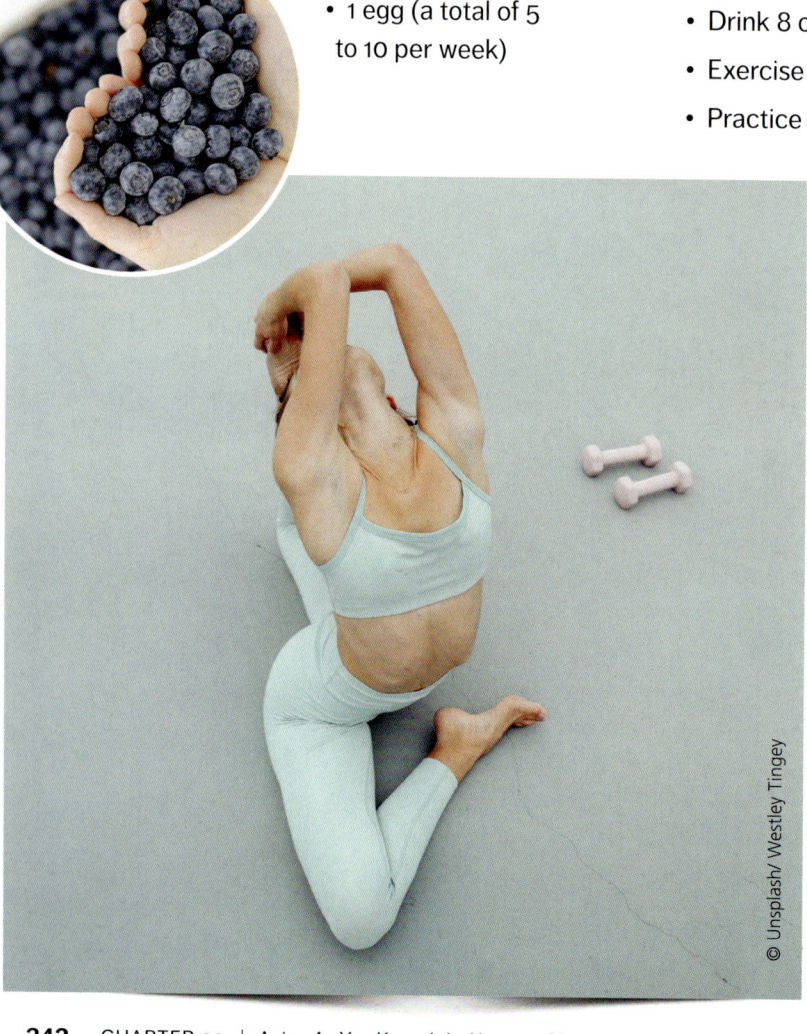

None of the women completed all the tasks all the days. That was expected, according to the researchers. Improvements in biological age were seen among women who adhered to the program an average of 82 percent of the time. The relatively high level of adherence among patients was likely due in large part to the nutritional coaching provided.

Aging confers an outsize risk of illness. If we can age ourselves backward, we can reduce the risk of dying by 7 percent for every year you reverse your age. Age yourself back 7 years, and you can reduce your risk of dying by 50 percent!

We don't want you to focus just on aging from a purely physical perspective! It is important to be happy as well. People think of aging and tell us they don't want to be decrepit for an additional fifty years. But what if you could feel like you did as a twenty-year-old? And improve how you look? And have the wisdom you have gleaned? And feel exceptionally happy? We believe this is all possible.

You may recognize in the next diagram that the way to heal our planet is the same way to promote illness and reverse aging! It is the same way you will achieve a state of wellbeing!

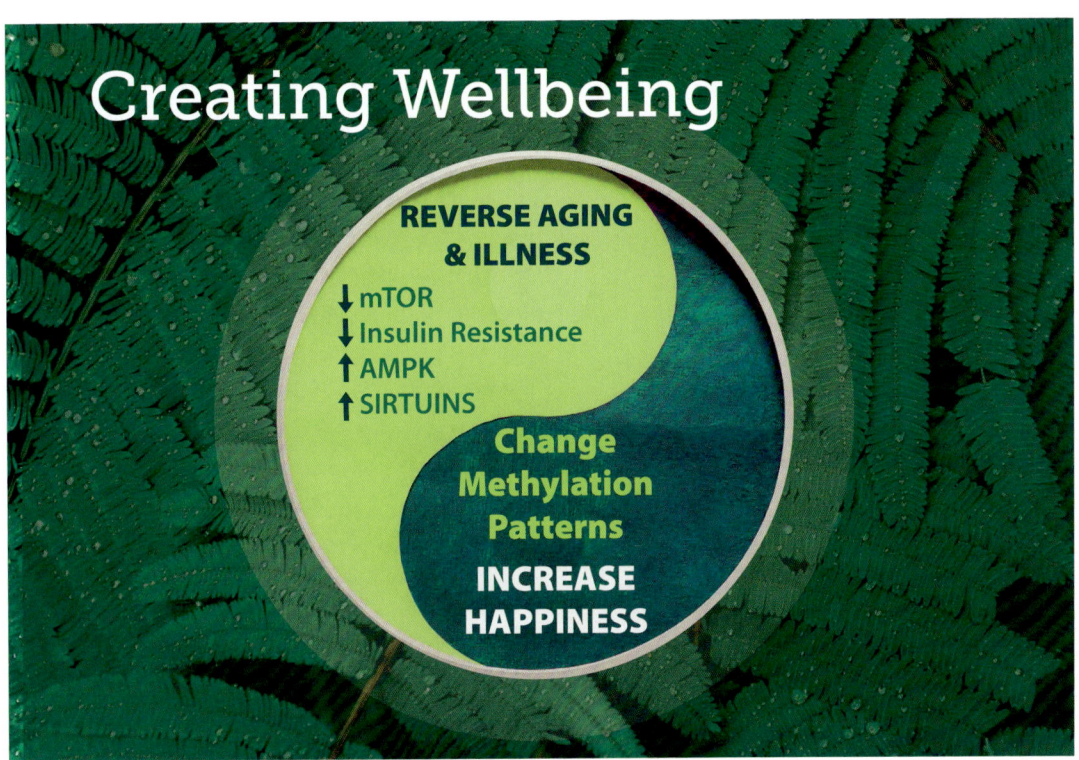

Wellbeing Begins with You

Your health and wellbeing is your highest good!

This might sound selfish, but it isn't. For you to feel healthy and happy, your spouse or partner needs to feel healthy and happy. Your kids can't be truly happy unless you are. Your community can't be healthy and happy unless everyone is healthy and happy. And we can't have healthier communities without improving our environmental footprint and overall wellbeing. The same goes for our country and our planet! It is when we fully realize that we live in a connected world that we understand we can and do make a difference. Each time we help ourselves, we start a ripple effect which will move us toward healing our planet.

Our Approach to **Modern Wellness**

After decades of treating patients using the principles of functional medicine, we feel we have a useful approach to modern wellness. We recommend the steps below as your way to ongoing good health as you age.

■ **Find a physician** who understands functional and integrative medicine and has an interest in aging.

■ **Measure your true biological age and your rate of aging.** Multiple "aging clocks" are available. We recommend a test that includes an advanced clock test, such as OMICmAGE from TruDiagnostic.

■ **Start off with a Transformational Wellness Plan.** Throughout this book we have shown you how to transform your health. We believe our Transformational Medicine approach should be the first step in improving your health and well-being. Consider low-cost options that include diet (specifically fasting–mimicking diets, intermittent fasting, and caloric restriction), lifestyle, exercise, sleep, and deep rest/meditation. Some low-cost supplements, such as DHEA and very low-dose lithium, appear to have promise. Drugs such as metformin may help some people, and low-dose rapamycin may hold promise. Expect lots of new options in the coming years.

■ **Consider minimally invasive ways to make you look and feel better.** Laser therapy continues to improve in cost and effectiveness. The benefits of the latest lasers is that they can literally reverse how you look in very short treatments with no burning or cutting, minimal side effects, and no real downtime.

Benefits of laser therapy include:
- It can help stop snoring. This improves sleep quality and can even help save your marriage!
- It can help reverse damage from sun exposure and aging.
- It can stimulate new hair growth or remove unwanted hair.
- It can help diminish unsightly veins.

The problem with lasers is that their results aren't permanent and may need to be repeated every one to three years.

■ **Renew your joints, ligaments, and tendons.** As we age, we often can maintain muscle strength, but our joints, ligaments, and tendons start becoming less elastic. They are more like a dried-out old tree than a young sapling. Techniques such as shockwave, prolotherapy, PRP, and stem cell injections, together with a rehab program, offer ways to make our joints young again, all without surgery.

The key is to start early in the degenerative process. Once a joint has deteriorated too much, these techniques won't help. Research the techniques and reputable practitioners carefully. This area is currently filled with scams, false claims, and unqualified practitioners.

■ **Recheck your biological age and rate of aging** every three to 12 months, depending on how aggressive you are being. If you aren't showing any improvement, it's time to course correct. Discuss this with your doctor.

■ **Remember, the goal of health is to improve your sense of wellbeing. Trying to reverse your age is a choice, not a mandate. If you find it stressful and not fun, you shouldn't be doing it. And if it's not imbuing a state of wellbeing, then you are going in the wrong direction.**

In this book, we've offered you lots of ways to improve your health and enhance your well-being. We wish you every success in your journey!

Sincerely,

Steve and Sandi

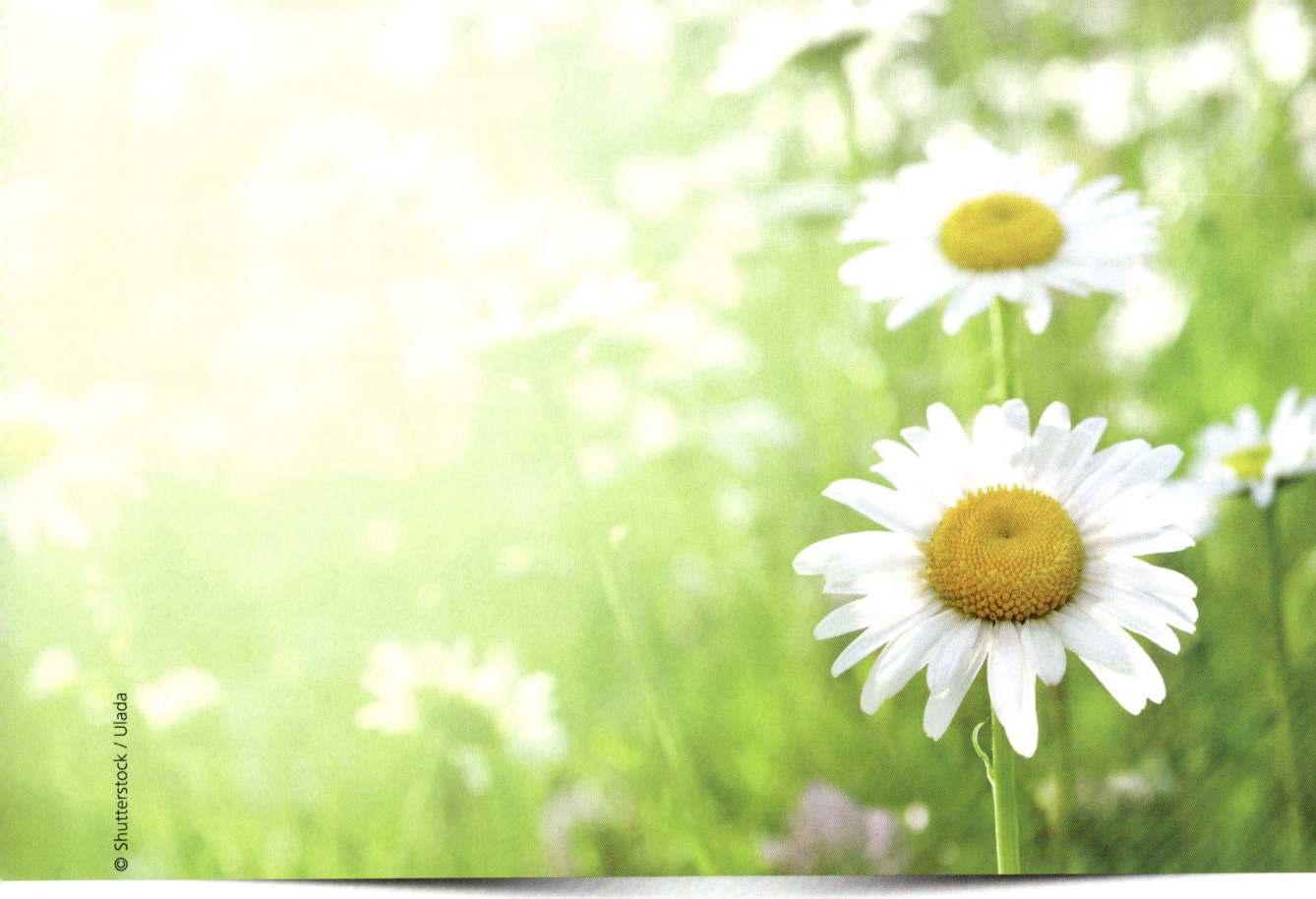

Acknowledgments

Sir Isaac Newton, the famous English scientist, once said, "If I have seen further, it is by standing on the shoulders of giants." We too are grateful to all the shoulders that have both held us up and inspired us over our lifetime. Especially to our incredible mentors, teachers, and supporters who have allowed us to create this body of work. We thank all of our contributing authors who helped enrich this book.

We would like to thank Jeff Bland, PhD, the father of functional medicine, who inspired us to understand medicine from a systems biology perspective. He helped us use science to understand disease from a root cause perspective, rather than using "a pill for every ill." To our phenomenal teachers of acupuncture, Sensei Shigeru Mii, Joe Helms, MD, and Nadia Volf, MD. To Rosalyn Bruyere, who pioneered the understanding of energy medicine.

We feel extremely privileged to have some of the preeminent leaders of functional and integrative medicine endorse this book. Thank you Doctors Brian Berman, Mark Hyman, Ben Kligler, Mimi Guarneri, Deanna Minich, David Perlmutter, Melinda Ring, Chris Suhar, and Aristo Vojdani for your kind words. Also, to Johnny G, who has inspired hundreds of thousands of people to exercise!

Thank you, Dean Kereiakes, MD, for all your support and guidance over the years. Dean is the consummate physician, a phenomenal clinician, an academic, and a researcher.

We would like to thank all those who served for years on the board of the Integrative Medicine Foundation: Tom Anderle, Nate Bachman, Dan Bailey, John Burns, Neil Bortz, Frederic Holzberger, Scott Kadish, Craig and Frances Lindner, and Heather Theders. We would also like to thank Steve and Molly Cobb, Dave Herche and Wendy Thursby, and Jill Kramer for their generous support. We also acknowledge all the members of the Bravewell Collaborative, whose philanthropic efforts helped raise the tide that floats all boats of the integrative medicine movement. We are also incredibly grateful to the leadership of The Christ Hospital, who understand that medicine needs to be more than a disease-care system and have created the Division of Modern Wellness to embrace a wellness-based system.

We could not have achieved this without you!

This book could not have existed without the deep insights and understanding of our editor Sheila Buff and the exceptional graphics and layout by Brenda Grannan (www.grannandesign.com). Both Sheila and Brenda remained extremely kind and gracious despite long delays in the writing of this book.

We have been lucky to have been buoyed for years by our amazing staff at AIM for Wellbeing. They know that healing begins when they answer the phone, or when a patient walks through our doors, and continues well after they leave. It is they who bring sunshine back into the lives of those that suffer.

We are also forever grateful to our extended families: Dennis and Phillip Amoils, Denise Bayvel and Carol Anne Mumby, and their spouses and children. We are lucky to have the most supportive friends, but too many to mention by name.

Finally, we would like to extend our deepest gratitude to our patients. When conventional medicine said this would never work, it was their enthusiasm, their gratitude, and their exemplary results that allowed us to forge on, knowing that integrative medicine has a place in the future.

References

Abeles SR, Jones MB, Santiago-Rodriguez TM, Ly M, Klitgord N, Yooseph S, Nelson KE, Pride DT. Microbial diversity in individuals and their household contacts following typical antibiotic courses. Microbiome. 2016 Jul 30;4(1):39. doi: 10.1186/s40168-016-0187-9. PMID: 27473422; PMCID: PMC4967329.

Abrams DI, Dolor R, Roberts R, Pechura C, Dusek J, Amoils S, Amoils S, Barrows K, Edman JS, Frye J, Guarneri E, Kligler B, Monti D, Spar M, Wolever RQ. The BraveNet prospective observational study on integrative medicine treatment approaches for pain. BMC Complement Altern Med. 2013 Jun 24;13:146. doi: 10.1186/1472-6882-13-146. PMID: 23800144; PMCID: PMC3717108.

Alba Sulaj, Stefan Kopf, Ekaterina von Rauchhaupt, Elisabeth Kliemank, Maik Brune, Zoltan Kender, Hannelore Bartl, Fabiola Garcia Cortizo, Katarina Klepac, Zhe Han, Varun Kumar, Valter Longo, Aurelio Teleman, Jürgen G Okun, Jakob Morgenstern, Thomas Fleming, Julia Szendroedi, Stephan Herzig, Peter P Nawroth, Six-Month Periodic Fasting in Patients With Type 2 Diabetes and Diabetic Nephropathy: A Proof-of-Concept Study, *The Journal of Clinical Endocrinology & Metabolism*, Volume 107, Issue 8, August 2022, Pages 2167-2181, https://doi.org/10.1210/clinem/dgac197

Ames BN. The metabolic tune-up: metabolic harmony and disease prevention. J Nutr. 2003 May;133(5 Suppl 1):1544S-8S. doi: 10.1093/jn/133.5.1544S. PMID: 12730462.

Ames BN. Prolonging healthy aging: Longevity vitamins and proteins. *Proc Natl Acad Sci U S A*. 2018;115(43):10836-10844. doi:10.1073/pnas.1809045115

Ames BN, Elson-Schwab I, Silver EA. High-dose vitamin therapy stimulates variant enzymes with decreased coenzyme binding affinity (increased K(m)): relevance to genetic disease and polymorphisms. Am J Clin Nutr. 2002 Apr;75(4):616-58. doi: 10.1093/ajcn/75.4.616. PMID: 11916749.

Amoils S, Kues J, Amoils S et al. The diagnostic validity of human electromagnetic field (aura) perception. *Journal of Medical Acupuncture.* 2002;13:25-28.

Angell M, Kassirer JP. Alternative medicine--the risks of untested and unregulated remedies. N Engl J Med. 1998 Sep 17;339(12):839-41. doi: 10.1056/NEJM199809173391210. PMID: 9738094.

Audette J. Acupuncture energetics: clues to an expanded view of somatovisceral homeostasis. *Pain Practitioner.* 2011;3:21.

Audette JF, Ryan AH. The role of acupuncture in pain management. *Phys Med Rehabil Clin N Am.* 2004; 15:749-772.

Belsky, J., Jonassaint, C., Pluess, M., Stanton, M., Brummett, B., and Williams, R. (2009). Vulnerability genes or plasticity genes? *Mol. Psychiatry* 14, 746–754. doi: 10.1038/mp.2009.44

Benson, Herb. *The Relaxation Response* (William Morrow, 2000).

Brandhorst S, Choi IY, Wei M, Cheng CW, Sedrakyan S, Navarrete G, Dubeau L, Yap LP, Park R, Vinciguerra M, Di Biase S, Mirzaei H, Mirisola MG, Childress P, Ji L, Groshen S, Penna F, Odetti P, Perin L, Conti PS, Ikeno Y, Kennedy BK, Cohen P, Morgan TE, Dorff TB, Longo VD. A Periodic Diet that Mimics Fasting Promotes Multi-System Regeneration, Enhanced Cognitive Performance, and Healthspan. Cell Metab. 2015 Jul 7;22(1):86-99. doi: 10.1016/j.cmet.2015.05.012. Epub 2015 Jun 18. PMID: 26094889; PMCID: PMC4509734.

Brandhorst S, Harputlugil E, Mitchell JR, Longo VD. Protective effects of short-term dietary restriction in surgical stress and chemotherapy. Ageing Res Rev. 2017 Oct;39:68-77. doi: 10.1016/j.arr.2017.02.001. Epub 2017 Feb 20. PMID: 28216454; PMCID: PMC5722209.

Buettner, Dan. *The Blue Zones: Lessons for Living Longer From the People Who've Lived the Longest* (National Geographic, 2009).

Buettner, Dan. *Thrive: Finding Happiness the Blue Zones Way* (National Geographic, 2011).

Caffa, I., Spagnolo, V., Vernieri, C. *et al.* Fasting-mimicking diet and hormone therapy induce breast cancer regression. *Nature* **583**, 620–624 (2020). https://doi.org/10.1038/s41586-020-2502-7

Campbell, Colin T. *The China Study: The Most Comprehensive Study of Nutrition Ever Conducted and the Startling Implications for Diet, Weight Loss, and Long-term Health* (BenBella Books, 2006).

Campbell DR, Kurzer MS. Flavonoid inhibition of aromatase enzyme activity in human preadipocytes. *J Steroid Biochem Mol Biol*. 1993;46(3):381-388. doi:10.1016/0960-0760(93)90228-o

Cao-Lei L, Massart R, Suderman MJ, Machnes Z, Elgbeili G, Laplante DP, Szyf M, King S. DNA methylation signatures triggered by prenatal maternal stress exposure to a natural disaster: Project Ice Storm. PLoS One. 2014 Sep 19;9(9):e107653. doi: 10.1371/journal.pone.0107653. PMID: 25238154; PMCID: PMC4169571

Cavalieri E, Rogan E. The 3,4-Quinones of Estrone and Estradiol Are the Initiators of Cancer whereas Resveratrol and *N*-acetylcysteine Are the Preventers. *Int J Mol Sci*. 2021;22(15):8238. Published 2021 Jul 30. doi:10.3390/ijms22158238

Cavalieri EL, Rogan EG. Depurinating estrogen-DNA adducts, generators of cancer initiation: their minimization leads to cancer prevention. *Clin Transl Med*. 2016;5(1):12. doi:10.1186/s40169-016-0088-3

Chlebowski RT, Anderson GL, Aragaki AK, et al. Association of Menopausal Hormone Therapy With Breast Cancer Incidence and Mortality During Long-term Follow-up of the Women's Health Initiative Randomized Clinical Trials. *JAMA*. 2020;324(4):369–380. doi:10.1001/jama.2020.9482

Cheng CW, Adams GB, Perin L, Wei M, Zhou X, Lam BS, Da Sacco S, Mirisola M, Quinn DI, Dorff TB, Kopchick JJ, Longo VD. Prolonged fasting reduces IGF-1/PKA to promote hematopoietic-stem-cell-based regeneration and reverse immunosuppression. Cell Stem Cell. 2014 Jun 5;14(6):810-23. doi: 10.1016/j.stem.2014.04.014. Erratum in: Cell Stem Cell. 2016 Feb 4;18(2):291-2. PMID: 24905167; PMCID: PMC4102383.

Cheng CW, Adams GB, Perin L, Wei M, Zhou X, Lam BS, Da Sacco S, Mirisola M, Quinn DI, Dorff TB, Kopchick JJ, Longo VD. Prolonged fasting reduces IGF-1/PKA to promote hematopoietic-stem-cell-based regeneration and reverse immunosuppression. Cell Stem Cell. 2014 Jun 5;14(6):810-23. doi: 10.1016/j.stem.2014.04.014. Erratum in: Cell Stem Cell. 2016 Feb 4;18(2):291-2. PMID: 24905167; PMCID: PMC4102383.

Cheng CW, Villani V, Buono R, Wei M, Kumar S, Yilmaz OH, Cohen P, Sneddon JB, Perin L, Longo VD. Fasting-Mimicking Diet Promotes Ngn3-Driven β-Cell Regeneration to Reverse Diabetes. Cell. 2017 Feb 23;168(5):775-788.e12. doi: 10.1016/j.cell.2017.01.040. PMID: 28235195; PMCID: PMC5357144.

Choi IY, Lee C, Longo VD. Nutrition and fasting mimicking diets in the prevention and treatment of autoimmune diseases and immunosenescence. Mol Cell Endocrinol. 2017 Nov 5;455:4-12. doi: 10.1016/j.mce.2017.01.042. Epub 2017 Jan 28. PMID: 28137612; PMCID: PMC5862044.

Chowdhury BA, Chandra RK. Biological and health implications of toxic heavy metal and essential trace element interactions. Prog Food Nutr Sci. 1987;11(1):55-113. PMID: 3303135.

Committee on Advancing Pain Research, Care, and Education, Institute of Medicine. *Relieving Pain in America: A Blueprint for Transforming Prevention, Care, Education, and Research* (National Academies Press, 2011).

Covasa M, Stephens RW, Toderean R, Cobuz C. Intestinal Sensing by Gut Microbiota: Targeting Gut Peptides. Front Endocrinol (Lausanne). 2019 Feb 19;10:82. doi: 10.3389/fendo.2019.00082. PMID: 30837951; PMCID: PMC6390476.

Danaei G, Finucane MM, Lu Y, Singh GM, Cowan MJ, Paciorek CJ, Lin JK, Farzadfar F, Khang YH, Stevens GA, Rao M, Ali MK, Riley LM, Robinson CA, Ezzati M; Global Burden of Metabolic Risk Factors of Chronic Diseases Collaborating Group (Blood Glucose). National, regional, and global trends in fasting plasma glucose and diabetes prevalence since 1980: systematic analysis of health examination surveys and epidemiological studies with 370 country-years and 2·7 million participants. Lancet. 2011 Jul 2;378(9785):31-40. doi: 10.1016/S0140-6736(11)60679-X. Epub 2011 Jun 24. PMID: 21705069.

De Silva A, Bloom SR. Gut Hormones and Appetite Control: A Focus on PYY and GLP-1 as Therapeutic Targets in Obesity. *Gut Liver*. 2012;6(1):10-20. doi:10.5009/gnl.2012.6.1.10

Dias BG, Ressler KJ. Parental olfactory experience influences behavior and neural structure in subsequent generations. *Nat Neurosci*. 2014;17(1):89-96. doi:10.1038/nn.3594

Dolinoy DC, Weidman JR, Waterland RA, Jirtle RL. Maternal genistein alters coat color and protects Avy mouse offspring from obesity by modifying the fetal epigenome. *Environ Health Perspect*. 2006;114(4):567-572. doi:10.1289/ehp.8700

Donadon MF, Martin-Santos R, Osório FL. The Associations Between Oxytocin and Trauma in Humans: A Systematic Review. *Front Pharmacol*. 2018;9:154. Published 2018 Mar 1. doi:10.3389/fphar.2018.00154

Dusek JA, Abrams DI, Roberts R, Griffin KH, Trebesch D, Dolor RJ, Wolever RQ, McKee MD, Kligler B. Patients Receiving Integrative Medicine Effectiveness Registry (PRIMIER) of the BraveNet practice-based research network: study protocol. BMC Complement Altern Med. 2016 Feb 4;16:53. doi: 10.1186/s12906-016-1025-0. PMID: 26846166; PMCID: PMC4743108.

van Eeden WA, van Hemert AM, Carlier IVE, Penninx BWJH, Lamers F, Fried EI, Schoevers R, Giltay EJ. Basal and LPS-stimulated inflammatory markers and the course of individual symptoms of depression. Transl Psychiatry. 2020 Jul 15;10(1):235. doi: 10.1038/s41398-020-00920-4. PMID: 32669537; PMCID: PMC7363825.)

Fitzgerald KN. *Younger You: Reduce Your Bio Age and Live Longer, Better*. Hachette Go, 2022.

Fitzgerald KN, Campbell T, Makarem S, Hodges R. Potential reversal of biological age in women following an 8-week methylation-supportive diet and lifestyle program: a case series. Aging (Albany NY). 2023 Mar 22; 15:1833-1839. https://doi.org/10.18632/aging.204602

Fuhrman BJ, Pfeiffer RM, Wu AH, et al. Green tea intake is associated with urinary estrogen profiles in Japanese-American women. *Nutr J*. 2013;12:25. Published 2013 Feb 15. doi:10.1186/1475-2891-12-25

Gasser P, Holstein D, Michel Y, Doblin R, Yazar-Klosinski B, Passie T, Brenneisen R. Safety and efficacy of lysergic acid diethylamide-assisted psychotherapy for anxiety associated with life-threatening diseases. J Nerv Ment Dis. 2014 Jul;202(7):513-20. doi: 10.1097/NMD.0000000000000113. PMID: 24594678; PMCID: PMC4086777.

Gore AC, Chappell VA, Fenton SE, Flaws JA, Nadal A, Prins GS, Toppari J, Zoeller RT. Executive Summary to EDC-2: The Endocrine Society's Second Scientific Statement on Endocrine-Disrupting Chemicals. Endocr Rev. 2015 Dec;36(6):593-602. doi: 10.1210/er.2015-1093. Epub 2015 Sep 28. PMID: 26414233; PMCID: PMC4702495.

Grundy SM, Cleeman JI, Daniels SR, Donato KA, Eckel RH, Franklin BA, Gordon DJ, Krauss RM, Savage PJ, Smith SC Jr, Spertus JA, Costa F; American Heart Association; National Heart, Lung, and Blood Institute. Diagnosis and management of the metabolic syndrome: an American Heart Association/National Heart, Lung, and Blood Institute Scientific Statement. Circulation. 2005 Oct 25;112(17):2735-52. doi: 10.1161/CIRCULATIONAHA.105.169404. Epub 2005 Sep 12. Erratum in: Circulation. 2005 Oct 25;112(17):e297. Erratum in: Circulation. 2005 Oct 25;112(17):e298. PMID: 16157765.

Guttman Y, Nudel A, Kerem Z. Polymorphism in Cytochrome P450 3A4 Is Ethnicity Related. *Front Genet*. 2019;10:224. Published 2019 Mar 19. doi:10.3389/fgene.2019.00224

Haggans CJ, Hutchins AM, Olson BA, Thomas W, Martini MC, Slavin JL. Effect of flaxseed consumption on urinary estrogen metabolites in postmenopausal women. *Nutr Cancer*. 1999;33(2):188-195. doi:10.1207/S15327914NC330211

Hahn J, Cook NR, Alexander EK, Friedman S, Walter J, Bubes V, Kotler G, Lee IM, Manson JE, Costenbader KH. Vitamin D and marine omega 3 fatty acid supplementation and incident autoimmune disease: VITAL randomized controlled trial. BMJ. 2022 Jan 26;376:e066452. doi: 10.1136/bmj-2021-066452. PMID: 35082139; PMCID: PMC8791065.

Helms, Joseph. *Getting to Know You: A Physician Explains How Acupuncture Helps You Be the Best You* (North Atlantic Books, 2007).

Hoffman C, Rice D, Sung HY. Persons with chronic conditions. Their prevalence and costs. JAMA. 1996 Nov 13;276(18):1473-9. PMID: 8903258.

Hossack MR, Reid MW, Aden JK, Gibbons T, Noe JC, Willis AM. Adverse Childhood Experience, Genes, and PTSD Risk in Soldiers: A Methylation Study. Mil Med. 2020 Mar 2;185(3-4):377-384. doi: 10.1093/milmed/usz292. PMID: 32976583.

Hölzel BK, Carmody J, Vangel M, Congleton C, Yerramsetti SM, Gard T, Lazar SW. Mindfulness practice leads to increases in regional brain gray matter density. Psychiatry Res. 2011 Jan 30;191(1):36-43. doi: 10.1016/j.pscychresns.2010.08.006. Epub 2010 Nov 10. PMID: 21071182; PMCID: PMC3004979.

Huang AW, Wei M, Caputo S, Wilson ML, Antoun J, Hsu WC. An Intermittent Fasting Mimicking Nutrition Bar Extends Physiologic Ketosis in Time Restricted Eating: A Randomized, Controlled, Parallel-Arm Study. Nutrients. 2021 Apr 30;13(5):1523. doi: 10.3390/nu13051523. PMID: 33946428; PMCID: PMC8147148.

Inchauspé J. *The Glucose Goddess Method: The 4-Week Guide to Cutting Cravings, Getting Your Energy Back, and Feeling Amazing.*

Inchauspé J. *Glucose Revolution: The Life-Changing Power of Balancing Your Blood Sugar.* Simon & Schuster/Simon Element, 2022.

Johnson MW. Classic Psychedelics in Addiction Treatment: The Case for Psilocybin in Tobacco Smoking Cessation. Curr Top Behav Neurosci. 2022;56:213-227. doi: 10.1007/7854_2022_327. PMID: 35704271.

Johnston CS, Kim CM, Buller AJ. Vinegar improves insulin sensitivity to a high-carbohydrate meal in subjects with insulin resistance or type 2 diabetes. *Diabetes Care*. 2004;27(1):281-282. doi:10.2337/diacare.27.1.281

Kabat-Zinn, Jon. *Wherever You Go, There You Are* (Hyperion, 2005).

Kaszkin-Bettag M, Beck S, Richardson A, Heger PW, Beer AM. Efficacy of the special extract ERr 731 from rhapontic rhubarb for menopausal complaints: a 6-month open observational study. *Altern Ther Health Med.* 2008;14:32-38.

Kawano H, Yasue H, Kitagawa A, Hirai N, Yoshida T, Soejima H, Miyamoto S, Nakano M, Ogawa H. Dehydroepiandrosterone supplementation improves endothelial function and insulin sensitivity in men. J Clin Endocrinol Metab. 2003 Jul;88(7):3190-5. doi: 10.1210/jc.2002-021603. PMID: 12843164.

Kawano H et al. Vitamin D receptor genetic polymorphisms and prostate cancer risk: a meta-analysis of 36 published studies. *Int J Clin Exp Med.* 2009;2(2):159-175.

Kim SH, Chunawala L, Linde R, Reaven GM. Comparison of the 1997 and 2003 American Diabetes Association classification of impaired fasting glucose: impact on prevalence of impaired fasting glucose, coronary heart disease risk factors, and coronary heart disease in a community-based medical practice. *J Am Coll Cardiol*. 2006;48(2):293-297. doi:10.1016/j.jacc.2006.03.043

King MC, Marks JH, Mandell JB; New York Breast Cancer Study Group. Breast and ovarian cancer risks due to inherited mutations in BRCA1 and BRCA2. Science. 2003 Oct 24;302(5645):643-6. doi: 10.1126/science.1088759. PMID: 14576434.

Klok MD, Jakobsdottir S, Drent ML. The role of leptin and ghrelin in the regulation of food intake and body weight in humans: a review. Obes Rev. 2007 Jan;8(1):21-34. doi: 10.1111/j.1467-789X.2006.00270.x. PMID: 17212793.

Knoops KT, de Groot LC, Kromhout D, Perrin AE, Moreiras-Varela O, Menotti A, van Staveren WA. Mediterranean diet, lifestyle factors, and 10-year mortality in elderly European men and women: the HALE project. JAMA. 2004 Sep 22;292(12):1433-9. doi: 10.1001/jama.292.12.1433. PMID: 15383513.

Konkolÿ Thege B, Horwood L, Slater L, Tan MC, Hodgins DC, Wild TC. Relationship between interpersonal trauma exposure and addictive behaviors: a systematic review. BMC Psychiatry. 2017 May 4;17(1):164. doi: 10.1186/s12888-017-1323-1. PMID: 28472931; PMCID: PMC5418764

Kris-Etherton P, Eckel RH, Howard BV, St Jeor S, Bazzarre TL; Nutrition Committee Population Science Committee and Clinical Science Committee of the American Heart Association. AHA Science Advisory: Lyon Diet Heart Study. Benefits of a Mediterranean-style, National Cholesterol Education Program/American Heart Association Step I Dietary Pattern on Cardiovascular Disease. Circulation. 2001 Apr 3;103(13):1823-5. doi: 10.1161/01.cir.103.13.1823. PMID: 11282918.

Kroenke K, Mangelsdorff AD. Common symptoms in ambulatory care: incidence, evaluation, therapy, and outcome. Am J Med. 1989 Mar;86(3):262-6. doi: 10.1016/0002-9343(89)90293-3. PMID: 2919607.

Kyrou I, Chrousos GP, Tsigos C. Stress, visceral obesity, and metabolic complications. Ann N Y Acad Sci. 2006 Nov;1083:77-110. doi: 10.1196/annals.1367.008. PMID: 17148735.

Lenoir C, Rollason V, Desmeules JA, Samer CF. Influence of Inflammation on Cytochromes P450 Activity in Adults: A Systematic Review of the Literature. *Front Pharmacol*. 2021;12:733935. Published 2021 Nov 16. doi:10.3389/fphar.2021.733935

Liu WM, Hall NK, Liu HSY, Hood FL, Dalgleish AG. Combination of cannabidiol with low-dose naltrexone increases the anticancer action of chemotherapy *in vitro* and *in vivo*. Oncol Rep. 2022 Apr;47(4):76. doi: 10.3892/or.2022.8287. Epub 2022 Feb 18. PMID: 35179218.

Lustig, RH. *Metabolical: The Lure and the Lies of Processed Food, Nutrition, and Modern Medicine.* Harper Wave, 2021.

Maloh J, Wei M, Hsu WC, Caputo S, Afzal N, Sivamani RK. The Effects of a Fasting Mimicking Diet on Skin Hydration, Skin Texture, and Skin Assessment: A Randomized Controlled Trial. J Clin Med. 2023 Feb 21;12(5):1710. doi: 10.3390/jcm12051710. PMID: 36902498; PMCID: PMC10003066.

Malvandi AM, Shahba S, Mehrzad J, Lombardi G. Metabolic Disruption by Naturally Occurring Mycotoxins in Circulation: A Focus on Vascular and Bone Homeostasis Dysfunction. *Front Nutr.* 2022;9:915681. Published 2022 Jun 24. doi:10.3389/fnut.2022.915681

McFarlin BK, Henning AL, Bowman EM, Gary MA, Carbajal KM. Oral spore-based probiotic supplementation was associated with reduced incidence of post-prandial dietary endotoxin, triglycerides, and disease risk biomarkers. World J Gastrointest Pathophysiol. 2017 Aug 15;8(3):117-126. doi: 10.4291/wjgp.v8.i3.117. PMID: 28868181; PMCID: PMC5561432.

Michaëlsson K, Baron JA, Byberg L, Höijer J, Larsson SC, Svennblad B, Melhus H, Wolk A, Warensjö Lemming E. Combined associations of body mass index and adherence to a Mediterranean-like diet with all-cause and cardiovascular mortality: A cohort study. PLoS Med. 2020 Sep 17;17(9):e1003331. doi: 10.1371/journal.pmed.1003331. PMID: 32941436; PMCID: PMC7497998.

Morris MC, Tangney CC, Wang Y, Sacks FM, Barnes LL, Bennett DA, Aggarwal NT. MIND diet slows cognitive decline with aging. Alzheimers Dement. 2015 Sep;11(9):1015-22. doi: 10.1016/j.jalz.2015.04.011. Epub 2015 Jun 15. PMID: 26086182; PMCID: PMC4581900.

Musanabaganwa C, Wani AH, Donglasan J, Fatumo S, Jansen S, Mutabaruka J, Rutembesa E, Uwineza A, Hermans EJ, Roozendaal B, Wildman DE, Mutesa L, Uddin M. Leukocyte methylomic imprints of exposure to the genocide against the Tutsi in Rwanda: a pilot epigenome-wide analysis. Epigenomics. 2022 Jan;14(1):11-25. doi: 10.2217/epi-2021-0310. Epub 2021 Dec 8. PMID: 34875875; PMCID: PMC8672329.

Naviaux RK. Metabolic features of the cell danger response. Mitochondrion. 2014 May;16:7-17. doi: 10.1016/j.mito.2013.08.006. Epub 2013 Aug 24. PMID: 23981537.

Naviaux RK. Perspective: Cell danger response Biology-The new science that connects environmental health with mitochondria and the rising tide of chronic illness. Mitochondrion. 2020 Mar;51:40-45. doi: 10.1016/j.mito.2019.12.005. Epub 2019 Dec 23. PMID: 31877376.

Nardon M, Venturelli M, Ruzzante F, Longo VD, Bertucco M. Fasting-Mimicking-Diet does not reduce skeletal muscle function in healthy young adults: a randomized control trial. Eur J Appl Physiol. 2022 Mar;122(3):651-661. doi: 10.1007/s00421-021-04867-2. Epub 2022 Jan 16. PMID: 35034194.

Newman M, Curran DA. Reliability of a dried urine test for comprehensive assessment of urine hormones and metabolites. BMC Chem. 2021 Mar 15;15(1):18. doi: 10.1186/s13065-021-00744-3. PMID: 33722278; PMCID: PMC7962249.

Newman M, Curran DA, Mayfield BP. Dried urine and salivary profiling for complete assessment of cortisol and cortisol metabolites. J Clin Transl Endocrinol. 2020 Nov 27;22:100243. doi: 10.1016/j.jcte.2020.100243. PMID: 33354516; PMCID: PMC7744704.

Newman MS, Curran DA, Mayfield BP, Saltiel D, Stanczyk FZ. Assessment of estrogen exposure from transdermal estradiol gel therapy with a dried urine assay. Steroids. 2022 Aug;184:109038. doi: 10.1016/j.steroids.2022.109038. Epub 2022 Apr 26. PMID: 35483542.

Newman MS, Mayfield BP, Saltiel D, Stanczyk FZ. Assessing estrogen exposure from transdermal estradiol patch therapy using a dried urine collection and a GC-MS/MS assay. Steroids. 2023 Jan;189:109149. doi: 10.1016/j.steroids.2022.109149. Epub 2022 Nov 19. PMID: 36414155.

Newman M, Pratt SM, Curran DA, Stanczyk FZ. Evaluating urinary estrogen and progesterone metabolites using dried filter paper samples and gas chromatography with tandem mass spectrometry (GC-MS/MS). *BMC Chem.* 2019;13(1):20. Published 2019 Feb 4. doi:10.1186/s13065-019-0539-1

DiNicolantonio JJ, O'Keefe JH, Wilson WL. Sugar addiction: is it real? A narrative review. Br J Sports Med. 2018 Jul;52(14):910-913. doi: 10.1136/bjsports-2017-097971. Epub 2017 Aug 23. PMID: 28835408.

Nguyen T, Nioi P, Pickett CB. The Nrf2-antioxidant response element signaling pathway and its activation by oxidative stress. J Biol Chem. 2009 May 15;284(20):13291-5. doi: 10.1074/jbc.R900010200. Epub 2009 Jan 30. PMID: 19182219; PMCID: PMC2679427.

Palumbo S, Mariotti V, Iofrida C, Pellegrini S. Genes and Aggressive Behavior: Epigenetic Mechanisms Underlying Individual Susceptibility to Aversive Environments. *Front Behav Neurosci.* 2018;12:117. Published 2018 Jun 13. doi:10.3389/fnbeh.2018.00117

Pant A, Gribbin S, McIntyre D, et al. Primary prevention of cardiovascular disease in women with a Mediterranean diet: systematic review and meta-analysis. Heart. 2023;heartjnl-2022-321930. doi:10.1136/heartjnl-2022-321930

Patel J, Pallazola VA, Dudum R, Greenland P, McEvoy JW, Blumenthal RS, Virani SS, Miedema MD, Shea S, Yeboah J, Abbate A, Hundley WG, Karger AB, Tsai MY, Sathiyakumar V, Ogunmoroti O, Cushman M, Savji N, Liu K, Nasir K, Blaha MJ, Martin SS, Al Rifai M. Assessment of Coronary Artery Calcium Scoring to Guide Statin Therapy Allocation According to Risk-Enhancing Factors: The Multi-Ethnic Study of Atherosclerosis. JAMA Cardiol. 2021 Oct 1;6(10):1161-1170. doi: 10.1001/jamacardio.2021.2321. PMID: 34259820; PMCID: PMC8281019.

Pingli Wei, Caitlin Keller, Lingjun Li,. Neuropeptides in gut-brain axis and their influence on host immunity and stress. Computational and Structural Biotechnology Journal,Volume 18,2020, 843-851. https://doi.org/10.1016/j.csbj.2020.02.018.

Pollan M. *How to Change Your Mind: What the New Science of Psychedelics Teaches Us About Consciousness, Dying, Addiction, Depression, and Transcendence* (Penguin, 2018).

Rahmani J, Montesanto A, Giovannucci E, Zand H, Barati M, Kopchick JJ, Mirisola MG, Lagani V, Bawadi H, Vardavas R, Laviano A, Christensen K, Passarino G, Longo VD. Association between IGF-1 levels ranges and all-cause mortality: A meta-analysis. Aging Cell. 2022 Feb;21(2):e13540. doi: 10.1111/acel.13540. Epub 2022 Jan 20. PMID: 35048526; PMCID: PMC8844108.

Reding KW, Han CJ, Whittington D, et al. Risk of Breast Cancer Associated with Estrogen DNA Adduct Biomarker. *Cancer Epidemiol Biomarkers Prev*. 2020;29(10):2096-2099. doi:10.1158/1055-9965.EPI-20-0133

Rees K, Takeda A, Martin N, Ellis L, Wijesekara D, Vepa A, Das A, Hartley L, Stranges S. Mediterranean-style diet for the primary and secondary prevention of cardiovascular disease. Cochrane Database Syst Rev. 2019 Mar 13;3(3):CD009825. doi: 10.1002/14651858.CD009825.pub3. PMID: 30864165; PMCID: PMC6414510.

Reuben SH. Reducing Environmental Cancer Risk: What We Can Do Now: 2008–2009 Annual Report, President's Cancer Panel. Bethesda, MD: National Cancer Institute; 2010.

Sapolsky, Robert. *Why Zebras Don't Get Ulcers* (Holt, 2004).

Samavat H, Kurzer MS. Estrogen metabolism and breast cancer. *Cancer Lett*. 2015;356(2 Pt A):231-243. doi:10.1016/j.canlet.2014.04.018

Schiffer L, Barnard L, Baranowski ES, et al. Human steroid biosynthesis, metabolism and excretion are differentially reflected by serum and urine steroid metabolomes: A comprehensive review. *J Steroid Biochem Mol Biol*. 2019;194:105439. doi:10.1016/j.jsbmb.2019.105439

Schulz LO, Chaudhari LS. High-Risk Populations: The Pimas of Arizona and Mexico. Curr Obes Rep. 2015 Mar;4(1):92-8. doi: 10.1007/s13679-014-0132-9. PMID: 25954599; PMCID: PMC4418458.

Sekhar A, Kuttan A, Borges JC, Rajachandran M. Food for Thought or Feeding a Dogma? Diet and Coronary Artery Disease: a Clinician's Perspective. Curr Cardiol Rep. 2021 Jul 19;23(9):127. doi: 10.1007/s11886-021-01557-5. PMID: 34279741.

Shah BR, Xu W, Mraz J. Cytochrome P450 1B1: role in health and disease and effect of nutrition on its expression. *RSC Adv*. 2019;9(36):21050-21062. Published 2019 Jul 4. doi:10.1039/c9ra03674a

Smerdová L, Šmerdová J, Kabátková M, et al. Upregulation of CYP1B1 expression by inflammatory cytokines is mediated by the p38 MAP kinase signal transduction pathway. *Carcinogenesis*. 2014;35(11):2534-2543. doi:10.1093/carcin/bgu190

Soin A, Soin Y, Dann T, Buenaventura R, Ferguson K, Atluri S, Sachdeva H, Sudarshan G, Akbik H, Italiano J. Low-Dose Naltrexone Use for Patients with Chronic Regional Pain Syndrome: A Systematic Literature Review. Pain Physician. 2021 Jul;24(4):E393-E406. PMID: 34213865.

Song M, Fung TT, Hu FB, et al. Association of Animal and Plant Protein Intake With All-Cause and Cause-Specific Mortality. *JAMA Intern Med.* 2016;176(10):1453–1463. doi:10.1001/jamainternmed.2016.4182

Spiegel K, Leproult R, L'hermite-Balériaux M, Copinschi G, Penev PD, Van Cauter E. Leptin levels are dependent on sleep duration: relationships with sympathovagal balance, carbohydrate regulation, cortisol, and thyrotropin. J Clin Endocrinol Metab. 2004 Nov;89(11):5762-71. doi: 10.1210/jc.2004-1003. PMID: 15531540.

Srinivasan A, Dutta P, Bansal D, Chakrabarti A, Bhansali AK, Hota D. Efficacy and safety of low-dose naltrexone in painful diabetic neuropathy: A randomized, double-blind, active-control, crossover clinical trial. J Diabetes. 2021 Oct;13(10):770-778. doi: 10.1111/1753-0407.13202. Epub 2021 Jun 1. PMID: 34014028.

Stanhope KL, Schwarz JM, Keim NL, Griffen SC, Bremer AA, Graham JL, Hatcher B, Cox CL, Dyachenko

A, Zhang W, McGahan JP, Seibert A, Krauss RM, Chiu S, Schaefer EJ, Ai M, Otokozawa S, Nakajima K, Nakano T, Beysen C, Hellerstein MK, Berglund L, Havel PJ. Consuming fructose-sweetened, not glucose-sweetened, beverages increases visceral adiposity and lipids and decreases insulin sensitivity in overweight/obese humans. J Clin Invest. 2009 May;119(5):1322-34. doi: 10.1172/JCI37385. Epub 2009 Apr 20. PMID: 19381015; PMCID: PMC2673878.

Svetkey LP, Stevens VJ, Brantley PJ, Appel LJ, Hollis JF, Loria CM, Vollmer WM, Gullion CM, Funk K, Smith P, Samuel-Hodge C, Myers V, Lien LF, Laferriere D, Kennedy B, Jerome GJ, Heinith F, Harsha DW, Evans P, Erlinger TP, Dalcin AT, Coughlin J, Charleston J, Champagne CM, Bauck A, Ard JD, Aicher K; Weight Loss Maintenance Collaborative Research Group. Comparison of strategies for sustaining weight loss: the weight loss maintenance randomized controlled trial. JAMA. 2008 Mar 12;299(10):1139-48. doi: 10.1001/jama.299.10.1139. PMID: 18334689.

Taubes, G. Rare form of dwarfism protects against cancer. Discover, March 26, 2013.

Thomas MP, Potter BV. The structural biology of oestrogen metabolism. *J Steroid Biochem Mol Biol*. 2013;137:27-49. doi:10.1016/j.jsbmb.2012.12.014

Veenendaal MVE, Costello PM, Lillycrop KA, de Rooij SR, van der Post JA, Bossuyt PM, Hanson MA, Painter RC, Roseboom TJ. Prenatal famine exposure, health in later life and promotor methylation of four candidate genes. Journal of Developmental Origins of Health and Disease. 2012 Dec;3(6):450-7

Wei M, Brandhorst S, Shelehchi M, Mirzaei H, Cheng CW, Budniak J, Groshen S, Mack WJ, Guen E, Di Biase S, Cohen P, Morgan TE, Dorff T, Hong K, Michalsen A, Laviano A, Longo VD. Fasting-mimicking diet and markers/risk factors for aging, diabetes, cancer, and cardiovascular disease. Sci Transl Med. 2017 Feb 15;9(377):eaai8700. doi: 10.1126/scitranslmed.aai8700. PMID: 28202779; PMCID: PMC6816332.

Welsh JA, Sharma A, Abramson JL, Vaccarino V, Gillespie C, Vos MB. Caloric sweetener consumption and dyslipidemia among US adults. JAMA. 2010 Apr 21;303(15):1490-7. doi: 10.1001/jama.2010.449. PMID: 20407058; PMCID: PMC3045262. *JAMA. 2010;303(15):1490-14977.*

Winkler N, Ruf-Leuschner M, Ertl V, Pfeiffer A, Schalinski I, Ovuga E, Neuner F, Elbert T. From War to Classroom: PTSD and Depression in Formerly Abducted Youth in Uganda. Front Psychiatry. 2015 Mar 3;6:2. doi: 10.3389/fpsyt.2015.00002. PMID: 25788887; PMCID: PMC4348469.

Wolever RQ, Abrams DI, Kligler B, Dusek JA, Roberts R, Frye J, Edman JS, Amoils S, Pradhan E, Spar M, Gaudet T, Guarneri E, Homel P, Amoils S, Lee RA, Berman B, Monti DA, Dolor R. Patients seek integrative medicine for preventive approach to optimize health. Explore (NY). 2012 Nov-Dec;8(6):348-52. doi: 10.1016/j.explore.2012.08.005. PMID: 23141791.

Yang CZ, Yaniger SI, Jordan VC, Klein DJ, Bittner GD. Most plastic products release estrogenic chemicals: a potential health problem that can be solved. Environ Health Perspect. 2011 Jul;119(7):989-96. doi: 10.1289/ehp.1003220. Epub 2011 Mar 2. PMID: 21367689; PMCID: PMC3222987.

Younger J, Parkitny L, McLain D. The use of low-dose naltrexone (LDN) as a novel anti-inflammatory treatment for chronic pain. Clin Rheumatol. 2014 Apr;33(4):451-9. doi: 10.1007/s10067-014-2517-2. Epub 2014 Feb 15. PMID: 24526250; PMCID: PMC3962576.

Zahid M, Beseler CL, Hall JB, LeVan T, Cavalieri EL, Rogan EG. Unbalanced estrogen metabolism in ovarian cancer. *Int J Cancer*. 2014;134(10):2414-2423. doi:10.1002/ijc.28565

Zahid M, Gaikwad NW, Ali MF, Lu F, Saeed M, Yang L, Rogan EG, Cavalieri EL. Prevention of estrogen-DNA adduct formation in MCF-10F cells by resveratrol. Free Radic Biol Med. 2008 Jul 15;45(2):136-45. doi: 10.1016/j.freeradbiomed.2008.03.017. Epub 2008 Apr 8. PMID: 18423413; PMCID: PMC2494714.

Zahid M, Saeed M, Beseler C, Rogan EG, Cavalieri EL. Resveratrol and N-acetylcysteine block the cancer-initiating step in MCF-10F cells. Free Radic Biol Med. 2011 Jan 1;50(1):78-85. doi: 10.1016/j.freeradbiomed.2010.10.662. Epub 2010 Oct 8. PMID: 20934508; PMCID: PMC4425208.

Zhong VW, Van Horn L, Greenland P, Carnethon MR, Ning H, Wilkins JT, Lloyd-Jones DM, Allen NB. Associations of Processed Meat, Unprocessed Red Meat, Poultry, or Fish Intake With Incident Cardiovascular Disease and All-Cause Mortality. JAMA Intern Med. 2020 Apr 1;180(4):503-512. doi: 10.1001/jamainternmed.2019.6969. PMID: 32011623; PMCID: PMC7042891.

Index

Locators in **bold** refer to figures.

A

abuse. *See* trauma
ACCTION Pain Taxonomy, 241
ACE healing treatment, 32–33, **32–33**, 292–293, **292–293**
acupuncture
    authors' personal experiences, 28, 29–30
    body healing through, 89, 281–285, 292–293, **292–293**, 327
    for chronic pain evaluation, 257–261, **258–259**, 269
    professional training for, 284
addictions, 57, 73–74, 76–78, 87
adrenal fatigue, 207–211
adrenal glands, **185**, 186, 189, 190. *See also* cortisol
adult-onset diabetes. *See* diabetes (type 2)
Advanced Allergy Therapeutics (AAT), 180
adverse childhood experiences (ACE), 71–75. *See also* trauma
aging
    biological and chronological, 42–43, 341–343, 344
    metabolism's role in, 96–101, **97**
    reversing, 23, 340–343
Akkermansia muciniphila, 230
alcohol, 74, 118, 132, 206, 210–211, 272
allergies
    about, 160–161, **160**
    to food, 121, 162–163, 167, **167**, 172–173, 180
    hygiene hypothesis, 162
    to molds, 164
    seasonal, 176
    treatment, 158, 163, 176, 180
allodynia, 241, 257
American Heart Association (AHA) diet, 126
Amoils, Maya, 320–321, 323, 325–330
AMP kinase (AMPK), **235**, 236–238
ancestral foods, 128
androgens, 186–187, 213
andropause, 190–192, 203
Angell, Marcia, 17
antecedent factors, 49, 51–52
antibiotics, 118, 124, 238
antidepressants, 86, 88, 91, 92, 270
antioxidant supplements, 147–148
apoptosis (programmed cell death), 109–110
apple cider vinegar, 229
artificial sweeteners, 133, 134, 229

Autoimmune Protocol (AIP) diet, 174
autoimmunity, 157–165
    about, 160–161
    allergies and, 158, 160–164
    cardiovascular health and, 308
    chronic illness web, 168–169, **168**
    chronic pain and, 257
    conventional versus functional approach, 158–159, 163
    environmentally induced, 157–158, 159, 164–165, 238
    gut dysfunction and, 159, 161–163
    stress and, 64
autonomic nervous system, 65
autophagy, 109–110, 143, 236–237, 238

B
beef, 129, 131, 133, 153–154
benign prostatic hyperplasia (BPH), 193–194, 203
bioidentical hormones, 203–204
biomechanics, 244–246, 252–256, **253–256**
biopsychotypes, 260–261, **262–267**, 268
biotensegrity, 244–246, **245**, 252–256, **253–256**, 278
biotoxins. *See* environment and environmental toxins
Bland, Jeffrey, 19, 332
blood glucose testing, 222, 231
Blue Zones, 100–101, 127, 128
The Blue Zones (Buettner), 100–101
body healing therapies, 275–301
    ACE healing treatment, 32–33, **32–33**, 292–293, **292–293**
    acupuncture, 89, 281–285, 292–293, 327. *See also* acupuncture
    approach (overview), 272–273, 276–279, 301
    energy healing techniques, 90–93, 269–270, 290–293, 327
    manipulative therapies, 280–281, 292–293
    massage and bodywork, 245, 287–290, 327
    for mind-body connection, 89, 91
    patient's role in, 297–300
    prolotherapy, 285–286
    psychedelic drugs, 77–78, 86–88, 335
    stem cell therapy, 286–287, 341
    supplemental therapies, 293–295
    supplements, 88–92, 106–107, 145–150, 165, 181, 204–205, 295–297
bodywork, 245, 268, 287–290, 327
brain-gut axis, 123–124
BRCA genes, 193, 323
breast cancer, 192–194, 196, 214–216, **214**
broccoli, 106, 128–129, 142, 204, 213, 327

broken heart syndrome, 270
Buettner, Dan, 100–101, 127
bypass grafts, 318

C
Campbell, T. Colin, 140
cancer
    conventional versus integrative approach, 238, 320–321, 322–329
    diet changes for, 238
    hormones and, 192–196, **195**, 205, 214–216, **214**, 220
    Maya's journey, 320–321, 323, 325–330
    prevention, 194, 214–216, 236–237
    resources, 328–329
    risk factors, 87, 98, 192–194, 196, 205
    staging, 321–322
    stress and, 64, 87, 98
cannabidiol (CBD), 296–297
cardiac (calcium) score, 310
cardiovascular health, 303–318
    artery health, 304–307
    inflammation and, 98, 101, 306, **307**, 308, 309, 313–314
    risk factors, 304, 307, 308
    testing for arterial damage, 313–315
    testing for heart disease, 309–312, **309**
    treatment, 315–318
CBD (cannabidiol), 296–297
celiac disease, 159, 162, 173
Cell Danger Response, 182
cell membrane integrity, 99
central nervous system, pain and, 241–243, 257
central sensitization, 257
chicken and eggs, 132, 151–152
The China Study (Campbell), 140
chiropractic treatment, 280–281, 292–293, **292–293**
cholesterol, 305–307, 309, **309**
cholesterol deposits (plaques), 304, 306
cholesterol-derived hormones, 186, 187–188, **189**
cholesterol-lowering drugs, 317–318
chronic fatigue syndrome (CFS), 108, 255–256
chronic illness web, 168–169, **168**
chronic inflammation, 97–101. *See also* inflammation
chronic inflammatory response syndrome (CIRS), 164
chronic pain, 239–273
    about, 240–243
    acupuncture evaluation, 257–261, **258–259**
    biomechanical evaluation, 252–256, **253–256**
    biopsychotypes, 260–270
    central sensitization evaluation, 257

evaluation and treatment overview, 243, 246, 272–273. *See also* body healing therapies
immunity and, 257
lifestyle analysis, 271–272
mind-body diagnoses, 270–271
neuromusculoskeletal exam, 247–248
pain generators exam, 248–250, **248–249**, **251**
perspective shifts, 244–246
research, 32–33, **32–33**, 292–293, **292–293**
risk factors, 243
as Transformational Moment, 301
trauma and, 271, 299–300
complex regional pain syndrome (CRPS), 250, 276
continuous glucose monitor, 231
conventional medicine
for autoimmune diseases and allergies, 158, 163
background, 14–17, **15**
for cancer, 321
for chronic pain, 243
lab testing, 36, 37–38, 40, 49, 64, 188
medical diagnosis, 36, 37–38, 51–52, 63
new directions for, 20, **20**. *See also* Transformational Medicine®
training directives, 26
coronary artery disease. *See* cardiovascular health
coronary catheter angiogram, 310
coronary computed tomography angiography (CCTA), 311
cortisol (stress hormone)
about, **185**, 186, 187, 188–189, **189**
balancing, 207–208
gut dysfunction and, 124
sleep disorders and, 39, 60
stress and, 60, 62, 65–67, **67**, 189, **189**, 190, 191
craniosacral therapy (CST), 288–289
crises, as Transformational Moment, 13, **13**, 26, 68, 85, 92–93, 301
cruciferous vegetables, 106, 128–129, 142, 213, 327
cultured and fermented foods, 129, 132
curcumin, 148–149
custom orthotics, 254, **254**
cytokines, 62–63, 97, 98, 99, 241

D

DASH diet, 136
degeneration, **97**, 100–101
dehydroepiandrosterone. *See* DHEA
depletion, 64–65
depression
alcohol use and, 74, 272
chronic illness web, **168**
gut dysfunction, 123
hormones and, 92, 196, 197, 205, 208
pain and, 32–33, **32–33**, 241, 246, 257, 270, 276
stress and, 61, 64
symptoms, 68
trauma and, 72–73, **75**, 77–78
treatment with bodywork, 287
treatment with drugs, 77–78, 86–88, 91, 92, 270
treatment with energy healing, 290
treatment with supplements, 88, 91, 147, 149, 205
dermatome pain patterns, 248–249, **248–249**, **251**, **258**, 259–260
detoxification, 102–110
about, 102–103
detox diet and supplements, 106–107, 145–148
for hormone balancing, 194–195, **195**, 212
impairment of, 103–105, 108
for insulin resistance, 230
process of, 105, **107**, 109–110
tipping point, 160, **160**
DHEA (dehydroepiandrosterone)
about, **185**, 188–190
balancing, 200, 204–205
for menopause, 209
polycystic ovary syndrome and, 213
precautions, 205
stress and, 60, 62
diabetes (type 1), 164, 218–219
diabetes (type 2)
about, 219, 223
cardiovascular health and, 308, 314
genetics and epigenetic factors, 47
path to, 221–223. *See also* insulin and insulin resistance
treating, 227–232
diagnosis. *See* expanded medical diagnosis
diet, 125–154
about, 8, 126–127, 130–135, **135**
aging and, 342–343
for cardiovascular health, 315
detox diet, 106–107, 145–146
fasting and time-restricted dieting, 143–145, 146, 227–228, 229, 237–238
finding the right diet, 126, 128–129, 136–142, **137**, **139–140**
food labels, 134–135, 151–154
for gut health, 129
for immunity, 173–177, 179
for inflammation, 91, 98–99
for insulin resistance, 227–229, 237–238
for metabolism, 145–149

portions of food, 135, **135**
Standard American Diet, 8, 98, 234–238, **235**, 334–335. *See also* SAD Situation; SAD Syndrome
supplements versus food, 149–150
what to avoid, 128, 132, 133
digestive enzymes, 114–115, 118
dihydrotestosterone (DHT), 207
DNA methylation. *See* methylation
dry needling, 284
dysautonomia, 65, **168**, 276
dysbiosis
  about, 116–118
  autoimmunity and, 164–165
  chronic illness and, 168, **168**
  endometriosis and, 212
  hormones and, 212
  markers for, 314
  neurological disorders and, 123
  treating, 118

E

Earth's health, 336–337, **336**
Eastern healing systems, 29–30, 269
educating children, 336–337
EGCG (green tea extract), 147–148, 207, 211, 237, 328
eggs, 132, 151–152
ego dissolution, 87–88
elimination diet, 173–174
emotional trauma. *See* trauma
endocrine disruptors, 193, 196, 204, 211, 215, 224
endometriosis, 211–212
endothelial function testing, 311–312
energy healing, 90–93, 269–270, 290–293, **292–293**, 327
enriched foods, 134. *See also* processed foods
environmentally induced autoimmunity, 157–158, 159, 164–165, 238
environment and environmental toxins
  autoimmunity and, 157–158, 159, 164–165
  detoxification of, 102–110
  diet and, 145
  epigenetics and, 46–48, **46**, **48**
  healing the environment, 336–337
  histamine and, 165
  toxin overload, 9, 160, **160**, 161, 335
epigenetics. *See also* methylation
  about, 41–43, **44**
  influences on, 46–48, **46**, **48**
  psychedelic drugs and, 78
  reversing aging through, 341

trauma and, 71–75, **75**
erectile dysfunction (ED), 189, 190–191, 312
estradiol
  about, 187, 194, 206
  as hormone therapy, 203, 210
  lab testing, 191, 208
  menopause and, 208–209
  testing for, 208–209
estrogen disruptors, 193, 196, 204, 211, 215, 224
estrogen dominance, 211, 212
estrogens
  about, **185**, 186–187, 188–190
  byproducts, 192, 194–195, **195**, 209, 214–216, **214**
  detoxification, 194–195, **195**, 212
  menopause and, 190, 191, 192–193
  stress and, **189**
  testing for levels of, 191–192
estrogen therapy, 192–193, 196, 201–204, 210
exhaustion, **58**, 60–65, 66, 90–92, **168**, 257
expanded medical diagnosis
  about, 36–37
  "conventional" versus, 36, 37–38, 50–52, 63
  of functional disorders, 40–41, **40**
  genetics and epigenetic factors, 41–48, **44**, **46**, **48**, 51
  mind-body connection, 52. *See also* stress curve
  normal lab results explained, 37, 38, 40
  personalized medicine and, 44–48
  tipping points, 49–50, 52–53
extracorporeal magnetotransduction therapy (EMTT), 295
extracorporeal shockwave therapy (ESWT), 294–295

F

fasting and fasting-mimicking diet, 143–145, 146, 179, 227–228, 229, 237–238
fatigue. *See* exhaustion
fats (healthy), 98, 131
fermented and cultured foods, 129, 132
fiber, 130, 131, 228–229
fibromyalgia, 108, **168**
Field, Tiffany, 287
fish, 152–153
fish oil, 145, 149, 165
Fitzgerald, Kara, 341–343
Flexner, Abraham, 14
FODMAP elimination diet, 177
FODMAP foods, 176–177
follicle stimulating hormone (FSH), 190, 191, 202, 209

food allergies, 121, 162–163, 167, **167**, 172–173, 180
food and nutrition. *See* diet; supplements
Food Rules (Pollan), 130
food sensitivities, 121–123, 161–163, 172–177, 180
fortified foods, 134
free radicals, 99–100
frequency specific microcurrent (FSM), 294
fruit juice, 133, 143
Fuller, R. Buckminster, 244–246
functional medicine, 19–20, **19–20**. *See also* expanded medical diagnosis

G

genetics and genomics, 44–48, **44**, **46**, 341. *See also* epigenetics
Glaser, Ronald, 81–82
GLP-1 drugs, 231–232
The Glucose Goddess Method (Inchauspé), 231
glucose/insulin loop, 236
Glucose Revolution (Inchauspé), 231
glucose testing, 222, 231
gluten-free diet, 174–175
gluten sensitivity, 123, 131, 162, 163, 172–175
glycocalyx, 119, 312
goiter, 197
Graves' disease, 197
green tea extract (EGCG), 147–148, 207, 211, 237, 328
gut-associated lymphoid tissue (GALT), 119, 159
gut health and dysfunction, 111–124
    about, **112**, 113–116
    antibiotics and, 238
    autoimmunity and, 159, 161–163
    chronic illness web, **168**
    diet for, 129
    hormones and, 124, **185**
    immunity and, 119–123, **120**, 159, 161–165, **168**, 172–173, 174
    inflammation and, 118, 120, 123, 124, 162
    insulin resistance and, 221, 225–226
    microbiome, 116–118, 123–124, 129, 157–159, 221, 225–226
    neurologic disorders and, 123–124

H

Hashimoto's thyroiditis, 197, 216
headaches, 249
healing therapies. *See* body healing therapies
health crises, as Transformational Moment, 13, **13**, 68, 85, 301
heart attack, 101, 304, 306
heart imaging, 309–310
heavy metals, 102, 104
Helms, Joseph, 260
herniated disk, 249, **249**, **251**, 280
histamine, 62, 165–167, **168**
histamine intolerance (HIT), 167, 175–176
hormone replacement therapy (HRT), 192–193, 196, 201–204, 210
hormones, 183–198. *See also* insulin and insulin resistance
    about, 184–189, **185**, **189**, 197
    adrenal fatigue, 207–208
    balancing steps, 200–207, **214**
    bioidentical hormones, 203–204
    cancer and, 192–196, **195**, 205, 214–216, **214**, 220
    detoxification, 194–195
    diagnosing imbalances, 187–188
    gut dysfunction and, 124
    in midlife, 189–193, 201–204, 208–211. *See also* sex hormones
    sleep disorders and, 39
    stress and, 56, 57, 60–63, 65–67. *See also* cortisol
    thyroid conditions, 196–197
How to Change Your Mind (Pollan), 77
hygiene hypothesis, 162
hyperalgesia, 257
hyperthyroidism, 197
hypoglycemia, 227, 229
hypogonadism, 202
hypothalamic-pituitary-adrenal (HPA) axis, 185–186, **185**, 196
hypothyroidism, 196–197, 216

I

illness
    epigenetics of, 41–43, 46–48, 51, 72–74
    expanded medical diagnosis and, 36–53. *See also* expanded medical diagnosis
    mind-body connection, 52
    road to illness, 39, 40–41, **40**, 52, 56, 64. *See also* metabolism; Stress Curve; trauma
immunity, 155–169
    about, 156–157
    allergies and autoimmunity, 157–165. *See also* autoimmunity
    chronic illness web, 168–169, **168**
    chronic pain and, 257
    gut dysfunction, 119–123, **120**, 159, 161–165, 172–173, 174
    histamine and, 165–167
    illness development and, 52

inflammation and, 97, 158–160, 164. *See also* autoimmunity
  normalizing function of, 178–182
  stress and, 61, 81–82
  supplements for, 149, 165
  toxin overload, 160, **160**
Inchauspé, Jessie, 231
inflammation
  about, 96–99, **97**
  cardiovascular health and, 98, 101, 306, **307**, 308, 309, 313–314
  chronic, 97–98
  dietary causes of, 98–99
  gut health and, 118, 120, 123, 124, 162, **168**
  histamine and, 165–167
  immunity and, 97, 158–160, 164. *See also* autoimmunity
  lab testing, 99
  stress and, 60–63
  supplements for, 147, 148–149, 181
  testing for, 309
innate vitality, 9–10
insulin and insulin resistance, 217–232
  about, **185**, 218–220
  cardiovascular health and, 314
  diet for, 237–238
  endocrine disruptors and, 224
  hormone balancing and, 201, 203, 210
  path to diabetes, 221–223
  polycystic ovary syndrome and, 213
  stress and, 63
  treating, 227–232
  weight management and, 219, 224–226, 231
integrative medicine, 17–20, **18**, **20**, 21, 26–27, 30–33, **32–33**
intermittent fasting, 144, 227
irregular periods, 211
irritable bowel syndrome, **168**

J
Johnson, Bryan, 23, 340
juices, 133, 143

K
karma, 74–75
Kereiakes, Dean, 315
ketogenic (keto) diet, 140–142, **140**, 227, 237
Kiecolt-Glaser, Janice, 80–81
kinases, 234–237, **235**
kinetic chains, 245–246
Kroenke, Kurt, 16–17

L
labels on foods, 134–135, 151–154
lab testing
  normal lab results, 37, 38, 40, 64, 188
  systems approach to, 50
Langevin, Helene, 284
laser therapy, 344
leaky gut syndrome
  autoimmunity and, 164–165
  chronic illness and, **168**
  endometriosis and, 212
  hormones and, 212
  immunity and, 120–123, **120**, 159, 161–163, 172–173, 174
  repairing, 121
  small intestinal bacterial overgrowth, 118
  symptoms, 122–123
lipoproteins (LDL and HDL), 305–307, 309, 313
liver detoxification, 102, 109, 147, 230
The Longevity Diet (Longo), 237–238
Longo, Valter, 140, 143, 227–228, 237–238
love, for healing, 334, 335–336
low-carb diet, 138, **139–140**, 140–142, 227
low-dose naltrexone (LDN), 181–182, 297
low FODMAP diet, 176–177
low histamine diet, 175–176
low level laser therapy (LLLT), 295
low protein diets, 140–142, **140**
Lupien, Sonia, 57
Lustig, Robert, 332
luteinizing hormone (LH), 202
lymphatic drainage, 290

M
malabsorption, 113, 115, 118
maldigestion, 113
manipulative therapies, 280–281, 292–293, **292–293**
manual lymphatic drainage, 290
marijuana, 296–297
massage, 245, 268, 287–290, 327
mast cell activation syndrome (MCAS), 62, 167
mast cells, 165–167, **166–167**
Maya's Way, 329
meats, 129, 131, 133, 151–154
medical diagnosis. *See* expanded medical diagnosis
medical marijuana, 297
Mediterranean diet, 126, 136–137, **137**, 142, 315
menopause, 189–193, 201–204, 208–211
mental health, 68, 70–75, 76–78, **168**. *See also* depression
metabolic syndrome, 221

metabolism, 95–110
    about, 96
    detoxification, 102–110, **107**, 145–148. *See also* detoxification
    hormones and, 196–197
    imbalances of, 96–101, **97**. *See also* inflammation
    SAD and lifestyle, 237–238
    supplements, 147–149
methylation
    markers of, 314, 324
    methylation patterns, 42–43
    psychedelic drugs and, 78
    supporting, 48, 342–343
    trauma and, 72–73, 74–75, **75**, 78
microbiome, 116–118, 123–124, 129, 157–159, 221, 225–226
midlife sex hormones, 189–193, 201–204, 208–211. *See also* sex hormones
migraine headaches, 249
Mii Sensei, 29–30
mind-body connection, 52, 268, 270–271
MIND diet, 136, **137**
mineral deficiencies, 114–115, 116
mitochondrial dysfunction, 108
Modern Wellness, 4, 20, 21–23, 339–344
modified Mediterranean diet, 136, **137**, 315
molds, 164
Mosconi, Lisa, 196
mTOR (mechanistic Target of Rapamycin), 234–238
multiomics, 45–46
Mutwa, Credo, 27
myalgic encephalomyelitis/chronic fatigue syndrome (ME/CFS), 108, 255–256
myocardial infarction (MI), 101, 304, 306
myoneural release, 290

N

N-acetylcysteine (NAC), 147, 181
nature vs. nurture debate, 71–72
Naviaux, Robert K., 182
nerve pain, 248–250, **251**, **255–256**
neurohormones, 186
neuromuscular therapy, 290
neurotransmitters, 123–124
normal lab results, 37, 38, 40, 64, 188
nutrition. *See* diet

O

obesity. *See* weight management
omega fatty acids, 98, 129, 131–132

organic foods, 131–132, 151–152, 154
Oriental medicine, 29–30, 269
Ornish Program, 315
orthotics, 254, **254**
osteoporosis, 210–211
oxidative stress, **97**, 99–100

P

pain. *See* chronic pain
pain generators, 248–250, **248–249**, **251**
Paleo diet, 138, 174
pancreas, **185**. *See also* insulin and insulin resistance
PCSK9 inhibitors, 317–318
PEA (palmitoylethanolamide), 296
peptides, 226
perineural injection therapy (PIT), 286
peripheral neuropathy, 181, 321
peripheral sensitization, 243
personalized medicine, 44–48
Peyer's patches, 119
physical trauma. *See* trauma
PI3 kinase, **235**, 237
pituitary gland, **185**, 186, 196
placebo, 297–298
plaques (cholesterol deposits), 304, 306
plastics, 104, 223
platelet-rich plasma (PRP) therapy, 287
Pollan, Michael, 77, 130
polycystic ovary syndrome (PCOS), 212–213, 222
portions of food, 135, **135**
post-traumatic stress disorder (PTSD), 72–73, 87, 271
precision neuromuscular therapy, 290
prediabetes, 219, 222, 314
premenstrual syndrome (PMS), 211
PRIMIER study, 32–33, **32–33**, 292–293, **292–293**
probiotics, 118, 124, 129, 230
processed foods, 98, 128–129, 133, 178, 220, 228
progesterone
    about, **185**, 186, 187
    cancer risk, 193, 196
    menopause and, 209
    testing for levels of, 192
progesterone therapy, 203
Prolon® fasting-mimicking diet, 143, 227–228, 229, 237–238
prolotherapy, 285–286
proprioceptive exercises, 8–9
prostate cancer, 193–194, 196, 214–216, **214**
protein intake, 138, 140, 211, 229
psychedelic drugs, 77–78, 86–88, 335

psychological transformation, 82–85
psychosomatic disorders, 40, 64
PULS testing, 315

R

radicular (nerve) pain, 248–250, **251**, **255–256**
rapamycin, 234–238
reflex sympathetic dystrophy, 276
regenerative therapy, **20**, 285–287
resolvins, 296
resveratrol, 148
Rolfing, 89, 245, 285, 289
"rusting," **97**, 99–100

S

SAD (Standard American Diet), 8, 98, 234–238, **235**, 334–335
SAD Situation, 74–75, **75**
SAD Syndrome, 332–337, **333**
Sapolsky, Robert, 57
seasonal affective disorder (SAD), 147
seasonal allergies, 176
self-care, 298–299, 342–343
self-love, 73, 76–77, 83, 326, 334, 335–336
self-purification. *See* detoxification
Selye, Hans, 56–57
sex hormones
    about, **185**, 186–187
    balancing, 201–213, **214**
    endocrine disruptors, 193, 196, 204, 211, 215, 224
    estrogen byproducts, 192–193, 194–196, **195**
    measuring, 191–192
    in midlife, 189–193, 201–204, 208–211
    stress and, 188, **189**
Shoemaker, Ritchie, 164
SIMTAP Study, 32–33, **32–33**
Sinclair, David, 340–341
sleep disorders, 39
sleep hygiene, 160, **160**, 178, 257, 344
small intestinal bacterial overgrowth (SIBO), 118, 123
smoothies, 144
Snyderman, Ralph, 17
societal dysfunction, 74–75, **75**, 334, 335–337
specialized pro-resolving mediators (SPMs), 296
spiritual transformation, 85
Standard American Diet (SAD), 8, 98, 234–238, **235**, 334–335. *See also* SAD Situation; SAD Syndrome
statins, 317–318
stem cell therapy, 286–287, 341
stents, 318
steroid pathways, 188

stomach acid, 113–114
Stress Curve, 55–68
    about, 56–57
    acute-to-chronic trajectory, 57–64, **58**
    cancer and, 64, 87, 98
    cardiovascular health and, 308
    chronic pain and, 271
    hormone balancing, 207–208, 209, 213, 216. *See also* cortisol
    illness development, 52, 56, 64
    overload, 160, **160**
    as Transformational Moment, 92–93
    transforming, 68, 89–93. *See also* stress transformation tools
    weight management, 225
stress transformation tools, 79–93
    about, 80–81
    diet, 91
    drugs for, 81–88, 91–92
    healing therapies, 89–92
    lifestyle habits, 80–81, 89–92
    mind-body techniques, 91
    seizing the moment, 92–93
    supplements, 88–92
sugars
    gut malabsorption and, 118
    immunity and, 178
    insulin resistance and, 218, 219–220, 228–229
    SAD Syndrome and, 334–335
sun exposure, 146–147, 178
supplements
    for depression, 88, 91, 147, 149, 205
    for detoxification, 106–107, 145–148
    as food or drug, 149–150
    for hormone balancing, 149, 204–205
    for immunity, 149, 165
    for inflammation, 147, 148–149, 181
    for metabolism, 147–149
    for nutritional deficiencies, 146–147
    for pain, 295–297
    quality of, 148
    for stress, 88–92
    transformational experience, 150
systemic mastocytosis, 165
systems biology approach
    about, 18–20, **18–19**
    chronic illness web, 168–169, **168**
    to lab testing, 50
    to SAD Syndrome, 332–337
    to supplements, 150

T

tai chi, 299
tensegrity, 244–246, **245**, 252–256, **253–256**, 278
testosterone, 186, 188–192, **189**, 200, 205–207, 213
testosterone therapy, 203–204, 206–207
Thrive: Find Happiness the Blue Zones Way (Buettner), 127
thyroid hormones, **185**, 187, 196–197, 216
time-restricted eating, 144–145, 227
TMJ syndrome, 290
TNM system, 321–322
toxins. *See* environment and environmental toxins
Transformational Medicine®
    AIM story and, 2–3, 26–31, 34
    complex web of chronic illness, 168–169
    development of, 17–20, **18**, **20–21**
    goals of, 12–14, **13**, 21, 23
    medical diagnosis, 36–53. *See also* expanded medical diagnosis
    research, 31–33, **32–33**, 292–293, **292–293**
    supplement program, 150
    for wellbeing and health, 4–10, **6**, 22, 150, 344
trauma, 69–78
    chronic pain and, 271, 299–300
    epigenetics and, 72–74
    healing from, 76–78, 335–336
    karma and, 74–75
    mental health and, 68, 70–75, 76–78, **168**
tribal thinking, 74–75
trigger points, 249–250, **255–256**, 256, 258–260, **258**, 284, 287
turmeric, 148–149, 181, 296
type 1 and type 2 diabetes. *See* diabetes

U

ulcers (stomach), 114

V

vitamin D, 146–147, 164–165, 178, 314, 329
vitamin deficiencies
    gut health and, 115–116
    supplements for, 146–147
    testing for, 116
Vojdani, Aristo, 157, 159

W

weight management
    drugs for, 231–232
    epigenetics and, 47, 48
    food portions for, 135, **135**
    inflammation and, 98–99
    with insulin resistance, 219, 224–226, 231
wellbeing
    about, 5–10
    future of, 2–4
    Modern Wellness, 4, 21–23, 339–344
    self-care and, 343
    as Transformational Medicine goal, 12–14, **13**
wellbeing (anabolic) steroids, **185**, 187, 188–189, **189**, 200, 201–213
wheat, 123, 162, 163, 173–175, 177
Why Zebras Don't Get Ulcers (Sapolsky), 57
willing openness, 297–298
Women's Health Initiative (WHI), 192–193, 201, 203
wound healing, 81–82

Y

Yamanaka factors, 341
yoga, 299
Younger You (Fitzgerald), 341

Z

zero-sum game, 74–75
zinc, 114, 115–116, 328

Appendix

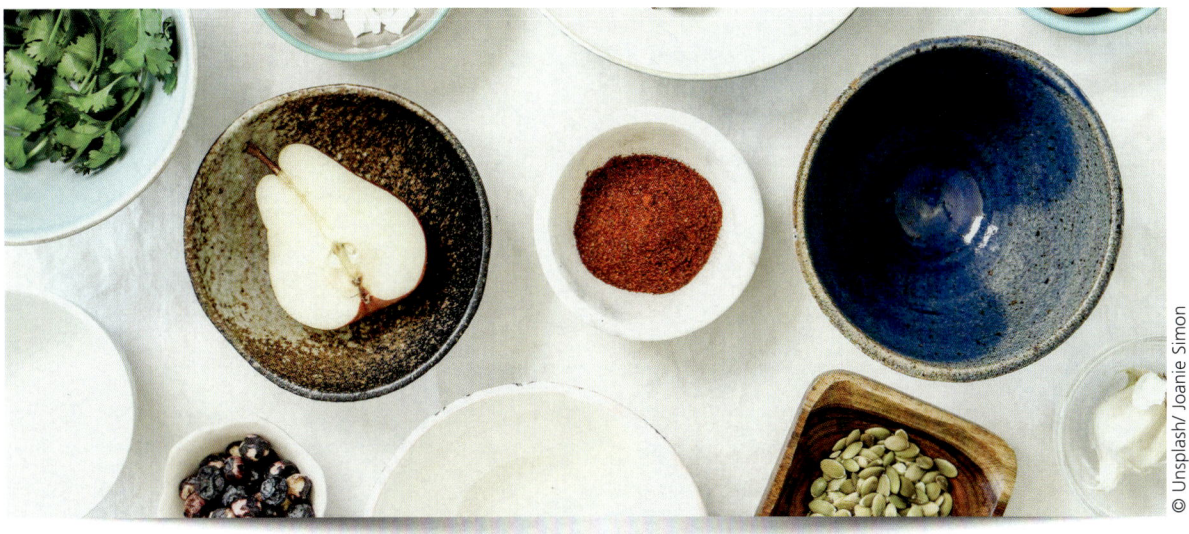

We recommend only using these diets on a temporary basis to help control symptoms.

Comprehensive Elimination Diet

The Comprehensive Elimination Diet is a dietary program designed to clear the body of foods and chemicals you may be allergic or sensitive to, and, at the same time, improve your body's ability to handle and dispose of these substances.

It is called this an "Elimination Diet" because you will be removing certain foods, and food categories, from your diet. The main rationale behind the diet is that these modifications allow your body's detoxification machinery, which may be overburdened or compromised, to recover and begin to function efficiently again. The dietary changes help the body eliminate or "clear" various toxins that may have accumulated due to environmental exposure, foods, beverages, drugs, alcohol, or cigarette smoking.

In our experience, this process is generally well tolerated and extremely beneficial. We hope that you will experience it that way too. There is really no "typical" or "normal" response. A person's initial response to any new diet is highly variable, and this diet is no exception. This is due to physiological, mental and biochemical differences among individuals; the degree of exposure to, and type of "toxin"; and other lifestyle factors.

Most often, individuals on the elimination diet report increased energy and mental clarity, a decrease in muscle or joint pain, and a general sense of improved well-being. However, some people report initial reactions especially in the first week as their bodies adjust to a different dietary program. Symptoms you may experience can include changes in sleep patterns, lightheadedness, headaches, joint or muscle stiffness, and changes in gastrointestinal function. Most of these symptoms rarely last more than a few days.

We realize that changing food habits can be a complex, difficult and sometimes confusing process. It doesn't have to be. We have simplified the information to make it a "do-able" process for you. Please read this information carefully.

Guidelines: Foods to Include and Exclude

Eat only the foods listed under "Foods to Include." If you have a question about a particular food, check to see if it is on the food list. You should, of course, avoid any foods (listed or not) to which you know you are intolerant or allergic. Some of these guidelines may change based upon your personal health conditions and history.

A few other suggestions that may be of help:

- You may use leftovers for the next day's meal or part of a meal, e.g., leftover broiled salmon and broccoli from dinner as a part of a large salad or for lunch the next day.

- It may be helpful to cook extra chicken, sweet potatoes, rice, beans, etc., that can be reheated for snacking or another meal.

- If you are drinking coffee or other caffeine-containing beverages on a regular basis, it better to slowly reduce your caffeine intake as this will prevent caffeine-withdrawal headaches. For instance, try drinking half decaf/half regular coffee for a few days, then slowly reduce the total amount of coffee.

- Select fresh foods whenever you can. If possible, choose organically grown fruits and vegetables to eliminate pesticide and chemical residue consumption. Wash fruits and vegetables thoroughly.

- Read oil labels. Use only those that are obtained by a "cold pressed" method.

- If you select animal sources of protein, look for free-range or organically raised chicken, turkey, or lamb. Trim visible fat and prepare by broiling, baking, stewing, grilling, or stir-frying. Cold water fish (e.g., salmon, mackerel, and halibut) is another excellent source of protein and the omega-3 essential fatty acids, which are important nutrients in this diet.

- Drink at least two quarts of plain, filtered water each day.

- Strenuous or prolonged exercise may be reduced during portions of this program (or even during the entire program) to allow the body to heal more effectively without the additional burden imposed by exercise. Adequate rest and stress reduction are also important to the success of this program.

Remember that anytime you change your diet significantly, you may experience fatigue, headache, or muscle aches for a few days. Your body needs time as it is "withdrawing" from the foods you eat daily. Your body may crave some foods it is used to consuming. Persevere. Those symptoms generally don't last long, and most people feel much better over the next few weeks!

Read Ingredient Labels Carefully! Things to watch for:

- Corn starch in baking powder and any processed foods

- Corn syrup in beverages and processed foods

- Vinegar in ketchup, mayonnaise and mustard is usually from wheat or corn

- Breads advertised as gluten-free may contain spelt, kamut, rye

- Many amaranth and millet flake cereals have corn

- Many canned tunas contain textured vegetable protein, which is a form of soy

- Look for low-salt versions which tend to be pure tuna, with no fillers

- Multi-grain rice cakes may not be just rice. Purchase plain rice cakes

Typical Foods to Include and Exclude on an Elimination Diet Program

	Include	Exclude
Fruits	• Whole fruits, unsweetened, frozen or water-packed, canned fruits and diluted juices	• Oranges and orange juice
Dairy and dairy substitutes	• Rice, oat, and nut milks such as almond milk and coconut milk	• Dairy and eggs: milk, cheese, eggs, cottage cheese, cream, yogurt, butter, ice cream, frozen yogurt, non-dairy creamers
Grains and starch	• Brown rice, oats, millet, quinoa, amaranth, teff, tapioca, buckwheat, potato flour	• Corn, wheat, barley, spelt, kamut, rye, triticale
Animal protein	• Fresh or water-packed fish, • wild game, lamb, duck, organic chicken and turkey	• Pork, beef/veal, sausage, cold nuts, canned meats, frankfurters, shellfish
Vegetable protein	• Split peas, lentils, and all dried beans other than soybeans	• Soybean products: soy sauce, soybean oil in processed foods, tempeh, tofu, soy milk, soy yogurt, textured vegetable protein
Nuts and seeds	• Sesame, pumpkin, and sunflower seeds, walnuts, hazelnuts, pecans, almonds, cashews, nut butters such as almond or tahini	• Peanuts and peanut butter
Vegetables	• All raw, steamed, sautéed, juiced or roasted vegetables	• Corn, creamed vegetables
Oils	• Cold-pressed olive, flax, walnut, safflower, grapeseed, sesame, almond, sunflower, canola, pumpkin, and coconut oils	• Butter, margarine, shortening, processed oils, salad dressings, mayonnaise, and spreads
Sweeteners	• Brown rice syrup, agave nectar, stevia, fruit sweeteners, blackstrap molasses	• Refined sugar, white/brown sugars, honey, maple syrup, high fructose corn syrup, evaporated cane juice, sucanat
Condiments	• Vinegar, all spices, including salt, pepper, basil, carob, cinnamon, cumin, dill, garlic, ginger, mustard, oregano, parsley, rosemary, tarragon, thyme, turmeric	• Chocolate, ketchup, relish, chutney, soy sauce, barbecue sauce, teriyaki, and other condiments

Reintroduction of Food

Once you have been on the elimination diet and you notice that you are feeling better in several ways you may start reintroducing new foods. The length of time that you need to be on the elimination diet will be determined by your unique body, it's state of health and how you respond.

Your physician will also guide you through this part of the process.

Please only reintroduce one new food at a time. Ingest it 2-3 times in the same day and assess your response to it in the next 48 hours.

Reactions you may experience could be related to:
- your digestion or bowel function
- joint or muscle aches
- headache
- nasal or chest congestion
- skin rash
- kidney or bladder function
- energy level

If you have such an experience with a particular food, it is advisable to avoid it for a longer period before trying to reintroduce it again. You will thus slowly reintroduce foods back in to your diet.

The end result of this process should be a good outcome. We hope you can turn this into a positive experience that will motivate you to making healthy eating choices in your future.

(The information used in this document has been supplied by The Institute for Functional Medicine)

Inspired by the Elimination Diet Food Plan, the Institute for Functional Medicine (www.ifm.org)

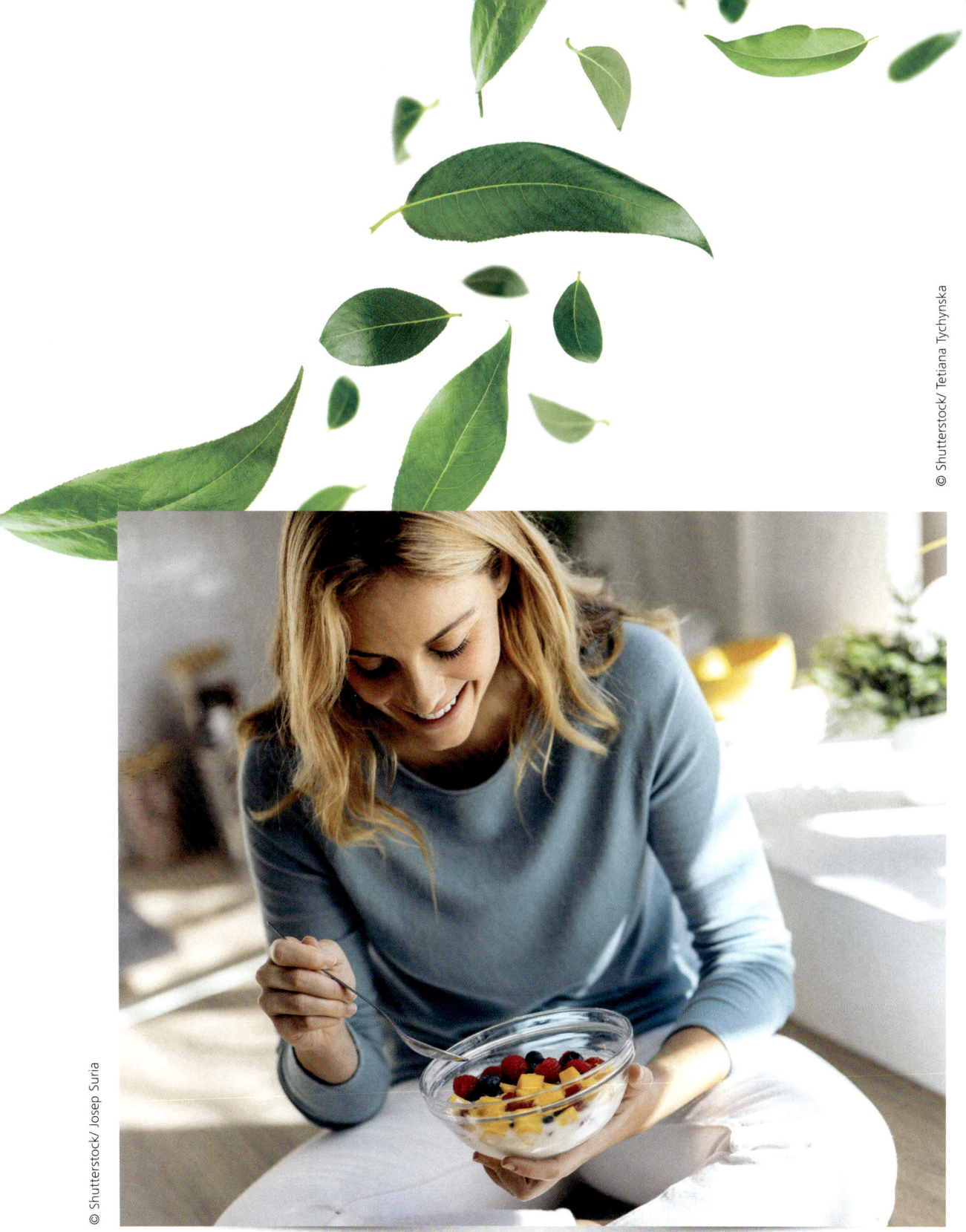

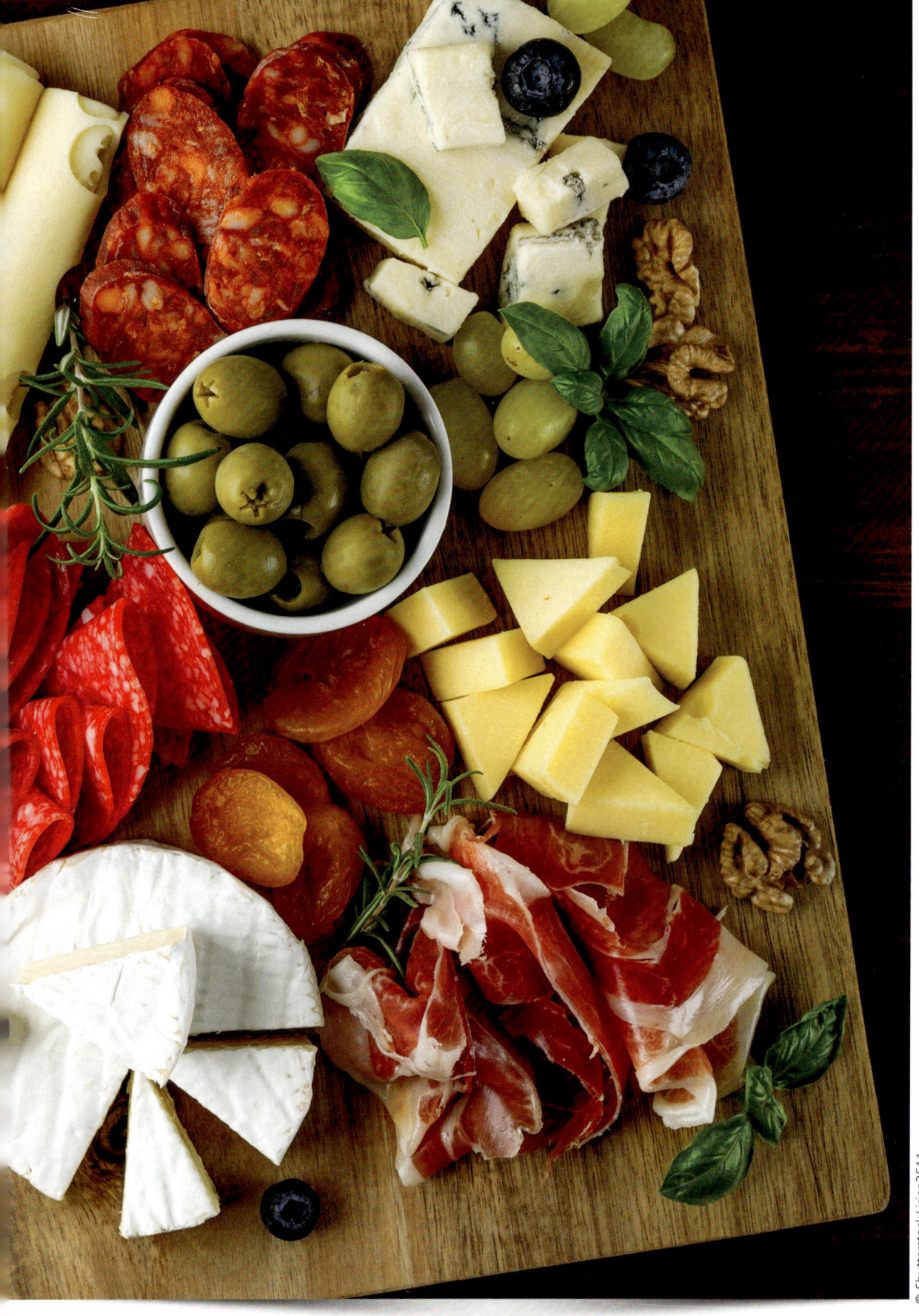

Histamine Guide

Histamines are chemical messengers typically associated with allergy-like symptoms such as runny eyes and nose, sneezing, hives, and itching. Humans naturally produce histamines on a daily basis. Typically, our bodies are able to balance histamine production and breakdown to keep circulating blood levels within normal limits. Enzymes, such as HTM and DAO, help break down histamines so they do not create problems.

A variety of situations can increase histamine production: chronic/extreme stress, hormone fluctuations, environmental reactions, bacterial imbalances, dietary triggers, medications and supplements, genetics, exercise, and poor sleep. High amounts of circulating histamines create a "boiling pot" effect: the more you add to the pot, the more likely it will boil over. For this reason, symptoms may be delayed until your "threshold" of tolerance is met.

Histamines in food are usually contributory, not causal to histamine overload. Symptoms are many and varied; no two people present intolerance in the same way. Histamines are found in a plethora of foods. The more a food is aged (either through fermentation or ripening), the greater the histamine content.

The best way to determine histamine intolerance is through exclusion of dietary histamines for a minimum of 2 weeks, however up to 6 weeks may provide the full benefit. It may be recommended to omit wheat, caffeine and sugar during this time given that these foods can cause adverse reactions and disrupt the nervous system. Discuss reintroduction with your registered dietitian or health care provider.

High histamine foods	Fermented and aged foods such as aged meats, cheeses, olives, canned meats and fish, sauerkraut, kimchi, fermented vegetables, wine, beer, cider, kombucha tea
Histamine liberators*	Citrus, tomatoes, spinach, ripe avocado, ripe bananas, nuts, fish

*These are not high in histamines, but can stimulate the release of histamines in the body

Remember: Diet is just a piece to the histamine puzzle. Be sure to manage other areas of your life that could be impacting histamine production, such as stress, environment, water, medications and supplements, hormones and GI health. It is important to treat the underlying condition.

Foods to Eat on a Low Histamine Diet
- Fresh meat, poultry and fish
- Fresh fruit
- Fresh vegetables
- Gluten-free grains: whole grain rice, oats, quinoa, corn, millet
- Healthy oils (olive oil, coconut oil)

Anti-Histamine Foods and Beverages
- Watercress, pea sprouts, onions
- Chamomile tea, peppermint tea
- Peaches, apples, pomegranate
- Mung bean sprouts
- Black rice bran
- Capers, turmeric, ginger, peppermint, tarragon, thyme, holy basil, moringa, garlic
- Black cumin oil

High Histamine & Histamine-Releasing Food and Beverages

Beverages	• Alcohol: Red wine, champagne, white wine, beer
	   ○ Both contains histamines and inhibits enzyme activity.
	• Chocolate, cocoa, cola drinks
	• Coffee, tea (including black, green and herbal teas)
	   ○ Coffee and tea inhibit enzyme activity (DAO-blockers).

Aged, smoked, canned and processed meat, poultry, and fish	• Sardines, mackerel, herring, tuna, crab, anchovies • Salami, ham, pepperoni, hot dogs, bratwurst, cured bacon
Leftover meat, poultry and fish	After meat and fish is cooked, the histamine levels increase due to microbial action that occurs as the meat sits. • Purchase frozen meat and fish to reduce histamine intake. • Freeze meat after cooking to reduce histamine production. • Avoid bone broth as it is high in histamines.
Picked and canned foods Fermented foods Soured foods	• Sauerkraut, pickles, relish, kombucha, kimchi • Fermented soy: soy sauce (including coconut aminos), tamari, miso, tempeh • Olives (brined or stored in vinegar) • Soured foods: sour cream, soured milk, buttermilk, soured bread
Aged dairy	• Cheese, especially aged cheeses like Swiss, cheddar, parmesan, goat cheese • Raw milk cheese (included flora content = higher histamine content) • Fermented milk: yogurt, buttermilk, kefir
Fruit	• Dried fruit • Banana • Strawberries • Papaya • Raspberries • Pineapple • Citrus • Mango • Avocado • Plums • Cherries
Vegetables	• Tomatoes, tomato products (ketchup, salsa) • Common: Spinach, eggplant. Less common: pumpkin, mushrooms • Canned vegetables and commercially prepared salads
Legumes	• Chickpeas • Peanuts • Soybeans (including edamame)
Nuts and Seeds	• Walnuts, cashews, sunflower seeds
Eggs	• Especially egg whites (small quantity cooked in food is okay)
Herbs, spices, baking ingredients	• Cinnamon, chili powder, cloves, anise, nutmeg, curry, cayenne, thyme • Baking powder and other chemical leavening agents • Yeast (breads, baked goods, condiments with yeast)
Artificial food colors and preservatives	• Tartrazine, benzoates, sulfites, MSG, nitrites, food coloring

* The above list is compiled from information available to date. Not all foods have been tested for their histamine content. It is also important to note that the histamine content in the same foods can vary based on stages of maturation, storage, and preparation.

* Information from: Am J Clin Nutr 2007;85:1185-96 and The Institute for Functional Medicine.